D1765130

Understanding Disease

The Pathological Society of Great Britain & Ireland
Oxford 1949

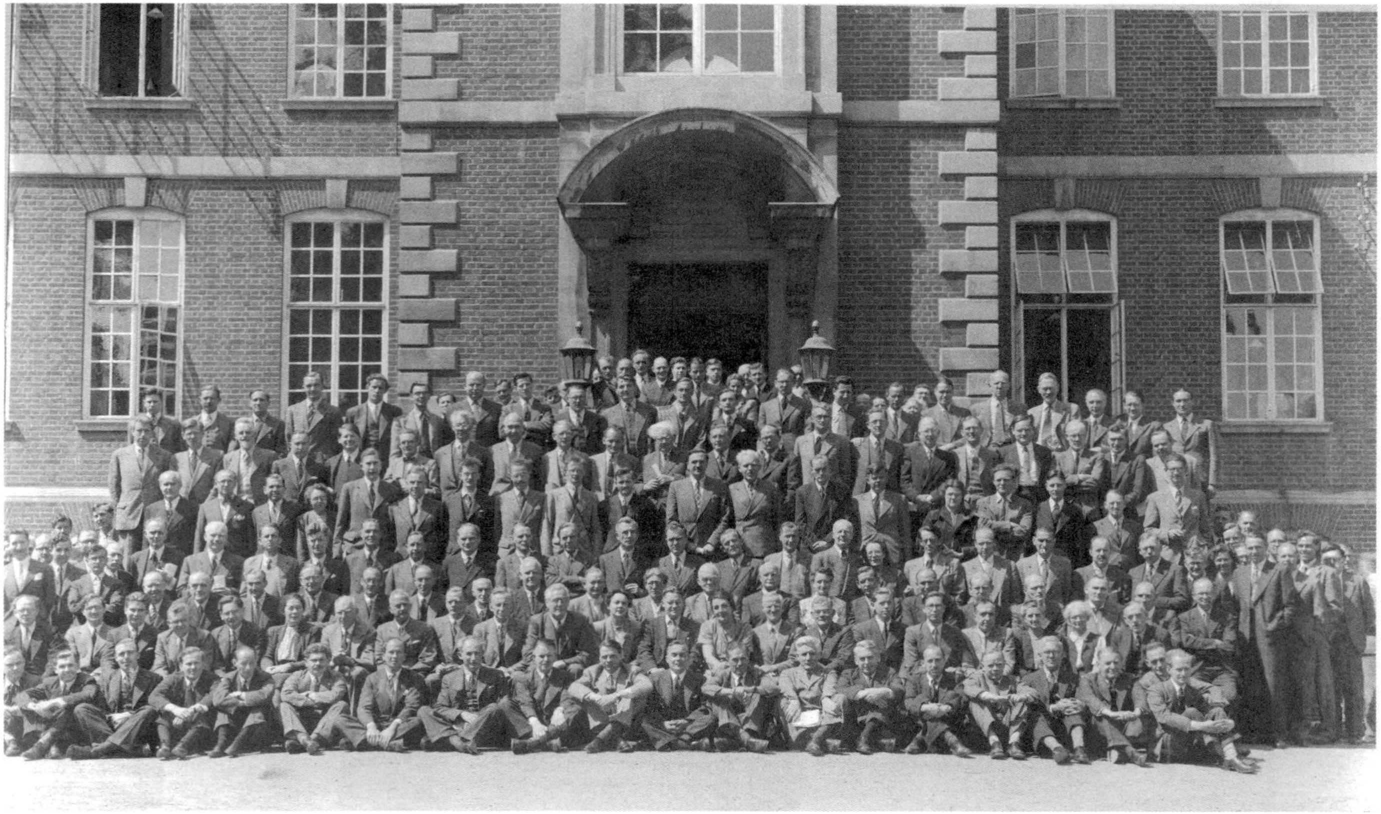

Understanding Disease

A Centenary Celebration of The Pathological Society

Editors
Peter A. Hall and **Nicholas A. Wright**
on behalf of The Pathological Society of Great Britain and Ireland

The Pathological Society

John Wiley & Sons, Ltd

Copyright © 2006 The Pathological Society of Great Britain and Ireland
Published by John Wiley & Sons Ltd
The Atrium, Southern Gate
Chichester, West Sussex PO19 8SQ, England
Telephone (+44) 1243 779777

Email (for orders and customer service enquiries): cs-books@wiley.co.uk
Visit our Home Page on www.wileyeurope.com or www.wiley.com

All Rights Reserved. No part of this publication may be reproduced, stored in a retrieval system or transmitted in any form or by any means, electronic, mechanical, photocopying, recording, scanning or otherwise, except under the terms of the Copyright, Designs and Patents Act 1988 or under the terms of a licence issued by the Copyright Licensing Agency Ltd, 90 Tottenham Court Road, London W1T 4LP, UK, without the permission in writing of The Pathological Society of Great Britain and Ireland. Requests to the Society should be addressed to The Pathological Society of Great Britain and Ireland, 2 Carlton House Terrace, London SW1Y 5AF, England, or emailed to admin@pathsoc.org.uk, or faxed to +44 (0)207976 1267.

Designations used by companies to distinguish their products are often claimed as trademarks. All brand names and product names used in this book are trade names, service marks, trademarks or registered trademarks of their respective owners. The Publisher is not associated with any product or vendor mentioned in this book.

This publication is designed to provide accurate and authoritative information in regard to the subject matter covered. It is sold on the understanding that the Publisher is not engaged in rendering professional services. If professional advice or other expert assistance is required, the services of a competent professional should be sought.

Other Wiley Editorial Offices

John Wiley & Sons Inc., 111 River Street, Hoboken, NJ 07030, USA

Jossey-Bass, 989 Market Street, San Francisco, CA 94103-1741, USA

Wiley-VCH Verlag GmbH, Boschstr. 12, D-69469 Weinheim, Germany

John Wiley & Sons Australia Ltd, 42 McDougall Street, Milton, Queensland 4064, Australia

John Wiley & Sons (Asia) Pte Ltd, 2 Clementi Loop #02-01, Jin Xing Distripark, Singapore 129809

John Wiley & Sons Canada Ltd, 6045 Freemont Blvd, Mississauga, ONT, Canada, L5R 4J3

Wiley also publishes its books in a variety of electronic formats. Some content that appears in print may not be available in electronic books.

British Library Cataloguing in Publication Data

A catalogue record for this book is available from the British Library

ISBN-13 978-0-470-03220-6 (HB)
ISBN-10 0-470-03220-0 (HB)

Typeset in 9.5/11.5pt Times Roman by Thomson Digital
Printed and bound in Great Britain by Antony Rowe Ltd, Chippenham, Wiltshire
This book is printed on acid-free paper responsibly manufactured from sustainable forestry in which at least two trees are planted for each one used for paper production.

Contents

Editor Biographies

Peter A. Hall trained in Medicine at St Bartholomew's Hospital, University of London and intercalated a BSc Degree in Immunology with Leslie Brent at St Mary's Hospital. After house jobs he entered Pathology at the London Hospital before moving on to become an ICRF Clinical Research Fellow at the Barts' Oncology Unit and subsequently the Lincoln's Inn Laboratories where he completed both an MD and then a PhD with Nick Wright. In 1990 he became Senior Lecturer at the RPMS and was appointed to the Chair of Histopathology at St Thomas's in 1991. In 1993 he moved to take the Chair of Pathology in Dundee and in 2001 he became the Musgrave Professor of Pathology at Queen's University Belfast. He has also worked as an NHS Consultant and in the Middle East. He is the author of more than 200 papers and reviews on aspects of molecular pathology. He has been General Secretary of The Pathological Society since 2003.

Nicholas A. Wright was trained in medicine at Kings College, University of Durham. After house jobs in Newcastle he entered pathology at the University of Newcastle, becoming a senior lecturer in the same Department in 1976. In 1977 he moved to Oxford as Nuffield Reader in Pathology, and in 1980 became Professor of Histopathology at the Royal Postgraduate Medical School (RPMS) at Hammersmith Hospital. In 1987 he also became Head of the Histopathology Unit at the ICRF Laboratories at Lincoln's Inn Fields. In 1998 he was appointed Dean of the RPMS, and then Deputy Principal of the Imperial College School of Medicine. In 2001 he moved to be the Warden of Barts and the London, Queen Mary's School of Medicine and Dentistry. He is Head of the Histopathology Unit at Cancer Research UK's London Research Institute, where his research centres on gut biology, colorectal cancer and stem cell biology. He was the first President of The Pathological Society of Great Britain and Ireland and was Knighted in January 2006.

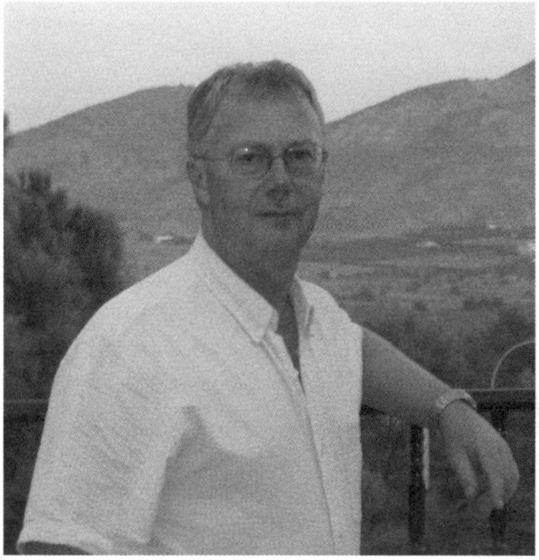

Peter A. Hall

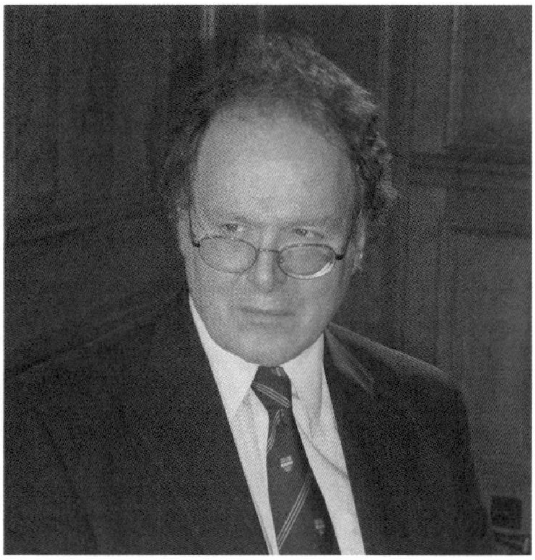

Nicholas A. Wright

List of Contributors

Professor Ingrid V. Allen Professor Emeritus of Neuropathology, Queen's University Belfast

Professor Alastair D. Burt Treasurer of The Pathological Society, Dean of Clinical Medicine, Professor of Pathology and Consultant Pathologist, School of Clinical and Laboratory Sciences, University of Newcastle-upon-Tyne, Tyne and Wear

Professor J. Gerald Collee Emeritus Professor of Bacteriology, Department of Medical Microbiology, University of Edinburgh

Professor J. Henry Dible (deceased) Royal Post Graduate Medical School and Hammersmith Hospital, DuCane Road, London

Professor Paola Domizio Professor of Pathology Education, Barts and the London, Queen Mary's School of Medicine and Dentistry, Department of Histopathology, Royal London Hospital, 80 Newark Street, London

Professor Brian I. Duerden Inspector of Microbiology and Infection Control, Department of Health, and Professor of Medical Microbiology, Department of Medical Microbiology, Cardiff University Medical School, Cardiff

Professor Chris W. Elston President of the British Division of the International Academy of Pathology, Consultant Pathologist, Department of Histopathology, Nottingham City Hospital NHS Trust, Nottingham

Professor Christopher D.M. Fletcher Professor of Pathology, Harvard Medical School and Director of Surgical Pathology, Brigham & Women's Hospital. 75 Francis Street, Boston MA, USA

Dr Patrick J. Gallagher Reader in Pathology, University of Southampton. Consultant Cardiovascular Pathologist, Southampton University Hospitals, Southampton

Professor Kevin C. Gatter Nuffield Department of Clinical Laboratory Sciences, University of Oxford, Oxford

Professor Peter A. Hall General Secretary of The Pathological Society and Musgrave Professor of Pathology, Queen's University Belfast, Royal Victoria Hospital, Institute of Pathology, Grosvenor Road, Belfast

Professor C. Simon Herrington Editor in Chief of the Journal of Pathology, and Professor of Pathology, Bute Medical School, University of St Andrews

Dr Jason L. Hornick Associate Pathologist, Brigham & Women's Hospital, Assistant Professor of Pathology, Harvard Medical School, Boston, USA

Ms Julie Johnstone The Pathological Society of Great Britain and Ireland, 2 Carlton House Terrace, London

Professor Nick R. Lemoine Director, Cancer Research UK Clinical Centre, Institute of Cancer, Barts and The London, Queen Mary's School of Medicine and Dentistry, University of London, Charterhouse Square, London

Professor Alan C. Lendrum (deceased) Professor of Pathology, University of Dundee, Ninewells Hospital and Medical School, Dundee

Professor David A. Levison President-elect of The Pathological Society, Professor of Pathology and Consultant Pathologist, University of Dundee, Ninewells Hospital and Medical School, Dundee

Professor A. Munro Neville Formerly Associate Director, Ludwig Institute for Cancer Research and Emeritus Professor, Imperial College London Department of Oncology, 8th Floor, Cyclotron Building, Du Cane Road, London

Professor John J. O'Leary Professor of Pathology, The University of Dublin, Trinity College Dublin and Consultant Pathologist St. James's Hospital and The Coombe Women's Hospital, Dublin, Ireland

Mrs Roselyn A. Pitts The Pathological Society of Great Britain and Ireland, 2 Carlton House Terrace, London

Professor Neil A. Shepherd Secretary of the British Division of the International Academy of Pathology, Consultant Pathologist, Department of Histopathology, Gloucestershire Royal Hospital, Gloucester and Visiting Professor, University of Cranfield, Bedfordshire

Dr Eric Sidebottom Freelance Medical Education & Research Consultant and Medical Historian, The Sir William Dunn School of Pathology, University of Oxford, Oxford

Dr Elizabeth Soilleux Nuffield Department of Clinical Laboratory Sciences, University of Oxford, Oxford

Professor Sir James C.E. Underwood Past President of the Royal College of Pathologists, Joseph Hunter Professor of Pathology, School of Medicine and Biomedical Sciences, University of Sheffield, Honorary Consultant, Sheffield Teaching Hospitals NHS Trust, Sheffield

Professor Eric Walker Emeritus Professor of Pathology, Department of Pathology, University of Aberdeen

Professor Sir Nicholas A. Wright President of The Pathological Society, and Warden, Barts and the London, Queen Mary's School of Medicine and Dentistry, and Histopathology Unit, London Research Institute, Cancer Research UK, London

Introduction

Peter A. Hall and Nicholas A. Wright

The Centenary of an organisation such as The Pathological Society should not pass without being appropriately marked. It is in an effort to do this that we have collected together a series of chapters that cover diverse aspects of the Society's history and the history of pathology. We have also included the thoughts and reminiscences of current and past members. We have endeavoured to cover the major events and themes of the Society and hope that there is something of interest for all members. We thank all who contributed the articles to be found in this work and all who have worked so hard to ensure that this project came to a timely fruition. The Society's Administrative staff, Roselyn Pitts and Julie Johnstone, played a huge part in gathering key information and helping with untold numbers of questions about Minutes, Meetings and the paraphernalia of the Society. This project could not have been completed without their hard work and enthusiasm. Miss Andrea Baier, Mr Jeremy Theobald and Miss Louise Ryan of Wiley have worked tirelessly to help with the production issues and the completion of this project in the completely ridiculous timescale set by the Editors. Getting this work published in the Centenary Year would not have been possible without their efforts and those of others within Wiley. Of course it goes without saying that the rush was the fault of the Editors: *we have known for nearly 100 years when the Centenary would be!*

The first chapter is a short biography of the first Secretary of the Society, James Ritchie. This is followed by a reprint of the first 'History of the Society' that was written by J. Henry Dible and published in the *Journal of Pathology and Bacteriology* in 1957 [*J. Pathol. Bacteriol.* 1957; 73 (Suppl.), 1–35]. At the Committee meeting of July 1981, held at Ninewell's Hospital in Dundee, it was proposed that the article by Dible describing the first 50 years of the Society be reprinted and published in a monograph, along with a 75th Anniversary appreciation that had been written by Alan Lendrum. It was reasonably recorded in the Minutes 'that it was hard to predict likely sales'. Six months later (January 1982, Churchill College, Cambridge) the Committee took a less enthusiastic approach and decided not to republish Dible's article of 1957, and to publish only the new Lendrum appreciation. By July of that year enthusiasm had waned further and it was now decided not to publish the Lendrum article as a stand-alone pamphlet but rather for it to appear in the *Journal of Pathology* with an introduction by the then General Secretary, McEntegart. Sadly this never happened, perhaps because the Society was in turmoil after the untimely death of its Treasurer and Editor of the *Journal of Pathology*, W.G. Spector. Consequently the 75th Anniversary appreciation, which takes the story of the Society from the end of the Dible history through to the beginning of the 1980s, languished in the Society archive and has never before been seen in print. We thank the family of the late Alan Lendrum for permission to publish his insightful commentary.

The next chapter considers the finances of the Society and is written by Munro Neville: the first of three contemporary Treasurers who happened to be Scots and have unimpeachable credentials as men of extreme prudence! The evolution of the Society over the past 25 years is the theme taken over the following three chapters, which provide perspectives on the meetings, people and events of the 1980s (by Walker), 1990s (by Levison) and the recent years of the Society (by Hall and Burt). Scattered through the volume are to be found short vignettes and anecdotes proffered to the editors by Society members. We have published as many as we could find space for. They appear unedited and provide an interesting, and sometimes amusing, perspective on the changing nature of the Society and its meetings.

The next two chapters consider the linked issues of the fortunes of the Society's Journal and the waxing and waning of academic pathology. The *Journal of Pathology and Bacteriology* has an impressive pedigree and is now available back to its inception online. In 1969 it became the *Journal of Pathology*, with the foundation of the *Journal of Medical Microbiology* and later *Reviews in Microbiology*. In recent years the *Journal of Pathology* has regained its pre-eminence as one of the premier pathology Journals, a position that we guard jealously and are very proud of. This history and the achievements of the Journal are discussed by the current Editor in Chief, Simon Herrington. In contrast to the upward trajectory of the Journal, academic pathology in these islands has been under threat. In Chapter 9, Nick Wright has written a discussion of the aetiology and pathogenesis of this and considers the macroscopic and microscopic features, the functional consequences, the prognosis and various remedies.

For most of the history of the Society there was an active microbiology component to the Membership. Sadly, for much of the last three decades there has been some degree of tension between this group and the more numerous tissue pathologists. This came to a head towards the end of the 1990s and in 2002 this group amicably moved away from the Society and joined the Society for General Microbiology. The huge contribution of microbiology to the Society's affairs and this later amicable separation are detailed in a chapter by Brian Deurden and Gerry Collee. Our relationship with another group, the Royal College of Pathologists, is covered by James Underwood (former President of the Royal College of Pathologists and former Meetings Secretary of The Pathological Society) who provides a potted history of the College.

Change is something we all experience but few of us truly enjoy and it is the theme of the next five chapters. Many have reservations about some aspects of modern educational theory and it has certainly had an effect on pathology in medical education. The changing role of pathology in the undergraduate curriculum is the theme taken by Paola Domizio, who is both a pathologist and Professor of Medical Education. There has also been radical change in the training of pathologists: change that continues apace. This is discussed by Patrick Gallagher and leads to a discussion of the changing work patterns of pathology by Chris Elston, Alastair Burt and Neil Shepherd. One of the most important changes in diagnostic practice as well as in research has been the impact of antibodies. Elisabeth Soilleux and Kevin Gatter concisely review this revolution and define the state of the art, circa 2006! Neuropathology has similarly changed and the history of this important sub-speciality is reviewed in Chapter 16 by Dame Ingrid Allen.

But what of the future? Further change will ensue without question. There are those who view the march of molecular biology to be central to the future of the discipline, whereas others might view the conventional H&E-stained histological section to be the cornerstone of current and all likely future practice. Chapter 17 considers whether H&E will be replaced by 'chips' or whether H&E will hold sway! Readers will have their own views! John O'Leary has taken the ideas a step further; he has placed himself 20 years in the future and considers the state of pathology as the Society moves towards its 125th birthday. This is a challenging chapter and argues that the range of skills we need must widen considerably for pathology to survive. The Society is committed to raising the profile of pathology, fostering the discipline and working with other organisations to promote the understanding of disease. Certainly the Society faces challenges and as we celebrate our Centenary we hope that his volume provides perspectives on the past and stimulates some thought and debate about our future.

1 James Ritchie (1864–1923): The First General Secretary of the Society

Eric Sidebottom

INTRODUCTION

As a biographer of James Ritchie I was naturally keen to see for myself the minutes of the early meetings of the Society written, perhaps, in Ritchie's own hand. Accordingly I arranged to visit 'Head office' and was delighted to find that the 'appropriate archive boxes' had all been carefully laid out for me. But alas, on opening them, no old Minute books were to be found – only 'middle-aged' records. The disappearance of the early records, temporarily we hope, has caused some difficulties for the present officers of the Society, especially the Secretary, who has written:

> 'the minutes ... oh what a saga. We have turned everything upside down, all the living officers, past and present have been contacted, and we have gone through the archives of the diseased ones (a singularly appropriate typo for a pathologist to make!) ... the upshot ... no sign of them. Moreover the Charity Commissioners now want sight of them.'

Fortunately James Ritchie's key role in founding the Society is set out clearly (although it should be noted, rather briefly) in Chapter 2 of this volume, the reprint of Henry Dible's history of The Pathological Society originally published in a supplement to the *Journal of Pathology and Bacteriology* in 1957. Unfortunately the details I had hoped to discover to embellish Dible's account will have to await the rediscovery of the old Minute books.

In summary I should like to quote from Robert Muir's obituary in the *BMJ* (Muir, 1923a):

> 'The unstinted way in which Ritchie devoted his powers to any work he undertook is strikingly illustrated by his services to The Pathological Society of GB & I. He was one of its secretaries from the foundation (in 1906, with AE Boycott), and when the Journal of Pathology and Bacteriology was adopted as its official organ (in 1907) he became assistant editor, and, on the death of Sir German Sims Woodhead, editor. The work which he did, both on the scientific and business sides, was invaluable; for along with his critical ability, always used with courtesy and tact, he had a special knowledge of the technical side of publishing, which was of great advantage. I am sure that all members of this society will acknowledge that to him the success and efficiency of both society and journal were largely due, and will always gratefully remember the debt they owe to him.'

As I have been unable to unearth much new information about Ritchie's role in The Pathological Society, this account will cover the whole of Ritchie's professional life (again about which there is surprisingly little documentary evidence).

RITCHIE'S BACKGROUND

James Ritchie was born in 1864 at Duns, Berwick, Scotland, the only son of an eminent clergyman of the United Presbyterian Church, a man of fine culture and great kindliness, characteristics clearly passed on to his son. After attending Edinburgh High School Ritchie entered the arts classes at Edinburgh University in 1880 and graduated with an MA in 1884. He had the uncommon skill of a mastery of shorthand, which enabled him to take down lectures verbatim, a gift that he used not only for his own benefit but also as a service to friends. He went on to study medicine where, en route, he won many distinctions and graduated with honours in 1888. He was appointed as house surgeon to Professor John Chiene and elected as one of the Presidents of the Royal Medical Society of Edinburgh, a much-coveted honour among young graduates. He then proceeded to study Public Health and graduated with a BSc in 1889. Soon after this, with Professor Chiene's blessing, he was invited to move to Oxford as assistant to Mr Horatio Symonds (who had himself trained in Edinburgh).

Obviously junior hospital posts in the 1890s were very different from today's 'house jobs' because it was reported that Ritchie had a considerable amount of leisure. He spent much of this time on bacteriological and pathological work and this work was submitted as an MD thesis entitled 'Some aspects of antiseptic action' to Edinburgh University in 1895. The thesis was awarded a gold medal. Ritchie was clearly fortunate in that the two most eminent medical professors in Oxford at the time of his arrival quickly got to know him and appreciate his talents. Sir Henry Acland, who had been Regius Professor of Medicine since 1857 and was in his late 70s, nevertheless encouraged his early research in bacteriology and provided him with laboratory space. He also invited him to give practical instruction in bacteriology; the first classes were held in 1894. John Burdon Sanderson, Professor of Physiology when Ritchie arrived but successor to Acland as Regius Professor in 1895, also encouraged him to offer formal pathology classes and campaigned in the University to appoint him to the newly created lectureship. At this time Burdon Sanderson was responsible for the hospital post-mortems and Ritchie assisted with these. The post-mortems were usually done at 2 pm and they provided excellent teaching material. Boycott later, in an obituary (1923), wrote in the Lancet about the new teaching arrangements:

> 'regular classes started in 1896. Six or eight or ten men, mostly those who had taken a BA in physiology and were stopping up for a fifth year to do anatomy with Arthur Thomson used to meet Ritchie at four o'clock on three afternoons a week in the two small rooms in the University museum assigned for the use of the Regius Professor of Medicine, and received, till dinnertime, instruction in the theory and practice of pathology under the ideal conditions of intimate personal contact with a great teacher...... always ready to spend any amount of time helping lame (but generally enthusiastic) dogs over the fearful beginnings of practical bacteriology and post-mortems'.

RITCHIE'S APPOINTMENT AT OXFORD

The University technically made its first appointment in pathology from 1 January 1897, but because this was a backdated appointment the formal decision was actually made at a meeting of the Common University Fund (the precursor to the General Board) early in March. James Ritchie received the good news from the Secretary of the Fund, Mr Gamlen, on 5 March and responded immediately, accepting the new post (Ritchie, 1897) (Figs 1.1 and 1.2). Although Ritchie was the man appointed to this first University post in pathology, the background to the appointment was the work done by two Regius Professors of Medicine, Sir Henry Acland (1815–1900) (Fig. 1.3) and Sir John Burdon Sanderson (1828–1905) (Fig. 1.4). Both had longstanding interests in pathology and bacteriology. Acland had, from the mid 1800s, assembled collections of physiological and

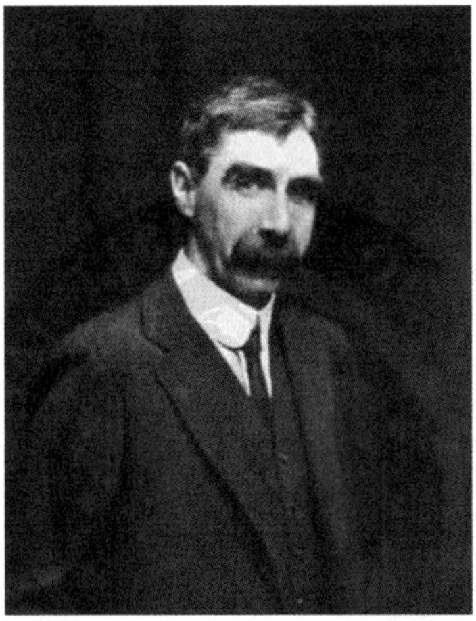

Figure 1.1 Photograph of Ritchie from the collection at the National Library of Medicine in the USA.

pathological specimens to illustrate normal development and the changes found in disease. These were exhibited in the University Museum of Natural History, which Acland himself had largely been responsible for persuading the University to build (Acland and Ruskin, 1859). He had also rigorously investigated the outbreaks of cholera in Oxford and its surroundings in 1854 and published his detailed findings (Acland, 1856). This led him to campaign for better water supplies and improved public health measures.

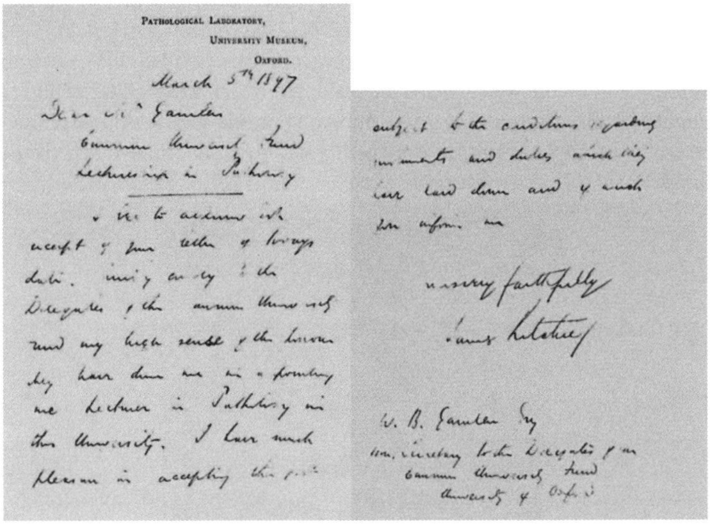

[Transcript: I beg to acknowledge receipt of your letter of today's date. Kindly convey to the Delegates of the Common University Fund my high sense of the honour they have done me in appointing me Lecturer in Pathology in this University. I have much pleasure in accepting the post subject to the conditions regarding emoluments and duties which they have laid down and of which you inform me.
Yours very faithfully
James Ritchie]

Figure 1.2 Ritchie's letter of acceptance of the University Lectureship.

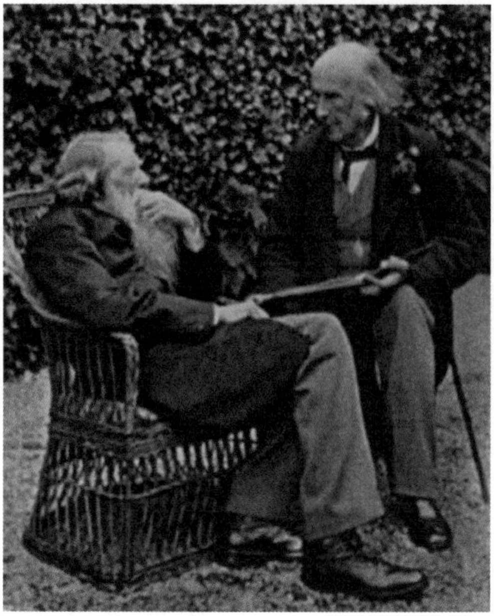

Figure 1.3 The now famous photograph of Ruskin (left) and Acland taken in 1893 by Acland's daughter Angie. This was the last meeting of the lifelong friends; they both died in 1900.

Burdon Sanderson's reputation in pathology resulted primarily from his own pioneering experimental investigations of contagious diseases and infective processes. In 1865 he demonstrated the particulate nature of the infective agent in cattle plague (Burdon Sanderson, 1866) and in 1867 he confirmed Jean Villemin's experiments on the inoculability of tuberculosis in animals (Burdon Sanderson, 1867). Although he was generally considered one of the leading exponents in England of the germ theory of disease, there was an ambiguity in his views. Although he demonstrated that bacteria were invariably present in septicaemia and pyaemia, he avoided the conclusion that

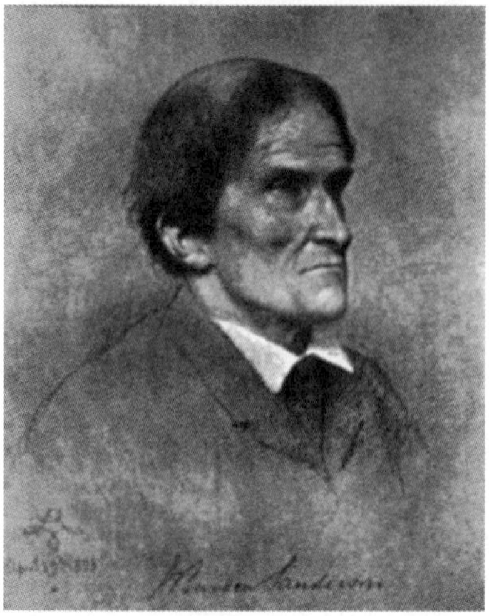

Figure 1.4 Sir John Burdon Sanderson.

the bacteria were directly causative; and as late as 1877 he held that 'there is but one case [splenic fever] in which the existence of a disease germ has been established'. His cautious attitude toward the germ theory resulted from the conflicting nature of the evidence then available, and from his own tendency toward theoretical scepticism (Burdon Sanderson, 1877). This caution obscures his position as one of the leading proponents of the germ theory. Burdon Sanderson, with Ritchie's assistance, gave the first systematic course of lectures in pathology and bacteriology in 1895/6.

Without the active support of these two eminent men Ritchie probably would have remained a little-known clinician. His story, which is not well known to present-day pathologists, reads superficially like a fairy tale. In his obituary of Ritchie, Robert Muir (1923b) wrote of:

> 'a character unusually lovable, a personality wonderfully proportioned and interesting, zest in all he had in hand, common sense and humour, and above all helpfulness to all and essential goodness – these were his in rare degree. He had a profound conviction that there is good and not evil at the heart of things but no trace of the facile optimism which sees only what it cares to see.'

When Ritchie arrived in Oxford in 1890 there was no formal instruction in pathology but when he left in 1907 there was not only a highly regarded teaching programme but also a fine new Pathology Institute.

LIFE AS A LECTURER

Ritchie's classes were popular; with an average of 10 students a year attending, the space in the museum soon became inadequate. Although the University was apparently reluctant to grant extra resources for the teaching of pathology, fate took a kind hand and a recent graduate, at first anonymous but soon revealed to be Dr Ewan Fraser, one of Ritchie's first students, offered £5000 towards a new pathology teaching laboratory provided that the University matched this money. At this time Ritchie was still engaged in general medical practice and in his memoirs Sir Arthur McNalty (1970), noted that on one occasion Ritchie, with his characteristic bushy black eyebrows and moustache, passing by on a bicycle wearing a bowler hat and a black morning coat with coat-tails flying, called out in a broad Scots accent 'McNalty, tell the class I shall be a wee thocht late, I am just off to a midwifery case'.

Ritchie almost certainly needed to do general practice to make enough money to have a reasonable standard of living for his family. His salary as a lecturer was £100 per year (supplemented by £50 towards the expenses of teaching). At this time an average general practitioner would earn about £500, a similar sum to a university professor. It is interesting to note therefore that in a document 'Memorandum as to pathology' written in 1901 to the Delegates of the Common University Fund, Frances Gotch, the Professor of Physiology, and Arthur Thompson, Professor of Anatomy, writing on behalf of the Regius Professor, who was indisposed at that time, made a plea to appoint Ritchie to a Professorship at a minimum salary of £500 (Gotch and Thompson, 1901). The document sets out eloquently the case for recognising the importance of pathology in Oxford and the virtue in confirming Ritchie as the appropriate person to lead the new department.

> 'Pathology has during the last 20 years developed in a manner unprecedented in the history of medical science and become a subject of national importance. In all the important universities in Europe and America there is at least one chair of Pathology and in every university in Great Britain except Oxford there is a professor in the subject.'

This document was considered by the Delegates of the Common University Fund at the same meeting on 7 March as a resolution from the Board of the Faculty of Medicine proposing that a Professor of Pathology should be appointed for 5 years at a salary of £500 to direct the new Pathology

Laboratory that was then approaching completion. However the Senior Proctor proposed, and the Vice-Chancellor seconded, an amendment that a Readership at a salary of £300 be created. The amendment was carried on a division and Oxford remained the only university medical school in the UK without a Professor of Pathology. It is also relevant to note that the Board of the Faculty of Medicine, at a meeting held on 9 March 1901, while admitting to being greatly indebted to the Delegates of the Common University Fund for constituting a Readership in Pathology at a salary of £300, felt that it could not agree to impose the restriction on private practice that had been proposed originally for the professorship until such time as the stipend accruing from the appointment reached a minimum of £500. The Board at the same time recommended that Ritchie should be appointed to the Readership.

THE NEW DEPARTMENT

The new Department of Pathology (Fig. 1.5) was built on a site adjacent to the museum and was formally opened on 12 October 1901 (incidentally, Virchow's 80th birthday; a congratulatory telegram was sent to him from the opening) by Sir William Church, President of the Royal College of Physicians. In Ritchie's obituary, Robert Muir (1923b) comments on the new building:

> 'It was carefully and ingeniously planned under Ritchie's direction and was a wonderful example of what could be got for money thoughtfully expended. Situated in quiet and beautiful surroundings and embowered in greenery, it was – I speak from experience (Muir spent a term working in the new department) – an ideal place for research work. Its freedom from dust was a feature that struck one who came from Glasgow.'

The building served pathology well until 1927 when the larger and grander Sir William Dunn School of Pathology was opened. It then passed to the University Department of Pharmacology, which occupied it until 1991, and thence to Chemistry.

After being appointed as University Reader in 1901 Ritchie was subsequently given the personal title of Professor in 1905 and appointed to a fellowship at New College. At this time it must have seemed externally as if 'everything in the garden was wonderful' for Ritchie; he had established pathology as a major subject in the medical curriculum and he had presided over the building of a much admired teaching and research institute. However a letter written by the Regius Professor, Burdon Sanderson, to the Vice-Chancellor on 22 October 1904 shows that this was not

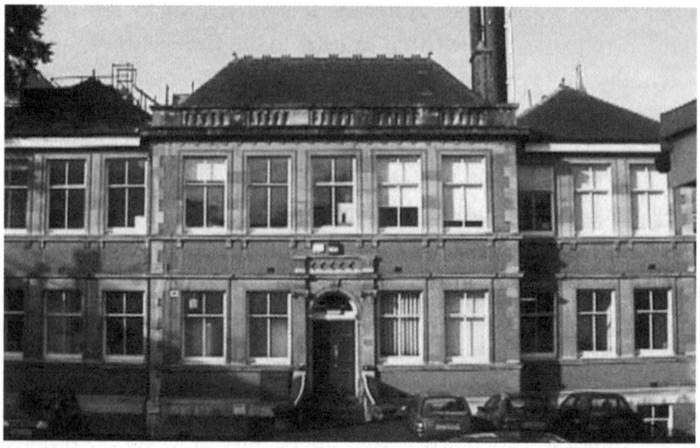

Figure 1.5 The first University Department of Pathology opened in October 1901 (photograph 2001).

so and Ritchie was still 'hard-up' and looking for a more remunerative post elsewhere (Burdon Sanderson, 1904).

In a long letter, after setting out the aim of medical studies in the university,

> 'not to instruct students in the practice of their profession but rather by a thorough scientific training to render them capable of making the best use of the opportunities which the great hospital schools of the metropolis afford,'

the Regius went on to outline how Ritchie had set up a complete course of pathology

> 'under very unfavourable conditions in certain rooms in the museum temporarily fitted up as laboratories.'

It continues:

> 'However since the completion of the new pathological laboratory in Oct 1901 the progress of the department has been in the highest degree satisfactory. The Director has given his time and energies unsparingly to the work of perfecting the internal arrangements and resources of the laboratory. It is now, though by no means the largest, perhaps the best arranged Pathology Laboratory in the UK; in which respect it excited the admiration of the experts who had the opportunity of seeing it at the recent meeting of the BMA.'

The letter eventually comes to its main point:

> 'Dr Ritchie finds that the demands which are made on his time by his office are more than he can meet without serious injury to his health. The emoluments of the readership are so inadequate that he is obliged to depend for his income on professional practice. While on the one hand his laboratory work requires his whole time, on the other his professional obligations compel him to be at the disposal of the public. Having determined to make scientific investigation the main business of his life he finds it necessary, unless his income can be increased, to seek some appointment more remunerative than the one he now holds. And I have reason to believe that he has at the present moment the refusal of an academic post which although by no means lucrative, would be sufficient for his purpose.'

Burdon Sanderson concludes by saying that the resignation of Ritchie would be a serious calamity to the Oxford Medical School; no one comparable would be available to replace him. As a result of the Regius Professor of Medicine's plea the University granted Ritchie an additional £100 for 2 years. In June 1905 he was given the personal title of professor and in February, 1906 his Readership was renewed for a further 5 years. But clearly none of these enticements was sufficient to prevent Ritchie from 'returning home' when the firm offer came from Edinburgh.

RITCHIE'S DEPARTURE FROM OXFORD

Another scheme to try to retain Ritchie in Oxford had also been devised by Burdon Sanderson and his scientific colleagues. Burdon Sanderson had apparently decided as early as 1903 that he should retire from the Regius' chair but the only widely favoured candidate was Sir William Church, President of the Royal College of Physicians, and he was not remotely interested. Burdon Sanderson then conceived the idea that Ritchie should combine the roles of Professor of Pathology with that of the Regius (as Henry Harris was to do more than 70 years later). This suggestion however was bitterly opposed by the Oxford graduates medical establishment in London who met on 5 January 1904 and forcefully set out their opinions in *The Times*. They regarded the chair as essentially clinical rather than scientific and a link with the London medical establishment. They had the ear of the Prime Minister, Arthur Balfour, and he effectively blocked Ritchie's nomination.

It seems likely that Ritchie decided to leave Oxford when the University refused to appoint him to a full Professorship and his remuneration was accordingly less than he felt he deserved and indeed needed. He now had a family and lived, presumably in some style, at 28 Beaumont St. It was therefore not such a surprise to his Oxford colleagues when in 1907 Ritchie accepted the invitation to become the Director of the Laboratory of the Royal College of Physicians in Edinburgh. Muir (1923a) wrote 'his departure from Oxford was of great regret to all who knew him. What he did during his stay was a wonderful achievement and the School of Pathology in Oxford will ever be his memorial.' Thomson (1923) wrote: 'In the interests of the School he worked with untiring energy, often sacrificing his own personal claims for the common good.'

Shortly before Ritchie's resignation a second Lecturer in Pathology had in fact been appointed. He was Ernest Ainley-Walker, who was to have a considerable, though low key, impact on the teaching of pathology in Oxford and indeed, as its first Dean in 1922, on the development of the whole medical school. After Ritchie's departure Ainley-Walker headed the Department until, later in the year, Georges Dreyer, a Dane, was appointed to the newly created Chair of Pathology. It is ironic that the creation of the Chair, which would probably have kept Ritchie in Oxford, was approved very shortly after his resignation.

As Superintendent of the laboratory of the Royal College of Physicians in Edinburgh Ritchie again had more time to pursue research and most of his modest output of scientific publications is from this period, but his heart (and indeed his major talents) was in teaching, writing and administration and it appears that he drifted back to these areas. Boycott (1923), in his obituary of Ritchie in the *Lancet* wrote 'by what would now be called some sort of inhibition, he became almost incapable of carrying out any long laboratory investigation'.

The origin of the Chair of Bacteriology in Edinburgh is not without interest. Robert Irvine left a share in the company owning Christmas Island to the University, with instructions that a Chair of Bacteriology should be established when the funds were sufficient. The unexpected prosperity of the island (due to the export of phosphates – from guano) enabled this to be done in 1913 and Ritchie was the obvious choice for the Chair. This appointment brought him back into the mainstream of teaching and he quickly became more involved in the affairs of the Medical School. He continued to act as Superintendent of the College of Physicians Laboratory until 1920. He was also appointed as a manager of the Edinburgh Royal Infirmary, Chairman of its House Committee and a member of the University Court during this time.

WHY HAS RITCHIE BEEN FORGOTTEN?

Looking back to his fundamental importance in the introduction of pathology teaching in Oxford University, his impact in Edinburgh University and his undoubted talents as a teacher and inspiration to the young, I find it surprising that Ritchie's name is not more widely known and appreciated. As well as being a dedicated and stimulating teacher, Ritchie was a more than competent clinician. He was clearly not, however, highly regarded as a research scientist and his publication of research papers is sparse. (see Appendix at end of chapter). Charles Webster (1986) has described all the heads of the Oxford pre-clinical departments in the early 1900s (Gotch, Thompson, Gunn and Ritchie) as minor figures in a scientific context, but he also said that Ritchie was 'a figure of initiative, imagination and ability'. In his defence it should be said that Ritchie's contribution to the leading textbooks of his time was very substantial. The Manual of Bacteriology, written with Robert Muir and first published in 1897, ran to seven editions in his lifetime and continued to bear his name until an 11th edition in 1949. The Textbook of General Pathology, co-edited with Marcus Pembrey and published in 1913, also had a long and distinguished history since Geoffrey Hadfield (1954), in reviewing the first edition of Florey's textbook of general pathology, commented:

> 'The last British treatise confined to general pathology and written by a panel of experts was published in 1913 under the editorship of M. S. Pembrey and James Ritchie. It was greatly treasured by a former generation of pathologists, but is now outmoded and out of print. It is therefore most gratifying to find, after a gap of 40 years, that Pembrey and Ritchie now have, in this product of the Oxford school, a modern equivalent and a worthy successor which preaches the same sound doctrine and is based upon the deep conviction that "the student must try to grasp what is known of the general principles underlying the pathological changes that he will be called upon to diagnose and treat.'

It is gratifying to my efforts to promote Ritchie to find Florey described in *any* context as a 'worthy successor to Ritchie'!

A cartoon (Fig. 1.6), reproduced from the menu of the 1896 Medical School Dinner, with the towering figures of Acland and Burdon Sanderson and the smaller caricatures of James Ritchie and Arthur Thompson, Professor of Anatomy, suggests that Ritchie was already a respected part of the teaching establishment even *before* he had been appointed to the Lecturership.

Perhaps Ritchie was just 'too nice' to push himself upwards. Although undoubtedly modest, what evidence we have does not sound as if he was a dull man. Arthur Thomson (1923) wrote:'In lighter vein his pawky Scottish humour just bubbled over. When on occasions in debate he took the floor at meetings of the Oxford Medical Club, his incisive criticism and brilliant repartee, often delivered in the broadest Doric, never failed to arouse the attention or stir the feelings of those who were privileged to hear him. Of Ritchie I never heard a man say an ill word – a tribute few can claim.'

Reynolds (1923), one of his Edinburgh students, wrote: 'Although the name of Ritchie will go down in the history of Edinburgh University as a great scientist, worker and teacher, it is even

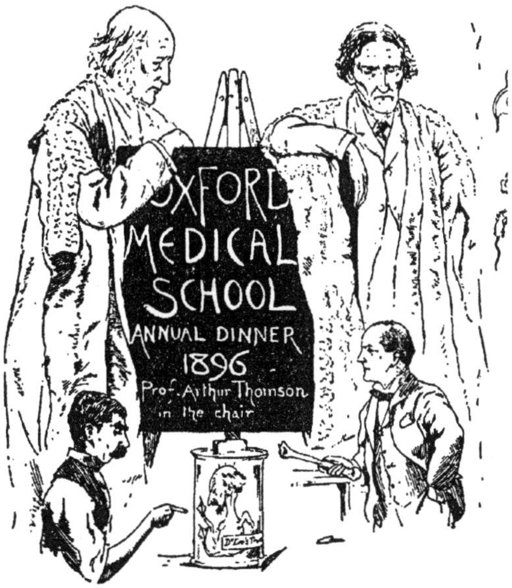
XFORD
MEDICAL
SCHOOL
ANNUAL DINNER
1896
Prof. Arthur Thomson
in the chair

Sir Henry Acland *Sir John Burdon-Sanderson*
Prof. James Ritchie —
Menu: Oxford Medical Dinner, 1896, by C. W. Pilcher

Figure 1.6 This cartoon, reproduced from the menu of the 1896 Medical School Dinner, with the towering figures of Acland and Burdon Sanderson and the smaller caricatures of James Ritchie and Arthur Thompson, Professor of Anatomy, suggests that Ritchie was already a respected part of the teaching establishment even *before* he had been appointed to the Lecturership.

more for his personality....we will treasure his memory. The keen interest he had in each of his students made us feel that in him we had a personal friend who shared with us our joys and successes, our difficulties and sorrows. Nothing was too much trouble for him to do on our behalf. Although fully occupied by his professorial and other duties, he was never too busy to give us freely of his advice and help both as a man and a scientist. As with all truly great men, patience, simplicity and humility were outstanding features of his character.'

To complete the 'fairy tale' aspects of his life, James Ritchie married Lily Souttar from Aberdeen in 1898 and apparently had a very happy family life with his wife and three daughters who all survived him; or in the slightly ambiguous words of Robert Muir 'had a peculiarly happy family life that was for him a priceless possession'.

Less happy, however, was his relatively early death. Normally very fit and energetic he became unwell in the summer of 1922 and an exploratory laparotomy in October revealed an untreatable malignancy, probably carcinoma of the pancreas. He died in the following January, aged only 58.

Robert Muir's obituary (Muir, 1923b) ends with the fitting epitaph:

> 'he is of those who by their services have made men remember them. In truth he has deserved right well of his day and generation.'

RITCHIE'S MEMORY TO BE CELEBRATED IN A PATHOLOGICAL SOCIETY MEDAL

Just as I was finishing this manuscript the rumour leaked through to me that a proposal was afoot for the Society to create a 'Ritchie Medal' *to be given to a Member of the Society for distinguished services to the art and science of Pathology, to the promotion of the subject in the Medical and Scientific community and/or to the wider community* (this proposal was adopted by the Committee of The Pathological Society on 3 January 2006).

This is a fitting end to my campaign to publicise the talents and achievements of James Ritchie. He himself would surely have deserved the medal. I feel I can now lay down my pen!

APPENDIX: RITCHIE'S PUBLICATIONS

Books

1897 (with R. Muir) *Manual of Bacteriology* (ran to seven editions in Ritchie's lifetime).
1909 In Allbutt & Rolleston's *System of Medicine, vol. 2. General Pathology of Infection.*
1913 (with M.S. Pembrey) *Textbook of General Pathology.* Edward Arnold: London.

Papers

1896 *Edinburgh Medical Journal*, **42**. Short notes on two cases of opium poisoning.
1901 *J. Hyg.* **i**: 125. Artificial modifications of toxins, with special reference to immunity.
1902 *J. Hyg.* **ii**: 215, 251, 452. Review of current theories regarding immunity.
1909 *J. Pathol. Bacteriol.* **XIII**: 119. A case of pyaemia and meningitis associated with a pathogenic haplothrix bacillus. (with S. McDonald)
1910 *J. Pathol. Bacteriol.* **XIV**: 615. On meningitis with an influenza-like bacillus.
1911 *Q.J. Exp. Pysiol.* **4**: 127. Suprarenal glands in diphtheritic toxaemia. (with A.N. Bruce)
1912 *J. Pathol. Bacteriol.* **XVI**: 147. On the relation between complement and the immune body, especially in relation to complement deviation. (with J.P. McGowan)
1912 *J. Pathol. Bacteriol.* **XVII**: 99. The effect of concentration of constituents on a haemolytic reaction. (with J.P. McGowan)

1912 *J. Pathol. Bacteriol.* **XVII**: 492. An enquiry into whether lipoids can act as antigens. (with J. Miller)

1915 *J. Pathol. Bacteriol.* **XX**: 159. Clinical and experimental observations on the pathology of trench foot. (with J. Lorrain Smith and J. Dawson)

1915 *Lancet* **ii**: 595. Clinical and experimental observations on the pathology of trench foot. (with J. Lorrain Smith and J. Dawson)

REFERENCES

Acland, H.W. (1856) *Memoir on the Cholera at Oxford in Year 1854.* JH&J Parker: Oxford.

Acland, H.W. and Ruskin, J. (1859) *The Oxford Museum.* Smith, Elder: London.

Boycott, A.E. (1923) *Lancet* **10 Feb.**: 207.

Burdon Sanderson, J.S. (1866) Appendix to the Third Report of the Cattle-Plague Commission. *BMJ* **14 July**: 42.

Burdon Sanderson, J.S. (1867) On the communicability of tubercle by inoculation. *Tenth Report of the Medical Officer of the Privy Council 116.*

Burdon Sanderson, J.S. (1877) Lectures on the infective processes of disease. *BMJ* **20 Dec.**: 880 (continued in several of the following editions).

Burdon Sanderson, J.S. (1904) Letter in Oxford University Archives, UC/FF/54K/3.

Gotch, F. and Thomson, A. (1901) *Memorandum as to Pathology.* Oxford University Archives, UC/FF/54K/3.

Hadfield, G. (1954) *BMJ* **5 June**: 1308.

McNalty, Sir A. (1970) In *Oxford Medicine* (ed. K. Dewhurst). Sandford Publications: Oxford.

Muir, R. (1923a) *BMJ* **10 Feb**. 263.

Muir, R. (1923b) *J. Pathol. Bacteriol.* **XXVI**: 137.

Reynolds, F.E. (1923) *BMJ* **10 Feb.**: 264.

Ritchie, J. (1897) Letter in Oxford University Archives, UC/FF.100/1/1.

Thomson, A. (1923) *BMJ* **10 Feb.**: 263.

Webster, C. (1986) Personal communication in Seminar of 19 June 1896.

Fame at last

It was the early 1960s, and I was attending one of my first Path Soc dinners, not long after publishing my first paper in the Journal. The formidable lady sitting opposite turned out to be Zaide Milner, who ran the Journal. After scrutinising the name tags of her neighbours, she turned to me and said 'Ah, you're Dr Scheuer'. Fame at last, I thought, clearly the result of my outstanding paper on haemochromatosis. But I realised that my fame rested elsewhere when she continued 'You're the man whose name we mis-spelt in the running head'.

Peter Scheuer*

A matter of culture

I was interested to learn that the Centenary Meeting is to be held at Manchester in 2006. Fifty years ago, I attended the 50th anniversary meeting, also in Manchester, and gave my first paper there, on experimental *Clostridium welchii* food poisoning, with my distinguished chief, Stephen Elek, as co-author. I was utterly terrified at this daunting prospect but, with the kindly support of our departmental Head, Professor Theo Crawford (and bolstered also by barbiturates and boiled sweets!) I was relieved to survive the ordeal intact. The acoustics of the lecture theatre were such that one had to bellow loudly to be heard at the back (no amplification in those days), but the hilarity of the capacity audience when I explained that bacterial cultures were added to an otherwise ordinary lunch taken by our volunteers in the St. George's

Hospital Medical School refectory had the effect of banishing my fears. Papers were never so trying for me ever again!

Frederick Dische

Is it significant?

One tiny vignette I still think of with pleasure after many years involved a sublimely indifferent presenter and Nick Wright:
Presenter: There was a difference of x% between the 2 data sets, but it wasn't statistically significant...
Nick Wright: So there wasn't a difference, then?
Presenter: There was a difference of x% between the 2 data sets, but it wasn't statistically significant...
Nick Wright: So there wasn't a difference!!
Presenter: There was a difference of x% between the 2 data sets, but it wasn't statistically significant...
Nick Wright: So there wasn't a difference!!!!!!!!
Presenter: There was a difference of x% between the 2 data sets, but it wasn't statistically significant...
Chairman: Moving on...
Nick Wright: silly *%$@ (sotto voce, mopping his brow...)

James Going

*Peter Scheuer sadly died after this book went to press

2 A History of The Pathological Society of Great Britain and Ireland[1]

J. Henry Dible

ORIGINS

In June 1906, many pathologists in Great Britain and Ireland received a copy of a notice (Fig. 2.1) suggesting the formation of a Pathological Society of Great Britain and Ireland. The signatories to this were amongst those most eminent in their subjects in these countries. We find the professors of pathology at Cambridge (G. Sims Woodhead), Edinburgh (W. S. Greenfield), Glasgow (R. Muir), Aberdeen (D. J. Hamilton), Manchester (J. Lorrain Smith), Oxford (J. Ritchie), Liverpool (R. Boyce), Leeds (A. S. Grünbaum), Birmingham (R. F. C. Leith) and McGill (J. G. Adami) and others, as well as leading bacteriologists such as W. Bulloch, S. Delépine, J. W. H. Eyre and A. E. Wright. There were also men eminent in the services (W. B. Leishman, professor at the Royal Army Medical College) and in tropical medicine (David Bruce and Patrick Manson), physicians like Clifford Allbutt, W. Osler, H. D. Rolleston, A. E. Garrod and Arthur Hall, professors of physiology like Noël Paton and T. G. Brodie, and veterinarians like J. McFadyean.

The idea of the formation of such a society had no doubt been forming in more minds than one. Sir Robert Muir has written: 'Active steps towards the foundation of a new Society were, however, first taken by Lorrain Smith, at that time Professor in Manchester. I remember well his stating his views to me and outlining a general scheme, with all of which I was in cordial agreement. We approached teachers of Pathology and others throughout the country and received generally the promise of whole-hearted support. The older pathologists, such as Greenfield, Hamilton, McFadyean and Woodhead were cordially with us as well as the teachers in all the provincial schools including Oxford and Cambridge.' It is clear, however, that those who were most active in forming the new society were Lorrain Smith and Muir, together with Ritchie and Boycott (Fig. 2.2) and to this little group of fathers of the Society Sims Woodhead must be added on account of his connection with the *Journal*: these are the names that recur most often in the early Minutes. It is perhaps noteworthy that of the 54 subscribers to the circular less than a third were from London, and this immediately arouses questions that can best be answered by a glance at the position of pathology in this country at that time and the way in which it had developed.

FIFTY YEARS AGO

If we look back 50 years and ask ourselves why this movement took place at this particular time, we find that it occurred at a climax in a period of great and expanding activity in pathology and

[1] Reprinted from the *Journal of Pathology and Bacteriology* 1957; **73** (Suppl.): 1–35.

June, 1906.

Dear Sir,

It is proposed to form a Pathological Society for Great Britain and Ireland similar in character to the Physiological and Anatomical Societies. For this purpose we are asking the co-operation of all those who are actually engaged in Pathological teaching or research, and we would be glad to enrol your name as one of the original members if you can see your way to join.

The first meeting will take place at Manchester on July 14th. The times and places of subsequent meetings will then be arranged and a ommittee will be appointed to draft rules for the management of the Society.

If you decide to join the Society would you kindly send your name to Prof. Muir, University, Glasgow; or to Prof. Lorrain Smith, University, Manchester. The Agenda papers will be forwarded to those who send in their names.

We are, yours faithfully,

J. G. Adami	Arthur Hall	G. H. F. Nuttall
T. Clifford Allbutt	I. Walker Hall	W. Osler
F. W. Andrewes	D. J. Hamilton	A. C. O'Sullivan
E. F. Bashford	V. Harley	D. Noel Paton
R. W. Boyce	E. Klein	J. Ritchie
T. G. Brodie	W. S. Lazarus-Barlow	H. D. Rolleston
D. Bruce	W. B. Leishman	M. Armand Ruffer
W. Bulloch	R. F. C. Leith	J. Lorrain Smith
L. Cobbett	J. MacFadyean	L. G. Sutherland
G. Dean	J. J. MacKenzie	W. St. C. Symmers
S. Delepine	E. J. McWeeney	E. F. Trevelyan
J. Dreschfeld	P. Manson	R. S. Trevor
J. W. H. Eyre	C. J. Martin	W. B. Warrington
A. R. Ferguson	Sidney Martin	A. H. White
A. G. R. Foulerton	A. E. Moore	C. Powell White
A. E. Garrod	F. W. Mott	Cartwright Wood
W. S. Greenfield	R. Muir	G. Sims Woodhead
A. S. Grunbaum	G. Murray	A. E. Wright

Figure 2.1 A faesimile reproduction of the notice suggesting the formation of The Pathological Society of Great Britain and Ireland.

medical science generally. The nineteenth century, and especially its first three-quarters, was teeming with pathological activity, and we may well consider that in this period the science of pathology, if not founded, certainly came to recognition as a branch of science with a defined place, distinct from the clinical arts. This is supported by a consideration of the literary output of the time: Matthew Baillie's atlas was published in 1793, Cruveillhier's magnificent atlas between 1829 and 1842, Carswell's great work in 1838, Virchow's Cellular Pathology in 1858, Villemin's experiments on tuberculosis in 1868, Cohnheim's Lectures in 1877–8, Koch's work on the aetiology of tuberculosis in 1882, and Metchnikoff's Lectures on the Comparative Pathology of Inflammation in 1892. Such stimuli evoked a wide response, and this coincided with a great outburst of activity along the newer lines that were being opened up by the technical advances of the histologists such as Weigert (1843–1904) and experimentalists like Ehrlich (1854–1915), and also by the great improvements in bacteriological technique, which in the last quarter of the nineteenth century led to a spate of discoveries of causal organisms in infective disease. This upsurge of activity demanded

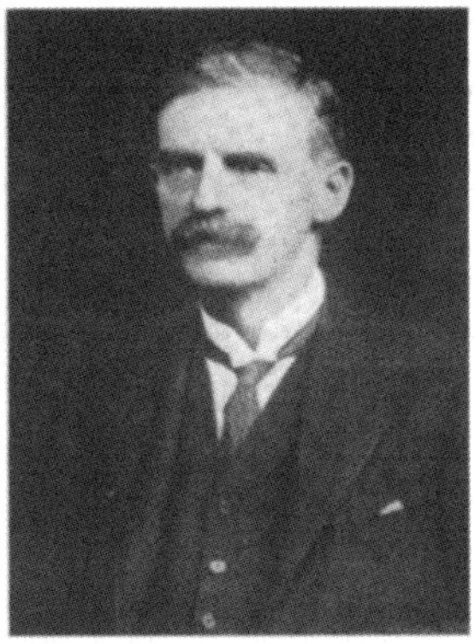

J. Lorrain Smith

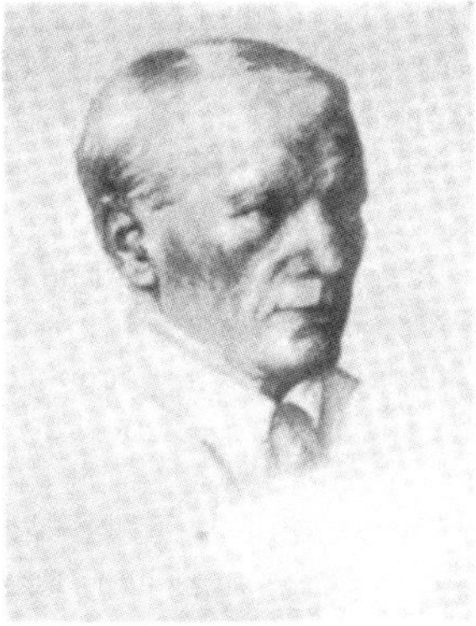

Robbert Muir

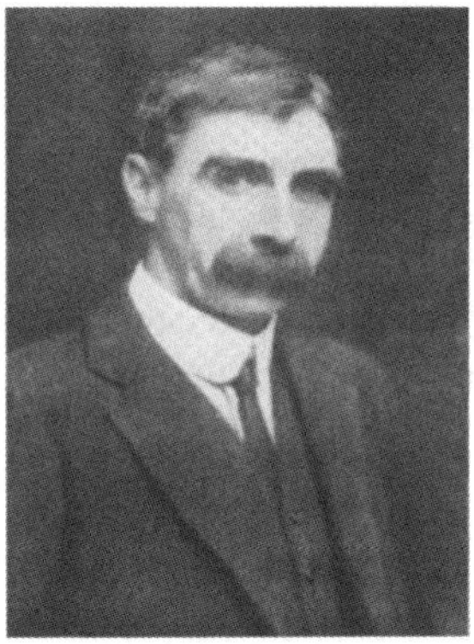

James Ritchie

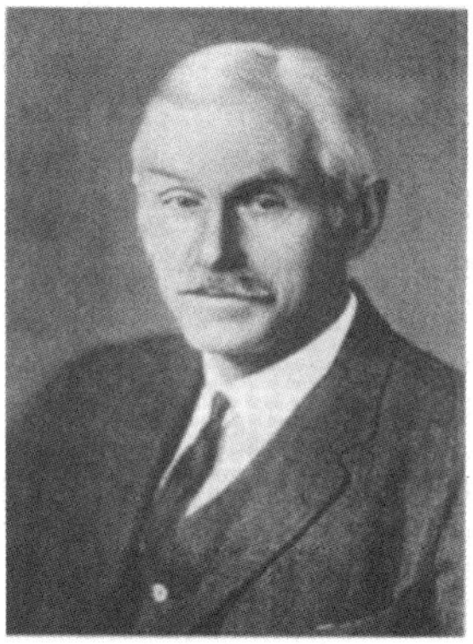

A. E. Boycott

Figure 2.2 The four 'fathers' of the society.

for its service more and more men with more specialised knowledge than had been available to the great clinical investigators like Hunter, Bright and Addison.

EARLY CHAIRS OF PATHOLOGY IN BRITAIN

What was happening in the medical schools and universities in this period? A superficial view suggests that there were two lines of evolution. In Scotland and in Cambridge, where there existed university medical schools of considerable age, pathology emerged as an additional subject and was incorporated into the curriculum in the traditional manner. Chairs were created and formal university teaching in the subject was begun. The English and Irish provincial universities followed the same general lines, though many of them were as yet in the process of evolution and their medical schools had not achieved full university status.

The first chair of pathology to be established in Great Britain was that of Edinburgh (1831) and to this was appointed John Thomson, a pupil of Sir Everard Home and therefore presumed to be a man imbued with the Hunterian tradition; he is perhaps best known as the father of Allen Thomson the anatomist. John Thomson was succeeded in 1842 by William Henderson who became a convert to homeopathy and in consequence was forced to resign his appointment to the Infirmary. Syme and others did their utmost to oust him from his university chair; it is a tribute to the liberality of university tradition that they failed, and he reigned until 1869. University College,

London, had also offered a chair of pathological anatomy in 1828 to Robert Carswell of Glasgow, but Carswell was busy with his work with the French physician, Louis, on tuberculosis and on his own Atlas of Pathological Anatomy and did not take up the appointment until 1831. After a few years in the chair Carswell found the financial struggle too great for him and eventually he became physician to the King of the Belgians ('Uncle Leopold') and was knighted by Queen Victoria. The chair then became a part-time appointment until A. E. Boycott was made Graham Professor in 1914. Fifty years after the Edinburgh innovation the second chair in the country, that of Aberdeen, was founded in 1882 through the liberality of Sir Erasmus Wilson, the first professor being D. J. Hamilton, FRS. In 1883, Cambridge appointed C. S. Roy and in 1894 Glasgow followed with Joseph Coats. Then came Manchester (Sheridan Delépine, 1891), Liverpool (Rubert Boyce, 1894), St Andrews (Robert Muir, 1898), Birmingham (R. F. C. Leith, 1899), and by the end of the century or within a few years of this chairs had been established in all the Scottish and in many of the English provincial universities.

In London the second chair to be established was at St Bartholomew's Hospital (F. W. Andrewes, 1912), followed by that at Guy's (P. P. Laidlaw, 1915). By such a criterion the London Schools generally, with the exception of University College, had lagged behind, and in this there is reflected an early difference in the relationship between pathology and the clinical subjects in London and in other parts of the country, which to some extent has persisted to the present day. The London medical schools at this time had no real university affiliation, but were appanages of the great London Hospitals, all of them independent and highly individual institutions, many with proud traditions stretching back over centuries; they were dominated by their honorary physicians and surgeons, often striking personalities with names that are famous, to whom pathology was part of their daily work, as it was to John Hunter.

They made notable contributions to the subject, as the names of Matthew Baillie (1761–1823), Bright (1789–1858), Hodgkin (1798–1866), Paget (1814–99), Brodie (1783–1862), Addison (1793–1860), and, rather later, of Bland-Sutton, Mott, Jonathan Hutchinson and Garrod will recall, but they left little room on their hospital staff for the pure pathologist, as distinct from the physician or surgeon interested in pathology – and, which largely settled the matter, there was no living for him. Pathology thus developed in London more as an ancillary to the clinical practice of the hospitals and less as a subject in its own right than it did elsewhere. This early difference in outlook and method of development goes far to explain the preponderance of Scottish and provincial names amongst the signatories to the memorandum that led to the formation of our Society.

Moreover, London, then as now, was well supplied with medical societies. There were several and they led a healthy and active independent existence until – as some think inadvisedly – they merged their identity into the Royal Society of Medicine.

THE PATHOLOGICAL SOCIETY OF LONDON

Pathology was catered for by The Pathological Society of London. This Society began some 60 years before ours, holding its first meeting on 1 February 1847, the President being C. J. B. Williams, MD, FRS, a pupil of Laënnec. Its 130 members were, except for three, entirely Londoners and included only one Professor of Pathology (W. H. Walshe, physician and also Professor of Pathological Anatomy in University College). The London Society flourished until a year after our foundation when, on 14 June 1907, it held its last meeting before becoming incorporated into The Royal Society of Medicine. Its ordinary members by then numbered 638 and its 30 Presidents were all, except for Burdon-Sanderson, the last but one, clinicians as we understand the term today. Twenty-two of them were Fellows of The Royal Society, which throws into relief one of the alterations in scientific values that has taken place during the last half-century. The last president, P. H. Pye-Smith, FRS, a consulting physician to Guy's Hospital, in a short final address said: 'When our Society was founded pathology was still the hand-maid of Medicine and Surgery as is shewn by the names I have cited. The science has now a far more independent position, and is the foundation or institute on which all scientific prevention and treatment of disease must rest.' These discerning remarks are worth quoting today when developments in state medicine have tended to obscure and to reverse the true relationship of pathology to medicine.

One notable name, absent from the signatories to the notice convening our Society, is that of S. G. Shattock. He, at the time, was the general secretary of The Pathological Society of London and editor of its Transactions, a position he had held since 1900, and he had been in some office in that Society since 1889. Under his editorship, from 1903 onwards, articles of his own in the Proceedings were usually given a Latin sub-title and were frequently accompanied by a summary in Latin as well: in this he succeeded in attracting a few imitators. A man of great parts and character, Shattock felt, like certain others, that the new society might be in competition with the London society and there was some lukewarmness from this direction at the time of its foundation. Shattock never became a member of our Society nor attended its meetings.

I have spent some time over this account of the beginnings of pathology in this country in order to show the background against which our Society was founded and grew up; in it will be discovered some of the reasons why The Pathological Society has in the past drawn its strength so largely from north of the Border and from the English provincial universities. This tradition is still with us.

MANCHESTER, 14 JULY 1906

The signatories to the memorandum met in the Physiological Theatre of the University of Manchester on Saturday morning, 4 July 5901, at 9.30 a.m. Professor Muir proposed that Professor Hamilton should take the chair, which he did, and after some opening remarks, supported by Professor Delépine, it was moved that: 'The Pathological Society of Great Britain and Ireland be constituted': this was carried by acclamation and so the Society came into being.

The Society then proceeded to the election of a committee to draw up a constitution and rules to be presented to the next meeting. Thirteen gentlemen were nominated and Drs James Ritchie, then pathologist to the Radcliffe Infirmary, Oxford, and A. E. Boycott, then assistant bacteriologist to the Lister Institute, were appointed secretaries, and C. Powell White (Pilkington Research Student at Manchester University) treasurer. A levy of five shillings was made to meet the current expenses. It was agreed that the next meeting should be in London, and also that the Society should offer to cooperate with the Physiological Society in presenting evidence from the pathological standpoint before the Royal Commission on Vivisection. The Society, which had thus been constituted, proceeded to public business; 17 papers and 31 demonstrations (by 17 demonstrators) were given. The first paper on the agenda was by James Ritchie, interestingly enough on 'Terminal thrombosis in amyloid degeneration'; it is easy to forget that Ritchie was a physician to the Radcliffe Infirmary before he became a leading bacteriologist. I have been told, however, by James Miller that he (Miller) actually gave the first paper ('Amyloid goitre and amyloid disease of the air passages'), as on Ritchie's name being called he was temporarily absent and Miller took his place. The members of the Society were entertained at lunch by Professor Dreschfeld, who had held the chair of pathology in Manchester from 1881 until 1891, as well as the position of physician to the Manchester Royal Infirmary. In 1891 he had moved to the chair of medicine and had been succeeded by Sheridan Delépine who was appointed the first professor of pathology and bacteriology. As the meeting had clearly been a large one, although the exact numbers are not now known because no record seems to have been kept, Dreschfeld's hospitality must have been considerable. (The old fashion of entertaining the Society to lunch lasted for many years, the latest record being at the invitation of the managers of the Royal Victoria Hospital on the occasion of the Belfast meeting in 1953.) On the Friday evening Henry Ashby and Mr Samuel Buckley entertained some members at the Clarendon Club and others were entertained by Dreschfeld. Mr Thorburn also gave an 'At home'. On the Saturday night the first dinner was held at the Queen's Hotel, where 81 were present, of whom 65 were members. Dreschfeld was in the chair. There were five toasts on the list, excluding 'The King'! The Pathological Society was proposed by Clifford Allbutt and the Victoria University by Osler; the Vice-Chancellor and Mr Thorburn replied. Thorburn became a famous surgeon and received a knighthood, but he will be affectionately remembered in the Society for his speech at this first dinner, when he said (and I have this on the authority of Sir Robert Muir): 'You have today lighted a candle, which will bear marvellous fruit'.

SECOND MEETING 1907

The Society's second meeting was held at the Lister Institute on 12 January 1907. As at this meeting it was decided to constitute the membership of the Society from those who had responded to

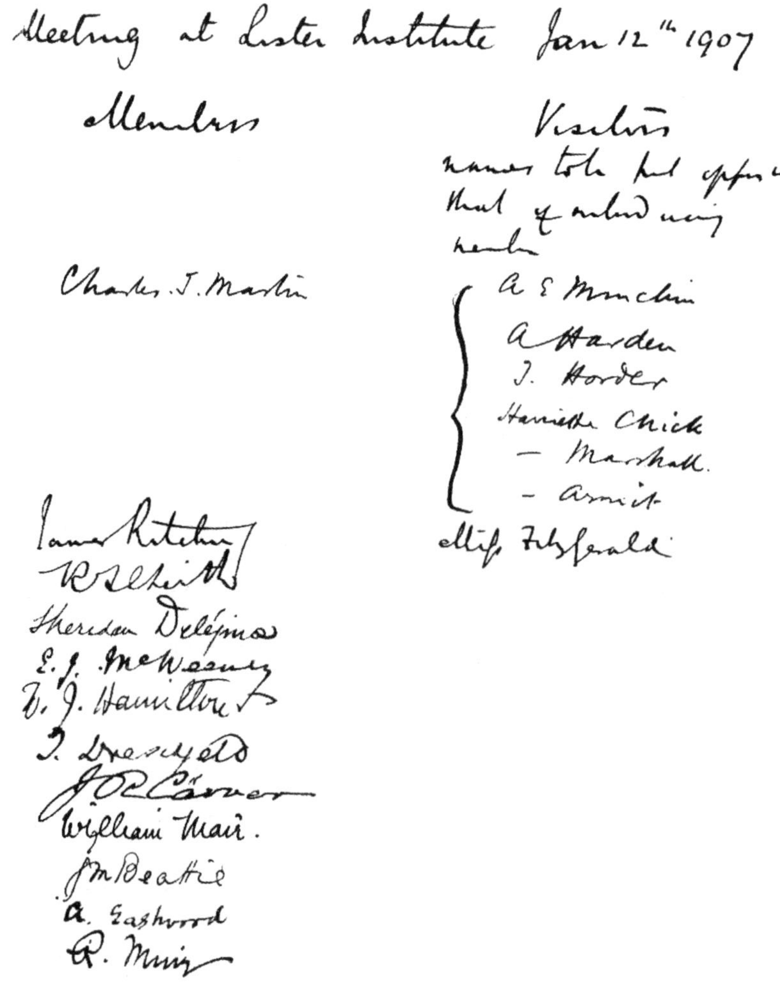

Figure 2.3 Fascimile reporduction of the signatures in the attendance book at the first official meeting.

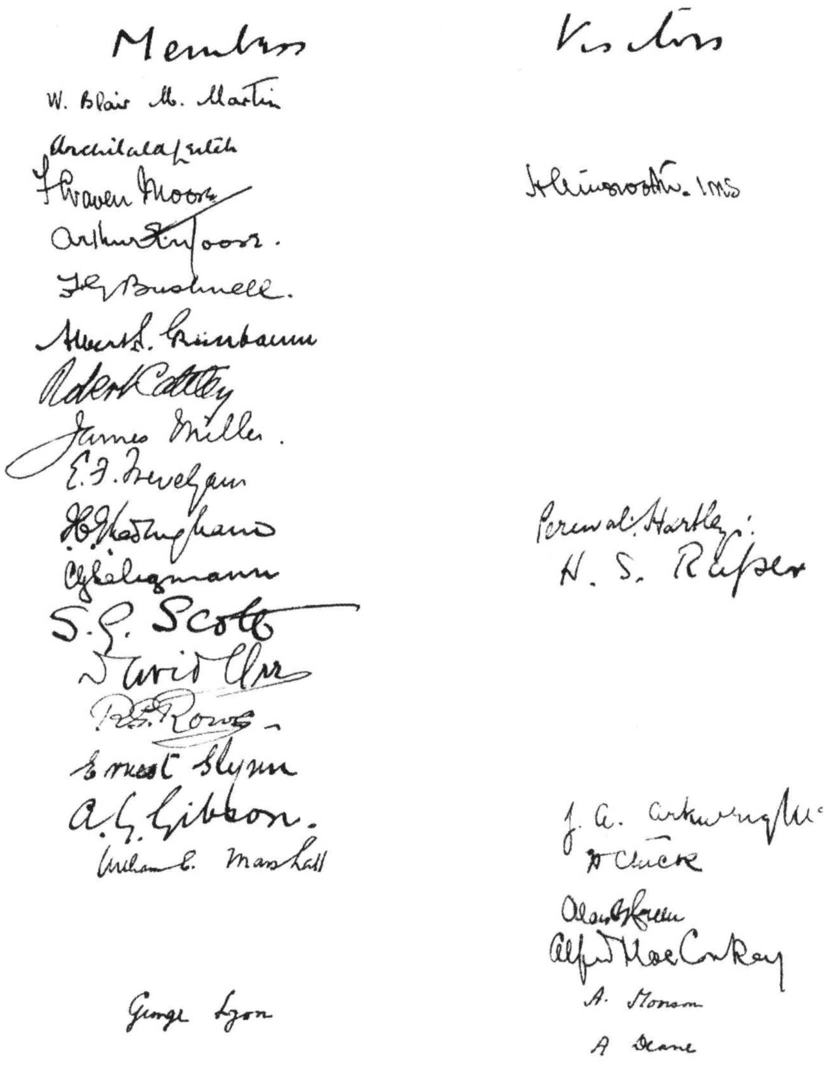

Figure 2.3 *(Continued)*

the circular of invitation issued in June 1906, this may be regarded as the first official meeting. The signatures in the attendance book are reproduced in Fig. 2.3. It was decided to adopt, with certain modifications, the draft rules and constitution that had been drawn up by the ad hoc committee; this committee was continued until the Statutory Meeting of 1907. The annual subscription was fixed at one guinea.

RULES

The rules of the Society and its constitution are known to all members and are embodied in the list that is published yearly, so I will not go into them except to mention that under rule 23 'the

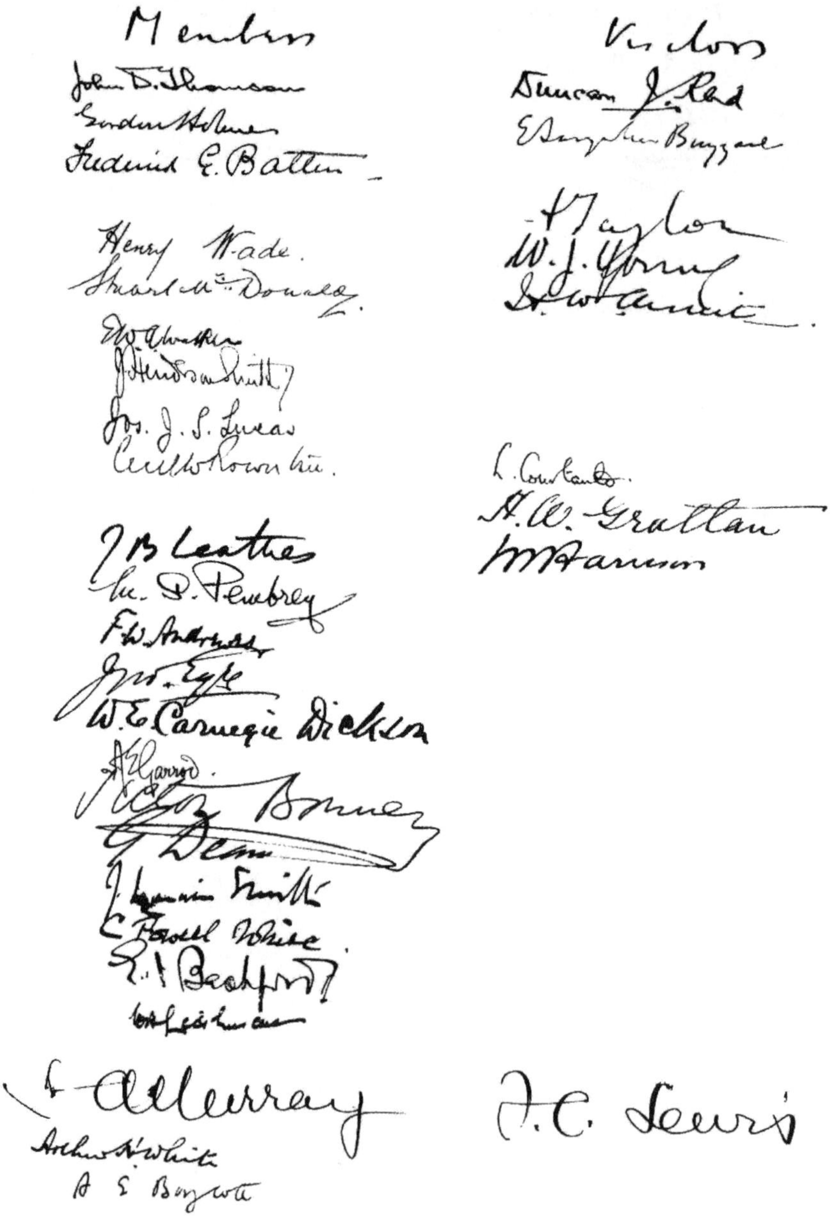

Figure 2.3 (*Continued*)

Chair shall be taken by the head of the laboratory in which the meeting is held, or by some member delegated by him for the purpose'; thus the Society has never had a permanent Chairman or President, which is sometimes a little confusing to those unfamiliar with its constitution. It has usually been the custom at places of meeting where there are Professors of both Pathology and Bacteriology for them to divide the duties of Chairman between them.

JOURNAL OF PATHOLOGY AND BACTERIOLOGY

The ad hoc committee next proceeded to investigate the possibility of securing an official publication, and in March 1907 recommended the formation of an Association with a capital of £550 to acquire from Professor Sims Woodhead the *Journal of Pathology and Bacteriology*, which he had founded in 1892 in conjunction with Young J. Pentland the Edinburgh publisher. It was agreed that Professor Woodhead was to be paid £275 in cash, and that £275 in shares in the Association was to be assigned to him. It was further agreed that the principles on which the Association should be conducted should be:

'(1) That not more than 4 1/2 per cent. interest should be paid on the capital.
(2) That out of the profits a sinking fund be furnished to redeem the capital of the Association (the shares being redeemed at par) and that ultimately the Journal should be handed over to the Society free of debt.
(3) That otherwise the profits of the Journal should be devoted to the conduct and development of the Journal and especially to the payment for illustrations.
(4) That the Journal should be supplied to the members of The Pathological Society at cost price, *i.e.* about 17/6d.
(5) That the shares in the Association be held only by members of The Pathological Society.'

The Journal was to continue to be published under the editorship of Sims Woodhead (see Fig. 2.4), with Ritchie and Boycott as assistant editors, and a committee consisting of Beattie, Leishman,

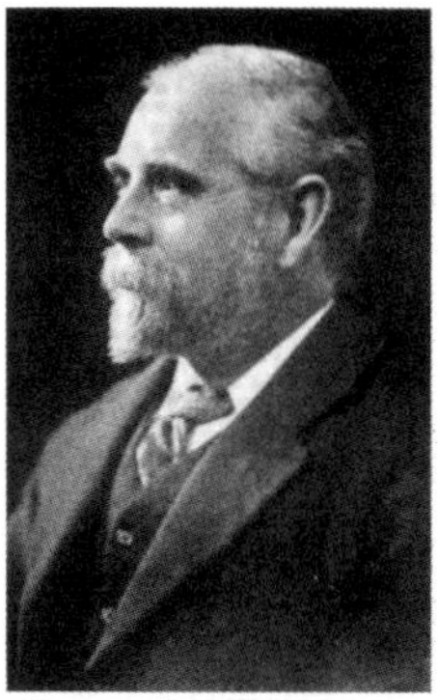

German Sims Woodhead

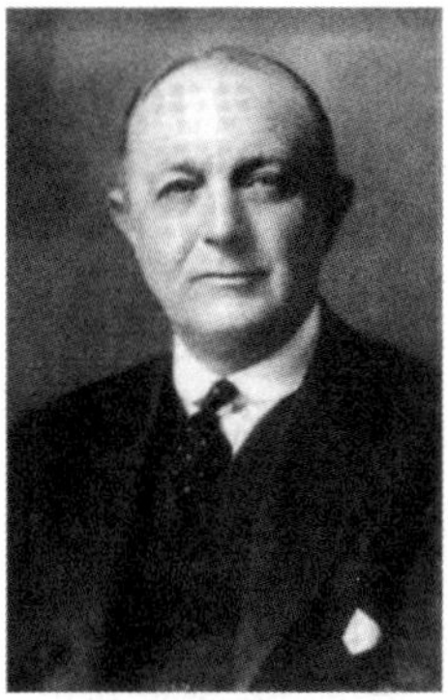

H. R. Dean

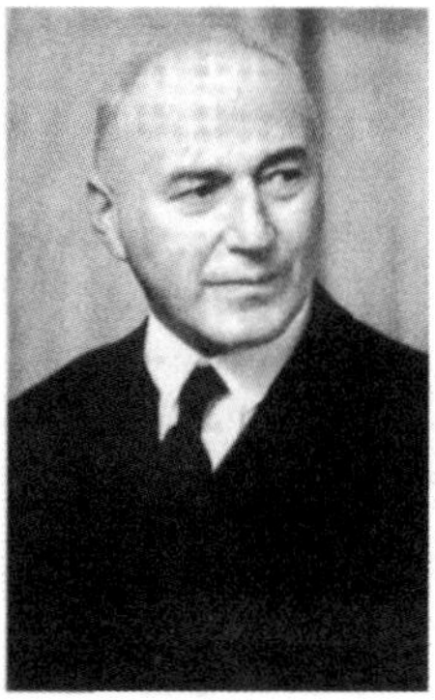

Robert Grant

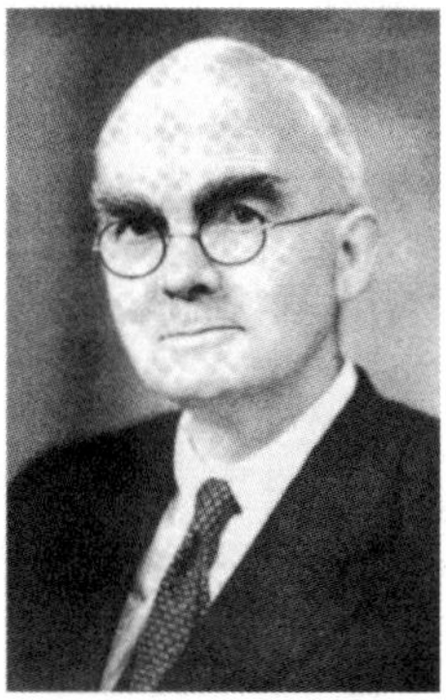

Matthew J. Stewart

Figure 2.4 Major contributors to the *Journal of Pathology and Bacteriology*.

Robert Muir and Lorrain Smith. One might feel today that rather a hard bargain had been driven, but it is evident from the Minutes that the members of the Association envisaged a considerable period of financial stringency. However things turned out well and by 1914 they were ready to transfer the Journal to the Society.

In the Editorial of October 1907, in announcing the new affiliation of the Journal, the Editor stated:

> 'As heretofore, no papers will be received that have appeared, or which are to appear, in other Journals. Records of personal research and not historical *résumés* are specially desired; and in all cases preference will be given to articles not overburdened with abstracts from literature. Illustrations must in all cases be confined to new features... Although the Editors reserve to themselves the right of editing articles submitted for the Journal, they will not hold themselves responsible for any statement made in the articles published.'

These forthright pronouncements gave some warning of the Editor's determination to be master in his own house, a decision from which he never departed and which outlived him as a tradition.

Amongst other matters the Committee also considered the admission as members of laboratory attendants engaged in scientific work, and found that 'there was nothing in the rules which necessarily prevented the admission of these gentlemen'. W. A. Mitchell of Cambridge was an original member of the Society and in the list of those approved at this meeting it is interesting to find the name of Richard Muir, a man outstanding for his technical work, and a considerable medical artist. Nominated as honorary members were Lord Lister, Metchnikoff, Roux, Laveran, Ehrlich, Koch, Golgi, Welch and von Recklinghausen.

1907–1913

The first statutory meeting under the rules was held in July 1907, at Edinburgh, and the Society in the form in which we have known it since was finally under way. The subscription was fixed at 'twenty-five shillings, including the price of the *Journal*'. Meetings followed at the Royal Army Medical College and Cambridge (1908), Leeds and Glasgow (1909, where there were 34 papers), Guy's Hospital and Bristol (1910) and Birmingham and Oxford (1911). A notable happening at the Oxford Committee meeting was: a 'sub-committee consisting of J. Lorrain Smith, J. C. G. Ledingham and A. E. Boycott was appointed "to consider and report upon the possibility of establishing some form of employment bureau for laboratory assistants".' At this meeting a record, which may never be exceeded, was the presentation of eight papers by a single member (H. G. M. Henry)! Sir W. Osler presided at the Society's dinner in University College. In 1912 the Society met at Liverpool and Newcastle-upon-Tyne. At the Liverpool meeting in January 1912 it was reported that an association of laboratory assistants in pathology and bacteriology was in the process of formation amongst the assistants themselves. The Committee recorded its sympathy with the project and its willingness to assist and encourage the objects of the Association. At about this period the Society was being asked repeatedly to send representatives to various congresses at home and abroad and in every instance declined. In 1913 meetings were held at St Bartholomew's Hospital and Sheffield. C. Powell White resigned from the office of treasurer and was succeeded by J. C. G. Ledingham. J. Bordet was elected an Honorary Member.

1914

The 1914 meetings were at the Royal Army Medical College and Cambridge. There was a special committee meeting in Manchester in May, to which Professor Sims Woodhead was invited, to consider the affairs of the Journal. At this meeting the Committee learnt that the 'proprietors' of the Journal would be in a position to transfer it to the Society during 1914, and therefore decided to give notice at the July meeting that at the next statutory meeting, which it was anticipated would be in the summer of 1915, the Society should resolve to accept the Journal, and to empower the Committee to appoint for a period of three years an Editor and Assistant Editors, who should be eligible for re-election, and to alter the rules accordingly. An important provision was that the Editor and Assistant Editors should be responsible *to the Committee* for the conduct of the Journal and for keeping its accounts. This delegation of responsibility to a small organisation created an arrangement that has worked extremely well and benefited both the Journal and the Society generally. It was decided that there should be a payment of 18 shillings a year to the Journal account from each member's subscription, and that the Journal account should be kept separate from the general accounts.

During the spring of 1914 approval was given for the formation of a subcommittee for a collective investigation of the subject of enlarged thymus, especially in relation to deaths from violence, and for the payment by the Society of the expenses of any necessary printing. E. Emrys Roberts (Cardiff) and C. McNeil (Edinburgh) formed the subcommittee. It appears that this subcommittee was unable to act during the war, and it was resuscitated in March 1920. The last meeting before the outbreak of the 1914–18 war was held in Cambridge in June 1914. It was a beautiful hot summer, as lovely as summer can be in Cambridge: I can feel it now, and it seems that as we walked with our friends amongst those shady backs leading down to the river there was a heavy oppression in the air as of a gathering thunderstorm. The lights were about to go out in Europe; we never saw them again. The Society held its customary meeting, authorised the committee to accept the Journal from the 'proprietors', heard the notice of motion anent the conduct of the Journal and the alteration in rules and adjourned at 2 p.m. on Saturday 27 June. It did not meet again for five years.

1919–1920: TYPE CULTURES AND LABORATORY ASSISTANTS

In July 1919 the Committee met in Edinburgh to gather up the threads. Perhaps the most fruitful of its labours was a discussion on the formation of a collection of standard cultures. It was resolved to communicate with the Director of the Lister Institute expressing the hope that the Institute would be able to undertake the formation and maintenance of such a collection, and offering facilities for communication with the general body of members by means of the circulars of the Society. This was the first step in the establishment of the National Collection of Type Cultures. At the general meeting H. R. Dean raised the question of the supply of reliable dyes and other special reagents, which had become difficult during the war and for which we had previously so largely depended upon Germany; a subcommittee was appointed to go into this matter. At the next Committee meeting, which was in Manchester in January 1920, the final legal formalities for the transfer of the Journal, which had been held up since 1914, were completed. A. Norman and W. Mitchell also attended this meeting and explained the constitution and objects of the Laboratory Assistants' Association and the proposed scheme of examination and certification. J. A. Murray, J. C. G. Ledingham and A. E. Boycott were appointed a subcommittee to make further enquiries, in conjunction with the officers of the Association, and to report. This year the Society held a spring meeting at Charing Cross Hospital. Here the scheme of examinations of the Laboratory Assistants' Association was explained and approved, and J. A. Murray and F. W. Andrewes were nominated as members of the examining council. At this meeting members were invited by the Charing Cross Hospital medical students to accompany them on their specially chartered steamer to see the Boat Race, an invitation that many accepted. At the summer Committee meeting Ritchie was appointed Editor of the Journal, with A. E. Boycott and H. R. Dean (see Fig. 2.4) as Assistant Editors: the Status Lymphaticus Subcommittee was reconstituted and enlarged to nine members.

Dean was elected a secretary in place of Ritchie, and until 1937 remained the active secretary: up to this time the Minutes are in Boycott's handwriting, which becomes progressively smaller as the years pass. Now they appear in Dean's unmistakable bold black vertical writing. Ritchie made a statement on the negotiations he had had with Messrs Oliver and Boyd of Edinburgh for the printing and publication of the Journal.

The full details of the reasons for this change do not appear in the Minutes, but it is evident that whilst the printing of the Journal was done in Edinburgh by Messrs Morrison and Gibb, the business of publishing was in the hands of the Cambridge Press. I have learnt from Mr Robert Grant (see Fig. 2.4) that, early in 1920, the Cambridge Press refused to continue the production, publication and financing of the Journal, and thereby placed the Editors in a serious quandary. Boycott and Ritchie approached Messrs Oliver and Boyd and had an interview with Mr James Thin (the senior partner) and Mr Robert Grant of that firm. The latter asked Boycott, was there a Pathological Society and how many members were there? The answer was 'Yes', and he thought there would be 100–150 members or thereby.

The next question was, could the Society finance the Journal? The answer was 'No; there were no funds and no provision had been made by Sims Woodhead for this unforeseen difficulty'. The upshot was that Mr Grant suggested that the production of the Journal should be entrusted to Messrs Oliver and Boyd, who would pay the outstanding debt to the Cambridge Press and return the property of the Journal without expense to the Society, the one condition being that its production and publication should be entrusted to Oliver and Boyd.

Boycott and Ritchie consulted with others and a few days later asked Mr Grant to draft an agreement embodying his proposals. The Committee was unanimous on the advisability of such a change and the new publishers took over from 1 June 1921.

MESSERS OLIVER AND BOYD AND THE JOURNAL

It is not an overstatement to say that this decision to associate the Journal with Messrs Oliver and Boyd was a most fortunate one for the Society. In this old-established Edinburgh house, with its traditions of fine work, the Journal under the splendid editorships of Ritchie, Boycott and Stewart became one of the best produced and most valuable medical journals of its kind, and probably supreme in its particular sphere. How much is owed to the Editors our members can readily appreciate: they may less easily learn how much is owed to Mr Robert Grant, the active head of Messrs Oliver and Boyd for the first 32 years of the Society's association with this firm. The Journal became a special interest of Mr Grant's and he also acted as its financial adviser, very much to our material advantage, and the sound financial position of the Journal is greatly due to his care and good advice. At the time this change was made the Journal 's finances were causing the Committee anxiety and it was decided at the Leeds meeting in January 1921 that the subscription must be raised at the summer meeting to £2. In due time this was done and the allocation to the Journal from members' subscriptions was increased to 35 shillings. The subscription remained unaltered for 35 years: a remarkable achievement! At this meeting the Stains Subcommittee reported a profit of £30 5s 1d from the distribution of stains they had procured and approved; this was handed to the Treasurer. In January 1922, the Society was in Glasgow. Here the Committee decided to prepare an index of the Journal and also to consider publishing reviews of books on pathology and bacteriology. The summer meeting was at University College Hospital. At this meeting notification of Sims Woodhead's death was communicated and a Minute recorded his high standing in British pathology and his especial service in the matter of the Journal; this was in due course transmitted to Lady Sims Woodhead. It was decided that a medallion should he engraved and appear on the title page of the Journal that he had founded. In 1922 Boycott resigned from his Secretaryship, which he had held since the Society was founded; M. J. Stewart was elected to the vacancy.

1923–1924

The January meeting of 1923 was in Sheffield, the summer one in Oxford. Ritchie was ill and a message was sent to him from Sheffield. By the time the Oxford meeting was reached he had died, and Boycott was appointed Editor, assisted by M. J. Stewart (see Fig. 2.4) and C. Price Jones. A further change was that Ledingham resigned from the treasurership and E. Emrys Roberts was appointed to succeed him. At this meeting the Committee Minutes briefly record: 'a member had suggested that the Society should meet in two sections (a) pathology, (b) bacteriology. The suggestion met with unanimous disapproval'. The Society dined at Queen's College and was entertained at lunch on Saturday by the President and members of the Oxford Medical Society. The winter meeting at Newcastle-upon-Tyne was a small one, only 17 communications being given. It was enlivened, however, by a brisk debate on a motion that A. Renshaw proposed should be forwarded to the Board of Agriculture: 'That this Society considers that the time has now arrived when full facilities should be granted to accredited pathologists to investigate Foot and Mouth Disease'. This referred to the official policy of stringent segregation and slaughter. After some discussion the following amendment was moved: 'That this Society, while in sympathy with the prosecution of research by individual members is not disposed, as a Society, to offer advice to a Government Department'. The amendment was carried by 21 votes to 3. This is an example, out of several that have occurred in the Society's history, of instances in which political action of some sort or another has been proposed. The Society has invariably declined to take such action and there can be little doubt that in so doing, and in remaining strictly a scientific society, it has acted wisely.

At its meeting in July 1924, the Committee nominated E. E. Glynn as treasurer: Emrys Roberts had died early in the year and Ledingham had acted in the interval. The practice concerning the printing of members' degrees and other qualifications was considered and 'it was agreed that decorations and "chief" degrees should be printed in the annual list of members. The selection of degrees or decorations in each case was left to the discretion of the secretaries.' This practice has continued with occasional oversights until today: the exclusion of diplomas and the like here finds its authorisation: there have sometimes been some heart-burnings, especially amongst junior members, but most will agree that the function of the Society's list is not to advertise the qualifications of its members. An interim report of the Status Lymphaticus Subcommittee was submitted by M. J. Stewart and it was resolved that it should be forwarded to the Medical Research Council and to the Editor; it was also presented at the general meeting and subsequently published in the Journal in 1925. The Subcommittee was authorised to co-opt additional members, up to ten, and to pay them an honorarium of £25 per annum. A final report eventually appeared in the Journal in 1931 above the names of M. J. Young and H. M. Turnbull.

At the general meeting of 1924 Boycott gave notice that at the next statutory meeting he would move 'that the ordinary membership of the Society be limited to 400'. Boycott also spoke during Private Business of the services to pathology of S. G. Shattock, who had died during the year, and the secretaries were instructed to send a letter of sympathy to the relatives. In this short tribute Boycott referred to Shattock's refusal to have anything to do with the Society, upon which I have already commented.

1925

In January 1925, the Committee met in Glynn's room in the Thompson Yates Laboratories in Liverpool. Boycott's proposal to limit the size of the Society was discussed and after a Boycott short debate he withdrew it: the principal opposition came from R. Muir, who urged the great advantages to young pathologists of membership of the Society and this, he pointed out, involved the receipt of the Journal – 'a very good journal' – which he thought it of great importance that they should read. A letter was considered suggesting the appointment of committees (a) to draw up a bacteriological classification, and (b) to consider the classification of the streptococci. The Committee decided to take no action. In the summer of 1925 the Society met in Dublin – which up to the present it has not again visited. The Committee decided to prepare and circulate some account of the Pathological and Bacteriological Laboratory Assistants' Association. It was reported that Mervyn Emrys Roberts, whose candidature for an Epsom College Foundationship had been supported by the Society, had been elected.

1926

In 1926 the Society met at the Lister Institute in January and in Aberdeen in July: this was the last occasion of a meeting at the Lister, the increase in size of the Society causing the severance of this old link. At the January Committee meeting it was reported that for the first time the Society's funds showed a debit balance. The treasurer, Glynn, suggested that the Public Trustee should be asked to act as Trustee for the Society and he and the Editor were empowered to consult the Public Trustee. There was also a loss of £29 on the Journal account, due to the cost of the index to the first 25 volumes. It was decided to support the candidature of John Wyon, the son of the late G. A. Wyon of the Pathology Department at Leeds, for an Epsom scholarship. Boycott criticised the cost of the dinner at this and the previous meeting of the Society.

1927

At the Committee meeting at the London School of Medicine for Women, in January 1927, it was decided to advise the Society to appoint the Public Trustee as trustee for the funds and property of the Society and that he be authorised to invest its funds in Trustee securities: this was duly agreed by the Society in General Meeting the next day. As a result of the excellent response to the Wyon fund, Stewart suggested that the Society should become a subscriber to Epsom College and it was decided to advise the Society in this respect; consent was also given to this. There was some discussion on the order in which papers should be grouped on the agenda, Dean saying that he had difficulty in classifying them under the headings of Morbid Anatomy and Bacteriology: as an alternative it was suggested that the papers might be placed in the order in which they were received. The majority favoured the existing method subject to the exercise of the secretaries' discretion.

A summary of several letters from S. C. Dyke concerning a proposed association of practising pathologists, from which the Association of Clinical Pathologists ultimately evolved, was received. The Society was entertained to lunch by the Council of the London School of Medicine for Women.

The Society at this time had been asked to take action with the Physiological Society in requesting its members not to accept posts in medical schools, or in universities or research institutions, in which on principle restrictions were imposed on the use of animals for experimental purposes. Representatives of the Society met those of the Physiological and Biochemical Societies and pointed out that there were difficulties in accepting this simple proposition, arising from the fact that many members of the Society held appointments as hospital pathologists. The conclusion of the matter was that the Society passed a resolution that, 'any further restriction on such use of animals would be detrimental to the progress of medical science'.

1928

At the meeting at St Thomas's Hospital in January 1928, it was reported to the Committee that the treasurer, E. E. Glynn, was gravely ill and steps were therefore taken to deal with the account that had been held in his name. Stewart reported that the matter of financial support for the candidature of John Wyon for a scholarship at Epsom had been brought to a successful conclusion: it was decided to subscribe 200 guineas to the general funds of Epsom College and that the votes derived from this should be used, at the discretion of the Committee, either for the benefit of members of the Society or their dependants who might be candidates for pensions or scholarships, or put at the disposal of the Council of Epsom College. The Committee also formed a provisional subcommittee to consider the formation of a National Committee in connection with the International Society for Microbiology. It was further decided to support the inclusion of a section of bacteriology in the International Botanical Conference to be held in Cambridge in 1930. The question of holding more than two meetings a year was debated, but the general sense of the Committee was against this. At the summer meeting, in view of the serious nature of Glynn's illness, it was decided to proceed with the election of a treasurer and E. H. Kettle was appointed.

1929

The list of honorary members, originally nine, had by the beginning of 1929 shrunk to four and in this year L. Aschoff, Theobald Smith, T. Madsen and G. Schmorl were added. At the Committee meeting in January of that year it was decided that at the Cambridge meeting in the following July the Committee, instead of meeting on the afternoon of the first day as had been customary, should dine together on the previous evening and meet afterwards for business: this pleasant custom has endured. The Cambridge meeting was held in the new Department that had just been built under Dean's direction in Tennis Court Road. On this occasion, on a ballot for members of the Committee, J. G. Greenfield and P. Hartley tied for third place. Hartley wished to retire, but the Society decided to vote again. On a second ballot they again tied. Hartley then proposed the election of Greenfield, which was approved unanimously.

1930

In 1930, the Society met at the Middlesex Hospital in January and at Manchester University in June. E. E. Glynn's death was reported at the Manchester meeting. The Journal had incurred a loss of £184 for the year and a decision was taken to ask the Editors to endeavour to reduce its cost, and at the same time to send a letter to members pointing out the position and asking them to curtail the length of their papers. W. W. C. Topley was appointed an Assistant Editor in place of H. D. Wright.

FINANCIAL DIFFICULTIES OF THE JOURNAL, 1931–1933

It is evident that the Committee, when it met in January, was seriously troubled about the deficit on the account; £900 was owing to the publishers and the Society's bank overdraft was £550. It was decided to sell securities to realise £550. The Editor stated that the size of the Journal would be reduced and that the next issue would contain about 110 pages. The position was again considered in the summer when it was decided to increase the price to outside purchasers from £2 to £3 per annum. The Editor was also asked to enquire of the publishers about a possible reduction in their charges and to examine the charges of other publishers. This enquiry was the beginning of quite a rumpus. At the Committee meeting in January 1932, Boycott reported that as a result of the Editors' efforts a loss of £759 in 1930 had been converted to a profit of £159 in 1931; with the increased price to outside purchasers he thought that there should be a further profit of £400 per annum. Messrs Oliver and Boyd had agreed to reduce their charges to 23/28ths of the charge made by them in 1920. Boycott also said that he had investigated the prices of other publishers, but that the facts were not very easy to ascertain owing to different methods of preparing estimates. Some members of the Committee, however, were not satisfied and Boycott was pressed, and agreed, to make further investigations and to obtain competitive prices. At the summer meeting in Oxford the Editor estimated a surplus of £500 or more on the Journal if its size was not increased. A detailed comparison with other firms' printing and publishing costs showed that, by transferring the Journal from Oliver and Boyd to one of the two other firms considered, a saving of £150 a year might be effected. After a long discussion the Committee decided in favour of this, by 9 votes to 6, Boycott and Stewart dissenting. When the Committee met in the January following (1933), its members had in their hands letters of resignation of office from Boycott and Stewart. Upon this B. H. Kettle, who had proposed at the previous meeting the transfer of the Journal from Messrs Oliver and Boyd, said: 'In common, I think, with every member of the Committee I was very distressed to learn of the resignations of Boycott and Stewart. I proposed the resolution at the last meeting of the Committee that we should change our publishers, because as Treasurer I felt it my duty to conserve the funds of the Society; but as a member of the Committee I feel I have an equally important duty to the Society, which is to do all I can to preserve its unity and strength which depends so largely upon the maintenance of good fellowship and good will. Had I realised that the editors felt so strongly in this matter I should certainly not have proposed the resolution and, if I had proposed it, I do not think I should have received the support of the Committee. The action of the Committee has had results which I for one did not contemplate for one moment and I therefore beg to propose that the resolution to change the publishers from Oliver and Boyd to the Oxford Medical Press, which was passed at the last meeting of the Committee, be rescinded.'

Kettle's resolution, which was seconded by Dean, was put to the meeting by the chairman and passed unanimously. The decision of the Committee was communicated to Boycott and Stewart, who had retired during the discussion, and who then rejoined the other members. Boycott said that he was glad to hear of the decision and wished to thank the Committee for the consideration that had been shown to Stewart and himself. After Stewart had spoken in the same sense they withdrew their resignations as editor and assistant editor. Boycott, however, went on to say that he had found the work of the Journal more and more arduous and that he did not think that he would be able to continue in the office of editor for any very long period. The chairman expressed the appreciation of the Committee of the work that had been done by Boycott and Stewart for the Journal and the pleasure felt at the withdrawal of their resignations. Thus the matter ended.

1931–1932

In detailing this incident, which is of some importance in the history of the Society since it confirmed the association with the publishing firm of Messrs Oliver and Boyd, an association that has continued to the present time, I have passed over certain other matters that have thereby lost their chronological order. Stewart reported in January 1931 that Bryan Strangeways, another candidate supported by the Society for an Epsom scholarship, had been successful. C. C. Okell was appointed an Assistant Editor at the Oxford meeting (1932) in place of W. W. C. Topley. At the same meeting J. W. McLeod asked the opinion of the Committee on the formation of a bacteriological section of the Society. McLeod's argument was that non-medical bacteriologists needed a society for the discussion of bacteriological problems that were not concerned with pathology. It was a question whether a separate Bacteriological Society should be formed, or whether there should be a section of The Pathological Society for the discussion of communications of this nature. There was no vote, but the majority of the members of the Committee appeared in favour of the view, which had been expressed before at meetings of the Committee, that it was important that all members of the Society should have an opportunity to hear all papers on the programme.

It was suggested that if a society of non-medical bacteriologists was formed the new society might be invited to hold its meetings at the same place as, and just before or just after, the meetings of The Pathological Society.

The programme at Oxford was very full, 41 papers being presented. With the approval of the Committee the Chairman proposed to the meeting that the time allotted to each paper should be reduced from fifteen to ten minutes, that members who were also showing demonstrations on the same subject as their communication should volunteer to limit themselves to their demonstration, and that papers on kindred subjects should be discussed together. With this guillotine in operation the meeting was able to adjourn at 12.50 p.m. on the Saturday. The Oxford meeting, the first in the new department built for Dreyer, was memorable for two incidents. One was the fact that the benches in the lecture theatre had been freshly varnished shortly before and, the weather being exceedingly hot, the varnish softened so that members adhered *a posteriori* when attempting to rise; by the end of the meeting all the benches were firmly plastered with agenda papers! The second, and more pleasurable, was that Dreyer had provided a large barrel of cider in the hall of his department, which was greatly appreciated and freely resorted to.

1933

At the July 1933 meeting in Leeds the Committee returned to the problem of the growing list of communications. It was agreed that in order that the meeting should end at 1 o'clock on the Saturday, and so as to allow fifteen minutes for papers as well as ample time for discussion, preference should be given to the first 24 papers on the programme, and that any in excess of this should be printed, but taken only if time permitted. This admirable solution proved in subsequent years a source of embarrassment to the secretaries and to be clearly incompatible with an earlier desire that papers on related subjects should be grouped on the programme. They did their best to combine the latter principle with a reasonable concession to priority of notice, and inevitably they met with some criticism. The matter arose more acutely in 1955 and I shall refer to it again.

1934: BOYCOTT RESIGNS

The 1934 January meeting was at St Mary's Hospital. Boycott, on medical advice, resigned his editorship that he had held since 1923, and M. J. Stewart was appointed in his place. There is no doubt that during his tenure Boycott rendered great service to the Society and advanced the status of the Journal very materially. As an editor he was meticulous, authoritative and autocratic. His methods did not pass without criticism and he was apt, in the interest of what he considered to be a better presentation, to alter the author's wording and occasionally, it must be said, his meaning. This sometimes involved a clash of opinion! Another of Boycott's foibles was his addiction to corresponding by postcard; often these bore the tersest of messages. In reply to a long letter of detailed explanation on some disputed point about a paper one might receive a postcard: 'Yes. A. E. B.' Mr Robert Grant has written to me: 'As an Editor he had his own ideas of punctuation and sometimes his alterations made difficulties with his contributors. One of our Readers made an alteration in Boycott's punctuation, and that resulted in a postcard to me: "Please instruct your compositors to follow in future *my* copy, even out of the window".' Sometimes he had a grave objection to printing an initial letter in place of the first Christian name. That resulted in another postcard: 'Please ascertain if "J" stands for James, John or Jemima'. Boycott had an extreme aversion to commas and struck them ruthlessly out of the manuscripts that came to him. I myself had as good a conceit of my ability to write English as Boycott, and would reinstate most of mine at the proof stage! These amusing trivialities in no way qualify the fact that Boycott was a great editor and left a permanent stamp on the Journal.

The Summer meeting of 1934 was held at the Queen's University of Belfast. Stewart resigned his office as one of the secretaries and J. H. Dible was appointed in his place; G. K. Cameron was appointed to fill the vacancy for an assistant editor. G. F. Nuttall was elected an Honorary Member. The Society was entertained to tea by the honorary staff of the Royal Victoria Hospital and on Saturday afternoon enjoyed various pleasant excursions to the Giant's Causeway and the Mourne mountains, or played golf on the links of the Royal County Down Golf Club as guests of the Belfast members. The July 1934 issue of the Journal was published in honour of Sir Robert Muir, FRS, to celebrate his 70th birthday, and was contributed entirely by his pupils.

1935

In 1935 the Society met in London (King's College Hospital) and at Liverpool University. K. Landsteiner, Peyton Rous and F. B. Mallory were added to the list of Honorary Members. At the Liverpool meeting a paper was given by one member whose claims to cure cancer and other diseases by the injection of vaccines had received prominence in the daily press and who had been strongly criticised to the Committee for the general character of his recent communications. As soon as he rose to speak there was a considerable and pointed exodus of a number of members from the theatre; having delivered himself, he publicly announced his resignation from the Society and walked out of the room: this dramatic gesture was succeeded by a prolonged silence, until the Chairman without comment called for the next paper.

1936

In 1936 the January meeting was at St Bartholomew's Hospital Medical School, and the July one at Dundee. At the latter meeting Sir Robert Muir was elected an Honorary Member. About this time, at the suggestion of Ainley Walker, the Committee decided to recommend the institution of a class of Senior Members to which those of twenty-five years' standing, who had retired from active work, might be elected at a nominal subscription of 10s., without being entitled to receive the Journal. As at the time there were 45 original members in the Society and some 90 members who might he considered eligible for Senior Membership, some anxiety was felt lest this suggestion should lead to a considerable drop in income. The matter was discussed at subsequent Committee meetings, but the fears proved groundless and in 1950 the subscription for senior members was abolished. The increasingly large number of members whose subscriptions were in arrear also engaged the Committee's attention: there were some 150 in arrear for a year or longer, and the Treasurer was authorised to obtain and pay for such assistance as he might need to collect subscriptions.

1936–1937: ARREARS OF SUBSCRIPTIONS

The meetings in 1937 were at the London School of Hygiene and Tropical Medicine, and in Cambridge. At the former the rule regarding Senior Members was approved, together with a new rule authorising the Committee to remove from membership anyone whose subscription was two years in arrear. Kettle had died in 1936 and Dean had carried on the duties of Treasurer in the meantime. Dean's investigation into the financial position showed that, in March, 390 members were in arrear and that a sum of £792 was consequently owing to the Society. As a result of energetic action, involving the sending of 369 letters between March and the end of June, £588 of the arrears had been collected, but £195 10s was still owing. Dean mentioned that he had received great assistance from W. A. Mitchell in dealing with the accounts. These now showed a balance that would enable the Society to invest £400. It was proposed and agreed that a new rule should be introduced whereby newly elected members must send a Banker's Order to the Treasurer, and the secretaries were instructed to draft such a rule. J. McIntosh was asked by the Committee if he would accept nomination to the office of Treasurer and agreed to do so. C. C. Okell resigned his Assistant Editorship and H. D. Wright was appointed. Dean announced that he proposed for the future to hand over the active duties of the secretaryship, which he had performed since 1919, to J. H. Dible.

In 1938 meetings took place at the Middlesex Hospital and Edinburgh University. McIntosh's acceptance of the office of Treasurer led to the Committee's meetings and supper in London usually being held in the pleasant surroundings of the Board Room of the Middlesex Hospital, an innovation that was continued later by Scarff. This was the last meeting held at the Middlesex, for reasons which now begin to appear.

In January a special meeting was held between representatives of the Society and those of the Pathological and Bacteriological Laboratory Assistants' Association, which had decided to revise its constitution and seek conversion into a limited company. The Association regarded the maintenance of the existing association with the Society of paramount importance and suggested that representatives of the Society might be on the Board of Directors. Further, a change of title was proposed incorporating the term 'technician'. Mr Denyer for the Association submitted draft Articles of Association.

1938: DEATH OF BOYCOTT

At the July meeting the death of A. E. Boycott was announced and Stewart spoke of Boycott's outstanding personality, his scientific achievements, his devotion to biological science, and his notable service to the Society as Editor of the Journal. Boycott was certainly an outstanding figure in the Society. Tall, cadaverous, with side-whiskers which moved up or down his face according to his whim, an incisive way of speaking, extremely and sometimes devastatingly logical and never moved to wrath or swayed by emotion – or so it seemed – his personality was felt at all the meetings at which he was present. An ascetic and an intellectual he tended to be contemptuous of some of the pleasures that appeal to many other men. He was a firm and merciless critic, at times perhaps a little harsh in dealing with a junior member giving his first paper, but not so of malice. He would find the recipient of his criticisms later and explain his point and make suggestions for avoiding the pitfall. He was a great supporter of the Society and had been in office from its inception until he resigned his editorship from ill-health in 1934. After being away ill for some time he reappeared at the St Bartholomew's meeting in January 1936 and read a paper – his last. The warmth of his reception then probably surprised him, but the Society felt more at home with him present again amongst its number; it was the flicker of a dying fire. With Boycott's departure the spirit of criticism, formerly so much abroad in the Society, seemed to suffer some decay; it was sustained by J. A. Murray and J. Cruickshank but nevertheless, or so it seems to one who has grown old in the Society, we are today more ready to accept the authority of the spoken statement and the didacticism of the lantern slide, and less apt to probe the facts behind and to question the validity of the conclusions, than we were 30 years ago.

The January meeting of 1939 was held at the Royal Free Hospital and London School of Medicine for Women, and the summer one in the University of Birmingham.

The draft Articles of Association of the Institute of Medical Laboratory Technology (as it was later named) were discussed by the Committee and various suggestions made. A clause providing for the payment of examiners was objected to by Dean, who received unanimous support.

J. A. MURRAY

At this meeting J. A. Murray was nominated as an Honorary Member. The Secretaries' letter to him drew the following characteristic reply:

2 Belgrave Gardens, NW8
14 Jan 1939
'My dear Dible,
Please convey to the Committee my sincere thanks for the kindly feeling which led to their proposal to put me down for the high compliment of Honorary Fellow of the Society.
It is with the greatest regret that I ask them not to proceed any further with it.
I think it is indecent to disturb a dead body that is not doing any harm.
Yours v. truly,
JAMES A. MURRAY.'

At the general meeting R. D. Passey suggested that in view of the large size of the Society the meetings in London might be held in some central institution instead of the various hospital laboratories as had been customary. The matter was referred to the Committee for consideration. At the summer Committee meeting Dible reported upon enquiries he had made about the possibility of meeting at the Royal Society of Medicine or the Royal College of Surgeons. The former institution would charge about £20, to which would have to be added the cost of hiring microscopes. The Royal College of Surgeons would willingly take the Society, but there might be some difficulty owing to examinations at the time of the winter meeting. After a discussion in which it was stated that the theatre at the Royal College of Surgeons was not suitable, and that there would be difficulties there for demonstrations, it was decided to continue to use such London medical schools and institutions as could provide the accommodation necessary.

1940–1941

The January meeting for 1940 was to have been held at Guy's Hospital. Owing to the war the Secretaries, who decided not to follow the precedent of the 1914–1918 war and suspend the activities of the Society, arranged a one-day meeting at Cambridge as an emergency measure after consulting with the Treasurer and Editor. This action was subjected to some criticism, but was endorsed unanimously by the Committee. The candidates approved by the Committee at this meeting were subsequently, in August 1940, by resolution of the Committee, offered temporary membership of the Society on the understanding that their names would come up for election at the first general meeting that could be held. Sixteen papers were read and 100 persons lunched and 95 dined at Trinity Hall. The summer meeting of 1940 had been arranged to be held at Trinity College, Dublin, but this proving impracticable an invitation from Florey to meet in Oxford was accepted and notices were sent out accordingly. These too had to be cancelled, owing to other difficulties arising out of the war, and no meeting could be held until one was arranged by Stewart for a single day in Leeds, in March 1941.

In the interim a special meeting of the Committee had been held, also in Leeds, in the January of that year. The Committee at each of these meetings numbered only six. A pleasing incident was the receipt of a letter from Dr William J. Deadman, Chairman of the Ontario Association of Pathologists, expressing sympathy with the Society in the difficulties and dangers to which its members were exposed as a result of the war and offering to arrange an exchange of duties, or any other form of relief for those of us who might be forced on medical grounds to seek temporary respite. This letter was read to the Society and was much appreciated. At the Leeds meeting W. G. MacCallum was elected an Honorary Member.

It was decided at the special Committee meeting in January that the March 1941 meeting should be deemed the statutory meeting for 1940, which had not been held, and that a notice should be printed in the Journal to this effect. In view of the uncertainties of the times the Committee then put forward certain resolutions to provide for possible eventualities. These read: 'In the event of no meeting of the Society being held in a given year:

(1) The officers and committee shall be continued in office;
(2) when an election does take place, only the three members of Committee senior in order of election shall retire;
(3) the Committee shall have power to fill casual vacancies in its membership;
(4) the Secretaries shall have power to decide that any given meeting is a statutory meeting;
(5) the Committee shall have power to elect new members and to transact any necessary business.'

The motion was adopted. Thus battened down, the Society prepared to ride out the storm. This meeting was attended by 70–80 members.

In July 1941, a meeting was held in Glasgow. Sir Henry Dale, FRS, was elected an Honorary Member. Seventeen papers were given and 56 persons were present at the dinner. It was decided to hold a meeting in Cambridge in the spring.

1942–1943: LABORATORY ANIMALS

In March 1942, the Society met in Cambridge, once more customarily for the two days: there was a good attendance, with 172 members and visitors signing the book. In Private Business a motion was discussed from D. McClean and A. A. Miles that the Society should institute a Benevolent Fund from a portion of its capital and from further monies accruing, as well as from a special voluntary levy upon members. This aroused considerable feeling and a letter was received from six Manchester members disapproving of the resolution and urging that the funds of the Society should be used for scientific purposes exclusively and for the needs of the Journal. The motion was lost by 38 votes to 25. A motion by H. J. Parish and W. B. Gye 'That the Society urges the Medical Research Council and the Agricultural Research Council to take up the question of large scale breeding of stocks of healthy experimental animals as a matter of national importance and urgency' was carried. This may be regarded as the stimulus that ultimately produced the Laboratory Animals' Bureau under the aegis of the Medical Research Council. At the dinner in the hall of Trinity Hall, A. Norman, on behalf of the Pathological and Bacteriological Laboratory Assistants' Association, presented the Society with a Chairman's walnut gavel, engraved with the names of the presidents of the Association since its foundation in 1912. H. R. Dean accepted the gift on behalf of the Society and thanked the members of the Association for a token of the happy and fruitful cooperation which had existed between the two bodies. In July 1942 the Society met in the Physics Laboratory, the Royal Fort, Bristol. The meeting was a small one, only 13 papers being given.

The Committee held a special meeting at the Middlesex Hospital in January 1943 to consider letters from the Inter-Departmental Committee on Medical Education ('Goodenough Committee') and a memorandum from H. R. Dean on the same subject. The Secretaries were instructed to compose a memorandum embodying the main conclusions of the meeting and J. Shaw Dunn, H. R. Dean and J. H. Dible were nominated to give evidence before the Inter-Departmental Committee. A memorandum from the Association of Scientific Workers on the provision of laboratory animals by Government Departments was also considered. The Committee recalled the earlier action by the Society in initiating this matter, but held that in view of the shortage of workers of all types throughout the country it was not practicable for such a scheme to be proceeded with during the war. This matter was again raised at the April 1943 Committee meeting since, as a result of pressure from the Association of Scientific Workers that asked the Society's support in this matter, the Medical Research Council had called a meeting with that body, the Agricultural Research Council and the Ministry of Supply, and Dible had been asked to attend as the Secretary of the Society resident in London. The two Councils had declined to take action during the war and, having heard the details of the discussion, the Committee reaffirmed its former decision to take no further action at this time. The Society was also asked by the Association of Scientific Workers to participate in the organisation of a Central Bureau for the coordination and registration of medical research. The Committee was unanimously of the opinion that a case had not been made for the establishment of the suggested bureau and register. At the Committee's General Meeting that followed the first matter was raised again, and the Committee's decision reported: it was, however, moved by the Chairman, and carried by 51 votes to 31, that 'the Society recommends that the Committee shall appoint a representative to the Committee established by the Association of Scientific Workers to investigate the matter of the breeding and supply of experimental animals'. Eventually a conference was convened at University College at which the Society was represented by A. A. Miles and H. J. Parish. A. W. Downie was elected an assistant editor at the April Committee meeting. The summer meeting of 1943 was held at Manchester: it was moderately attended, with 78 members and 27 visitors signing the book. The Society decided to collaborate in an appeal for funds for the presentation of a laboratory to a Moscow hospital, which it was agreed Dean should sign as a secretary of the Society.

1944

In March 1944, the Committee met for supper under war-time conditions in considerable discomfort at Schmidt's restaurant in Soho and subsequently moved to the London School of Hygiene for its business. From a discussion on the nomination of newly qualified candidates for membership, which was becoming increasingly common, it was agreed that except in very special circumstances it was undesirable that candidates who had been qualified for only one or two years should be put forward for membership. This was expanded at a subsequent Committee meeting and at the general meeting, a year later, it was confirmed that: 'Candidates for membership should be persons who had been engaged for some years in research or teaching in pathology, or who had held for some years recognised appointments as pathologists, and also persons who had a comparable training and experience in any of the allied sciences; accordingly it was undesirable that beginners or "trainees", and persons with a very limited experience in pathology, should be nominated for membership of the Society'. It was at this time decided that the summer meeting of 1994 should be held at Cardiff. In fact it did not prove possible to hold another scientific meeting until a year later when, in the spring of 1945, the Society met at St Thomas's Hospital Medical School. In the interim, however, a joint meeting with the Biochemical Society at the Royal Society of Medicine was held that December for discussions on 'Oestrogens and malignant disease' and, 'Viruses in relation to cancer, with special reference to the milk factor'.

RUMOURS OF A NATIONAL HEALTH SERVICE

At this time there were considerable stirrings arising from the obvious intention of all political parties to promote a more extended National Health Service. The Royal Colleges established a Committee of Consultants to advise their representatives in discussions with the Ministry of Health, and Dible was invited to represent the Society on this Committee. At about this time also the Vice-Chancellor of the University of London asked the members of the Committee who were resident in London and available to undertake the classification of the pathologists in the London area. This was done, although the list supplied contained a number of omissions to which attention was drawn, and it was therefore plainly stated that the draft sent to the Vice-Chancellor could only be regarded as provisional. The object of this survey was stated in Parliament to be to determine, for the purposes of the Government, the number of specialists available in the area. The General Medical Council also approached the Society regarding the possible formation of a register of specialists. The Committee agreed that the Society should take action in this regard, in order to be in a position to advise on the qualification of individuals for recognition should the duty of compiling a register devolve upon the General Medical Council. The Association of Clinical Pathologists had also been approached and a Committee was appointed to meet jointly with the Clinical Pathologists. The Committee of the Royal Colleges to which I have already referred, and upon which the Society was represented, continued to meet and to consider the steps that should be taken to plan a Consultant Specialists Service. Two further activities of the Committee at this period were the nomination of representatives to serve on the Medical Research Council's Committee on Medical Mycology and the setting up of a Joint Standing Committee, with the Association of Clinical Pathologists and the Institute of Medical Laboratory Technology, for the consideration of matters of mutual interest concerning technicians.

The Committee held another special meeting in July 1944 at which it was reported that Government restrictions on travel made it necessary that the Cardiff meeting should be abandoned. Under the emergency powers conferred on it at the General Meeting on 28 March 1941, the Committee left it to the discretion of the Secretaries to arrange for a meeting in January 1945 if possible, Birmingham being suggested as the venue. Candidates for membership were approved on the assumption that a meeting would be held in January, but it was decided that they should be deemed to be elected if no such meeting could be held. The report of the subcommittee appointed to draft a reply to the General Medical Council on the qualification of pathologists for registration was submitted and adopted. The preamble is interesting: 'The Committee resolved, that should it be found necessary to compile a register of specialists in pathology, and should this duty lie with the General Medical Council, to recommend... etc.'. The multiple qualifications illustrate the uncertainty of the position at the time. The Government were groping their way and no one knew where such a statutory duty might lie, if indeed it lay anywhere. The General Medical Council was as uncertain as the rest of us. It is not necessary to quote here the full text of the Committee's considered report, since at the moment the issue is not before us, but the main points that were emphasised may be mentioned: experience in general medicine and surgery by whole-time resident appointments; a minimum of five years' study in the laboratories of a medical school or a hospital approved for this purpose by the University in the region, with one year of the five in a University Department of Pathology; no insistence on a diploma, but recognition to be given to time spent in acquiring this.

Information was also received on the formation of the Biological Council and the Society for General Microbiology, and a representative from the Society was appointed to the former. The hope was expressed that it would be possible at times to arrange meetings of the Society and the Society for General Microbiology upon consecutive days.

1945

On 2 January 1945, the Committee met again and learnt from the Secretaries that it had not been possible to meet in Birmingham and that it had been agreed by correspondence to postpone the meeting until March and if possible to hold it in London. The Treasurer reported that the state of the Society's finances had improved very materially during the war owing to increased sales of the Journal and the diminution in general expenses consequent on the restriction of meetings. The shortage of paper was, however, a serious problem to the Editor and publication was beginning to fall seriously into arrear.

The March meeting was eventually held at St Thomas's Hospital Medical School and was attended by 137 members and 56 guests. In Private Business the Committee's recommendation regarding the qualifications of candidates for election was communicated. Attention was drawn to the desire that had been expressed that symposia upon current problems of special interest might be organised and members were invited to suggest subjects.

The January 1945 issue of the Journal was dedicated to H. M. Turnbull, FRS, on his 70th birthday: it included a reproduction of his portrait by Wilhelm Kaufmann.

The postponed Cardiff meeting was held in June 1945. The Committee considered the possible employment at some period of a paid Editor. The amount of work devolving upon the Editor had exercised some members for a considerable time and various suggestions had been made on earlier occasions of ways of providing Stewart with assistance, but none of these had been very effective. Stewart declined any honorarium for himself, but warned the Society that paid assistance might be required after the war when the size of the Journal would increase. At this meeting A. W. Downie desired to resign from his Assistant Editorship, but he was asked to continue until the end of the year.

Dible raised the question of the limitation of the size of the Society, which had been previously raised by Boycott in 1925 and rejected. The reasons that impelled him to do this again were that the growth of the Society made it difficult to find accommodation for the London meetings and that it would become more and more difficult in the future to continue the traditional form of the meetings unless some limitation was imposed. There seemed little support for frank limitation and the discussion that followed divided itself along two lines, one group of members favouring a division of the programme at the winter meeting into sections and the other the holding of three meetings a year as a possible solution. It was agreed that the latter should be tried in 1946 and that the Society should be recommended to meet at the Westminster Hospital in January, in Liverpool in April and in Aberdeen in July. At the general meeting G. H. Whipple was elected an Honorary Member.

1946

These pious resolves were upset by the clash between the Grand National and the projected Liverpool Spring meeting, so that when the Committee met again in January it was proposed to change the venue of the March meeting to Sheffield. The Committee also decided to recommend a donation towards the University education of J. Gray, the son of an old member of the Society. A suggestion was received from the Association of Clinical Pathologists that the Society should engage with the Association in negotiations on the salaries of whole-time pathologists in the National Medical Service. It was agreed without dissent that: 'since the primary objects of the Society were scientific it was not its function to engage in negotiations of this kind'. The Committee made a grant towards the expenses of the Biological Council and appointed W. G. Barnard as its representative. R. W. Scarff proposed the formation of a histological consultative panel for the Society and the formation of a reference collection: a subcommittee was appointed to consider the question and to report. At the Sheffield Committee meeting in March, the Histological Consultative Panel was constituted, and this absorbed the older panel of advisers that had been in existence for some time under the aegis of the National Radium Commission, as well as a panel supported by the British Empire Cancer Campaign. Scarf was appointed Secretary to the panel, which has since done much useful work. At the General Meeting in Sheffield the Secretaries reported a gratifying response to the appeal on behalf of the son of the late J. Gray.

At the Aberdeen meeting in July 1946, the Secretaries reported a deficit of £5 16s on the Sheffield meeting, due to members failing to honour their obligations to dine or use the accommodation reserved on their behalf. The deficit was paid by the Society, but on subsequent occasions similar difficulties were encountered and as a result the Secretaries later were forced to demand payments in advance: this has now become customary. A suggestion was received at this meeting from the Association of Clinical Pathologists for the production of a joint Journal. This the Committee declined, the Editor stating that he would be willing to advise authors to submit their papers to a Journal published under the auspices of the Association of Clinical Pathologists if it appeared that they were better suited to such a publication than to the Journal.

1947

When the Committee met at the London School of Hygiene and Tropical Medicine in January 1947, the protracted discussion on the qualification of members was brought to a conclusion: it was decided that unless there were exceptional considerations a candidate should not be recommended for membership unless he had been three years qualified and completed two whole years in pathological work. J. W. Howie was elected an assistant editor. At this meeting the question of a spring meeting in Liverpool was again canvassed and owing to the local difficulties the Committee decided to abandon it. The Conference on Experimental Animals, which had reported at the Sheffield meeting, announced that it had concluded its labours and was left with a deficit of £50. The Society decided to contribute £5.

At the July Committee meeting (1947) an invitation was received from N. Goormaghtigh to hold the next summer meeting in Ghent: this was cordially welcomed and the Secretaries were asked to make arrangements. This meeting was later cancelled owing to the refusal of the Treasury to allow the necessary currency. Stewart, at short notice, arranged for the meeting to be in Leeds.

1948

In 1948 the January meeting was held at St Bartholomew's Hospital Medical College and the July one at Leeds. At the latter the Committee discussed at length the difficulties, arising from the increase in membership, of continuing to hold meetings of the type traditional in the Society. The Barts' meeting had been attended by over 300 individuals and was very overcrowded. Of the various remedies discussed the Committee considered that the experiment of meeting in two sections was the most practicable and should be given a trial. At the general meeting H. M. Turnbull and Oswald T. Avery were elected Honorary Members.

JAMES McINTOSH

At this meeting, in the course of the Secretaries' report, J. H. Dible paid a tribute to James McIntosh, who had died during the course of the year. McIntosh was a much admired and personally loved member of the Society, the former for his great ability and important contributions to the advancement of pathology throughout his whole working life, and the latter for his personal qualities. A strong and vigorous personality, quick to anger and a man of strong likes and dislikes, McIntosh was generous and kind in the extreme. His vigorous qualities were a great asset at the meetings of our Society and with him departed one of the more vivid personalities of the Society's middle period. He was Treasurer from 1939 to 1948.

At the meeting in December 1948 the Committee received a welcome invitation from a new quarter. Dr M. Straub of Rotterdam wrote suggesting that the Society should hold an additional meeting in Holland in the month of April. This was cordially received and Straub was nominated a member of the Society. The scientific sessions at the December general meeting were held in two sections for the first time. Pathological papers were given at University College Hospital Medical School and bacteriological papers at the London School of Hygiene and Tropical Medicine, where the demonstrations were also taken. At this meeting 39 new members were elected, a record to that date; but at the following winter meeting 50 new members were elected: these figures show the very rapid growth of the Society and emphasise the seriousness of the problem of accommodation. During the course of the Society's dinner at the Mecca Restaurant, A. Norman, on behalf of the Institute of Medical Laboratory Technology, presented the Woodhead Medal of the Institute to H. R. Dean.

1949

The Summer meeting of 1949 was held at Oxford. The Committee dined at Worcester College. At this meeting, for the third time in the Society's history, an attempt was set on foot to limit its size, E. T. C. Spooner giving notice that he would move a resolution on the matter at the next Committee meeting when the item could be on the agenda. It was decided to support British Abstracts to the extent of £300 a year for three years. R. W. Scarff was nominated to the Board of Directors and G. R. Cameron to the Committee dealing with Section A covering pathological subjects. The Committee also learnt that a large meeting of representatives of societies interested in the standardisation of biological dyestuffs had met at the Royal Society of Medicine under Dible's chairmanship. As a result 'The British Dyestuffs Commission' had been constituted with Sir John Simonson as its Chairman and Dr W. B. Sandiford as its secretary. The Committee also approved a British National Committee for the International Society of Geographical Pathology. Dr Straub attended the general meeting and issued a personal invitation from the Netherlands Pathological Society for meetings in Amsterdam and Leiden on 14 and 15 April 1950, which was enthusiastically received. The Oxford programme was a large one, consisting of 31 communications and 19 demonstrations; the sections of Pathology and Bacteriology met separately. Many members were accommodated in Colleges and the Society's dinner was held in Hertford College.

1950: EMBARRASSING GROWTH OF THE SOCIETY

In 1950 the Society grappled for the third and perhaps the last time with the problem of its size (Fig. 2.5). The Secretaries reported to the Committee that in their examination of the possibilities of meeting in some central hall they had investigated the Beveridge Hall of London University, the Friends' House, the Royal Society of Medicine, the Royal Geographical Society, the Royal Institute of British Architects, the Royal College of Nursing, the Royal Institution, the Scala Theatre, the Royal Horticultural Society, Imperial College, and other Institutes of the University of London, but none of these had been available or suitable for the winter meeting. The matter was lengthily debated and it was widely agreed that much was lost by splitting the Society's meeting into two sections. The main problem concerned the London meetings and Dible gave it as his opinion that if the membership of the Society was limited to 800 it would be possible to continue the traditional character of its meetings, although in London it might be necessary, in the absence of

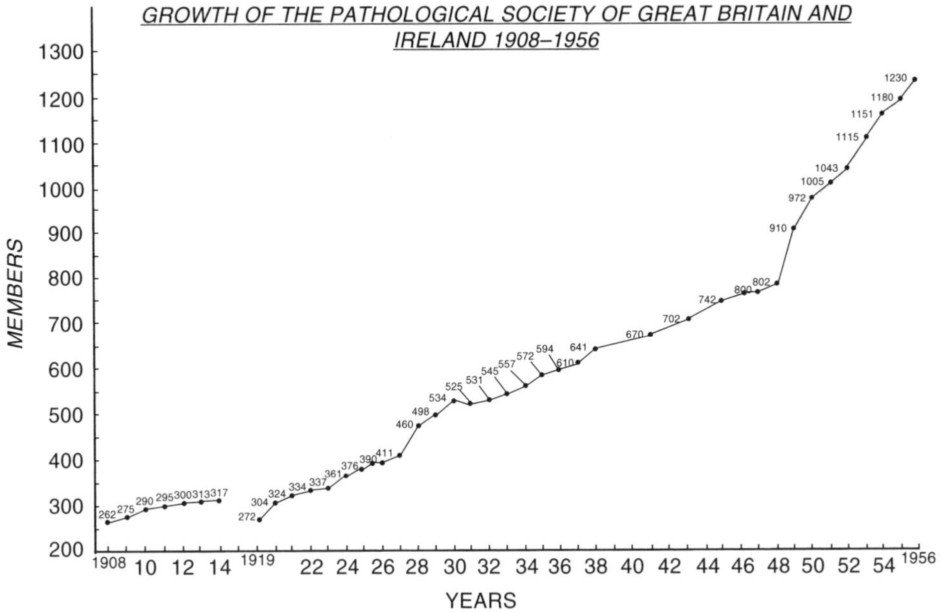

Figure 2.5 Growth of the Society.

a large hall, to meet in two sections. Spooner proposed, and Downie seconded, a motion that 'the number of new members elected each year be limited to 20 until the membership of the Society is reduced to 800 at which it should remain. The election of new members to be by ballot of those proposed after the nominations have been approved by the Committee.' Their motion was carried by 11 votes to 4. The Secretaries were also asked to arrange for three meetings a year, if possible. At the following general meeting the Secretaries gave notice that this motion would be presented for decision by the Society at the Statutory meeting in the summer. Thus the matter remained until the Committee met in Dundee in July. Then a memorandum from Dean setting out the arguments against limitation was considered and a number of members of the Committee spoke of objections to the proposal that had been made to them. Spooner, who was absent, had sent a letter in which he said he would agree to withdraw the motion if the Committee were of a like mind, and in effect the Committee decided to ask permission of the Society to withdraw the motion for limitation of its size at the private business meeting on the following day. This was its fate. The writer of this record of the Society, who from his experience as one of its secretaries had proposed in 1945 the limitation of the Society's size, believes that this act was not in the best interests of the Society. A compact Society of reasonable size is able to transact scientific business in an admirably informal manner; this is of great value to those engaged in the prosecution of research who desire to communicate and obtain criticism of work that is in hand but not at the moment in its final form. Such a proving ground is impossible in a Society of large size in which personal criticism is more difficult. Moreover, the very size of the Society in later years has imposed physical restraints upon its meetings that can only be escaped from by corresponding limitations, the most obvious of which is the splitting of the Society into sections. In the laudable desire to keep the Society open to all aspirants for membership, its members have imposed upon themselves limitations that they have repeatedly exclaimed against.

At this meeting the Committee received a request from the Royal College of Physicians to act as a 'Specialist Association', and to classify its members for the information of the Advisory

Committee on Distinction Awards: the invitation was declined. A request from a member for support of a claim for recognition as a consultant was also refused.

AMSTERDAM

The Society met in Amsterdam on Friday, 14 April and in the University of Leiden on Saturday 15 April 1950. Papers were presented by members of the Society and by members of the Netherlands Pathological Society. The meeting was an enjoyable and memorable one, and by the kindness of the Society's Dutch hosts visits were made to the battlefield of Arnhem and the cemetery of the Airborne Division at Oosterbeek, as well as to De Hoge Veluwe and the van Gogh museum. The kind hospitality of the Society's Dutch hosts will be long remembered by those who were present and marked the good fellowship between Dutch and British pathologists that it is hoped will long endure.

At its meeting in Dundee in July 1950, the Committee decided against a meeting in March 1951. The number of assistant editors was increased from two to four, the two senior assistant editors to be ex officio members of the Committee. Here, at the general meeting, it was agreed to circulate the audited accounts and balance sheet prior to the statutory meeting and also that Senior Members should in future pay no subscription. The members of the Society were entertained to tea by the kindness of the College Council.

At the December meeting, a statement was made to the Committee that vacancies in its number were repeatedly filled by the same individuals so that new blood was not introduced: a regulation was suggested to obviate this. On looking into the matter it was found that over the preceding seven years only one member had in fact been elected twice: the Committee agreed however that, without making any rule in the matter, it was not desirable for a retiring member to allow his name to he proposed for election until a reasonable period, such as two or three years, had passed. The general meeting, which was at St Thomas's Hospital, was divided into two sections: 'A' of Morbid Anatomy, Experimental Pathology and Cancer Research, and 'B' of Bacteriology, Serology and Virus Infections.

1951

The January 1951 issue of the Journal was published in honour of Sir Alexander Fleming, FRS, and the April issue in honour of Professor Carl Browning, FRS, in each case on the occasion of the member's 70th birthday.

The summer meeting of 1951 was held in the large Arts Theatre of Liverpool University, which accommodated the whole company comfortably. The Committee considered criticisms that had been made of the style of presentation of papers by some contributors and the illegibility of much of the tabular matter shown on slides. S. L. Baker wrote: 'The worst type of paper, of which we usually have one or more at each meeting, takes the form of an inaudible soliloquy in front of a series of invisible tables'. The Secretaries were instructed to draft a memorandum on this subject, discouraging the reading of papers and making suggestions for improving presentation and for the amount of tabular matter that could be shown intelligibly on a lantern slide. This resulted in the leaflet that it is now the practice to send to all members who submit the title of a paper. An interesting project for a Science Centre for London, under the aegis of the Royal Society, was made known. The centre, it was suggested, might provide the societies invited to collaborate with a hall suitable for large meetings, as well as facilities for demonstrations and refreshments, the use of a committee room and possibly an office for secretarial purposes. The plan appealed very much to members of the Committee. The Royal Society initially refused to consider a request that

The Pathological Society should have an opportunity to participate. The matter had however been re-opened through the energetic action of certain members, in particular Dean, Wilson Smith and Florey, and the Royal Society had agreed to reconsider the matter. At this time it seemed that such a centre might provide a solution for the problems of the Society's London meetings, and possibly for some of those arising from the Journal. The matter does not seem to have been proceeded with.

1952

In consequence of criticisms of the Society's conservative financial policy, made during Private Business at the Liverpool meeting, together with a suggestion that accumulated capital might be employed in providing Research Studentships, Fellowships, Prizes and a hospitality fund, the Committee deliberated on its financial policy at the January 1952 meeting in Cambridge. The conclusion reached was that the Society's resources should be conserved in view of increasing expenses, especially with regard to the Journal and the probability that these would continue to increase in the future. The Society's officers were asked to prepare a memorandum giving a reasoned statement of the way in which the Society's monies had been used in the past, and of the financial position, for presentation to all members at the summer meeting. It was also decided to provide some funds for hospitality and social entertainment for the Society's Dutch colleagues and their wives who were expected at the Glasgow meeting, and Cappell was authorised to make certain expenditure for this purpose. The Cambridge meeting was extended over three days and embraced 51 communications. The whole Society met in the Anatomy theatre on the Thursday afternoon, and on the Friday and Saturday divided into sections that met in the departments of Anatomy and Pathology.

In July 1952 the Society met in Glasgow, again for three days: J. W. Howie resigned the senior assistant editorship that he had held since 1947. L. Foulds also resigned from the post of a junior assistant editor and D. H. Collins was appointed to the latter vacancy. The price of the Journal was considered and Stewart advised that the subscription should be raised: this was not acceded to by the Committee, but it was decided to increase the cost to outside subscribers to £4. H. J. Parish reported on the valuable work of the Laboratory Animals Bureau, on which he represented the Society. It was agreed to subscribe £10 10s annually to the funds of Epsom College and £40 per annum to assist in the schooling of Bryan Flaks. The memorandum setting out the financial position of the Society in relation to its resources, which had been drafted by Dible, was presented at Private Business during this meeting. Members of the Netherlands Pathological Society were present; the special arrangements for the entertainment included a dinner for the Dutch ladies in the University Rooms and a dinner for the visitors in the Faculty Hall of the Royal Faculty of Physicians and Surgeons of Glasgow. An excursion was arranged on the Sunday following the meeting to Loch Katrine and the Trossachs.

1953

In 1953 the January meeting was held in London in two sections: that of Pathology at the London School of Hygiene and Tropical Medicine and that of Bacteriology at the Wellcome Research Institute. At the January Committee meeting Stewart reported on the delay in publishing papers that had reached from six to eight months. The question of publishing additional volumes each year and also of increasing the subscription to the Society was considered: it was decided to review the matter at the July meeting. A sum of £100 a year for five years was voted for the assistance of the family of the late E. A. Home. It was decided to discontinue supporting the Biological Council since the Society gained little advantage from its activities.

At the Belfast Committee meeting in the summer Stewart again strongly urged an increase in the subscription owing to the growing losses on the Journal account. It was decided not to do this immediately, in view of the sound financial position of the Society as a whole, but as an interim measure to increase the proportion of members' subscriptions to the Journal account from 6s per member per part to 8s, a compromise that Stewart sturdily disapproved. A request was received from the Association of Clinical Pathologists that the Society should send representatives to an ad hoc committee set up by the Association to discuss the question of promoting a Faculty of Pathologists. The Committee decided that it was in no position to send representatives from the Society, but nominated three observers who might attend the Association's committee and who would be at liberty to express their personal opinions.

1954

In 1954 the January meeting was held in Birmingham and the July one in Edinburgh. At both of these meetings the Society was divided into sections. At the latter it was finally decided to withdraw the Society's financial support from British Abstracts, which had experienced various vicissitudes but was not in the Committee's view of sufficient value to pathologists to warrant the considerable expenditure the Society had incurred over the past four years. H. R. Dean and M. J. Stewart were elected Honorary Members at the Edinburgh meeting. At this meeting Dean resigned his secretaryship, which he had held since 1920. On the motion of the Chairman (A. M. Drennan) the Society recorded in the Minutes its gratitude and appreciation of his long service. A. W. Downie was appointed to the vacancy. The splitting of the Society into sections was adversely criticised by J. W. McLeod during the Private Business, and in this he was supported by A. C. Lendrum. It was suggested that more communications could be given in the form of demonstrations. The Chairman remarked that splitting was a penalty of the Society's size.

1955

In 1955 the January meeting was held in the Great Hall of the new Royal College of Surgeons buildings in Lincoln's Inn Fields. It was hoped that the space available would enable the division of the meeting into sections to be avoided and that in the splendid accommodation of this fine new building, with so many amenities available, a solution might be found to the chronic difficulties of the London meetings that became greater every year. These hopes were not entirely fulfilled, as the more formal arrangements dictated by so large a meeting destroyed some of the intimacy and facility for debate so valued in the Society. However, it seems that these difficulties are not insoluble and on future occasions the Society may he extremely glad to accept again the hospitality of the Royal College. Once more the Committee wrestled with the incompatibilities of meeting as a single body, providing adequate time for discussion, avoiding an extra session on Thursday, terminating the meeting at lunch time on the Saturday, and dealing with programmes and audiences of a size that made these desiderata impossible! In fact at this meeting, which occupied two days, 41 communications were given and the end was not reached until 5 p.m. on the Saturday evening.

STEWART RESIGNS

At the summer meeting in Bristol, Stewart informed the Committee of his desire to resign his editorship at the end of the year; at the same time Cameron resigned his post as a senior assistant editor, which he had held since C. L. Oakley undertook to discharge the duties of Editor for one year and to report. J. W. Orr was appointed an assistant editor. At the Private Business on the following day G. L. Montgomery voiced the Society's very real and deep appreciation of Stewart's long, unselfish and efficient editorship, by which he had made the Journal a model amongst scientific journals. He moved: 'That the Society do express its sorrow and regret at Stewart's retirement and offer him its sincere and warmest thanks for his great and outstanding service'. In replying, Stewart said that his labour as an Editor had been a labour of love. He referred to his long association with Boycott to whom he attributed many of the editorial traditions of the Journal, and to the help he had had from his assistant editors. At this meeting Pierre Masson was elected an Honorary Member.

1956

The Committee at its Bristol meeting had received a memorandum from a number of signatories regarding ways in which it was suggested that the meetings might be improved. These problems had exercised the Committee for some time and various shifts had already been tried or were under consideration to meet the points raised. As an outcome of this the Secretaries met the subscribers to the memorandum at the Westminster School in January 1956 and had a full and frank discussion in which all the matters were dealt with and the possibilities explored. On the Secretaries reporting this discussion to the Committee it was decided, as an experiment, to convene the summer meeting in Manchester in 1956 for the Thursday morning and to continue to meet as a single body until Saturday mid-day, but to divide the subjects on the agenda in a more formal manner than had been done at any previous meeting and, by taking these sections consecutively and as far as possible at stated times, to try to permit those whose interests lay only in special parts of the programme to attend these without inconvenience. Other suggestions, e.g. that contributors should be asked to submit summaries of their papers, or that the programme should be limited in size and that the secretaries should make a selection of the papers offered, were not supported. A. Macdonald resigned from the post of a junior assistant editor.

ROTTERDAM

A special meeting was held in Rotterdam by the invitation of the Netherlands Pathological Society on 13–14 April 1956. Twenty-seven papers were read, and 49 members of the Society and 45 of the Netherlands Society signed the book.

THE JUBILEE MEETING

The summer meeting in Manchester in 1956 marked the jubilee of the Society, which as I have recounted began its existence in the same lecture theatre of that University 50 years previously. This physiological lecture theatre, which is a striking reminder of the large views of the late Professor William Stirling, comfortably accommodated the whole Society (Fig. 2.6); a beautiful bouquet of carnations, presented by The Pathological Society of the Netherlands, adorned the lecture table. The meeting began at 10 a.m. on the Thursday, 12 July, and the papers were arranged in sections as had been decided previously. Forty-four scientific papers were given and ten demonstrations. In Private Business the increase in the subscription to £3 was authorised. At the close of the Private Business the writer gave a short account of the history of the Society based upon the present article. A telegram of greeting was sent to Sir Robert Muir, who returned a most appreciative reply. The customary Committee supper was enlarged on this occasion to include all those who had served

THE SOCIETY AT MANCHESTER, JUBILEE MEETING, 13TH JULY 1956

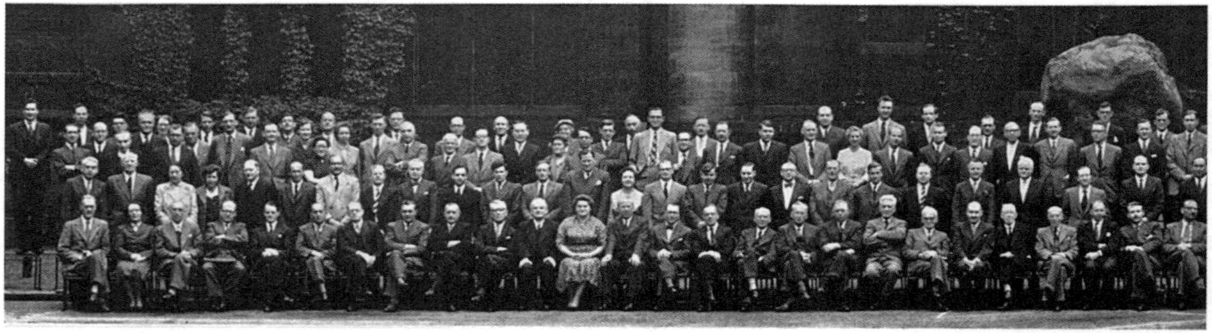

Photo by Guttenberg, Ltd., Manchester

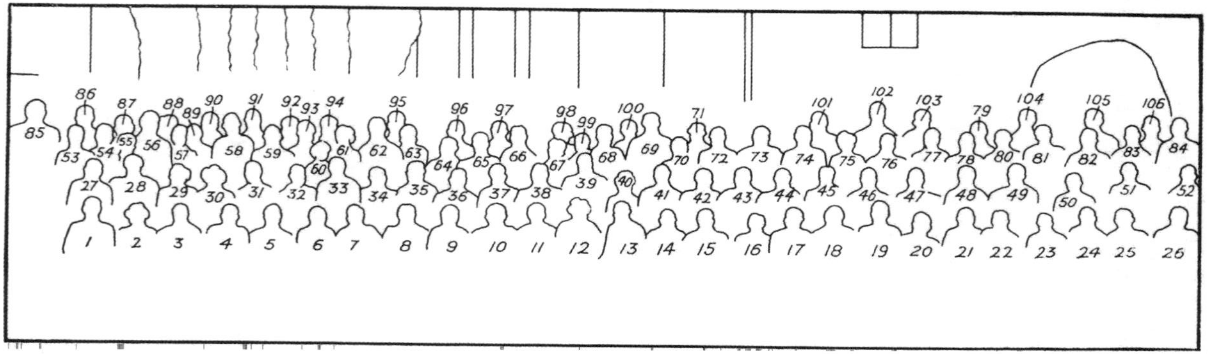

Figure 2.6 Members of the Sociity at the Jubile Meeting.

1. J. B. Duguid
2. Janet S. F. Niven
3. R. F. Ogilvie
4. F. O. MacCallum
5. A. C. P. Campbell
6. V. D. Allison
7. D. M. Pryce
8. T. Crawford
9. R. J. V. Pulvertaft
10. J. W. Orr
11. C. L. Oakley
12. Zaidéc Milner
13. D. H. Collins
14. C. V. Harrison
15. H. N. Green
16. W. D. Newcomb
17. S. L. Baker
18. H. B. Maitland
19. J. W. McLeod
20. M. J. Stewart
21. D. F. Cappell
22. C. H. Browning
23. W. Mair
24. A. F. J. Maloney
25. J. W. Czekalowski
26. B. J. Mansens
27. H. L. Sheehan
28. J. S. Faulds
29. Dorothy S. Russell
30. Elizabeth Travers
31. G. A. Dunlop
32. N. J. Brown
33. F. J. W. Lewis
34. A. G. Marshall
35. W. H. McMenemey
36. M. A. Epstein
37. J. C. Sherris
38. J. W. Stewart
39. R. W. Fairbrother
40. Joan Taylor
41. S. T. Cowan
42. R. E. O. Williams
43. J. W. Howie
44. K. S. Zinnemann
45. C. A. Green
46. J. F. Wilson
47. A. W. Branwood
48. A. C. Lendrum
49. H. E. Schornagel
50. D. MacKinnon
51. N. F. C. Gowing
52. I. Friedmann
53. J. Ball
54. L. Golberg
55. H. S. Baar
56. D. J. O'Brien
57. A. E. Chaplin
58. A. J. McCall
59. A. J. Watson
60. Pang Shu-Chao
61. H. Morag MacCallum
62. J. R. Anderson
63. I. Rannie
64. F. B. Smith
65. M. C. Berenbaum
66. S. Szutowicz
67. Edith K. Dawson
68. H. B. Stoner
69. H. J. Whiteley
70. D. Rivers
71. C. C. S. Pike
72. E. M. Ward
73. J. J. Bullen
74. A. E. Francis
75. Georgiana M. Bonser
76. A. G. Rickards
77. K. R. Dumbell
78. W. G. D. Caldwell
79. D. Hobson
80. F. Pick
81. T. D. S. Holliday
82. Th. G. Van Rijssel
83. B. E. Heard
84. A. G. Heppleston
85. F. C. Chesterman
86. L. M. Franks
87. G. E. Paget
88. Mary A. Head
89. W. Whitelaw
90. I. M. P. Dawson
91. J. B. Walter
92. R. J. C. Hari
93. Marry Catto
94. M. T. Parker
95. P. N. Magee
96. R. E. B. Hudson
97. H. B. Hewitt
98. Clara Stewart
99. J. O. Laws
100. I. Doniach
101. H. K. Weinbren
102. M. G. McEntegart
103. K. McCarthy
104. H. de C. Baker
105. H. Williams
106. G. Williams

Figure 2.6 *(Continued)*

during Stewart's tenure of office as Editor. Thirty-three were present, including Stewart and Mrs Stewart. On behalf of his colleagues Dean presented Stewart with a Georgian silver tea service as a memento of affection and regard, and of their appreciation of his devoted and distinguished work as Editor of the Journal for over 20 years, and both Stewart and Mrs Stewart replied.

On Thursday evening, 12 July, a reception to mark the anniversary of the Society's foundation was given by the Council of Manchester University in the Whitworth Hall. The Vice-Chancellor Sir John Stopford, FRS, and Lady Stopford received the guests.

The Society's dinner in the Students' Union departed on this occasion from the traditional custom, in that the remaining original members were invited to be present as guests, and of these W. Mair and Carl H. Browning were able to attend; other guests were the senior members of the Faculty of Medicine of the University. The chair at the dinner was taken by H. R. Dean; the health of the Society was proposed by Sir Geoffrey Jefferson, FRS, Emeritus Professor of Neurosurgery in the University of Manchester and replied to by Carl H. Browning, FRS, Emeritus Professor of Bacteriology in the University of Glasgow.

EPILOGUE

Thus ends this short account of The Pathological Society. If I have delved rather deeply into the day-to-day work of the Committee and its somewhat humdrum problems, I have done this deliberately

THE SOCIETY AT MANCHESTER, JUBILEE MEETING, 13TH JULY 1956

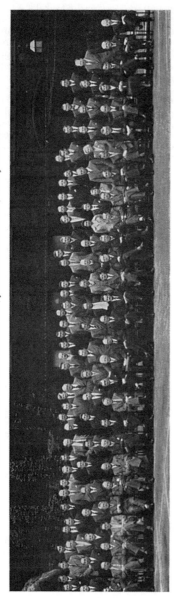

Photo by Guttenberg, Ltd., Manchester

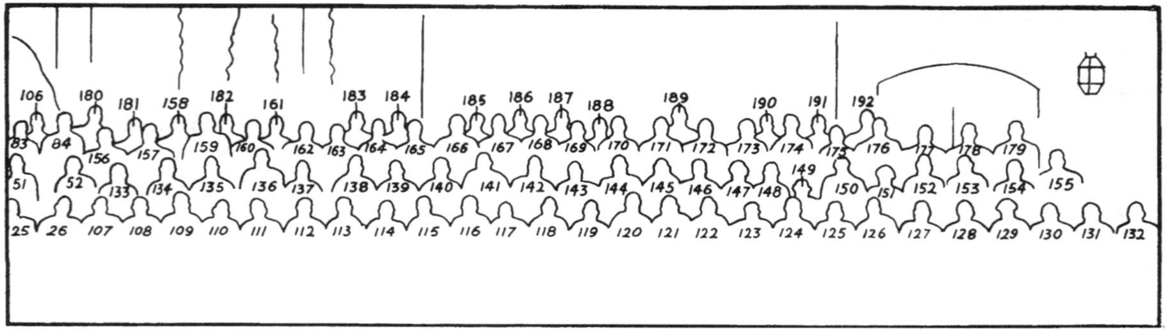

Figure 2.6 (*Continued*)

25. J. W. Czekalowski
26. B. J. Mansens
51. N. F. C. Gowing
52. I. Friedmann
83. B. E. Heard
84. A. G. Heppleston
106. G. Williams
107. R. W. Scarff
108. A. de Minjer
109. O. H. Dijkstra
110. J. H. Dible
111. J. Cruickshank
112. H. R. Dean
113. A. W. Downie
114. J. Mills
115. J. H. Biggart
116. H. Hamperl
117. J. E. Morison
118. J. C. Burne
119. P. O. Yates
120. R. F. Jennison
121. S. H. Jackson
122. R. Whitehead
123. F. A. Langley
124. J. P. Smith
125. T. S. L. Beswick
126. F. S. Mooney
127. J. Gough
128. A. C. Thackray
129. Isobel P. Beswick
130. R. Finlayson
131. E. M. Dunlop
132. G. P. McCullagh
133. S. D. Elek
134. Scott Thomson
135. T. E. Parry
136. E. G. Hall
137. K. B. Rogers
138. F. Whitwell
139. M. K. Alexander
140. J. D. A. Gray
141. E. M. Darmady
142. R. J. R. Cureton
143. R. Schade
144. B. Lennox
145. W. H. Hughes
146. E. W. Hurst
147. E. Florence McKeown
148. T. H. Flewett
149. Eileen O. Bartley
150. G. W. A. Dick
151. Mary Sharp
152. J. V. T. Gostling
153. J. S. Young
154. A. G. Stansfeld
155. G. A. C. Summers
156. W. J. Williams
157. R. A. Parker
158. J. S. Kennedy
159. R. C. Curran
160. D. C. Roberts
161. D. G. F. Harriman
162. H. Lederer
163. E. T. Ruston
164. D. McLean
165. R. M. Fry
166. J. H. Rack
167. D. L. Gardner
168. B. Cruickshank
169. J. B. Gibson
170. G. Grant
171. M. Symons
172. R. A. Caldwell
173. R. H. Mole
174. G. A. K. Missen
175. H. I. Winner
176. A. D. Thomson
177. H. A. Sissons
178. A. H. Cruickshank
179. W. St. C. Symmers
180. R. A. B. Drury
181. P. Pullar
182. M. Corridan
183. T. Bird
184. D. G. Scott
185. H. C. Moore
186. H. T. G. Strawbridge
187. H. N. Hadders
188. H. Urich
189. M. C. H. Dodgson
190. D. B. Brewer
191. K. R. Thornton
192. L. Michaels

Figure 2.6 *(Continued)*

so that members may have a record of what has been done. In our Society the business of keeping the wheels turning has always been accepted by the Committee, and thus valuable time at meetings has not been frittered away by tedious discussions on minor matters of business; this at times evokes criticism, but on reflection I believe the policy to have been wise. Our Society also, as far as it has been able, has refused to be drawn into political activities with all the entanglements and wrangling that these involve. This I am certain has been wise and by maintaining itself essentially as a scientific society ('The objects of the Society shall be to advance pathology... ') it has done well and enhanced its value and status.

I think it was Voltaire who said 'L'histoire ne peint que l'homme' and it is men who give colour and drama to history. In 50 years of a scientific Society's existence there is little that is likely to be stirring in a dramatic sense. The true history of the Society is the work of its members and this is to be found in the records of its meetings and in the volumes of the *Journal of Pathology and Bacteriology*. Let us agree that this is so, and that the incidents that have punctuated its progress are only the bricks in an edifice that is just beginning. But even so we eventually come back to the men; the figures who conceived the building and raised the scaffolding; the architects and founders of our Society: Lorrain Smith, Robert Muir, James Ritchie and A. E. Boycott, and others who coming quickly afterwards contributed so much to its structure and its present status, especially H. R. Dean and M. J. Stewart (Table 2.1).

On this our 50th birthday we have a right to be proud of an honourable and honoured past, and in praising the great men, 'our fathers that begat us', we are certain that the present and future generations will uphold the traditions that the past 50 years of the Society's existence have seen established under their guidance.

Table 2.1 Officers of the Society from 1906 to 1956

Data	Secretaries	Treasurer	Editor[a]	Assistant editors
1906	Ritchie Boycott	Power White		
1913		Ledingham		
1920	Boycott Dean		Ritchie	Boycott Dean
1922	Dean Stewart			
1923		Emrys Roberts	Boycott	Stewart Price-Jones
1924		Glymn		
1927				Stewart Wright
1928		Kettle		
1930				Stewart Topley
1932				Stewart Okell
1934	Dean Dible		Stewart	Okell Cameron
1937		McIntosh		Cameron Wright
1943				Cameron Downie
1947				Cameron Howie
1948		Scarff		
1952				Cameron Oakley
1954	Dible Downie			
1956			Oakley	Collins Orr

[a] The Journal, from its foundation in 1892 until the Society acquired it in 1920, was owned by Sims Woodhead who edited it, assisted from 1907 by Ritchie and Boycott.

I am especially grateful to Sir Robert Muir for information about the earliest days of the Society. The facts recorded have been derived from the Minute Books. The manuscript has been read by Carl Browning, H. R. Dean and the late M. I. Stewart. The portrait of Sir Robert Muir (in Fig. 2.2) is reproduced from a wash drawing by his sister Miss Anne D. Muir, RSW. (J. Henry Dible)

3 A 75th Anniversary Tribute to the Society[1]

Alan C. Lendrum

Firstly, I would thank the Committee for deciding to entrust me with this oration, on the grounds that to be trusted is a greater compliment than to be loved. However, I am at least able to open with a quotation from a real historian. Lord Acton, in a similar situation, said 'I shall never again enjoy the opportunity of speaking my thoughts to such an audience as this, and on so privileged an occasion a lecturer may well be tempted to bethink himself whether he knows of any neglected truth'. And so, fellow members and others, let me offer a neglected truth. A startling example of this neglect occurs in the first four pages of the current Bulletin of our College. The truth is, the findings in one necropsy may be sufficient for the clinician concerned, but to the pathologist, as a student of the processes of disease, the value of one necropsy depends on 99 other necropsies of the same disease. For the young or the immature pathologist, this is where the museum proves of value if it is huge and the curator is a true disciple of Heraclitus, of Virchow and, more recently, of Sir Francis Walshe, who said, almost in Virchow's words, 'The idea of process enters far too little into our thought'. Despite the fact, as Lancelot Whyte maintained, that Europeans lack a vocabulary of change, there is hope, for a man can alter his way of thinking, even after the age of 50.

Our Society did, in its 50th year; it unexpectedly decided to take note of the event, and asked its Secretary to be its historian. No better choice could have been made, as J.H. Dible was dedicated to the well-being of the Society, steeped in its tradition, and no mean historian, as later confirmed by his fascinating book on Naploeon's Surgeon, Larrey. Henry Dible had a truly Hellenic regard for excellence, for the urbanity of Platonic Athens, and his history had no trace of smear or sneer. Some hot-heads could not understand his lack of passion for sudden change, and yet he was an enthusiast for the promising. His immediate warmth in the association with our Dutch colleagues certainly helped to create possibly the most humane international linkage in European history. For all of us, Henry Dible as the Secretary was the man with the oiled feather; for the younger members I would explain that this was how we used to silence squeaking hinges.

In Dible's account he quotes Pye-Smith's statement in 1907 that pathology 'is the foundation or institute on which all scientific prevention and treatment of disease must rest' and adds his own comment, 'These discerning remarks are worth quoting today when developments in state medicine have tended to obscure and to reverse the true relationship of pathology to medicine'. This apparently reactionary comment is recalled because, in a Committee discussion in 1976 on the MRCPath, two members insisted that the present examination laid too great an emphasis on routine pathology to the detriment of academic work, and quoted Payling Wright 'To confine a man to routine departmental work for a long period is seriously detrimental to his development as an investigator'. If, however, a man wished to follow Virchow as an investigator... of disease in the human being, he would find that the hospital service provides the opportunity to study the

[1] This article has not been published previously. It was written as a 75th anniversary tribute and presented to The Pathological Society Committee in July 1981 on the occasion of the summer meeting in Dundee. It is reproduced here with the permission of Professor Lendrum's family.

processes of disease in man. As J.W. Howie in 1959 well said of Sir Robert Muir, 'He regarded sound laboratory work as the scientific foundation of all clinical practice; and he was successful beyond all expectation in persuading many with great influence in the Universities and in Medicine that this was indeed the truth. For this we are all his debtors'. I might add here that Sir Robert rated... very highly... the pedagogic obligation. His heart was in it. This is no place to detail all the events in the Society's history as Dible did in his paper, but we might look at a few of the innovations in our time: of these, some were forced on us by extraneous events – others by intrinsic events. A few have proved good... but some... resemble the inhabitants of Corsica, immortalized by Gibbon... as easier to deplore than to describe. Let us take a peep into 1954's Minutes... not quoted in Dible's paper. A member suggested that a subject be announced and perhaps speakers be invited from abroad. This was rejected by the Committee unanimously; it was also said that the artificial stimulation of interest in special subjects was not likely to be as fruitful as the Society's normal activities.

1957

Two Honorary members' deaths recorded, M.J. Stewart, editor of the *Journal* for many years, and T. Madsen, elected 1929.

1958

A member spoke against valedictory addresses, thinking that reference to selected members was invidious. It was agreed that decisions be left to the Committee. Professor G.R. Cameron sent a letter suggesting a series of short addresses to commemorate Virchow's Cellular Pathology 1858. The Committee considered that this would 'introduce difficulties and that it might prove an embarrassing innovation'. The member with the distaste for obituaries suggested non-acceptance of a certain number of papers, the arrangement of symposia with a series of experts and the presentation of papers by invitation. The Minute says 'There did not appear to be any volume of support for these suggestions'.

J.H. Dible retires from Secretaryship. C.H. Browning elected Honorary member. The Committee agreed with the desirability of offering facilities as part of this country's contribution to the technical education of overseas students and felt that the Institute of Medical Laboratory Technicians should approach the heads of such departments as the Institute selected.

1959

Death of Sir Robert Muir. Among those members who have died since 1956 we have proof of the benefit of membership of the Society, and of a Scottish University – as Dible had. The prime examples are C.E. Dukes (Edinburgh) aged 86, C.H. Browning and J.W. McLeod (both Glasgow) aged 90, Win Boyd (Edinburgh) aged 94, Sir Robert Muir (Edinburgh) aged 95 and, the exception in many more ways than one, Parkes Weber (Cambridge) aged 99. Among the senior survivors we have a precious and unique member Walter Pagel, elected Fellow of the British Academy and almost certainly the only member ever to have attained such an intellectual eminence.

To return to 1959: Honorary members Sir F.M. Burnet and J.H. Dible elected; death of Honorary member Pierre Masson (elected 1955).

1960

Letter from Mary Barber stating that, with bacteriological papers always taken first, many bacteriologists were denied the opportunity of attending the dinner. Agreed to alternate as from 1961.

Scaiff said that a histological panel on bone tumour was necessary under a National Research Council investigation on methods of treatment. The British Empire Cancer Campaign (BECC) had agreed to finance this as a subcommittee of the main histological panel run by the Society and the BECC. Four members were nominated for the panel.

Third joint meeting in Holland held at Utrecht in May. Weather, wit and wisdom all in good measure.

1961

July, Aberdeen: J.W. MacLeod elected Honorary member. Death of two Honorary members H.R. Dean and Jules Bordet elected in 1913!

1962

January: A group from the Society, headed by J.W. Howie, to meet officers of the Association of Clinical Pathologists (ACP)... to send a memorandum to all members of both organisations on the matter of a possible College, for definite answers and willingness to support financially. If sufficient answers in favour, the officers of the two societies would arrange a public meeting to appoint office-bearers of the new College.

July, Leeds, with the Dutch: Downie gave an account of the meeting on 21 June to found this College. T. Crawford, Registrar of the new College, expressed the thanks of the Council for help, financial and otherwise, they had received from the Society.

1963

May: First joint meeting on invitation from the Norwegian Society, held in Oslo and in Bergen. Very different from war-time recollection were whale-steaks that might have been Aberdeen-Angus.

July, Glasgow: Honorary members W. Boyd, J. Cruickshank, O.M. Dijkstra, L. Kreyberg and Dorothy Russell were elected.

1964

May: Joint meeting in Groningen.

July, Birmingham: A request for abstracts of papers to be published quickly after the meeting was countered by the Editor's distaste for accepting unedited material. Two new honorary members Sir Howard Florey and Rebecca Lancefield were elected.

1965

Suggestion of a symposium on a specified subject, with invited speakers at each meeting and occupying not more than one session was accepted as worth a trial, preferably at a summer meeting. Sixteen years later we might feel that the current type of 'put-on show to entice the uninformed by a continued dialectic' scarcely merits the term symposium, and further degradation (of percentage unknown) has produced a clutch of minisymposia. New honorary members Sir Roy Cameron and Arnold Rich were elected.

1966

R.W. Scarff elected honorary member. Death of J. Cruickshank.

1967

The Society to have two journals: *Journal of Pathology* and *Journal of Medical Microbiology*. Oakley thought that the Committee should consider more than two meetings in the year. Honorary membership accorded to Harry Goldblatt.

1968

Intimation that the College would appreciate an approach from the Society to define areas of common interest and useful collaboration between the College, the Society and the ACP. Death of honorary members Lord Florey and A.R. Rich. Honorary membership accorded to D.F. Cappell and J.W. Orr.

1969

B. Lennox, Lexicographer, wished for some kind of introduction to symposia, to help non-specialists. W.G. Spector elected treasurer. Abstracts of papers given to be published in a form suitable for citation. Honorary membership for Sir Christopher Andrewes, A.W. Downie and Sir Graham Wilson. Death of Sir Henry Dale (lion. member 1941).

September, Special Committee Meeting: Symposia should be a recurrent feature, when appropriate, speakers to be invited and subsidised. From time to time host university department to be encouraged to mount a symposium of broad general interest with contributions from its own staff and possibly outside participants. Joint meetings with other societies or groups should be encouraged. Secretaries to meet representatives of the specialist panels financed by the BECC to consider improvement of communication between the panels and the Society.

Specialist groups: To ask members 'What groups should be established'. Groups to meet for not less than one hour, during the demonstration session, with the aim of educating the general membership in the group's expertise by occasional papers or symposia. A group could be associated with an existing group outwith the Society. This secular reformation recalls the danger to an institution that keeps changing its character, and the fact that being up-to-date may merely mean chasing the contemporary fads.

1970

Maximum number of honorary members raised from 20 to 30 without restriction therein on the number of UK residents. The Society's account was transferred to a prominent London firm of investment advisers. The Society agreed to sponsor a microbiology Teaching Group. Death of honorary member R.W. Scarff.

1971

Middlesex Hospital Immunology Group to have discussion in Edinburgh in July on the case for clinical immunology as a fifth laboratory discipline in the NHS. Honorary membership of the Dutch Society was granted to C.V. Harrison, A.C. Lendrum and G.L. Montgomery. Death of honorary member J.H. Dible.

In view of rising costs, List of Members to be published in full every three years, with list of changes issued in intervening years. The treasurer reported a modest surplus.

1972

Professor Dustin proposed a joint meeting with the Belgian Society in Brussels in 1973.

Working party's recommendations on Future Editorial Policy: Editorial Board of *Journal of Pathology* enlarged to 15–20 members; part or whole-time editorial assistant of good calibre to help with both journals. For next three years at least, W.G. Spector to be Chairman of the Editorial Board. Thanks to improved financial situation the treasurer hoped to pay off the debt to Messrs Constable by end of 1972. Death of honorary member C.H. Browning.

July, Leeds: Oakley expressed his gratitude to fellow editors and to Miss Milner for great help and friendliness over the years – 1950–56 as assistant editor of *Journal of Pathology and*

Bacteriology, 1956–68 as editor, 1969–72 as editor of *Journal of Pathology* and 1968–71 as editor of *Journal of Medical Microbiology.* At the dinner, W.G. Spector presented the President of the Royal College of Pathologists with the Society's gift to the College, a Georgian silver basket (by Henry Chorner, 1795) to be used at College dinners. W.G. Spector to be editor and D.W. Willoughby deputy editor of *Journal of Pathology*, with editorial board of about 20. Honorary membership for J.B. Duguid, G.L. Montgomery and C.L. Oakley.

1973

January: Secretary to write offering congratulations to Miss Mabel Fitzgerald, a member since 1908 who had recently at the age of 100 been given an honorary MA by the University of Oxford. She had qualified with distinction in physiology at the turn of the Century, but under existing regulations could not have a degree conferred on her because of her sex.

April, Brussels: 60–70 delegates from the UK attended a joint meeting with the Belgian Society.

July, Manchester: The Teaching Group had a well-attended discussion on 'What should we teach?'.

1974

Report on joint meeting of the Society, the ACP and the Royal College of Pathology. Agreed that a suitable diploma in pathology sponsored by the College was very desirable, particularly for overseas students.

The organisation of the coming Cardiff meeting was proving very complex. The Minute reads: 'It was left to Crane, Neville and Williams to sort out the jig-saw as they thought best' which you must agree is a puzzling metaphor.

July, Cardiff: Joint meeting with the Dutch Society. On the dinner, the Minute reads: 'The menu, printed in Welsh, Dutch and French, must surely have been unique in the Society's history' – certainly the understatement of the year.

A.M. Neville to succeed W.A.J. Crane as Meetings Secretary. The debt to Longmans has been cleared and some addition made to the Society's capital. A.G. Lendrum elected Honorary member.

1975

The Middlesex: A.M. Neville 'suggested that when the programme included a number of related papers in a particular field, an expert in that field should be invited to give an introductory background paper lasting 20–30 minutes. This would make it easier for non-specialists to understand the significance of the papers that followed'. This echoes exactly B. Lennox in 1969 and the Committee agreed it was worth a trial. Editor reported that the *Journal of Pathology* had a 60% rejection rate over the year and that about one in four of the papers now came from overseas. The *Journal of Medical Microbiology* rejections were down, but still over 55%. Death of honorary member C.L. Oakley.

1976

Society representatives to College Standing Committees: Histopathology, R.C. Curran; Medical Microbiology, A.A. Glynn; Lab. Technician, J.C. Sloper.

Qualification for membership: 'With greater emphasis on the MRC Path examination, pathologists of quite senior standing might now have few or no publications to their name'. Agreed other criteria were relevant. 'In general, however, membership should not be offered to those below the Senior Registrar grade'.

July, Newcastle: The extroversion of the Society grows apace. At the symposium on capillary abnormalities of the glomeruli, taking part were Dr Liliane Morel-Maroger and her Parisian team. Death of Honorary members G.H. Whipple, D.F. Cappell and O.H. Dijkstra.

1977

Charing Cross: Symposium jointly with Association of Clinical Pathologists, celebrating their 50th year, on Techniques in Pathology. This cordial union led to four mini-symposia.

July, Aberdeen: The Dutch Society elected P.M. Bakker to follow C.A. Wagenvoort as their representative on the Committee. A new feature was a social function on the Thursday afternoon, a visit to Crathes Castle and its famous garden. A symposium on The Autopsy had a demonstration of direct colour television from the autopsy.

Sir James Howie was elected honorary member. M.G. McEntegart to succeed B. Moore as general secretary. Death of honorary member Harry Goldblatt.

1978

Barts: A.M. Neville observed that all the available accommodation at Barts had been taken up, and clearly met a need. A book exhibition by H.K. Lewis was on display during the meeting. The Editor of the *Journal of Pathology* said that the first solicited review article was now passed for press.

July, Southampton, Joint meeting with the Dutch Society: The contribution to the European Congress of Pathology had been repaid plus 10% interest. Request from Dr Foster for help towards the cost of a permanent home for the Colchester Collection of Historical Instruments; agreed to give £100, on request. Thursday afternoon to H.M.S. Victory in Portsmouth. Death of honorary member, J.W. McLeod. Edith K. Dawson and R.A. Willis elected to honorary membership.

1979

Charing Cross: Letter of thanks from M.T. Parker for the Society's support to the VIIth International Symposium on Streptococci. Inaugural C.L. Oakley Lecturer, C.S.F. Easmon, spoke on 'Experimental Staphylococcal Infection in Mice'. The Lectureship is funded by an endowment from the 6th European Congress of Pathology.

July, Leicester: Congratulations to Professor H. Smith on his election as Fellow of the Royal Society. Agreed to sponsor, along with the Pharmacological Society and the College, the J. Barnes Memorial Lecture in Toxicology. Agreed that the Meetings Secretary should approach A.C. Lendrum to prepare and deliver an account of the 25 years of the Society's life since that given by J.H. Dible on the occasion of the 50th Anniversary. Elected to Honorary membership: Sir Theo Crawford and Dame Janet Vaughan. The treasurer reported that the Society's assets had doubled in the past five years. The *Journal of Medical Microbiology* is attracting more papers, about half from overseas, but papers on virology have fallen to almost nil, due probably to the proliferation of virology journals.

1980

Oxford: The Editor announced that from May the *Journal of Pathology* would be printed by Ballantyne Spotiswoode in Colchester. Longmans will continue as publisher. This brings to an end a tradition as old as the Society, Constable having been associated with the original publisher Oliver and Boyd since about 1890.

Agreed that abstracts would be stringently edited and published. Meanwhile, the Committee Minutes every six months become more voluminous! The Standing Advisory Committee on Laboratory Staffing and Organisation supported in principle the suggestion of a forensic NHS commitment per region. The second Oakley Lecture was given by B.I. Duerden on 'The identification and occurrence of bacteroides species in the normal human flora and from clinical infections'. 265 Members and guests signed the attendance book; 16 members acted as Chairmen of sessions; and in all there were 100 papers and 8 demonstrations, the total membership now standing at 1668.

May, Joint Meeting in Groningen: The Society presented to our hosts an engraved silver plate, and received from them a Commemorative Medallion. The agenda was overcrowded and some papers overlong, otherwise successful.

July, Glasgow: The Committee discussed the question of sponsorship of another journal with more slant towards histopathology. The Officers of the Society were empowered to negotiate with possible publishers and to report back. Agreed to make a donation of £750 towards the 4th International Meeting on Future Trends in Inflammation at the Royal College of Surgeons, refundable if a profit is made. Death of honorary members William Boyd and R.A. Willis. Elected to honorary membership: Sir Ashley Miles and Sir Thomas Symington.

1981

Middlesex: Teaching Group debated the motion 'Poor Recruitment is due to Poor Teaching at the Undergraduate Level'. (Question: Had any of the speakers studied the paper on students' aspirations, *BMJ* 1976; **11 Sept.**: 631?) 3rd Oakley Lecture by D.N. Slater, 'Expectations in Diabetic Mellitus – Pancreas Transplantation': in all, 116 papers.

Death of honorary member J.B. Duguid. Two travel fellowships awarded to attend the joint meeting with the Canadian pathologists in June in Toronto.

REFERENCES

Arnott, M. (1981) *Bull. R. Coll. Pathol.* **35**: 1–4.

Dible, J.H. (1957) *J. Pathol. Bacteriol.* **73 Suppl.**: 1–35.

Dible, J.H. (1970) *Napoleon's Surgeon.* W. Heinemann Medical Books: London.

Walshe, F.M.R. (1948) *Harveian Oration: The Structure of and its Place Among the Sciences.* E. and S. Livingstone: Edinburgh.

Whyte, L.L. (1960) *The Unconscious before Freud.* Basic Books: New York (Anchor Books: New York, 1962).

Anti-freeze

My first contribution to the Path Soc was as a young lecturer in Edinburgh. It was the Winter Meeting at Bart's starting on 2nd January (!) 1969, and it was my first ever scientific meeting. The title, 'The vasculature of Brown-Pearce carcinoma in growth and regression', conveys little of what the Communication and demonstration involved. The B-P carcinoma was maintained in rabbit testes, being passed from generation unto generation by intra-testicular needle inoculation. The late Andy Shivas, then Senior Lecturer and part-time tympanist in the Edinburgh Department, had read about the use of latex casts to demonstrate blood vessels in anatomical preparations, and set me to work on the B-P carcinoma. After three months of careful, if somewhat kitchen-sink, methodology, I had produced a series of (five) casts. When viewed through a stereoscopic microscope with the cast floating in water, these were rather impressive – at least to me. They were a striking brick-red colour and their tubes and fronds looked like something from the Great Barrier Reef. One of my more senior colleagues was less impressed, asking me on at least one occasion if I was still playing with my rubber balls. On the strength of a few complete casts, however, Dr. Shivas submitted a poster. Had it been simply a poster with photographs I would have been spared several problems, but my mentor thought that I should take 'normal' and 'tumour-bearing' casts to the meeting. Remember, the casts would collapse if taken out of the supporting water. I found two suitable glass jars with screw-top lids to transport them to London and took the casts home ready for my journey on New Year's Day. When I went to pick them up from the window-sill in the porch ('You're not bringing those into the house!'), both my casts were frozen solid. I couldn't risk rapid heating as the cast might have deformed, so it was a slow thaw on the radiator.

With one eye on my testes (as it were) and one on the clock (I was running late for the train by this stage), I watched as the ice slowly melted. With fluidity restored and the prospect of carrying these jars through the Arctic conditions prevailing around Edinburgh's Waverley station, I decided that a sensible precaution would be to add some anti-freeze. There then followed a long and, at times, cold journey in which a bag containing the precious casts was maintained in a strictly level position in one hand, while I held a suitcase containing a microscope wrapped in underwear and socks in the other. At last, the casts were in situ at Bart's. I had carefully changed the 'transport medium' for clean water and invited Dr Shivas to inspect the casts prior to the session. As he stared down the microscope he declared, 'Well I never, some of these vessels have even got a bluish tinge – like venous sinusoids!'. I didn't have the nerve to tell him that was the anti-freeze!

Mike Dixon

A moving experience

One of the most moving experiences (!) for several members of the Society was at the 1994 Winter Path Society meeting hosted by the The London Hospital. Earlier in the week there had been the traditional Committee Dinner which was hosted at the Reform Club by Colin Berry. A sizeable proportion of the group were struck down by a very unpleasant gastroenteritis during the course of the meeting. This was subsequently shown by one of our microbiological colleagues to have been due to a real virus which had been lurking in the oysters (who had the audacity to go on to publish this in a clinical microbiology journal!). I will always remember the moment that I was personally struck by this nasty virus. I had been asked to mark the posters and was halfway through this task when I had to exit stage left; I left a rather dumbfounded young investigator mid-sentence! Not all of those that had attended the dinner were so afflicted. Based on preliminary observations of those that had been there, Nick Wright proposed a hypothesis that alcohol in excess afforded protection against the effects of the micro-organism. To my knowledge this has never been formally tested. In spite of the evidence base however, it appears that many members of the Society have adopted a strategy of using alcohol as a 'prophylactic' at Society meetings.

Alastair Burt

4 The Society's Finances – A Perspective

A. Munro Neville

One of my most vivid early memories of Society Meetings, when still a very new member, occurred at noon, usually on the second day of the Meeting. Several senior figures, not only of the Society but of pathology in general, quietly rose from their seats at or near the front and left the Meeting in ones and twos. Indeed, the speaker was still at the podium! Then, around three o'clock, most returned again in dribs and drabs. The readily observable red noses could not be totally accounted for by either the cold at the Winter Meeting or the sun at the Summer Meeting. Eventually, I discovered that they had been attending the *Journal of Pathology and Bacteriology* Editorial Board lunch and that such refection was their sole compensation for serving as Associate Editors.

Next day, there followed the AGM when it was announced with neither aplomb nor apology that the Society was compensating the publishers to produce and distribute the Journal. It was not until the early 1970s that losses on the Society's publications were reversed and this debt repaid. It is interesting to read in the historical records that this was by no means the first time that the publication of the Journal had resulted in the Society incurring debts to publishers. Such was the case on several occasions in the 1920s and again in the 1930s.

The position of Treasurer throughout the life of the Society has been the least visible of the Society's posts. If successful, it provides the bedrock for advancement and future development. Without a positive balance in the coffers no new initiatives, positive responses to members' suggestions (even if the Committee were prepared to implement them) or proposals to advance the objectives of the Society and pathology in general would be feasible.

From the late 1970s, pathology entered a further phase in its development brought about largely by the discovery of new methods in immunology, genetics and cell biology. Attendance at Society meetings was rising. The research quality was also improving and the results most exciting. It was essential to adapt and encompass these opportunities and provide a forum and leadership for this significant research challenge. Yet the Society's assets some 75 years after its founding were only of the order of £200 000 and had remained at this rather static level over a prolonged period, despite a modest surplus being recorded from time to time. It was vital for the Society to meet these challenges. Accordingly, it had to adopt a more business-like attitude and approach to all aspects of its affairs – scientific, clinical, financial and administrative. Thus, attention focused on finances first because without the wherewithal further advances and initiatives would not be feasible.

Seldom, if ever, are major bequests or donations made to the Society, although the generosity of members themselves at its inauguration in the early part of the century and then occasionally thereafter were contributions of great value. Regretfully, the pharmaceutical industry, through failure to understand the role that pathology could play and is playing in the development of modern techniques for diagnosis and therapy, has not been a traditional supporter. From time to time, members in their enthusiasm to suggest ways of improving the finances have suggested that funds be deployed in the Irish Sweepstake, the Lottery or Ernie's Premium Bonds. Wisdom, however, prevailed with the recognition that an integrated and long-term positive programme was needed that focused upon the Society's own resources and ingenuity rather than on outside assistance in the first instance.

The first decision in this new programme was to appoint, over the last quarter of the century, a series of Scottish Treasurers. Members came to regard their miserly spending attitudes with dismay. They exhibited a reluctance to part with any financial gains. By comparison, Scrooge (indeed even Aberdonians) appeared magnanimous. However, their parsimonious resolve in those early stages was crucial to the success later to be attained. The Society's publications in financial terms were performing poorly, being only marginally profitable through the 1970s. The *Journal of Pathology and Bacteriology* and more recently its successors, *Journal of Pathology* and *Journal of Medical Microbiology*, have always played an important role in the Society's finances but not always to its advantage, as has been alluded to previously.

The *Journal of Pathology and Bacteriology* was originally purchased in instalments from Professor Sims Woodhead for the sum of £550 in 1907 (a tidy sum in those days), having been founded and edited by him since 1892. Once the total sum had been repaid, ownership of the Journal passed to the Society. An Editor and Editorial Board were then appointed. The Committee of the Society at that time agreed that any profits were to be returned to the Journal, mainly to defray the cost of illustrations (a familiar tale). The Editorial Board was responsible to the Society's Committee and Membership for its affairs, including finances. Out of the annual dues of £2.00 paid by Members, £1.75 was transferred to the Journal. All seemed to be well initially with this arrangement but in time the Journal ran into financial trouble and was initially bailed out by the publishers but latterly even they were no longer prepared to foot the debts that were incurred in printing and distribution. Significant repayments had to be made on several occasions out of the Society's funds. In fact the debts were not fully repaid until 1974.

In 1967, it had been decided to separate the Society's publications into two, namely the *Journal of Pathology* and the *Journal of Medical Microbiology*. However, their publication had been left in the hands of the original publisher These journals were the window to the world presented by the Society and their value, both medically and financially, needed to be truly realised to a far greater extent. A new strategy was required because if a reliable profit could be achieved from their publication this would give the initial boost to the finances that was becoming so necessary. Accordingly the publication of the two journals was put out to tender. Following competitive bids, a different publisher was chosen for each journal and new profit-sharing five-year contracts renewable only in principle were signed. With this more professional approach the returns to the Society increased dramatically, with five- and even six-figure sums being received annually. The quality of the journals improved greatly due to the efforts of the Editors and their Boards, whose services were given freely or at minimal cost so that the profits in very large measure passed directly through to the Society coffers. A third journal, *Reviews in Medical Microbiology*, was started in 1990 by the *Journal of Medical Microbiology* publishers in association with the Society, which added small amounts of further revenue.

Could this improved state of affairs have been realised earlier in the Society's life? Probably not, because the *Journal of Pathology and Bacteriology* had lost much of its appeal and had been overtaken by and was in competition with other related publications. Additionally, having two journals enabled the Society to seek competitive quotes from several publishers for the respective contracts. This change in attitude of the Society to its publications and publishers provided the basis to tackle the next avenue of increasing revenue, namely an investment policy with the aim of long-term capital growth. This was undertaken with professional help together with financial planning advice from a different set of accountants and auditors.

It is interesting to compare and note *en passant* that a sound investment strategy bears resemblance to any new academic venture. Both typically take the first five years to get off the ground, the next five to see the early fruits of the endeavour, and thereafter hopefully to witness significant benefit. This is the case with the Society's investments, helped by the tax-free status of being a Charity and the progressive rise in the value of the market itself. From around £100 000 in the late 1970s and early 1980s, with the ability to add annually to the capital and the collective unwillingness of Treasurers to allow significant raiding of the potential nest egg too early, assets of the order of £6 million were achieved by the start of the New Millennium. The dramatic reversals of the stock market in 2001 made large inroads into this but the situation has improved dramatically and reserves are now (December 2005) around £5 million. Additional sources of income include Members' subscriptions and, since 1991, Meeting registration fees, although the latter are largely or totally consumed by the cost of the meetings in question. The results of these investment and fiscal policies are of fundamental importance to the Society, which now finds itself in a position such that, through judicious use of the interest received from the capital, it is capable of being self-sufficient and able to dispense some of the largesse to the benefit of pathology (as will be outlined later) while still retaining flexibility to meet new challenges as perceived from time to time.

Society history reveals, as recounted 50 years ago by Professor Dible and reprinted elsewhere in this book (Chapter 2), several most gratifying aspects of benevolence despite the Society's limited finances of the 1920s. Support for young dependents whose Member fathers had died prematurely, leaving the family in straightened circumstances, was provided on several occasions to support their education, mostly at Epsom College, Surrey. Additionally, not insignificant donations were made to the College itself to benefit the Member's children or put at the disposal of the Council of the College. This College was a notable source of future medical students throughout the country; most of them seem to have ended up at St. George's Hospital Medical School. Just imagine such an item on the AGM Agenda for the Business Meeting in 2006!

Although occasional sponsorship for pathologically related meetings by smaller bodies or societies has always been a feature of the Society's affairs, even early in its existence, today it is young investigators, usually pathologists, who are the main beneficiaries either of awards in recognition of their achievements or of support to further enable their research. The first significant new venture was the establishment of the C.L.Oakley Lectureship in honour of a former editor of the *Journal of Pathology and Bacteriology*. Building on this success, the Society extended its gifting to support intercalated BSc students in pathology each year, together with a rolling three-year PhD Fellowship programme with Society members acting as the sponsors and supervisors. More recently a scheme for clinical trainees has been instituted. The ready ability to travel to other prestigious laboratories or departments to learn new techniques and to return with them to their base is an area in which it has always been difficult to obtain funds. This has been a most important gap filled by the Society establishing a Travelling Fellowship Fund available to any UK-based scientist or clinician, not just Society members. In recent years, the Society has been able to recognise formally the accomplishments of more established investigators. One, the Doniach Award, is given to Senior Members who have made a substantial contribution to cellular pathology and the Society, while the other, the Goudie Lecture, is to someone not necessarily a Member who has made a seminal contribution to pathological science. These are wise policies with far-reaching consequences, albeit small in number compared to the country as a whole. However, their focus on laboratory science and medicine makes them unique and highly laudatory.

In the late 1970s–1980s, a dramatic increase in the size and complexity of the Meetings occurred that resulted in the officers no longer being able to attend to the Society's day-to-day affairs on an ad hoc basis. The smooth running of the Society and ensuring the best use of all its resources was achieved through leasing space for an administrative headquarters within the premises of the Royal College of Pathologists at 2 Carlton House Terrace. The events leading to this are considered in Chapter 5 by Eric Walker. This has ensured, at minimal cost, the interaction between both bodies for the benefit of all concerned. The lease has been extended (see Chapters 6 and 7) to 2024.

At this time of Centenary celebrations, the Society finds itself in a comfortable but not rich situation with the ability to carry out its current programme of activities largely, if not wholly, through the use of the annual proceeds derived from its current capital assets. The investment portfolio, while showing variations with time, will invariably rise with the market and keep ahead of inflation. However, to be complacent and rest solely on this source of income would be far from prudent. Nevertheless, it is gratifying to know that the Society is, at the time of its Centenary, able to offer substantial grants and awards to promote the discipline and help the Members.

Treasurers inevitably research other means of increasing revenues. Could Members, other than through their subscriptions or the proceeds from the *Journal of Pathology* (the sole Society publication having divested itself of the microbiology journals), be benefactors themselves? There is a marvellous reference in the historical notes to a 'Stains Subcommittee', which, with Members' help, had prepared, validated and distributed a series of special stains to other laboratories. Proceeds from this venture were donated to the Society. Looking ahead, is there a way in which a proportion of the profits from the sale of the monoclonal and other antibodies, cell lines, gene probes, array systems and the like, prepared by members and sold under licence by industry worldwide, could find their way to advance the Society's finances?

Academic medicine and pathology in particular are experiencing difficult times, here and all over the world, that may not be transient. The Society has a role to play in stimulating new endeavours and supporting the continuity of those of current value. The wise use of its funds, perhaps on occasions in a rather selfish, egocentric manner, will enable it to build on its achievements to date and fulfil a small but important role in all future aspects of pathology.

Close encounters

I had just finished my DPhil thesis and Florey, my supervisor, thought it might be a good idea if I presented my stuff at a forthcoming meeting of The Pathological Society that was due to take place in London. Both Florey and Fleming were at the meeting. I strutted my stuff – it was about a new trace technique for studying chemotaxis of leucocytes. After my talk Florey came over and asked if I'd like to meet Fleming. It was clear he wanted me to meet him and so I let him wheel me over to the man in the bow tie. He introduced me and went off immediately. I hoped Fleming might say something but as nothing emerged I ventured a few words. He made no answer, so I took that as my clue to clear off, which I did. I met Fleming again on another occasion, but couldn't get a word out of him then either. But that incident isn't graven in my mind as sharply as our first encounter.

Henry Harris

Exit stage right?

My first poster at Pathsoc – 'Granulomatous vasculitis: the cause of Crohn's disease'. We blew up a beautiful picture of a granulomatous vasculitis in Crohn's disease to full poster size. Muggins, a fresh-faced SHO, stood there and got torn to shreds, while senior authors made a rapid exit to the bar!

Marco Novelli

5 The 1980s: People, Events and Meetings

Eric Walker

INTRODUCTION

This is an informed but informal account of the Society in the 1980s. It is based largely upon my own recollections assisted by annotations, made at the time, in my copies of the abstract books of the Society's Scientific Meetings. The Minutes of the Committee and Business Meetings of that period were also trawled. The current General Secretary, Peter Hall, also perused those Minutes and added some additional perspectives.

The 1980s in The Pathological Society, as well as in other areas of society, were a period of extraordinary change. Looking back at this period, and in particular through the window of the Society records, the Minutes of Committee meetings and the record of work presented to Society meetings in the abstract books (all of which can be found in the Back Record of the *Journal of Pathology* available to all members online), it is quite extraordinary how much has indeed changed! Typical meetings in the 1970s and early 1980s attracted no more than 50–100 abstracts and not many more attendees. Indeed the first meeting with 150 abstracts was January 1981. Accurate numbers of attendees are hard to define because no registration was required, simply the signing of an attendance book. In the Minutes of the Society Committee a note is sometimes to be found of how many signed this but it is stated that the information is very inaccurate. At the Dundee meeting of July 1981 it is remarked that about 120 attended but that 'this was perhaps an underestimate'. The growth in the meetings during the 1980s is evidenced by the dramatic increase in the number of proffered abstracts (see Fig. 9.1 In Chapter 9).

As well as the increase in number of abstracts, the content of the abstracts changed and showed the impact of technology. Indeed, one might consider the growth in the meetings of the 1980s as the direct result of technology. Consider the topics covered in the Symposia: The cell surface and uses of animal models to study microbial pathogenicity (Oxford, January 1980); Ultrastructural aspects of diagnostic pathology (Manchester, July 1980); Cytofluorimetry (Dundee, July 1981); The Monoclonal Revolution (Cambridge, January 1982); Stereology and pathology (Sheffield, July 1982); Computers in pathology (Birmingham, 1983); Immunocytochemical innovations (Royal Postgraduate Medical School, January 1984); Chromosomes and cancer (Leeds, July 1984); Immunocytochemistry in diagnostic pathology and implications of molecular biology for pathology (Northwick Park, January 1985); Growth control and neoplasia (Cardiff, July 1985); Objective methods in pathology (Barts, January 1988). In addition, keynote and named lectures were dominated by technological advances, including the 11th Oakley lecture on 'Diagnostic immunocytochemistry: achievements and challenges' (Kevin Gatter, UCH/Middlesex, January 1989) and the Lucio Luzatto Lecture on 'Gene rearrangements in human pathology' (The London, January 1986). So much of the structured part of Society meetings in the 1980s related to technological advances.

This emphasis on methodologies and in particular antibody-based methods took the presentations of The Pathological Society meetings away from the traditional arena of experimental pathology into a more observational (dare one say 'translational') form of work – lectins, antibodies, flow cytometers and the applications of such technologies to clinical as well as experimental settings. The effect of technology was evident throughout this decade, often in odd ways. At the Committee Meeting of January 1980 held at Merton College, Oxford, a discussion is recorded about the problems of getting notices of the meetings to Members in the 'Dominions'. The cost of airmail delivery to all such members was considered prohibitive. It was decided to send a set of Notices to one such Member in Australia or in another Dominion who might then be able to distribute it to colleagues elsewhere! Forgetting the politically incorrect choice of term Dominion, the approach seems fanciful today only a quarter of a century later.

On the other hand, looking back it is clear that some things have not changed. The issue of Society membership was a matter of concern in the 1980s. In 1984 Membership fell below 1600 (to 1589 in fact). At the 1984 Annual Business Meeting held in Leeds (the current General Secretary's first attendance at a Society meeting by the way) it is recorded that the General Secretary said that 'heads of departments were asked to attempt to recruit new members from their junior staff'. Also at the winter meeting of 1981 held at the Middlesex Hospital there was a debate Chaired by P.G. Isaacson of the Teaching Group Meeting entitled 'Poor recruitment in pathology is due to poor teaching at the undergraduate level'. J.R. Anderson and C.S. Foster spoke for this motion and J.R. Tighe and J. Swanson-Beck spoke against. Given the changes in the undergraduate curriculum in more recent years, one wonders what those speakers would now think! Similarly the issue of recruitment into pathology was then, as now, an issue of considerable concern. The General Secretary (McEntegart) indicated that 39% of consultants were over 55 and that the ratio of Senior Registrars to such staff was 1:4. Interestingly it was agreed that the promotion of the Intercalated BSc in Pathology was a potential means of promoting the discipline as a career option.

In January 1981 the Society was asked to contribute financially to a project to make a film to be entitled 'What pathology is and what pathologists do'. Today, a quarter of a century later, this undoubtedly would be viewed as a good thing, with engagement of the public and the rest of the profession being perceived as being of huge importance. It is thus salutary to note that it is recorded in the Minutes that a senior person stated '...such a production is unnecessary and may even be unhelpful...'. The project was not supported!

MEETINGS: THE EARLY 1980S

At the heart of the Society's activities were the winter and summer meetings. There were people to meet, friends to greet, sessions to attend, presentations to be made or listened to, posters to view, discussions with those having like interests (sometimes with vigour but rarely heated), conversations and chat (a generic term that encompasses gossip). There was an ambience of intellectual action, reaction and, above all, interaction. Although there were dull moments there was never a dull meeting. In the background were occasions ranging from the Society Dinner to small self-selected groups – usually sharing special interests or training affiliations – where with food and drink one could socialise. Such meetings were informative, lively and enjoyable.

The first meeting of that decade, the 140th meeting of the Society, was held at the John Radcliffe Hospital in Oxford and commenced on Thursday 3 January 1980. This day and date were not arbitrary but determined by the arcane formula of the Thursday after the first Wednesday unless 1 January was a Wednesday. This was out of term for all potential host departments and fitted in with train services, especially from the north. The meeting ran through to Saturday, the last occasion it did so.[1] Accommodation was provided in Merton College and St Edmund's Hall. The

[1] In fact the July 1992 Meeting in Manchester did have a Symposium on the Saturday morning.

latter was the venue for the Society Dinner on the Friday evening, and the reception on Thursday evening was in the Ashmolean.

The Committee met in Merton College on the Wednesday evening. George Williams from Manchester as the senior and willing member was in the chair. This was common practice. The Society since its inception had seen no need for a President or a Chairman so there was no provision in the constitution. Among the matters discussed were freeing the Journal from the limitations of hot metal typesetting and the role of the Society in relation to specialist groups. Both of these were significant discussion points in the early 1980s. The Minutes end with '... many members of the Committee were by now hypothermic so the meeting was concluded at 7.00 p.m.'. This reflection on the ambient temperature in a college out of term in winter is not peculiar to Oxford. At a later meeting in the decade and with a different secretary a similar sentiment is recorded about Cambridge.

In the scientific sessions there were a total of 103 presentations covering an eclectic mix of things pathological, microbiological and immunological. There was an impressive joint symposium in association with the Royal College of Pathologists on 'The cell surface'. There was a paper entitled 'Did the Gonococcus acquire the ability to produce beta-lactamase in 1976?'. One abstract memorably began 'The commonest guinea pig is now the mouse', and the neuroendocrine group from the Hammersmith were beginning to flex their muscles. The techniques employed included histochemistry, immunocytochemistry and electron microscopy. There was nothing to pre-sage the deluge of monoclonal antibodies and nucleic acid probes of only slightly later years. The Business Meeting commenced at 8.40 a.m. on Saturday. Under 'any other business' a senior member, Bernard Lennox (the author of a seminal paper on vitamin B deficiency and brain haemorrhage), who could be delightfully waspish on such occasions, 'Regretted the absence from the session chairmen of a firm timekeeper and requested that the Society return to the clock'.

The summer meeting that year was in Glasgow, from Wednesday to Friday. Of significance were discussions on funding intercalated BSc students and also students on electives. Both of these were subsequently implemented. At the July Committee Meeting the problems of microbiology within the Society were raised (a theme that was to continue throughout the next two decades) and the idea of a Microbiology Meetings secretary to try to help this was mooted. This was implemented with the election of Charles Easmon at the following winter meeting. Interestingly, the Microbiology Meetings secretary did not become an Officer of the Society until 1983.

The winter meeting in 1981 was at the Middlesex Hospital, London, and was the biggest meeting yet with nearly 150 abstracts. Although the deaths of members are formally recorded at the Business Meeting it was a rare event for there to be a formal tribute. This, however, was such an occasion when Rupert Willis was remembered by Colin Bird, one of his students in the early 1960s. That year the summer meeting was at Ninewells Hospital Medical School, Dundee. Alan Lendrum, from the host department, delivered a tribute to mark our 75th Anniversary '... and, in particular, its activities, during the past 25 years since the last history was published by J. Henry Dible in 1957...'. The committee decided that Lendrum's contribution should be published and, true to their word, it now appears as Chapter 3 of this book, although the Introduction to this book indicates the slightly tortuous route that this took!

The winter meeting in 1982 was at Churchill College, Cambridge, and ran from Tuesday to Friday. A ticket for the Society Dinner was £12 10p, there was no registration fee and B&B was £15, with coffee, lunch and tea being £5 50p. The first day was devoted to a joint symposium with the Royal College of Pathologists, aptly entitled 'The Monoclonal Revolution'. The keynote speaker was Cesar Milstein and there followed some 20 related presentations. It was a meeting with a high impact factor. Behind the scenes, unbeknown to anyone at the meeting, events were unfolding that were to have a major effect on the organisation of the Society. The Committee Meeting had not been in decision-making mode. The General Secretary was about to retire, the Meetings Secretary had recently demitted office and, at the last minute, an apology had been received on the telephone saying that the Treasurer, Wally Spector, was unable to attend. He was also the Editor of the *Journal of Pathology* and a principal agenda item for discussion was the increasingly strained relationship between the Journal and its publishers. The message was inconvenient but not overly concerning, the impression being that he had acquired some seasonal virus. Decisions were put on hold until the next meeting.

On the last day of the Cambridge meeting it was bitterly cold and the weather forecast was ominous so the meeting was truncated to obviate travel problems. As the attendees (including Committee Members) were dispersing it became known that Wally had died.

There was a hiatus terminated before the end of January by Bill Crane, acting on the senior and willing member principle, convening an emergency Committee Meeting in Sheffield. It was quorate and it was decided to approach a particular member (Neville) to take over as Treasurer and another member (Walker) to chair a small working party to recommend the appointment of an Editor for the Journal and to negotiate a new contract with publishers. The decision to move publishers stemmed from some dissatisfaction with the former publishers (lost copy, lost parts of copy, issues published in the wrong order, etc.) that had led to a falling in the standing of the Journal. After a competitive 'beauty parade' with five established publishers, tenders were submitted and evaluated. In the course of this I phoned Dillwyn, who evinced some surprise when he was requested to send a member of his staff to Companies House (in Cardiff) to obtain a copy of one of the tenderers' annual accounts. This was forthcoming next day. The outcome was that Munro Neville became Treasurer, Dennis Wright became Editor and the new publisher was Wiley. Twenty-four years later Munro and Dennis are now retired but Wiley still publish the Journal. This episode had other long-reaching consequences for the Society. The need for central organisation and a permanent office was implanted in certain minds. The Society subsequently has eschewed secular pluralism.

The summer meeting of 1982 was in Sheffield. The Business Meeting, as was the custom then, was chaired by a member of the host department, Bill Crane. He spelt out the changes necessary for the well-being of the Society but those present were not notably receptive. In contrast, the scientific sessions were especially lively. The Hammersmith and Cardiff departments (orJulia's entourage and Dillwyn's bunch, as they were more usually known) were major contributors. Of note is that the annual Society subscription was then £10.

Unusually the winter meeting in 1983 was not in the golden triangle but in Birmingham. It was well attended and most of the academic departments were represented, but numerically Hammersmith was dominant and indeed may have set the record for the number of presentations at a single meeting. Sadly the Committee was informed of the death of Bill Crane, who had galvanised them to activity exactly a year previously. The summer meeting of 1983 was remarkably international. The contributing departments included those from The Netherlands, France, Greece, Portugal, USA, Nigeria, Ghana, Sweden and Norway. This was not attributable to any special effort on the part of the Society but may well relate to the venue, Edinburgh, which has always encouraged and nurtured such connections both at town and gown levels. Comments annotated on the programme indicate Andrew Wyllie's response to a question after his presentation: 'One can never exclude the possibility that something one hasn't thought of might occur'. Henry Harris, Oxford, delivered a keynote lecture 'Where is pathology going?' His message in essence was 'There is a requirement for intellectual input in pathology.' A comment from an unidentified voice as the audience left was: 'He obviously was not present at last year's symposium in Cambridge'. The Committee Dinner, presided over by the Godfather a.k.a. Alastair Currie, had overtones of Burns. An account of the meal overheard at next morning's scientific session had it that Committee Members were bemused and the guests were thrilled: 'He actually killed a haggis at the table before their very eyes and then delivered an epitaph'.

The winter meeting in 1984 was at the Hammersmith. An innovation was that the Minutes of the Business Meeting held the previous July were printed in the programme. This was part of the reorganisation to improve the communication of information to members. The 'in' joke on that occasion, mindful of the proximity of Wormwood Scrubs, was 'What kind of wright would set up shop beside a prison? A Nick Wright'. Of note from the Committee Minutes was the proposal by E.D. Williams for joint meetings with other bodies and organisations as a way of promoting pathology. This was soundly rejected but sadly the Minutes do not reveal the nature of the arguments. The increasing number of abstracts and the desire to allow as many presentations of proffered papers as possible led to presentations being reduced to 10 min!

In 1984 there were two summer meetings. In May, in Bergen, there was a joint meeting of The Pathological Society of Great Britain and Ireland with the Netherlands Pathological Society and the Norwegian Pathological Society. There were 31 members and 10 guests from the British Isles, 18 members and 7 guests from The Netherlands and 36 members and 4 guests from Norway. Harold Fox featured prominently in the programme. Incidentally it emerged that the fronts, beloved of weather forecasters, was a concept that originated in Bergen in the 19th century. Reindeer was on the menu of the Society Dinner. It was a lot better than swan! In July 1984, Leeds was the venue. There were 141 presentations. The Departments of Pathology and Microbiology gave a reception and buffet at Temple Newsam House and the Dinner was in the Senior Common Room. There was a large microbiology input to this meeting.

THE CHANGING FACE OF THE MEETINGS

In January 1985 the Society met at Northwick Park, London, debatably within the golden triangle. There were 190 presentations. The Oakley Lecture was delivered by Barry Gusterson. It was a well-attended, well-organised and friendly occasion but the Dinner venue, the Wembley Conference Centre, was soulless. Despite this, after the Society Dinner those present were given a piece of iced cake made by Miss Christine Bateman (Senior MLSO at Northwick Park) to celebrate the 150th Scientific Meeting of the Society. The summer meeting was at the University College of Wales College of Medicine, Cardiff. As expected of a meeting hosted by Dillwyn Williams it was lively, but what sticks in my mind was the Committee Dinner in which for the first time I tasted seaweed – in the form of laver bread, with bacon. Having previously taken this oceanic vegetable for granted it can be stated that this dish was not just novel but memorably tasty. It is worth trying. The reception was in Cardiff Castle, and was also memorable.

Winter 1986 was marked by the meeting at the London Hospital and there were more than 200 abstracts for the first time. The guest lecture was delivered by Luzzatto, entiled 'Gene rearrangements in human pathology'. There was a presentation of 'An autopsy study of mountaineering accidents in Scotland': one of the co-authors subsequently became Minister for Education and Sport in the devolved Scottish Assembly. The take-home message was 'wear a helmet'. Another presentation, adjudged at the time as an effective throwaway delivery with good timing, commenced 'This is a slightly dubious exercise but I undertook it anyway'. A penetrating query from the floor, emanating from a tall Welshman, was prefaced with 'An elegant contribution to the question but not to the answer'. Wordsmiths were to the fore at that session. This was also the first meeting at which markers of lymphocyte phenotype that worked in routine material were presented (abstracts from Andrew Norton and Kevin West), a trickle that became a flood! Nick Wright was the new Meetings secretary and he proposed the introduction of poster prizes of £100, £50 and £25. E.M. (Mary) Cooke took over from Colin Easmon as Microbiology Meetings secretary. The July meeting was in Dublin and held jointly with the Dutch Pathological Society. A symposium on 'New Developments in Pulmonary Pathology' was chaired by Michael Dunnill. The lymphoma phenotyping explosion continued and Quirke, Durdey, Williams and Dixon presented their seminal paper 'Local recurrence after surgery for rectal adenocarcinoma results from incomplete removal'. The dinner was held in the Incorporated Law Society Building and the delights of Dublin were savoured.

The January 1987 meeting was in Oxford with the Committee Meeting being held at Linacre College. Here it was reported that the first full-day Editorial Board meeting was held on 22 October 1986 in the Reform Club. It was noted that the Journal had some significant problems, including lack of copy and a high rejection rate, but that there had been a 40% increase in subscriptions in the previous 12 months. At this Meeting of the Committee the idea of introducing Registration Fees was raised but no action was taken. There was also a discussion on investing in property in South East England, and similarly no action was taken. For the Oxford meeting the accommodation and the Dinner were in St Edmund's Hall. The reception was held in the University Museum on Parks Road. The number of presentations was 252. The weighty symposium was 'Viruses in Human Cancer'. The contributors included Doll, Epstein and zur Hausen. This was the last meeting at which the small abstract book format was used. This last small abstract book contained gems, including the first report to the Society of Ag-NORs by the late John Crocker, as well as the use of Ki67 as a prognostic marker (Hall) and many presentations on the delights of antibody panels.

There was a large colourful introduction to the summer meeting in the form of a blue A4 printed programme replacing the previous white A5 programme. The meeting, in Southampton, was also large and colourful. The weighty symposium was 'Pathology of the Acquired Immunodeficiency Syndrome'. The contributors included Armes, Millard and Sebastian Lucas. At a discussion session the Chairman, a short Mancunian, declined to read the title and the list of authors of one poster on the grounds that this would take up half of the allocated discussion time of 4 min. Peacock, du Boulay and Kirkham asked if the 'Autopsy was a useful tool or an old relic?'. We now have a clearer view of what the rest of the profession think! At the Business Meeting there was a brief discussion about the desirability of setting up a central office in London to integrate administrative activities, including the organisation of Society meetings. Complaints were noted by several members regarding the Society Dinner in January 1987 when no grace was said, there was no loyal toast and no soft drinks were available: the meeting secretary (N.A. Wright) stated 'he would look into this'. There is no record of any action! Action did take place, however, on the River Boat Shuffle, which went down the Solent and up the Hamble to Buckler's Hard. A balmy evening, with chicken salad and large volumes of lubrication, and with the vessel being followed by seagulls feasting on the remnants of the picnic!

The 1988 January meeting was held at St Bartholomew's Medical School, London. The local organiser was David Levison, a future treasurer of the Society, and this may explain why the issue of Registration Fees was raised again. Again, no action was taken. Peter Toner proposed an Undergraduate Pathology Essay prize to stimulate interest in medical schools. Sadly it was not until 2005 that this was instituted! Action was taken more promptly on another matter, that of accommodation, where it was unanimously agreed that business would be best carried out from a central office. The then treasurer A.M. Neville was deputed to write to the President of the Royal College of Pathologists because it was known that space would become available in at 2 Carlton House Terrace. After a lull, nucleolar organiser regions were the subject of eight presentations in a variety of sessions prompting E.D. Williams to state that he was an 'AgNOR-stic'. Both the reception and the Dinner were in the Great Hall of the hospital. The dinner was £30 although coffee, lunch and teas were now cheaper at £4!

The summer meeting was in Newcastle. On the Wednesday morning an event waiting to happen occurred. There were concurrent sessions and they became out of sync. A paper was called 5 min ahead of its programmed time and no-one appeared to present it. A voice from the audience said 'They are speaking next door'. The chairman was indulgent and replied 'With your consent we shall wait'. Right on time there was a commotion towards the rear of the lecture theatre as the Hammersmith histochemical horde, led by Julia and urged on by the new Meetings Secretary, entered. The chairman exclaimed 'In the nick of time'. In the Committee Minutes the first mention of the University Grants Committee (UGC) Research Selectivity Exercise (a.k.a. RAE) was made. It was agreed to send a letter to the UGC suggesting that the Society be able to nominate members to specific subcommittees, and to ask that clinical workload not militate against departments and that cognizance be taken of the big cutbacks in pathology departments that had taken place in the past decade! The impact of the successive Research Assessment Exercise (RAE) is documented in Chapter 9.

The winter meeting in 1989 was at University College, London, hosted by Peter Isaacson. A reception was held in the Courtauld Institute (the old one in Woburn Square). The venue was unique, with *objets d'art* ranging from a Florentine dowry chest to Manet's 'Bar at the Folies-Bergere'; eclectic, with taste. The visual arts were reinforced by the performing arts – a musical duo (one was the host's daughter) that blended with the setting and contributed to the ambience. The heavyweight symposium, unsurprisingly, was 'Pathology of the T-cell'. The Oakley Lecture was delivered by Kevin Gatter on the subject of immunohistochemistry (see Chapter 15).

The July meeting in the last year of the 1980s was in Aberdeen. The local organiser was John Simpson. A striking feature was that the weather was perfect. The sessions were in the Zoology Building, which is situated alongside and has direct access to the Cruikshank Botanic Garden. Morning coffee and afternoon tea were more often than not taken in the open air. The heavyweight symposium was 'The New Genetics and Human Cancer' and contributors included Steel, Cowell and Andrew Wyllie. The guest lecturer was Enzinger. A poster with particularly fine illustrations was presented by Jennifer Young. At the Society Dinner the Meetings Secretary reported that with 288 presentations 'this was the largest summer meeting on record'. Interestingly, at the last Committee Meeting of this decade Rab Goudie posed the question 'should not the Society have a President.' It took another decade to get a clear answer.

CHANGING TIMES

Regarding the Society as a whole during the decade the membership was of the order of 1500: major themes, trends and developments are readily identified. The impact of new molecular biological methods on investigative pathology is clear from the scientific programmes. At the beginning of the decade immunocytochemistry was largely polyclonal: by the end this was almost entirely replaced and considerably extended by the advent of monoclonals. In the late 1980s came the polymerase chain reaction and in situ hybridisation. The joke at the time was that the election of the new Meetings Secretary in 1987 was an example of 'nick translation'. Under a succession of Meetings Secretaries the scientific programme evolved to deal with varied interests, and the increasing number of submissions, concurrent sessions, symposia, keynote speakers, posters and poster discussions became regular features.

Even the Society Dinner was shaken up. Up to the 1970s this was a pleasant but low-key function with one brief speech, 'the vote of thanks', usually delivered by a member who had been fingered a day or two earlier. There were no oratorical excesses. There were no prizes to give. Seating was more or less a free for all. Through a succession of small changes, some attributable to the Meetings Secretaries and some attributable to members, the occasion became what it is now: table plans were introduced so that names could be written in; poster prizes were awarded; the winner of the slide quiz received a crate of champagne that had to be distributed before the end of the dinner; and the speech became the responsibility of the Meetings Secretary. Last was the emergence of the sweepstake based on the duration of the speech. This was an unintentional but welcome consequence of the introduction of seating arrangements. Inevitably this had led to some mono-departmental tables, the noisiest of which was Southampton (closely pressed, on occasion, by Cardiff) and it was that table that started the sweepstake. Adjacent tables expressed an interest and at subsequent meetings the sweepstake became a general feature of the Dinner.

The major development in the 1980s was organisational. Up to that time the Society was run initially by two and subsequently by three officers and their respective and respected secretaries. The best known of these was Zadie Milner from Leeds, a lady of formidable mien who regularly attended the Business Meetings up to the early 1970s (see Vignette: Fame at last P. Scheuer p 11). When the officers changed, currently relevant papers were passed to their successors and earlier documents were sent to whichever officer had the large tin trunk. Such arrangements were appropriate for the earlier years of the Society but were patently not up to late 20th century requirements. Spector's untimely death crystallised the situation. Eventually, after due enquiry, consultation and discussion, the Committee agreed unanimously 'that the business of the Society should be conducted from a central office in London, preferably in the same building as the Royal College of Pathologists'. This was at the winter meeting in 1988. On 1 February 1989 the Society opened its central office in London at 2 Carlton House Terrace (2CHT), and the foundation Administrator, Jacqui Edwards, was installed. The proponent, indeed driver, of these necessary changes was Munro Neville and he implemented them. Three years later he was 'poached' to be Treasurer of the Royal College of Pathologists and the Society did not get a transfer fee. Was this perhaps a foretaste of the Bosman ruling?

The preceding paragraph harbours a mystery. Was the large tin trunk a society myth or was it a reality? Well, a large tin trunk and several associated cardboard boxes were subsequently retrieved from Bart's and eventually transported to 2CHT. It contained Minute books, attendance logs, journals and all sorts of odd papers that are now filed in the central office. It was only when this centennial publication was being discussed that it was recognised what was not in the trunk. This cannot be dealt with in an account of the 1980s because at that time these omissions were not recognised. Perhaps the subsequent contributions to this publication, relating to later years, will shed light on the matter.

Anyhow the trunk has again disappeared. It was last seen in the office in the early 1990s – nondescript and battered. At that time the office was in the basement and extensive building renovation works were going on at 2CHT. The contents of the trunk are certainly on file in the relocated office on the top floor of 2CHT but the trunk is not there. Possibly it was put in a skip or maybe it was incorporated in a floor or put behind a wall (builders do these things). On an encouraging note, the basement of 2CHT is about to be renovated as an educational centre. There is a remote chance that the large tin trunk may reappear.

Acknowledgements

Thanks to Jacqui Edwards for reminiscences over dinner and in true mandarin minder style subsequently providing notes of the conversation. Thanks to Ros Pitts for ready access to the minutes and numerous cups of coffee. Peter Hall added some material to early versions of this manuscript. The opportunity is taken to respond to Peter Hall's e-mailed question 'How did the officers manage before the central office was established in 1989?'. The answer is 'With *great* difficulty'.

Colin Bird's mandible

I was warned at an early stage of my career that the meetings of the 'Path Soc' were the academic equivalent of the Colosseum in Rome (at the height of the fashion for gladiatorial combats). The 1987 Path Soc meeting was hosted by Professor Gerry Slavin at Bart's. Being on the academic staff at Bart's I could no longer escape my fate and made my belated entry into the arena. To survive the ordeal I knew that I had to fortify my presentation (which was on polyposis) with a thumbs-up message and therefore slipped in a pre-publication and tightly embargoed aside on the location of the APC gene on chromosome 5. This produced a sudden sound (followed by a loud and long groan) from the auditorium. I later learned that the sound was caused by the mandible of Professor Colin Bird hitting the floor-boards. It transpired that Professor Bird's research group was a mere sword-stroke from the same discovery.

Jeremy Jass

6 The 1990s: People, Events and Meetings

David A. Levison

The 1990s was a decade of consolidation and steady development for The Pathological Society under the astute leadership of Eric Walker (Professor of Pathology in the University of Aberdeen), who was Chairman and General Secretary from 1992 to 2000. His diplomatic skills were constantly tested during his Chairmanship by a number of different issues and in particular the different needs and aspirations of the microbiologists and histopathologists in the Society. It is a great tribute to Eric's diplomacy that when the decision was eventually taken that the microbiologists would be better placed in another organisation, this was effected and perceived as a positive move for all parties and individuals.

The growing strength, influence and confidence of the Society in the 1990s was underpinned by its sound financial position (see Chapter 4). The credit for this belongs undoubtedly with the Treasurer up until 1993, Munro Neville, who had taken over as Treasurer in 1983 when the Society was in a weak financial position. Through a combination of astute investments, sound and perceptive negotiations with the College, a firm 'Scottish' attitude to finances and an ability to say 'No' when required, he made the Society strong financially and was responsible for our acquisition of the lease on our office accommodation on the top floor of 2 Carlton House Terrace. Munro's talents as a Treasurer were recognised by the College, who recruited him as their Treasurer in 1993. I took over as The Pathological Society Treasurer from Munro in 1993 and, thanks to the mechanisms and arrangements set up by him I (despite limited aptitude for financial matters – ask my wife), did not find the job too burdensome. One of the first things I did as Treasurer, on Munro's advice, was to open up negotiations with the College on extending the lease on the top floor of 2 Carlton House Terrace, which was due to run out in 1999. The negotiations were complex and protracted, but eventually we were able to agree a further 10-year extension to the lease at a very reasonable cost to the Society for excellent accommodation in central London. One of the few pieces of advice that I passed on in 2003 to my successor as Treasurer, Alastair Burt, was to start negotiations with the College over a further extension to the lease, which was due to run out in 2009. From Alastair's report to the Business Meeting of the Society in July 2005 it sounds as though the negotiations this time had extra layers of complexity to be navigated, but he has clearly achieved a very good deal for the Society, with concomitant advantages to the College, and an extension to the lease of a further 20 years. It is extremely useful to the Society to have this base within the same building as the College. The close physical association of the Society and the College has mutual advantages, with the two organisations having been able to respond in harmony to unforeseen crises on a number of occasions. Throughout the 1990s the College and the Society jointly financed and allocated elective bursaries, and our administrative staff benefited and continue to benefit from being linked to the larger College structure and robust pay scales.

We were also able, because of our strong financial position in the 1990s, to take a number of initiatives and set up a number of new schemes for the benefit of members of the Society and pathology in general. Such initiatives included the setting up of the Society's PhD Scheme, the

Trainees' Support Scheme and the Open Scheme. The PhD scheme began in 1995 and provides full funding for 3 years for a PhD student supervised by a member of the Society. The Society supports three students at any one time, with one new student starting each year as one finishes her/his 3 years of support. The scheme has proved very successful and popular with members of the Society. The annual call for applications for one of these studentships always produces a keen and top quality competition. The scheme during 1996–2001 has supported students in departments throughout the land, including Cambridge (twice), Guy's, King's and St Thomas's (twice), Dundee, Glasgow and Leicester, on research topics reflecting the wide research interests of Society members, producing several significant contributions to our understanding of matters ranging from the complexity of the p53 pathway to molecular mechanisms of renal carcinogenesis. Presentations from Society-supported PhD students are now a regular feature of the Society's Scientific Meetings. Specific Trainee support began in 1998 as the Clinical Trainees' Grant Scheme and continues rebadged as the Pilot Study Grant Scheme, a twice yearly competition for grants of up to £5000 for pump priming of a research project undertaken by a trainee. The Trainee Support Scheme has spawned the now established and successful Annual Trainees' Day at Winter Pathological Society Meetings and the embryonic Pathological Society Trainees' Subcommittee.

Part of the move to a proper business base and management of the Society was the move in 1993 to running the financial side of the main Scientific Meetings through the Society's Office and the Society's Administrator. It seems unbelievable now that until 1992 the financial responsibility for the meeting had rested with the host department, which was also responsible for managing the accounts and paying the bills entailed in running the meeting. I actually hosted one of the last meetings to be run under the old scheme (Winter 1992). I can tell this story now because so many years have elapsed, but we were never billed by the caterers for the Society Dinner that year, despite a series of reminders sent by me and the Society's Administrator over a 2–3-year period. By the time 5 years had elapsed, still with no bill, I transferred the Dinner money account from the host organisation to the Society because I reasoned that it had originally been collected for a Society event, and by that time I was the Treasurer of the Society!

The *Journal of Pathology* also grew in stature and influence throughout the 1990s (see Chapter 8). Its upward trajectory had been begun by Dennis Wright in 1983, and was continued and accelerated by Peter Toner through from 1993. Peter laid the foundations for the sound business and organisational basis on which the Journal currently operates. Throughout the 1990s the Society was also responsible for and owned the *Journal of Medical Microbiology*. The Editor-in-Chief throughout that period was Brian Duerden, and so successful was his stewardship of that journal that it formed the dowry taken by the microbiologists when they left the Society, and enabled all parties to feel that a fair and favourable business solution accompanied the parting of the ways of microbiologists and pathologists in the Society. Microbiology Meetings Secretaries through the 1990s were R.J. Williams (1991–1995) and Curtis Gemmell (1995–2001). They kept the microbiological section of the meetings alive through a difficult period for their subject and for the microbiological members of the Society, and they always contributed positively at Officers and Committee Meetings.

MEETINGS

The Pathology Meetings Secretaries through the 1990s were Nick Wright (1987–1992), James Underwood (1992–1996) and Michael Wells (1996–2000). All were very successful, all made innovations to improve meetings and they were not afraid to try new things. Between them they introduced many of the now established features of the Meetings, such as poster prizes, poster rounds in a variety of formats, plenary sessions, various named guest lectures and joint meetings with other societies, and all three entertained the Society royally in their own inimitable and unique styles at Society Dinners. The duration of the Meetings Secretaries speech at the Society Dinner had been the source of a small wager for some time. Legend has it that this started on the 'Southampton table' but during the 1990s (in part due to the efforts of William Roche) this evolved to involve all at the dinner, a pound being the stake and the best guess of the duration winning the pot! William's strategy for ensuring participation seemed to largely involve the (non-pc) use of pretty SHOs and SpRs to persuade the punters to part with a pound. On one occasion William actually won! Cries of 'fix' abounded but one is sure of complete probity in the process!

The Society ran a memorable series of meetings throughout the 1990s (see Appendix 6). Attendances peaked in the early 1990s with slightly reduced attendances in the latter part of the decade (see Fig. 9.1, Chapter 9). However, the quality of the meetings both scientifically and socially was maintained and enhanced throughout this period. The winter meetings had in fact become so large in the early 1990s that they could not be accommodated by any of the London Medical Schools with the exception of the Hammersmith Hospital. This led to meetings being hosted by one Medical School, e.g. Guy's/Thomas's, but held in another (the Hammersmith), and then to the series of winter meetings hosted by London Schools but held in the Queen Elizabeth II Conference Centre off Parliament Square. This location had advantages and disadvantages for the Society. Disadvantages included the cost of the premises, problems with audiovisual arrangements and dissociation from the Host Department. Advantages included adequate space, a prime location in central London (with great views of Westminster Abbey) and, in January 1994, a conducted tour and reception in the Houses of Parliament.

The first meeting of the new decade was held in January 1990 at the Hammersmith Hospital, with N.A. Wright both as host and as Meetings Secretary. An overriding memory of this and the next few winter meetings was the extreme cold! The walk from East Acton tube station to the Hammersmith past Wormwood Scrubb's was particularly cold, with a biting North wind reminding one of the trials and tribulations of polar explorers. The Stamp lecture theatre was not much warmer but it was the biggest Society Scientific Meeting to date and the first time with over 300 abstracts (327). There was a symposium on Cell Differentiation in Pathology and Werner Franke was guest lecturer (and I recall he had two carousels of slides!)

The summer meeting was held in Nottingham with rather stringent security as a consequence of threats from animal rights activists. Wishing to leave a little early and hoping to place his valise behind the registration desk, Peter Hall was slightly embarrassed to have it searched by David Turner's secretary who found (predictably) only dirty clothes! Nevertheless such security issues have actually only rarely been needed at Society meetings, even today. Hall and others. presented papers on the immunohistological detection of PCNA as a marker of proliferation, beginning a flood of interest in this strategy – interest enhanced perhaps by one of the other co-authors being a strikingly attractive blond! At the AGM in Nottingham the Meetings Secretary indicated that because the meetings continued to grow, and with increasing complexity and organisation, there was a need to defray the increasing costs of the meetings. Consequently, and after nearly a decade of discussion and debate, it was announced that there would be the introduction of a registration fee from July 1991.

As with January 1990, the January 1991 meeting in Cambridge was characterised by freezing conditions and profound wind-chill due to icy blasts coming across the Fens. A symposium on Aspects of Genetic Pathology presaged a splurge of papers on PCR and similar methodologies but in the 1990s much of the proffered papers still remained largely immunohistochemical and observational in nature. In July 1991 the Society gathered in Belfast for the first time in many years. The meeting was notable for the introduction of registration fees (£10 per day) and the introduction of camera-ready abstracts. The former had been a contentious source of debate in the Committee for a decade and the latter had been first proposed 2 years before by the Meetings Secretary, Nick Wright, who at the Belfast meeting demitted office to be replaced by James Underwood. The Belfast meeting was a highly successful social event, with an excellent programme, enjoyed by all who went. Of note was an afternoon trip in beautiful sunshine to the Giant's Causeway, followed by an abortive attempt to visit the Bushmill's Distillery. This was eagerly awaited after the exertions of the walk down to and back up from the Causeway. Sadly no-one had told the organisers that it was shut for their annual summer holiday!

In January 1992, a prompt return of the Society to the Royal Postgraduate Medical School and Hammermith Hospital was dictated by the size of the meeting and the inability of the host departments (University Medical and Dental School, Guy's and St Thomas's Hospitals) to provide large enough venues. Bert Vogelstein declined an invitation but Stanley Hamilton was an excellent replacement. A symposium organised by Peter Hall on the 'nucleus and cell proliferation' included luminaries such as Ron Laskey, Nick Wright, David Lane, Fiona Watt and Andrew Wyllie. This was associated with an odd misunderstanding. In the trade exhibition there were several displays of books. Bizarrely most were not on pathological issues, but on topics related to nuclear power, nuclear non-proliferation, nuclear this and that: all because the word nucleus in the symposium title had elicited an incorrect response! The summer meeting of 1992 was held jointly with the Dutch Pathological Society in Manchester. There was an abortive attempt at that meeting to return to the old tradition of running from Thursday through to Saturday. Although the meeting was a great success (with dinner at the Old Trafford cricket ground, including a visit to the square), the Saturday session (on developmental biology and pathology) was not well attended and one doubts if this timing will ever be repeated.

January 1993 saw the first use by the Society of the Queen Elisabeth II (QE2) Conference Centre in Westminster, with a meeting hosted by St Mary's Hospital Medical School. Although expensive, this venue was felt to be needed, but meetings in this venue (which continued for the rest of the decade) prompted diverse responses from love to hate. Juan Rosai made his first of three visits in 10 years as guest lecturer to the Society (the others being Dublin in 2002 and Bristol in 2003). Figure 6.1 shows the attendees at the January 1993 Committee Dinner. The summer meeting of 1993 was hosted by the Edinburgh pathologists led by C.C. Bird but held at Heriot-Watt University in blazing July heat. Discussion seminars were introduced at that meeting, as were invited lectures from the great and the good: E.D. Willliams spoke on Natural Selection and Pathology, and David Page (Vanderbilt University, USA) on breast pathology. Colin Bird had suggested previously to the Committee that the main poster prize be denoted as the Alistair Currie Prize. This was agreed by the Committee, the family were duly asked and having given their assent this was enacted (appropriately) from the Edinburgh Meeting.

The 1994 winter meeting at the QE2 Conference Centre was hosted by St Bartholomew's and the London Hospital Medical School and was notable for a discussion session where we asked 'Do falling autopsy rates matter?', a lecture by Gunter Kloppel on 'pancreatitis' and a symposium on 'The Pathology of Devices'. However, it will be a long remembered meeting, not because of these scientific offerings, nor for a Reception held in the Houses of Parliament (organised by Colin Berry) with an inspiring tour of the various Chambers, but rather because of the Committee Dinner and its dramatic results! This incident is documented in Chapter 10 (p. 121) and in the vignette by Alistair Burt (p. 56). Suffice it to say that I, as Treasurer, delayed paying the bill for the Committee Dinner pending an enquiry into an incident that was being investigated by the Communicable Diseases consultant for the City of Westminster! The Summer meeting of the Society in 1994 was held in Glasgow and it was fitting that the Society honoured a stalwart of the Membership and a long-serving Officer, R.A.B. Goudie, who lectured entertainingly and informatively on the History of Organ Specific Autoimmune Disease.

At about this time the Officers received a complaint from a notable senior London professor who described the Society meetings as 'elitist and singularly uninformative'. This individual also complained that there were an excessive number of 'case reports' that had flooded the meeting. It is recorded in the Minutes that the Meetings Secretary (J.C.E. Underwood) pointed out to the Committee that the complainer was actually the author of one of the 10 case reports (which

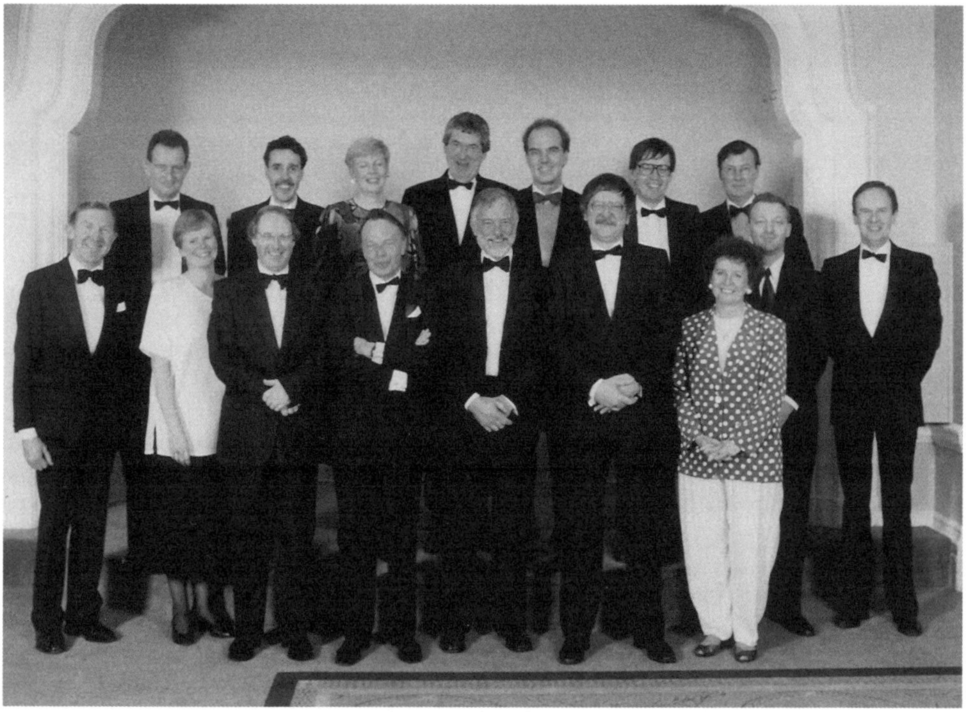

Figure 6.1 The Pathological Society Committee January 1993. *Front row*: Professor C.T. Doyle, Dr Rosamund J. Williams (Medical Microbiology Meetings Secretary), Professor B.I. Deurden (Editor of *Journal of Medical Microbiology*), Professor F. Walker (Chairman and General Secretary), Professor D.H. Wright (Editor of *Journal of Pathology*), Dr D.W.K. Cotton, Dr Anne-Marie McNicol, Dr S.P. Borriello, Professor J.C.E. Underwood (Meetings Secretary). *Back row*: Professor E.L. Jones, Dr J.G.M. Hastings, Mrs Jacqui Edwards (Administrator), Professor A.M. Neville (Treasurer), Dr N. Kirkham, Dr P. Quirke, Dr D. Lamb. (Missing are Dr M.J. Hill, Professor C.J.L.M. Meijer and Dr C. Wray).

represented less than 5% of the total abstracts at the January meeting)! Nevertheless this marked the beginnings of some concern that the progressive rise in attendance at Society meetings and submission of abstracts was beginning to slow and indeed reverse (see Fig. 9.1, Chapter 9). The genesis of this fall in attendance at the Society's meetings after a decade of growth is complex and diverse and certainly includes the effects of the 1992 and 1996 Research Assessment Exercise and the impact that this had on pathology within Universities. Staffing issues, financial stringencies and changes in training perhaps also contributed to this, and the long-term effects of these effects are still with us.

In January 1995 we congregated in Oxford where Judah Folkman argued for the central place of angiogenesis in cancer biology. Later that year we met with the Dutch Pathological Society in Amsterdam (Fig. 6.2) at a hugely successful meeting and again a luminary of the Society spoke, this time D.H. Wright on 'Burkitt's lymphoma: safaris, translocations, oncogenes and viruses'. During the last two decades poster presentations have been complemented by diverse strategies to promote their attendance and use. In Amsterdam poster rounds again surfaced! The 1996 winter meeting was hosted by King's College Hospital and again held at the QE2 Conference Centre. Guy Brugal (Grenoble) spoke on proliferation markers and a symposium asked 'Is quantitation only for research'? In Southampton in July, Peter Scheuer spoke on 'Thirty years of chronic hepatitis'. It is of note that the Committee Minutes record that at the Annual Business Meeting of 1996 the

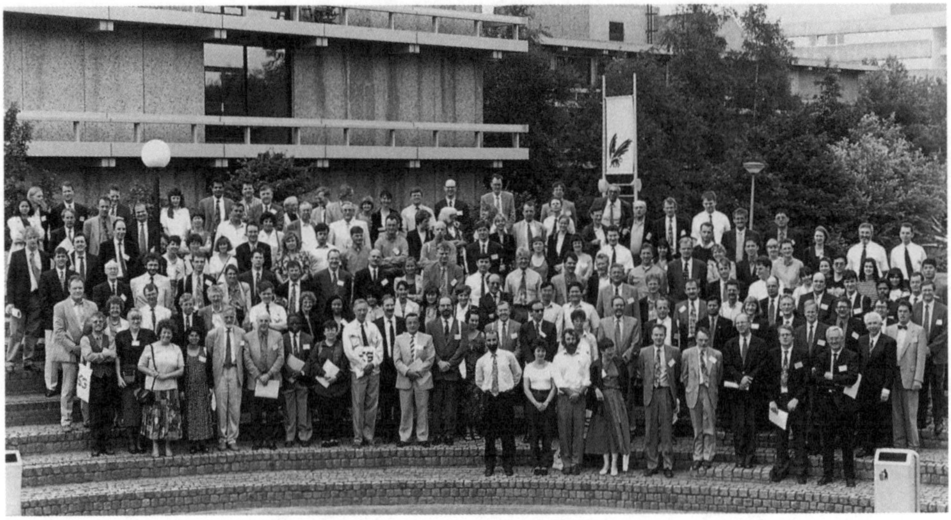

Figure 6.2 Delegates at the Summer Meeting of The Pathological Society held jointly with the Dutch Society in Amsterdam, July 1995.

Chairman and General Secretary, Eric Walker, indicated under 'any other business that: 'D.H. Wright as host is in fact the civilian advisor in Histopathology to the Royal Navy and hoped to exercise the privileges of rank during the Society's Dinner on HMS Warrior that evening. In this capacity he has the power to conduct marriages and bury the dead at sea. Any members who wished to avail themselves of these services should contact him directly'. It is not recorded if any such events occurred.

The winter 1997 meeting was hosted by the Royal Free Hospital Medical School (venue: QE2 Conference Centre) and the summer meeting was in Sheffield where the Royal College of Pathologists' Kettle Lecture was given by M.R. Stratton (Cambridge) on 'genetics and pathology'. D.J. Barker (Southampton) also spoke on the controversial subject of 'the fetal origins of adult disease', and there was a symposium on 'transgenic models and human disease'. The winter 1998 meeting (again at the QE2 Conference Centre), hosted by Imperial and Charing Cross Hospitals, was marked by the introduction of Plenary sessions, a successful experiment promoted by the new Meetings Secretary Mike Wells, and which continues to this day. Chris Fletcher (Boston and formerly of St Thomas's Hospital) gave an impressive exposition on 'Soft tissue tumours: the impact of cytogenetics and molecular analysis' and elegantly demonstrated the loss that UK pathology suffered when he left for the USA. In July the Society gathered in Leicester where the Kettle Lecture was given by Andrew Wyllie on 'apoptosis in cancer'. The Society Committee of the time recorded (summer 1998) that there needed to be more photographic records of the Society and its Meetings. Consequently disposable cameras were purchased, but sadly there is no record of their use!

After a meeting in Cambridge (winter 1999) with a reprise of cancer genetics and Peter Krammer's exposition of the roles of Fas/APO1/CD95 in cell death, the Society visited Dundee where the Royal College's Cameron Lecture was given by Salvador Moncada and a symposium on the molecular basis of cancer was (predictably perhaps) all about p53. It is a funny thing, but most of the things that stick in my mind about the Society's Meetings from the 1990s relate to the social rather than the scientific aspects of the meetings! For the Dundee meeting the Society Dinner was held in The Old Course Hotel in St Andrews and, during a protracted break between the main course and the sweet, Frank Carey suggested we take a stroll to enjoy the air and the ambience. Even at 10 p.m. it was still a beautiful sunny warm evening as we walked out onto the 17th fairway (the Famous Road Hole of the Old Course). A group of golfers were putting out on the 17th green – and the wine was slipping down very easily. Later that same evening the last bus due to take us back to Dundee broke down and refused to start. During the wait for a replacement bus I am afraid I used my position as Host of the Meeting and Society Treasurer to order beers for everybody on the bus. We had two visitors from Romania who were snoozing quietly, but promptly awoke when the word 'beer' was mentioned. We had encountered some communication problems with the Romanians until that moment, but not thereafter.

JOURNALS AND WEBS

Other important developments for the Society in the 1990s included the signing of a 10-year publishing deal for the *Journal of Pathology* with Wiley in 1994 and the setting up of the first version of the Society's website. There is always the potential for friction between a publisher and a Society that owns the journal title and selects and edits the content of the journal. I think that the Society has been fortunate to have been dealing with Wiley for some 25 years now. As Treasurer I had considerable difficulties with the various publishers of the other Society journal (*Journal of Medical Microbiology*) during the 1990s. This is reflected in the number of times the publisher was changed throughout the 1990s, and the often highly charged editorial board meetings when publishing issues were under discussion, despite the undoubted financial and scientific success of the Journal. Despite the inevitable differences we have had with Wiley, they are nothing compared to the real difficulties we have had with other publishers. Our relationship with Wiley undoubtedly has been mutually beneficial and continues to develop.

In early 1996 the matter of insurance for both journals became an issue. For example, what would happen if the journal(s) were to be sued or were deemed liable as a consequence of material published in them. Insurance was deemed prohibitively expensive, so the option of ring fencing the journals in a separate Foundation was investigated, thus keeping the Society free of liability. This was in fact set up in September 1996 but disbanded in January 1997 because of the adverse impact on Charitable status and liability to VAT and corporation tax!

In 1995 the internet was increasingly making an impact in academic life. Browsers such as Mosaic were in use and web pages from a small number of academic institutions and societies were appearing. The contents of the *Journal of Pathology* were first placed online on a website hosted by the University of Nottingham and written and organised by James Lowe. A proposal to start a website for The Pathological Society was received by the Committee in 1996 and it was agreed to host a site with the internet provider Netbenefit, with the domain name pathsoc.org.uk. The website was created and went live on 30 June 1996. The earliest website had rudimentary graphics and duplicate sets of pages that were 'text only' in recognition of the fact that many browsers still ran on text-only terminals. By early 1998 a graphical website was developed because by then most people were using Netscape as their browser of choice. We started archiving with the Internet Archive in 1997, so members may like to review what it looked like then (see http://web.archive.org/web/*/http://www.pathsoc.org.uk). It was agreed that Wiley would take over the development of the site in 2003, but this did not progress nearly as well as our dealings with Wiley over the *Journal of Pathology*. Eventually the Society had to terminate its collaboration with Wiley over this matter – a difficult exercise but firmly and effectively managed by Peter Hall, in fact so effectively managed that the Society's relationship with Wiley was in no way damaged and the Society emerged in a stronger negotiating position than ever before (and we got all our money back!). The development of the Society's new website is now being led by Jim Lowe and Peter Hamilton. The Society is fortunate to have individuals within its membership with the knowledge and skills to take on and develop such an important activity for a modern organisation.

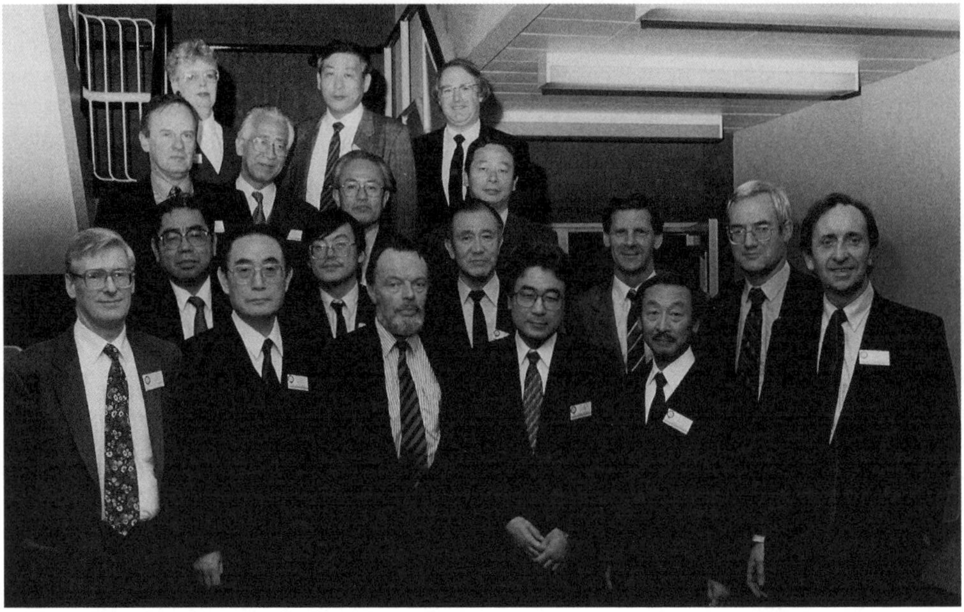

Figure 6.3 Officers and members of the Society with Japanese delegates in 1996.

THE COMMITTEE

A crucial element of the Society's functioning is its Committee, made up of Society members elected by their peers for a 3-year term. In addition, there are of course the Officers (see Fig. 6.3) who are similarly elected and serve for periods of 5 years. During the 1990s a range of weighty and not so weighty matters were considered by the Committee. For some considerable time a matter of great concern was discussion of whether the Committee Dinner should or should not be a black tie event! Indeed this matter swayed back and forth and eventually a vote on this issue went 15 against and 6 for continuing the tradition of black tie! Some traditionalists have ascribed the food poisoning incident at the Winter 1994 Meeting to divine retribution as opposed to a viral aetiology! It is noted that in 1996 a Committee wine tasting was held and a 1993 Cotes de Nuits Village and a 1994 Artea Sauvignon Blanc were purchased and laid down for future Committee Dinners. Regrettably none remains and the Committee has not repeated the experiment of wine tasting and laying down a cellar. The author views this with sadness.

More weighty matters considered by the Committee in the early 1990s included succession planning: for example, for Dennis Wright who had by 1993 served 10 years as Editor of the *Journal of Pathology*, and for Munro Neville who had similarly acted for a decade as Treasurer. Ultimately Peter Toner and David Levison were elected to these important positions. Nick Wright was replaced by James Underwood in 1991 as Meetings Secretary and in 1996 Mike Wells took over this role. One of the traditions of the Society that was challenged (unsuccessfully) several times during the 1990s is that the Society does not pay the expenses of Officers or Committee members for attending Officers' or Committee meetings that coincide with Scientific meetings. The rationale is that the Officers and Committee members would be at the Scientific meeting anyway, and should not be treated differently from ordinary members. However, the one perk/thank you that the Officers and Committee members do enjoy in repayment for their efforts on behalf of the Society is attending the Committee Dinner, which takes place after the Committee meeting and the evening before the start of the main meeting. This is usually a well-supported affair, but

I think apoplexy accurately describes what I experienced when I was presented as Treasurer with the bill for the Maastricht Committee Dinner in 2001. However, members will be pleased to know that strict guidelines now prevent a repeat of such extravagant 'thanks'.

Interactions with other organisations were also of concern to the Committee. The Society began to be much more outward looking in the 1990s – an example of this is the development of our relationship with the Japanese Pathological Society. Since 1995 a series of delegations from the Society have attended Japanese Pathological Society meetings to present posters and give oral presentations, and Japanese pathologists have attended and presented at our meetings in alternate years (Fig. 6.3). I think this was the beginning of the Society really starting to be outward looking. Closer to home, in March 1996 it was suggested that the British Division of the International and Academy of Pathology (BDIAP) move into 2 Carlton House Terrace and join with the Society in the use of the 3rd floor offices. The Minutes state that 'the IAP decided they could not afford this ... although the Society stated that the door was still open'. Of course this would actually have been difficult because the terms of the lease cannot be varied by the Society. But it is perhaps a shame that some development of this kind was not achieved, given the burgeoning interactions of the Society with the BDIAP (see below and Chapter 7). Other discussions with the IAP at the same time were in relation to joint meetings, and an initial overture was sadly hindered by financial considerations because it was felt that a joint meeting might cost ~£12 000 and the IAP thought that this was too much[1].

The issue of the Society's name exercised some during the 1990s and indeed on into this century. On several occasions the possibility of a Royal Charter was proposed. At the January 1992 Committee meeting there was a proposal to change the Society's name to the 'Pathology Society' and to seek a Royal Charter in time for the centenary in 2006. This was discussed at the summer Annual Business Meeting held in Manchester and after heated discussion the name proposals were royally (!) thrown out ... with Roche commenting 'that no one ever talked about the Royal Horticulture Society ... !'. The idea of a Royal Charter was also raised again in 1999 and in 2004, and similarly rejected on both occasions. It is minuted (July 2004) that the issue should not be reconsidered for at least a further 5 years (present Officers then having thankfully demitted office!!).

The Society and its Officers and Committee were brilliantly served (and indeed could not have functioned) throughout the 1990s by the Society Administrator Mrs Jacqui Edwards. Jacqui always kept us right and up to date, and provided us with the facts and figures needed for presentations at business meetings; she also kept a close eye on institutions and individuals who did not deal with the Society in the meticulous way that she always (rightly) expected. Jacqui was joined in 1999 and eventually succeeded on her retirement in 2001 by Ros Pitts, whom we also greatly appreciate. We wondered how we would find an adequate replacement for Jacqui, but (with Jacqui's recruiting skills) we did.

THE END OF THE 1990s: MICROBIOLOGY, MEETINGS AND THE PRESIDENCY

The issues that most exercised the Committee in the latter years of the 1990s were the increasing tensions within the Society in relation to the place of the microbiologists, the falling attendance at meetings and the potential need for a President. An Awayday to discuss such issues of relevance and in particular the meetings and governance was held in Birmingham on 8 December 1998. Among the points made at this was that 60% of microbiologists favoured leaving the Society and joining the newly formed clinical section of the Society for General Microbiology under

[1] Ironically the first joint meeting in July 2001 ran at a deficit of ~£48 000, covered entirely by The Pathological Society.

the auspices of the Federation of Infection Societies (FIS). This was presented as 'realignment not schism' and was recognised to be the beginning of an endplay that had in reality begun two decades before and that the 'time had come for an amicable separation'. The place of microbiology within the Society had been a major topic of debate for some time. For example, in the Committee Minutes of 1994 it is noted that there is a general feeling that microbiology and the rest of the Society may be pulling against each other and some discussion of realignment should occur. It is interesting to note that the Committee Minutes defined the numbers of microbiologists and pathologists separately only from 1994! This coincided with the use of a computerised membership records system and it was thus, of course, easier to establish these data from this point onwards, but it may also reflect an increasing tension and need for identity of the two groups.

Another view that was firmly held by those at the Awayday was that the Society needed to develop a higher profile and that a President might be a vehicle for doing this. A personal perspective on the genesis of this Office is given by Eric Walker, the then Chairman and General Secretary, in the vignette on p. 79, and the Office and its effects are discussed in Chapter 7. Mike Wells presented a paper on the future of meetings, pointing out the falling number of registrants and abstracts. The issue of the Society's constituency was discussed but no clear definition of this was provided. Various suggestions were made, including the idea of joint meetings with other organisations and a move to one meeting per annum. With regard to the former issue it was proposed that the Officers of the Society should meet with the Officers of the BDIAP to discuss the idea. Nick Wright, the incoming President, contacted the IAP who responded favourably to the idea of collaboration and all four officers of the IAP were invited to a dinner with the Officers of the Society; this was held on 19 May 1999. It is minuted that those present 'agreed that there were opportunities and benefits for all, and that a 4 day meeting every second year might be a way forward'. A Joint Meeting Programme Committee was suggested but sadly was not formed. In addition, letters were to be sent from the Secretaries of both Societies (Eric Walker and Eamon Sweeney) to their respective memberships. With regard to The Pathological Society membership, sadly there were very few replies but they were supportive (actually there were four replies – a 200% increase on any previous solicitation!). Consequently, at the 1999 Annual Business Meeting in Dundee the idea of joint meetings was put to the membership. This was approved, with the first planned for 2001.

With regard to the proposal to move to one meeting per annum, this was eventually agreed but why it was the winter and not the summer meeting that was viewed as the one to be stopped remains a mystery because perusal of the data on attendance and abstract submission (see Fig. 9.1, chapter 9) clearly makes the summer meeting the more obvious target for abolition? Commitments had already been made so the last ever winter meeting was planned for Maastrict in January 2001 (in fact it turned out only to be a suspension of the winter meetings, with restoration in 2005).

The end of the 1990s also saw the Society get both a logo and a Mission Statement and the *Journal of Pathology* undergo radical change. The idea of a logo developed out of conversations in Committee and in 1999 David Levison offered to approach the Duncan of Jordanstone College of Art (part of Dundee University), who held an undergraduate competition for the design of a suitable image. This is now to be found on all Society literature and is on the cover of this book. The Mission statement was the brainchild of Philip Quirke and was originally based upon a similar literary device used by the British Society of Gastroenterology. The original version was somewhat modified and substantially shortened in 2004 (see Chapter 7). Finally, the end of the century saw a determination to take the *Journal of Pathology* to a new level. The success of the 1998 Awayday prompted the Society and Peter Toner, with the help and involvement of the publishers, to hold a two-day meeting to discuss the Journal on 6 and 7 December 2000 at Beaconsfield. The outcomes of this are detailed in Chapters 7 and 8.

The final acts of the century were the alterations in Governance that had been promoted at the Birmingham Awayday and agreed at the 1999 AGM in Dundee. Eric Walker stepped down as

Chairman and General Secretary. Nick Wright and Mike Wells were duly proposed and elected as the first President and new General Secretary, respectively, with Simon Herrington being elected to replace Mike Wells as Meetings Secretary. The Society thus entered the new millennium. Further change was imminent and pathology was to be wracked by upheaval because of events in Bristol and Alder Hey!

Acknowledgements

James Lowe is thanked for his information regarding the website and Peter Hall for much of the information on the meetings gleaned from his readings of the Society Minutes.

On the Origin of the office of President

From its inception the Path Soc. was egalitarian and self-contained in a professional, Edwardian manner. This was reflected in the original minimalist constitution and in the conduct of the Annual Business Meeting which was chaired by a member of the host department and considered only matters 'properly the concern of the Society'. Dible, in his history of the first 50 years, comments ... thus the Society has never had a permanent Chairman or President, which is sometimes a little confusing to those unfamiliar with its constitution. Path Soc. as an entity saw little need to attempt to influence or be influenced by outside forces other than disease processes. This may be exemplified by the formation of the NHS in the late 1940s. This antedated the foundation of the Royal College of Pathologists by more than a decade. By way of the Royal College of Physicians the Department of Health consulted appropriate professional bodies including the Society about, *inter alia*, Merit Awards. The response was that the Society had no view on such matters. Over succeeding decades outside forces, notably government policies and paymaster directives, increasingly impinged on research, education and service, matters properly of concern to the Society.

Fast forward to the 1980s. The General Secretary was Rab Goudie. He was concerned that many communications to the Society were addressed to the Chairman and that when he responded as General Secretary many of the recipients felt they were being fobbed off by a lesser officer. Accordingly his title metamorphosed to 'Chairman and General Secretary'. His duties and responsibilities did not change, it was merely a change in the Society's addressee.

The priming of the events – in so far as such can be recognized – which ultimately led to the introduction of the Office of the President occurred in 1989 at the January meeting held at University College. A tongue in the cheek poster of little scientific merit drew the Society's attention to the upcoming 'research selectivity exercise' and indicated the potential effects on the Society and on academic departments of pathology. The subsequent poster discussion session was packed. The Chairman (Kevin Gatter) was relatively inexperienced and announced his intention not to discuss this particular poster. The audience became restive, there was prolonged murmuring then a loud clear voice (it was Tom Anderson's) said 'Why, Mr Chairman, do you think there are so many of us here?'. And so the poster was discussed and the episode was probably forgotten by the end of the meeting. Six years and two RAEs (as the research selectivity exercise became formally known) later, views and opinions among Society members had moved considerably. This was appreciated by the officers who were of the general view that changes of direction were essential and that this could be facilitated by changes in the constitution.

It was arranged to hold an away day (actually a 2 day away) meeting of the officers and a select cross section of the active membership. (This idea was first floated to me by Mike Wells in a conversation at Leicester railway station after the 1998 meeting but there may well have been antecedents of which I was unaware). Later that year such a meeting, organized by Jacqui, was held in Birmingham – we meant business. Remarkably clear proposals emerged one of which was that the Society should have a president. At the subsequent officers' meeting this was approved and it was left to the Chairman and General Secretary, assisted by the Administrator, to implement. The redraft of the constitution was on the agenda of the 1999 annual business meeting and was approved without dissent. Thereafter all that remained was to take soundings amongst the members. A single preferred name was clearly identifiable and that individual agreed to be nominated. By intent the old Chairman and General Secretary had intimated at the time of his nomination for a second term that he would be demitting office before his term was complete. By good fortune his demittance coincided with the election of the new President and the election of a New General Secretary.

Eric Walker

7 The Pathological Society in the 21st Century

Peter A. Hall and Alastair D. Burt

INTRODUCTION

3 July 2001: in the faded elegance of the Adelphi Hotel, Liverpool; in a large room, with a darkened stage and 200 expectant people. The lights dim. A hush falls. Slowly, almost imperceptibly at first, music comes from speakers at the corners of the stage. Familiar music. Everyone remembers the movie, not so many remember the name of Richard Strauss's Opus 30: *Also Sprach Zarathustra*. The music moves to a crescendo and then just like the opening of Kubrick's *2001 A Space Odyssey* there is a burst of light: fireworks and lots of them ... and what a way to start a meeting! 'Welcome to the 21st Century' boomed Chris Foster, Professor of Pathology at Liverpool University and local organiser of the 183rd Meeting of the Society. Of course it was not really the first meeting of the 21st Century, which had been held in Maastrict 6 months earlier (or for those who cannot count, a year before that at the Queen Elizabeth Conference Centre in London). But it felt like the first meeting of a new era because this was the first meeting to be held jointly with the British Division of the International Academy of Pathology (BDIAP). Furthermore, it was the first summer meeting with a new President: a new Office only created as the new millennium began (see Chapter 6 and the vignette by Eric Walker on p. 79). The first years of the new millennium, the last years of the first century of the Society, have seen big changes and significant challenges. Here we try to put some perspective into these events that will shape the early years of the second century of the Society.

THE PRESIDENCY

There was no raz-a-mataz Presidential campaign and the UN election watch was not needed to oversee the proceedings; there was only one person who could take on this role: Nick Wright. As the first President, he undertook a programme of steps to try to move forward the agenda for academic pathology. Perhaps most important here was the organisation of a residential meeting of diverse groups with an interest in academic pathology, ranging from Postgraduate Deans, cancer Czars, heads of Manpower Planning for the Royal College, researchers, teachers and other groups. The focus of this meeting was to raise the awareness of the fundamental issues facing the profession and to define a series of key action points. Many of these action points were ultimately achieved, although it is fair to say that several were never really addressed. The report can be found as Appendix 11 to this publication.

Wright proposed the abolition of the Association of Professors of Pathology (generally perceived as an ineffective group) and its replacement with an Academic Forum that was then made open to all with an interest in the future of academic pathology. As an annual event the Forum occurs at a lunchtime during one of the Scientific Meetings and acts as a platform for debate and discussion on matters of relevance to the profession. The President has given the Society a voice at a national level for Clinical Excellence Awards, among other issues, and has worked hard behind the scenes to get the PPP Clinician Scientists Award in collaboration with the College. There was considerable concern about the outcome of the 2001 Research Assessment Exercise (RAE) where academic pathology was concerned (see Chapter 9) and the President was able to interact directly with Sir Gareth Roberts to ensure that pathology and similar craft-based disciplines received fairer treatment at the 2008 RAE. This influence has been reflected further in the appointment of RAE Panel members for 2008 (Burt, Quirke and Wright are all members of Sub Panels and Wylie is a Panel Chair).

Perhaps the most important achievement of the President lay in an area that neither he nor others could have envisaged or really wanted: the issue of human organs and the alleged scandals relating to them. His introduction to this was sudden – being called late at night to appear on the BBC Radio 4 *Today Programme* on the morning following the publication of the Redfern Report on Alder Hey. The actuality of defending 'arrogant, condescending and uncaring' pathologists from John Humphrey *and* Sue MacGregor left a lasting impression, but he thought he gave as good as he received. There followed a long process of closed and open debate with the Retained Organ Commission, and on the publication of the Human Tissue Bill he led the Academy of Medical Sciences in their response, a document that was also endorsed by the Royal Society, the Council of Heads of Medical Schools and of course The Pathological Society. There followed briefings with a number of MPs, including Frank Dobson and Ian Gibson, and, after the Bill passed through the Commons, with a number of peers. The Human Tissue Act received Royal Assent on 15 November 2004 and a number of arguments were accepted and significant concessions achieved. The Society, through the actions of its President and in concert with other groups, had exerted some significant influence. All existing collections continue to be available for research and the use of tissue for educational purposes and for training for research does not require consent. Lord Jenkin of Roding, quoted by Hansard on 25 October 2004, stated in the Lord's:

> 'I was particularly impressed by a note that I received from the Council of Heads of Medical Schools. It made some strong points, and I shall refer to them. The Council simply said that it was impossible, in practice, to separate training for research from training for diagnosis. The Council considers the matter from the point of view of the role of the pathologist. Pathology is the hidden science at the heart of modern medicine. It is vital to the diagnosis and clinical management of disease. Pathologists are central to the delivery of quality clinical care in the NHS, and their work underlies much of the work that must be done subsequently by surgeons and other specialists. The Council also says something that accords with my experience as a Secretary of State for Health and Chairman of a Health Authority: "It is part of every doctor's role to advance medical knowledge through research and this is especially true in pathology. The techniques which pathologists use in the diagnosis of disease are also those which are used in research, and consequently it is simply not possible to make a distinction between training for research and training for diagnosis." The work that is done to decide the appropriate treatment for a patient's cancer and the work that is done to enable research to go forward into the appropriate treatment for a patient's cancer is, the Council says, indivisible. That is why it argues, as I argue, that there is a wholly artificial distinction in the Bill.'

Whether or not this vigorous activity counted against the President, he was unfortunately not accorded a position on the Human Tissue Authority!

Within the Society, the President proposed the establishment of the Doniach Lecture, now established in our calendar, and also of the Goudie Medal and Lecture, after one of his boyhood heroes. He was also, from the beginning, a fierce advocate of the re-introduction of the winter meeting, and was delighted when this was resurrected (see below). The President has also worked hard to advocate the importance of animals in research, an activity that has led to more trauma from *The Today* programme and some very interesting letters offering him differing degrees of bodily harm. Developing out of this area has come a realisation that the Society needs to engage actively with the public. The Society has promoted Public Lectures within our meetings and in other fora, and has sponsored a session in the September 2005 meeting of the British Association for the Advancement of Science entitled 'Pathology, Pathologists and the Public'. Quoting from the November 2005 Society newsletter, the President wrote:

> 'We had collected a panel of lay persons and pathologists, including the President-Elect of our College, Professor Adrian Newland and the chair was Gordon Cropper, who also chairs the College's Lay Advisory Committee. The BA issued a press release, as did the College, and yours truly got the names of all Irish medical correspondents and invited them. We also rather bravely, I thought, invited the pressure group, Parents for Justice, and they promised to come along. And indeed they did, although they didn't say much. We had rather hoped for some animated discussion with members of the public over issues such as organ retention, the Human Tissue Act and the way forward to regaining public trust, which we all believe we have lost. However: animated discussion we did have, but mainly between panel members and scientists attending the British Association, medical correspondents and local pathologists in the audience. The public listened, but did not engage. Not that the discussion wasn't good and lively and went on without a perceptible pause for nigh on two hours in which everything from the role of pathologists in patient communication to the future of tissue based research was covered, but a dialogue with the public it was not. So there you are. It raises several questions: do the public – whoever they are, care? Are we tackling a problem that does not really exist? Are we doing the right things or are there other ways of getting through?'

Clearly the issues are complex but it remains the Society's view that we must continue to endeavour to engage with the public and get the message across that pathology is important in medicine and science and that the events of Alder Hey, etc. do not reflect the reality of pathology or pathologists. Moreover, it seems highly likely that the media response in all likelihood may not reflect broad public opinion!

WINTER MEETINGS, STUDY GROUPS AND 'MEET THE ACADEMIC'

Over the years, the winter meetings were for many the main meeting of the year; some felt the summer meeting more of a social gathering. This was certainly the experience of one of us (A.D.B.) in their formative years who fondly remembers the 'Sleeper from Glasgow' where even as an intercalated BSc student he was given an introduction to both Scientific Meetings and Malt Whiskey (see the vignette by Roddy MacSween, p. 231). However, there was a perception that the withering of academic pathology in these islands meant that there was neither the interest nor the body of research that warranted two scientific meetings a year. This decision was taken in 1999 and arguably marked the nadir of the Society. In retrospect it was a rather strange decision because examination of the attendance at meetings (see Fig. 9.1 in Chapter 9) shows that the winter meetings were, in general, actually the better attended.

The last winter meeting was held in Maastricht in January 2001 jointly with the Dutch Pathological Society. Juan Rosai again entertained the Society with a Guest Lecture on 'Tumours and tumour like conditions of the accessory immune system' and there was a symposium chaired by Professors Quirke and Kluin on 'Exciting advances in molecular pathology'. Most notable (or perhaps infamous), however, was the Committee dinner at the Baluga Restaurant. The genesis of the decision to order Dom Perignon is lost in the mists of time but may perhaps reflect the view that the end of the winter meetings should be toasted: suffice to say the Treasurer was shocked!

The winter meetings were replaced, at the suggestion of the then General Secretary Mike Wells, with 'Closed Study Groups'. The idea was that the Society would sponsor workshops where a specific topic of interest would be debated by experts and a Consensus or Position Paper would be produced based upon the discussion and data presented. Such a document might then be published in the *Journal of Pathology*, forming the basis for providing an evidence base for clinical practice and research in that area. The first of these was held in January 2003 on the subject of 'Ploidy in Pathology' and organised by Mike Wells. Although this was undoubtedly of interest to those that attended, there was a feeling that the place of ploidy analysis was fairly limited and the data for its widespread adoption in pathology were scanty. As a consequence the output was not thought to merit a Supplement for the *Journal of Pathology*, although some of it was subsequently published in *Histopathology* (Baak and Janssen, 2004; Grabsch *et al.*, 2004; Hall, 2004; Fox, 2005). The second (and final) Closed Study Group was held in January 2004 on the subject of 'Molecular Pathology and Targeted Therapy in Cancer' and organised by Phil Quirke and Kenneth Hillan. Again this was successful in terms of the participants but no written output emanated and we did not achieve the goal of establishing a Position Paper in the area. These two meetings were an invaluable experiment but the fact that they were closed and their failure to achieve their goals led to a reassessment of what the Society should be doing with regard to winter meetings.

A general feeling had developed during the late 1990s and early part of this century that the Society was not doing enough for trainee pathologists. Phil Quirke and Massimo Pignatelli (who by 2002 was the new Meetings Secretary replacing Simon Herrington, who was now Editor of the *Journal of Pathology*) took this forward and with the help of James Underwood (who as President of the Royal College of Pathologists ensured that it was a joint activity with the College) developed the idea of a full day meeting focused on trainees and with the goal of promoting academic pathology. It was Phil Quirke's idea to call it 'Meet the Academics', which was described by Nick Wright as 'a phrase that seems more redolent of some soon to be extinct species'. Despite the name, such meetings proved popular and were run in January 2004 and 2005. The latter meeting occurred the day before the recreated Winter Scientific meeting (see below). In 2006 it was formally amalgamated with the winter meeting, although the newly created Trainees Subcommittee (also see below) may develop this concept further.

With new Officers (in 2002, Pignatelli; in 2003, Peter Hall replaced Mike Wells as Secretary as he moved to be Editor of *Histopathology*, and Alastair Burt replaced David Levison) and with Nick Wright at the helm there was a passionate view in favour of the reinstitution of the winter meetings. There was without doubt some nervousness that we would not be able to sustain this but it was pleasing to see that at the meeting at Bart's under the local Chairmanship of Jo Martin we had 74 proffered abstracts and attracted 143 registrants. This vindicated the resurrection of the Winter Pathological Society, which we hope will now continue to flourish. The Barts meeting also saw the first award of the Goudie Medal to David Wynford Thomas, who gave a lecture 'Modelling multi-step tumorigenesis in vitro: the importance of cellular context'. At this meeting one of the memorable events (apart from the science of course) was the Society Dinner in St Bartholomew's Great Hall. The regular sweepstake on the length of speech by the Meetings Secretary (which has become a regular tradition) was won by the President Nick Wright (by all accounts the first time he had ever won anything!). Fortunately he was persuaded by his wife to contribute the entire amount (£151.92) to the Tsunami Appeal.[1] As this book goes to press the Society, its Officers and Committee (see Fig. 7.1) are gathering in Cambridge with 139 abstracts and more than 200 registrants to begin the Centenary Celebrations. This brings to the authors fond memories of previous Oxbridge meetings with accommodation in cold, drafty rooms, with long treks to showers with a trickle of lukewarm water, fatty bacon breakfasts and very narrow beds. Not for the professors of today, some of whom need more comfort!

[1] On Boxing Day 2004 a tsunami devastated the coastline of much of the Indian Ocean, killing more than 250 000 people.

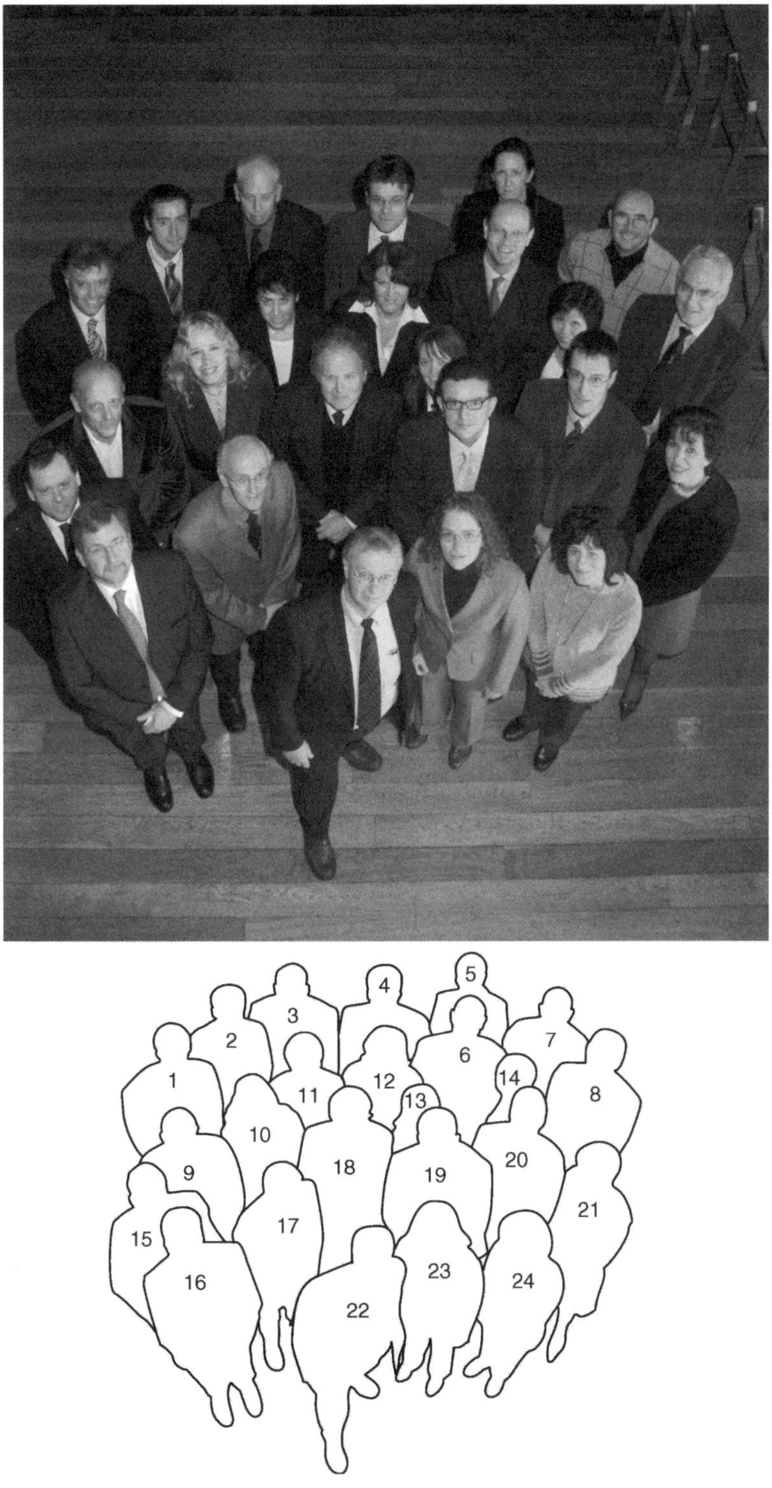

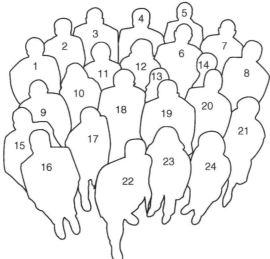

Figure 7.1 The Centenary Committee, Cambridge, 3 January 2006.

1 Prof. N.A. (Neil) Shepherd, Gloucester, BDIAP Representative – *co-opted*

2 Prof. P.W. (Peter) Hamilton, Belfast

3 Dr S.S. (Simon) Cross, Sheffield

4 Prof. M. (Marco) Novelli, London

5 Prof. A.M. (Adrienne) Flanagan, London

6 Dr M.J. (Mark) Arends, Cambridge

7 Prof. S. (Stewart) Fleming, Dundee

8 Prof. D.A. (David) Levison, Dundee, ***President-Elect (President from July 2006)***

9 Prof. P. (Paul) van der Valk, Amsterdam, NVVP (Dutch Pathological Society) Representative – *co-opted*

10 Dr K.A. Oien (Karin), Glasgow

11 Prof. E. (Elaine) Kay, Dublin, Irish Republic Representative – *co-opted*

12 Ms R.A. (Roselyn) Pitts, Pathological Society Administrator

13 Miss J. (Julie) Johnstone, Pathological Society Deputy Administrator

14 Dr J.W.M. (Jade) Chow, London

15 Prof. J. (James) Lowe, Nottingham, ***Webmaster – Advisor***

16 Prof. A.D. (Alastair) Burt, Newcastle-upon-Tyne, ***Treasurer***

17 Prof. A.H. (Andrew) Wyllie, Cambridge – Winter Scientific Meeting, Host

18 Prof. Sir N.A. (Nicholas) Wright, ***President***

19 Prof. M. (Massimo) Pignatelli, ***Meetings Secretary***

20 Prof. C.S. (Simon) Herrington, ***Editor-in-Chief, Journal of Pathology – Advisor***

21 Dr S. (Suha) Deen, Nottingham

22 Prof. P.A. (Peter) Hall, Belfast, ***General Secretary***

23 Dr H. (Heike) Grabsch, Leeds

24 Prof. P. (Paola) Domizio, London, Education Representative – *co-opted*

Other Committee Members (not present in photograph)

Dr B. (Brian) Angus, Newcastle-upon-Tyne
Dr J.J. (James) Going, Glasgow

Figure 7.1 (*Continued*)

SUMMER MEETINGS IN THE NEW CENTURY

The last meeting of the millennium was held in Nottingham and is noteworthy because it was here that the idea of a Society logo was born; the Minutes credit Phil Quirke with the idea. The Committee charged David Levison with taking the idea forward and the Duncan & Jordanstone College of Art (part of Dundee University) held an undergraduate competition. The winning entry was subsequently adopted by the Society and is on the front of this volume. The Liverpool meeting of July 2001 has already been mentioned. It was the first of a continuing and highly successful series of joint meetings with the BDIAP. Satellite meetings with other groups also were held, including the British Association of Gynaecological Pathology and the Association of Clinical Electron Microscopy, as well as diverse EQA groups. Joint meetings have proved very popular and several luminaries have proposed the idea of a Pathology Week in which the various societies and groups within these islands may work together to promote the subject.

The Liverpool meeting did have some notable events associated with it. For example, the dissolution of the 'Association of Professors of Pathology' and the decision to replace it with a regular Academic Forum open to all. Indeed, this happened on the same day that *The Times* published an Editorial on pathology and pathologists (see Fig. 7.2) in which they said of pathologists 'It is a life

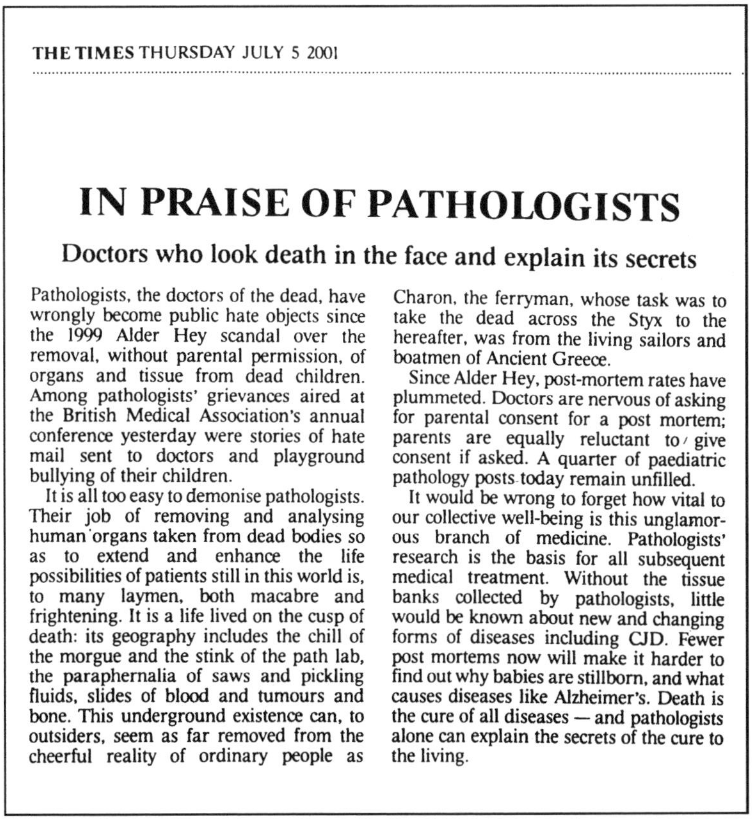

THE TIMES THURSDAY JULY 5 2001

IN PRAISE OF PATHOLOGISTS

Doctors who look death in the face and explain its secrets

Pathologists, the doctors of the dead, have wrongly become public hate objects since the 1999 Alder Hey scandal over the removal, without parental permission, of organs and tissue from dead children. Among pathologists' grievances aired at the British Medical Association's annual conference yesterday were stories of hate mail sent to doctors and playground bullying of their children.

It is all too easy to demonise pathologists. Their job of removing and analysing human organs taken from dead bodies so as to extend and enhance the life possibilities of patients still in this world is, to many laymen, both macabre and frightening. It is a life lived on the cusp of death: its geography includes the chill of the morgue and the stink of the path lab, the paraphernalia of saws and pickling fluids, slides of blood and tumours and bone. This underground existence can, to outsiders, seem as far removed from the cheerful reality of ordinary people as Charon, the ferryman, whose task was to take the dead across the Styx to the hereafter, was from the living sailors and boatmen of Ancient Greece.

Since Alder Hey, post-mortem rates have plummeted. Doctors are nervous of asking for parental consent for a post mortem; parents are equally reluctant to give consent if asked. A quarter of paediatric pathology posts today remain unfilled.

It would be wrong to forget how vital to our collective well-being is this unglamorous branch of medicine. Pathologists' research is the basis for all subsequent medical treatment. Without the tissue banks collected by pathologists, little would be known about new and changing forms of diseases including CJD. Fewer post mortems now will make it harder to find out why babies are stillborn, and what causes diseases like Alzheimer's. Death is the cure of all diseases — and pathologists alone can explain the secrets of the cure to the living.

Figure 7.2 The Times Editorial, 'In praise of pathologists', Thursday 5 July 2001. Reproduced with permission from The Times.

lived on the cusp of death: its geography includes the chill of the morgue and the stink of the path lab, the paraphernalia of saws and pickling fluids, slides of blood and tumours and bone'. A rebuttal of the views portrayed in this Editorial was indeed the first action of the Academic Forum, but sadly *The Times* chose not to publish a more reasoned description of pathologists!

Unfortunately some lax editorial control of the Liverpool meeting meant that there were three lectures on similar topics: Nick Wright gave a lecture entitled 'Adventures with the Y chromosome'; the Oakley Lecture by Marco Novelli was on 'Man and mouse as models in gastrointestinal pathology'; and Walter Bodmer spoke on 'The somatic evolution of colorectal cancer'. All were excellent, although there was a perception that all three in fact used varying combinations of the same slides! However, all was forgiven when we were entertained by the 'Bootleg Beetles' in a Liverpool theme evening.

The following year we collected in Dublin as the guests of Trinity College. As with previous meetings in Dublin, the quality of the meeting was surpassed only by the quality and extent of the hospitality! Notable consequences of this included Simon Herrington's fractured 5th metatarsal of his left foot, sustained after tripping down a step in a bar ('I forget which one' he said when asked). In addition there was an exceptional reception at the Guinness Storehouse, after which one of us (A.D.B.) lost his passport in a dingy Dublin pub; fortunately at the time A.D.B. was not Treasurer and did not have the Society credit card in his jacket!

The 2003 meeting in Bristol was the second joint meeting with the BDIAP and was a huge success in terms of registrants, with something for all tastes in the programme. Clearly a model to be followed! It also showed that these meetings could be financially viable. The role of the food in Society meetings should not be underestimated... especially with the succession of gastronomes who have populated the office of Meetings Secretary. The Italian background of the current holder of this office means that food is of crucial importance, so much so that the Officers and Committee members of both organisations were treated to a visit to the Edward Jenner museum in Berkley (Gloucestershire) and then a fine meal followed by more delicacies at the home of Bryan Warren. The culinary skills of Massimo and Bryan made for a considerable addition to the overall mass of those present! Sadly there was no Oakley Lecturer but the slot was usefully filled by Phil Quirke in his position as the Royal College of Pathologists' Manpower Lead when he spoke to the title 'Climbing out of the abyss'. The changing fortunes of pathology manpower are discussed elsewhere (see Chapter 13). Juan Rosai gave another lecture to the Society, this time on the subject of GISTs; and the First Doniach Lecture was given in the presence of Deborah Doniach (widow of the late Isreal Doniach) and her son, where Peter Isaacson explored the borderland between chronic inflammation and lymphoma and reviewed two decades of his seminal contributions to pathological science – a fitting first Doniach Lecture. Dame Julia Polak gave the second Doniach Lecture (which was commendably short!) on 'Stem cells and regenerative medicine' at a meeting held in Amsterdam in July 2004. Sadly, despite an excellent programme and a high number of registrants, the lecture theatres were relatively sparsely populated: perhaps people were drawn to the other diverse attractions of the city?

The third joint meeting with the BDIAP was in the North East. This again was able to attract the same impressive number of registrants that had been seen at Bristol (almost 500). One of us (A.D.B.) was the local organiser and had hoped to educate the entire country about the scenic beauty and cultural richness of the area. The Gods were against us, however, at least for some of the meeting, because Newcastle saw some of its wettest July days on record. The elation of London's successful bid for the 2012 Olympics turned to sadness on the Thursday of the meeting as the atrocities of 7 July in London unfolded. Another problem was that the Medical School in Newcastle had been so successful in research over recent years that it had transformed all of the space it used to have for poster demonstrations into laboratories. As a consequence we had a split site for the meeting, with lectures and posters some distance apart; this probably would have been acceptable had it not been for the heavens opening! The meeting was very successful, however, and one notable session (run by Hilary Russell and Peter Furness on research ethics) was packed with participants, with the audience literally sitting in the aisles!

The Third Doniach Lecture was given by Dillwyn Williams and the BDIAP awarded the Cunningham Medal and Lecture to Chris Elston, who spoke on 'The modern management of the patient with breast cancer: a celebration of the role of the pathologist'. It was wholly fitting that this inspirational lecture was given at a joint meeting because the subject matter spanned the range of interests of experimentalists and clinical pathologists, and advanced the thesis that pathology really is at the centre of translational research. At the Newcastle meeting, Karin Oien became the first Oakley Lecturer to deliver her lecture twice – or at least some of it twice – because it was interrupted by a fire alarm (and there was a real fire in a lift shaft!). Indeed the fire alarms had caused quite a lot of trouble because their testing earlier that day had caused near-apoplexy in the organisers of a stem cell symposium. In spite of all these irritations the meeting was well received and eventually the sun shone for those who stayed for the final dinner in Harry Potter land at Alnwick Castle.

FINANCES AND NEGOTIATIONS ABOUT ACCOMMODATION

As noted in Chapter 6, one of the key messages to one of us (A.D.B.) on taking up the Treasurership was to make an early approach to the College to secure a fruitful renegotiation of the lease at 2 Carlton House Terrace. It became clear, however, that things were changing in the College and there was significant pressure over space. The proposal we got was that yes we could extend the lease, but in return for downsizing the accommodation. In essence there was a request that we give up the existing 3rd floor Committee room in exchange for an extended lease. Having considered this, we believed that we could indeed give up this space without compromising our activities, but we used the opportunity to find further stability by seeking an extension of the lease until 2024. The process of renegotiation, however, did cause the Officers to consider whether the Society should move elsewhere; a very serious options appraisal was undertaken that included the consideration of moving the Offices out of the capital. There were some investment opportunities with a temporarily depressed property market in London that excited the Treasurer but there was an overwhelming feeling within the Committee that the advantages of staying at 2 Carlton House Terrace in close proximity to the College outweighed the opportunities (and risks) of delving into the property market. The detailed negotiations about the lease have taken some considerable time to sort out (and yet to be finally signed off) but in essence the Society has contributed a large one-off payment to the College towards its Appeal for renovation of the building and in return the Society will have the security of a lease on the Offices until 2024; as part of the deal, one of the rooms in the renovated College space will be named after the Society.

COMMUNICATIONS: THE NEWSLETTER, THE WEB AND THE JOURNAL

The introduction of the Newsletter was one of the suggestions of one of us (P.A.H.) in the early days as the new General Secretary. The first such Newsletter was produced by him in Microsoft Word and then printed. Subsequent editions were commercially typeset with editing and assistance from Julie Johnstone, the Deputy Administrator. Getting copy was always a problem. Persuasion, cajoling and sometimes strong-arm tactics were required but we managed to get some information and newsworthy material from Officers and other Society Members. We tried various devices to encourage readers and contributors: a spot-the-venue competition (won by the only entrant, J.C.E. Underwood, and hence recipient of a glorious Society tie) in Issue 1; caption competitions with no respondents (Issue 2) and one respondent (Issue 3); and eventually a recipe (Issue 4). Nevertheless, this twice yearly exercise in communication has, we think, been a success and we shall continue with it.

The early history of the Society website was discussed elsewhere (see Chapter 6). The idea of using the web to interact more effectively with the Society members, e.g. to distribute notices, to inform members of developments, to gain feedback and to manage our subscriptions, was very desirable. In 2002 we entered into a partnership with the publishers of our Journal to develop this concept. We were excited by the prospect of a professionally managed website that would link our activities and that of the Journal and be a really excellent portal that many might use as their home page. Sadly, after nearly 3 years and a lot of effort on the part of our Administrative staff, little was achieved. We were forced into terminating the contract and seeking full reimbursement, which we did indeed get! This done, we have now moved to other providers for these crucial services and there will be a new beginning to this for the Centenary year.

The history of the *Journal of Pathology* is considered elsewhere (see Chapters 2 and 8 in particular) but a few words are required because the Journal has been a topic of some debate in the early years of the century. There can be no doubt that it is highly successful and the last two decades have seen it develop into one of the most respected journals of its type. Furthermore, it is hugely successful as a financial enterprise and underpins our ability to support diverse schemes and projects. A central tenet of the relationship of the Society and the Editor-in-Chief, is editorial independence. Although the Society wholly owns the title and the Copyright, the Officers and Committee defer all editorial responsibility to the Editor-in-Chief, who sits as an advisor on the Society Committee and attends the key subcommittee (Finance and General Purposes) to ensure good communication. A consequence of this editorial independence is that the direction of the Journal is set by the Editor. This leads to a tension that some Members are concerned about, which is that the subject matter of the Journal is often distinct from the day-to-day needs of (for example) diagnostic pathologists. The Society recognises this and has debated it extensively *but* as our scientific flagship and key source of income we continue to feel that the need to have a strong internationally competitive scientific journal outweighs any other view.

MATTERS OF OMISSION AND THE CHARITIES COMMISSION

Another of the new Treasurer's and General Secretary's tasks has been dealing with the Charities Commission. As a registered Charity we are bound (and quite rightly so) by stringent rules. However, sometimes we did wonder ..! In 2004 it became apparent that the Commission had not been kept appropriately appraised of the Society's activities and in particular issues relating to the AGM and rule changes. Indeed it would appear that some of the last communications dated back to the 1950s when the mission of the Society included, among other things, 'the promotion of intercourse between pathologists!' In an effort to rectify this error of omission we sought the Minutes for the period in question for the Annual General Meetings and the Committee meetings. That crucial Minutes were missing in fact came to light when Eric Sidebottom tried to research key events in the Society's history for this very book! The matter of a 'lost trunk' is recorded in Chapter 5 by Eric Walker. We have searched high and low, spoken to all living past Officers and searched the archives of Dundee (where Lendrum worked and many of the relevant Minutes are cited in Chapter 3), but to no avail! Egg on face! But the Charities Commission seemed satisfied... until it became apparent that some years ago the fourth item of the Constitution was changed by previous Officers and the Committee: sadly the power to do this lies with the Privy Council, not with the Society, who can change the Rules but not the Constitution! More egg on face!! However, this error of commission is not in fact fatal and can be easily rectified.

There has been a sea change in the scrutiny under which Charities are placed. There are now very clear guidelines around the responsibilities of Trustees (which in the case of the Society means all Committee members). It behoves each of them to ensure that our financial standing, investment strategies (ethically correct) and expenditure are consistent with our overall Mission. To this end we now receive regular briefings from our investment advisors, Cazenoves, and wherever possible have them attend at least one Committee meeting per year. The coffers of the Society remain healthy, with our overall assets currently approaching £6 million. We shall return to this shortly!

THE AWAYDAY AND THE WAY FORWARD

The idea of an Away Weekend arose at the Committee dinner in January 2004. It began, as so many ideas do, as a glimmer of an idea over the port and after a brief gestation (perhaps 5 min!) was enunciated by the President in his speech as a challenge to the Officers and Committee to come up with a way forward (we will return to that phrase) for the Society. The General Secretary was charged with organising the event, which was held at the Templepatrick Hilton near Belfast on 4–5 November 2004. The choice of venue was dictated by cost, the ease of EasyJet flights and, crucially, the General Secretary's comfort.

A range of factors had prompted it. Although the Society has a long history of promoting pathology and in particular academic pathology, it was perceived as facing important challenges, including a shrinking and ageing Membership (see Fig. 7.3). The changes in the nature of academic life and the atrophy of academic medicine in general (and pathology in particular) have dramatically altered the environment in which it functioned (see Chapter 9). In many ways the Society had changed relatively little in the past quarter-century and the seriousness of the shifting landscape was felt possibly to warrant significant alterations in the way we function and support the interests of our Members. Although the Awayday of 1998 had led to some important changes and of course the Presidency, there was concern about what the Society was for. It was with that background that the two-day meeting was charged with answering the issue of where the Society needs to be in 5 and 10 years time.

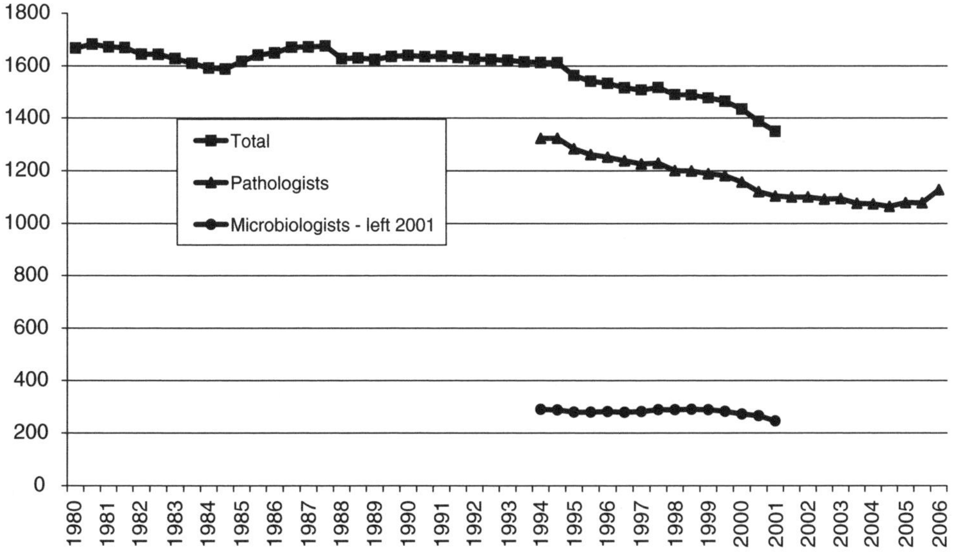

Figure 7.3 Change in membership over the last 25 years.

We hoped to address a series of questions that included: (i) How effectively does the Society achieve the goals defined in its Mission Statement and are these goals appropriate? (ii) How should the Society be involved in undergraduate teaching and education? (iii) How should the Society be involved in postgraduate teaching and education? (iv) How should the Society support and promote research? How should the Society be involved in research ethics? (v) How should the Society engage with the general public? (vi) How can the Society reverse the continued fall in Membership and alter the seriously skewed age profile. (vii) How should the Society manage its financial position and resources to accomplish the above? Other issues included a consideration of the linkages with other bodies, both National and International. In considering these issues we had to remain cognisant of our responsibilities as Trustees of a Charity. In addition we need to be very focused on the needs and desires of the Membership and pose the question: are we doing enough to encourage and support them? It was hoped that the output of this meeting would be a clear plan of how we can proceed over the coming years.

An obvious starting point was the Membership. So what did they think? We had tried to find out! Nick Rooney had undertaken a postal survey in the spring of 2004. However, the response rate of <7% and the fact that the majority of respondents were senior members means that the results lack any validity, although it was an improvement on the four responses solicited in 1998. This might reflect a number of issues but paramount among them was the fact that the Society might not be 'important' to Members. Another key element of any plan for the future was a SWOT analysis. At the Away Weekend this idea was developed by Stewart Fleming, who led a brainstorming session. We could identify some significant strengths, including a sound financial position, the Journal was a lucrative flagship and was a leading and highly respected Journal in the field of experimental pathology and disease. We have an academic focus with sound administration, a strong tradition, a history of good meetings and have good links with other bodies. Unfortunately significant weaknesses existed with a falling and ageing membership. It was argued that our Mission Statement lacks focus and that we lacked broad appeal and may be perceived as a parochial and tired 'meeting organisation' that lacked representation for trainees. In addition it could be thought that our financial programmes may not reach the whole Membership and that the Journal does not reflect the interests of the Membership. On the other hand, opportunities existed with increasing numbers of trainees in pathology, good relations with other bodies and a broad recognition of the crisis in academic medicine, with some action being taken to address it. The Presidency had been a success with burgeoning influence and of course translational research was the order of the day. Of course, equally, there were threats that included the crisis in academic medicine, poor public perception, perceived tension with clinical pathology, changes in the undergraduate curriculum that mean that pathology has no profile and no role models, and financial threats to the income from the Journal as a consequence of the Open Access movement.

From this rather stark base, those attending (see Table 7.1) then addressed a series of questions. Paola Domizio (who had been co-opted onto the Committee at the suggestion of the new General Secretary to champion educational issues) and Elaine Kay considered the issue of how the Society should be involved in undergraduate and postgraduate education. This was developed by Patrick Gallagher, who had been asked to join the group as a director of an SHO Training School, and Heike Grabsch (at the time a trainee) made an important contribution by presenting the views of trainees that she had derived from a questionnaire (which was much more successful than the Society's one!). How we should be involved in research was addressed by Marco Novelli and Karin Oien. Our involvement in ethics and with the general public was also considered, and there was general acceptance of the view that we needed to be more pro-active in these areas.

A further issue was our Mission Statement. The original Mission Statement developed by Phil Quirke stated 'Our mission is to enhance the capacity of our members to advance the science of disease by discovering, disseminating and applying new knowledge for the benefit of patients'.

Table 7.1 Attendees at The Pathological Society Away Weekend, 4–5 November 2004

Officers:	N.A. Wright (President)
	P.A. Hall (General Secretary)
	A.D. Burt (Treasurer)
	M. Pignatelli (Meetings Secretary)
Committee:	M.J. Arends
	B. Angus
	P. Domizio (Education Rep.)
	S. Fleming
	J.J. Going
	E. Kay (Irish Rep.)
	M. Novelli
	K.A. Oien
	N.A. Shepherd (BDIAP Rep.)
	P. van der Valk (Dutch Pathological Society Rep.)
Advisors:	C.S. Herrington, *Journal of Pathology*; Editor-in-Chief
	J. Lowe, Webmaster
Guests:	P.J. Gallagher, Southampton, SHO School Rep.
	H. Grabsch, Leeds, Trainee Rep.
	V. Howarth, Stockport, DGH Consultant
Admin:	R.A. Pitts (Administrator)
	J. Johnstone (Deputy Administrator)
Apologies:	N. Rooney and P. Quirke

Although valid, this was felt to be ambiguous and lacking in focus or clarity, and it could indeed be the Mission Statement for almost any Medical Charity. This lack of clarity is magnified when the coda to the Mission Statement were considered (they ran to nearly two pages!). Ideally a Mission Statement defines the goals and vision of the organisation and defines in a few words what it is about (the Mission Statement of the Coca Cola Organisation might simply be 'Beat Pepsi'). It allows those associated with the organisation to instantly understand these goals and share and identify in the ownership of the organisation. The statement should be the bedrock of the Society, from which all else flows. The key words that the group felt defined our values include the words Research, Academic, Teaching and Communication, and our key goal is 'understanding disease'. As a consequence we decided to make this our 'strapline' and a key element of our Mission Statement, which became 'The mission of The Pathological Society is to increase the understanding of disease'.

Another important element of this discussion related to our relationship with the other three organisations (Royal College of Pathologists, BDIAP, Association of Clinical Pathologists). What differentiated us from them? Why are we different? Why would someone want to be a member of our Society? We felt that people will become and remain members if they see that the Society adds value to their professional lives. To this end we need to have a clear identity and we will not succeed if we cannot be differentiated from the other societies. Perhaps, therefore, we need to accept that our role is academic, with the understanding of disease being the key goal and research and educational activities the means to this goal. We thus synergise with the other societies and provide a focus for a specific subset of pathologists. Hopefully our success in this endeavour will help to foster the view that this is an important aspect of pathology (in the broadest sense).

From the presentations and discussions over the two days a clear consensus emerged that there was a need for change. A four-point action plan was agreed: (i) the development of a new image with a clear profile; (ii) a commitment to provide tangible benefits to the members; (iii) building partnerships with other organisations to promote pathology; and (iv) enhancing the transparency of the Society with increased member involvement. The latter point led to the development of new Governance arrangements. Historically the Officers held most of the Society's power and decision-making functions. The Officer's Committee was rebranded as the Finance and General Purposes Committee, and new subcommittees that report to the Committee were proposed: an *Education subcommittee* was formed with the intention of it being the focal point for educational activities, undergraduate, postgraduate and lay; a *Trainees subcommittee* was to be formed to promote the interests of trainees; a *Research subcommittee* was to be created with the goals of bringing forward research programmes that support the Society's goals, reviewing the PhD and Pilot grant schemes and allocating the money designated for these schemes by Officers and Committee; and a *Programme subcommittee* was to be created to develop meetings and workshop programmes that support the Society's goals. All of these had been formed by the end of 2005 in time for the Centenary year.

The huge amount of work and discussion that went into this Away Weekend led to the drafting of a report that was presented to Committee in January 2005. This was developed into a full set of proposals entitled 'The Way Forward', which were circulated to Members in the spring of that year and formally adopted by the AGM in July 2005 (see Appendix 12). This was perhaps the biggest change in the Society in its 100-year history, and hopefully paves the way for the future.

THE FUTURE: *PUTTING OURSELVES ABOUT*

The past few years have seen huge developments in the Society. We may have reached a nadir with the ending of winter meetings... but the Presidency, the Beaconsfield Meeting, the Away Weekend, the Way Forward, the new Governance arrangements with the spreading of involvement and responsibility, the developments in Schemes and Awards, the Newsletter and the rebirth of the winter meeting and the development of joint meetings with the BDIAP have all helped in a process of developing the influence and impact of the Society. Our Centenary gives us the opportunity to do even more and the careful financial stewardship over the last 25 years puts us in a position to have an impact: *to make a splash*! As Officers of the Society, we honestly think that we have the potential to move the Society forward and to stimulate academic pathology: but we really need to be even more pro-active and make much more noise... *we need to put ourselves about*!

The Society is in a strong position. We have a sound administrative base and sound finances. Our Membership is once again growing (see Fig. 7.3) and 'The Way Forward' defines what we hope is a set of Governance arrangements and subcommittees that are more responsive to the challenges we face. We are optimistic that our renewed focus on trainees coupled with efforts to use our financial strength will have a positive effect on academic pathology: certainly when coupled with the new Academic Clinical Fellowships/Clinical lectureships post-Walport.[2] Although our contributions are financially modest compared with some organisations, they are ring-fenced for pathology. We aspire to link other organisations to promote pathology. The joint meetings with the BDIAP exemplify this but we hope that this develops further, perhaps with the development of 'a UK Pathology Week'. Finally we aspire to link with similar organisations in other countries: links to Japan already exist and we are developing associations with China. To take things forward, we believe we need to use our strengths and in particular our financial position for the benefit of the members and for the discipline. We are optimistic that this will have a positive effect. Perhaps

[2] In March 2005 a report was produced by the academic subcommittee of Modernising Medical Careers (MMC) and the UK Clinical Research Collaboration (UKCRC), providing recommendations for the future training of medically and dentally qualified academic staff. The subcommittee is chaired by Dr Mark Walport, Director of the Wellcome Trust, and has become known anecdotally as the 'Walport' report.

the Manchester Centenary meeting, where this publication will be first presented, marks a turning point. One wonders how they will trumpet the first meeting of the next century of the Society?

REFERENCES

Baak, J.P. and Janssen, E. (2004) DNA ploidy analysis in histopathology. Morphometry and DNA cytometry reproducibility conditions and clinical applications. *Histopathology* **44**: 603–614.

Fox, H. (2005) Ploidy in gynaecological cancers. *Histopathology* **46**: 121–129.

Grabsch, H., Kerr, D. and Quirke, P. (2004) Is there a case for routine clinical application of ploidy measurements in gastrointestinal tumours? *Histopathology* **45**: 312–334.

Hall, P.A. (2004) DNA ploidy analysis in histopathology. DNA ploidy studies in pathology – a critical appraisal. *Histopathology* **44**: 614–620.

Saddam Hussein and my first presentation

I'd been a lecturer in histopathology for two years and was really looking forward to giving my first oral presentation at Pathsoc in January 1991. I'd done a large study of small bowel lymphomas and had been preparing for months for the presentation. The fact that Pathsoc would be held in Cambridge was even better. I'd loved the city from the time I'd applied – unsuccessfully – to be a medical student there, though I knew that early January would be cold. Most of my slides were ready, but there were some finishing touches that I wanted to make. The few days between Christmas and New Year were the time I'd put aside to make the changes. After all, there would be very little routine work to be done and I'd have plenty of time to do what I needed.

On the 27th December, the first day back to work after the Christmas break, my then boyfriend was called up to serve in the first Gulf War. He was a psychiatrist, but also a major in the Territorial Army, and the government felt that they needed his services in the Gulf. The shock and despair hit me like a ton of bricks. Totally unable to concentrate on work, we decided that we should get married before he left for the Gulf on January 2nd. Instead of working on my presentation, the next few days were spent in getting a special licence and a reception organised. All the authorities were exceptionally helpful – Islington Council even opened up the Registry Office especially for us. On New Year's Eve 1990, we went to work in the morning and were married in the afternoon. And guess what – I hadn't spent a single moment on my presentation!

That evening we went to a friend's party as planned. The chicken drumsticks were a little undercooked, so it was no great surprise when I was forced out of bed the following morning by the symptoms of gastroenteritis. I spent the first day of married life alternating between the bed and the toilet. Still no chance to work on my presentation!

The following day, after tearfully waving my new husband goodbye as he went to war, I wearily travelled to Cambridge. I thought I might be able to look at the presentation on the train, but I was too tired and fell asleep. That night, with my presentation scheduled for the following morning, I retired early to my room, hoping to read through what I'd prepared. I hadn't had any chance to make the changes I'd wanted, but at least I still had something to say. I was staying in one of the older Colleges, and the facilities were primitive to say the least. A huge room with high ceilings and just one single-bar electric fire. It was cold outside. As night fell, the temperature plummeted, so much so that I put on every item of clothing I had with me, including coat, shoes and scarf, grabbed every blanket I could find and curled up in front of the fire. I spent the entire night that way, depressed, still unwell from the food poisoning, shivering uncontrollably and totally unable to sleep.

The morning couldn't come quickly enough. I felt exhausted, unprepared, nervous and still freezing cold. I was convinced I'd do the presentation badly – how could I do otherwise with all that had happened to me in the previous week – but by some miracle, the adrenaline kicked in and the talk went as planned. Afterwards, I was even complimented on how well organised my presentation was!

I've now done hundreds of talks and lectures, some of which have gone well and others less so, but to this day, nothing matches the emotional and physical trauma of my first ever Pathsoc presentation. A truly memorable experience!

Paola Domizio

Hubris

The late 1980s saw a huge growth in the size of the Society Meetings driven in part by burgeoning immunohistochemical methods. Much of this was directed at lymphoma pathology and the 1987 Winter Meeting at Bart's heard of the diagnostic utility of CD15 antibodies such as LeuM1 in the diagnosis of Hodgkin's disease. A senior lymphomaniac from University College argued strongly that LeuM1 was ***the*** diagnostic arbiter of Hodgkin's Disease. This seemed a little unlikely and Jane d'Ardenne, Alfred Stansfeld and I had presented a poster with evidence for lack of specificity and sensitivity.

'How then' Peter Isaacson pointedly asked in the poster discussion session 'would ***you*** diagnose Hodgkin's disease?'

Sadly mouth engaged before brain and I replied 'Why a good H&E and 20 years experience'!

I was put firmly in my place when Peter Isaacson retorted even more pointedly 'you do know that both can be quite hard to get'!

Peter Hall

How to write an Editorial that moves and shakes

(1) Become a reviewer and read great articles at least one year before everyone else (a real trip into the future), (2) Convince the editor (this is the easy bit) that the article that you have reviewed is a classic that should be fast-tracked but at the same time will be totally misunderstood by the few who bother to read it, (3) Insist that someone (guess who?) should be cajoled into writing an Editorial that will direct fishers and not swine toward the pearls, (4) Make sure that the title of the Editorial is a great deal funnier than the title of the article, (5) Include an Abstract with the Editorial (Abstracts are highly visible and imply – to the suggestible – the presence of a major research-based article), (6) Voila: 'Serrated route to colorectal cancer: backstreet or super highway? Journal of Pathology 2001;193:283'.

Jeremy Jass

8 The Journal of Pathology: Past, Present and Future

C. Simon Herrington

ORIGINS

The *Journal of Pathology* began life in 1893 as the *Journal of Pathology and Bacteriology*. It was founded by German Sims-Woodhead (Fig. 8.1) who, at the time, was Director of the Laboratories of the Conjoint Board of the Royal College of Physicians (London) and Royal College of Surgeons (England). He had moved to London in 1890 from Edinburgh, where he had previously been a medical student, then first assistant to Professor Greenfield and subsequently the first Superintendent of the Royal College of Physicians Laboratory. This explains the fact that the Journal was initially published in conjunction with his friend Young J. Pentland of Edinburgh. This was very much a private enterprise but found support from a number of illustrious figures from pathology history, including Virchow and Metchnikoff, who both contributed to the first issue (Metchnikoff, 1893; Virchow, 1893). The introduction to the first volume of the Journal makes interesting reading and still holds resonance today: 'It has been thought desirable, therefore, to found a Journal specially devoted to the publication of original contributions on General Pathology, Pathological Anatomy, and Experimental Pathology, including Bacteriology. These contributions will, of course, be mainly from British Laboratories and Hospitals; but the co-operation of many distinguished Continental, American, and Colonial Pathologists has been obtained, and papers written or edited by them will, from time to time, be placed before our readers' (Sims-Woodhead, 1893). Further details of Sims-Woodhead's contribution to pathology and to the Journal are given in an editorial written by Dennis Wright (Wright, 1986).

The Journal proved to be a significant financial burden to Sims-Woodhead and, when The Pathological Society of Great Britain and Ireland was founded in 1906, he offered to share its proprietorship with the Society. In March 1907, an Association was formed to acquire the Journal from Sims-Woodhead, who was paid a cash sum together with an allocation of shares in the Association. The new arrangements were announced in an editorial published in 1908 (Editorial, 1908). Further details of this transaction are recorded in the history written by J. H. Dible to mark the Society's 50th Anniversary (Dible, 1957).

A SOCIETY JOURNAL

Sims-Woodhead continued as editor, with J. Ritchie and A. E. Boycott as assistant editors and, in 1914, he was invited to a special meeting of the committee at which transfer of ownership of the Journal to the Society was discussed. The decision was taken to conclude this transfer in the Summer of 1915. However, the First World War intervened and the Society committee did not

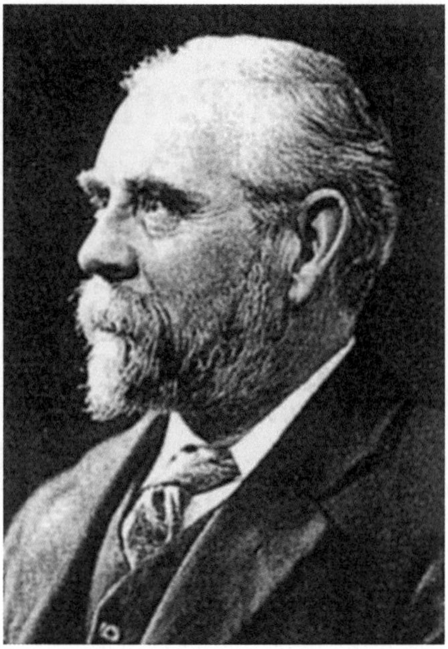

Figure 8.1 G. Sims-Woodhead, Founder and Editor 1893–1920.

meet again for 5 years. In January 1920, the Journal title finally passed to the Society, who have owned it ever since.

Coincident with this transfer of title, it was agreed that the editorship of the Journal should be determined by the Committee of The Pathological Society. As a result, the editorship passed, by mutual agreement and after some 27 years, from Sims-Woodhead to J. Ritchie (Fig. 8.2)

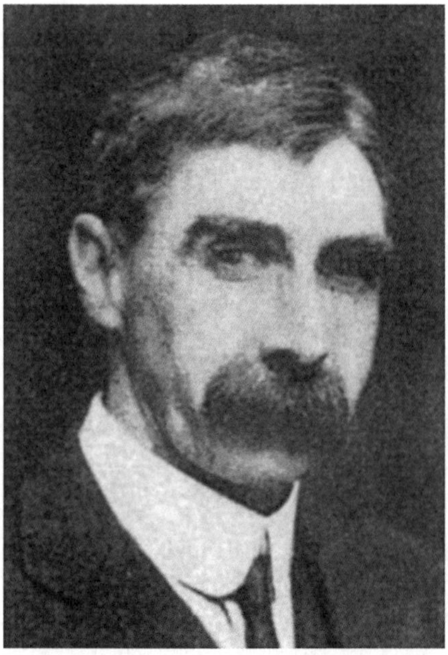

Figure 8.2 J. Ritchie, Editor 1920–1923.

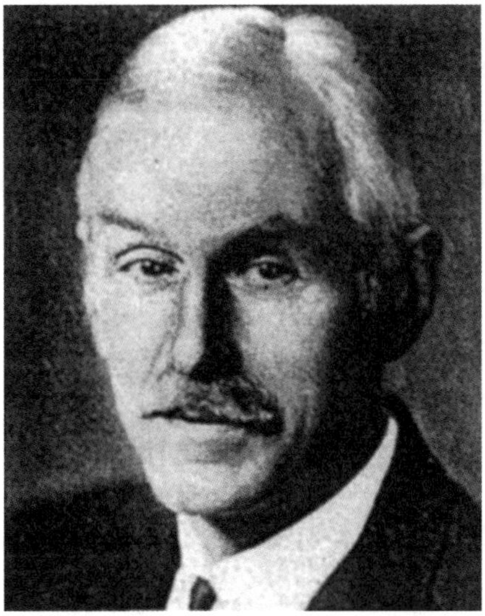

Figure 8.3 A. E. Boycott, Editor 1923–1934.

in the summer of 1920, with A. E. Boycott and H. R. Dean as assistant editors. At this time, the Journal was published by Cambridge Press but printed by Messrs Morrison and Gibb in Edinburgh. Early in 1920, however, the publishers refused to continue to finance and publish the Journal, precipitating a crisis and leading to a change in publishers to Messrs Oliver and Boyd, also of Edinburgh (Dible, 1957). In 1923, Ritchie died. A. E. Boycott (Fig. 8.3) was appointed editor, with M. J. Stewart and C. Price Jones as assistant editors. The first hint of the resurgence of financial difficulties was recorded in 1930, when the Journal had incurred a loss. The editors were asked to reduce costs and also to write to members asking them to curtail the length of their papers! This heralded a period of financial uncertainty. The amount owed to the publishers was greater than the level of the Society's overdraft and the editor was charged with trying to negotiate a reduction in the publisher's fees, as well as with the task of exploring other publishers. A significant turnaround was achieved by 1931, in terms of both conversion of loss into profit and negotiation of a reduced charge levied by the publishers. The Committee of the Society, however, asked for further investigation of alternative publishers and subsequently voted that the Journal be transferred to Oxford Medical Press. This prompted the resignation of both Boycott and Stewart, as a result of which the decision of the committee was rescinded. Boycott and Stewart withdrew their resignations but Boycott signalled that he did not feel he could continue as editor for much longer. Dible viewed this series of events as a significant landmark in the history of the Society (Dible, 1957) because it cemented the relationship between the Society and the publisher, which was still ongoing at the time that he wrote his article and, indeed, continued for many years to come. There is no doubt that the Journal's history is intimately intertwined with both its publishers and the Society, a principle that is still true today.

In 1934, Boycott resigned as editor on medical advice (he died in 1938) and M. J. Stewart (Fig. 8.4) was appointed in his place. By all accounts, Boycott had been a remarkable editor. He was described as 'autocratic' and said to have an 'extreme aversion to commas' (Dible, 1957), a subject that still has the capacity to induce heated debate.

The Second World War had a significant effect on both the Society and the Journal. Somewhat paradoxically, the Society's finances improved during the War, as a result of a reduced number of meetings, but the shortage of paper proved a cause for concern for the editor because this

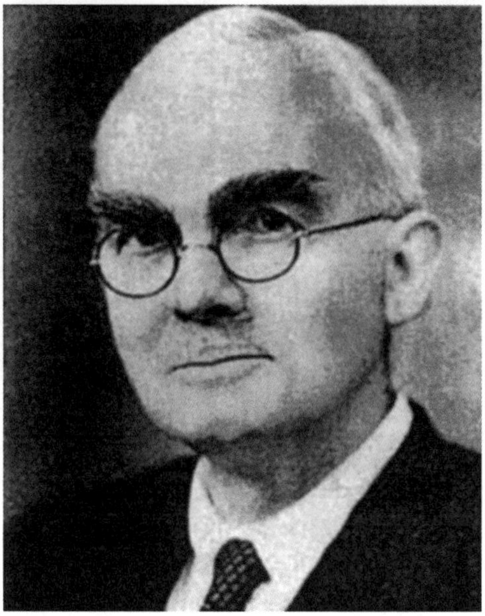

Figure 8.4 M. J. Stewart, Editor 1934–1955.

had produced a backlog of papers for publication. In 1953, the delay in publishing papers had reached 8 months and the publication of additional volumes, along with an increase in subscriptions, was considered. Stewart resigned as editor at the end of 1955 and was replaced by C. L. Oakley (Fig. 8.5).

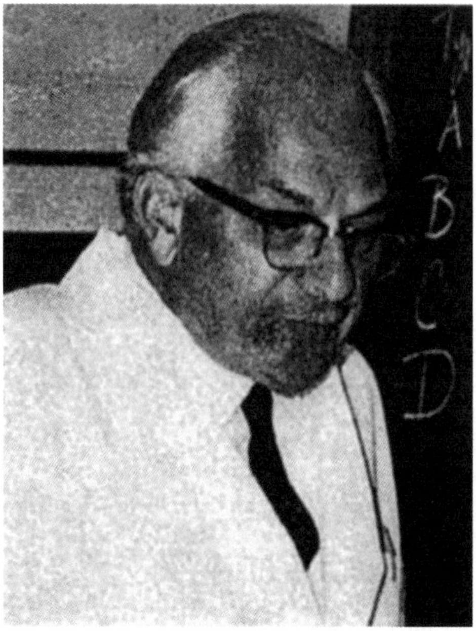

Figure 8.5 C. L. Oakley, Editor 1955–1973.

DIVISON OF THE JOURNAL

The next major event in the Journal's history was its separation into the *Journal of Pathology* and the *Journal of Medical Microbiology*. The latter is dealt with in Chapter 10 (Duerden and Collee, 2006) and the following discussion deals specifically with the *Journal of Pathology*. There is a record, in Lendrum's 75th Anniversary account of the Society, that this was agreed in 1967 (Lendrum, 1981) but it did not happen until 1969 (Fig. 8.6 A and B). This very significant change

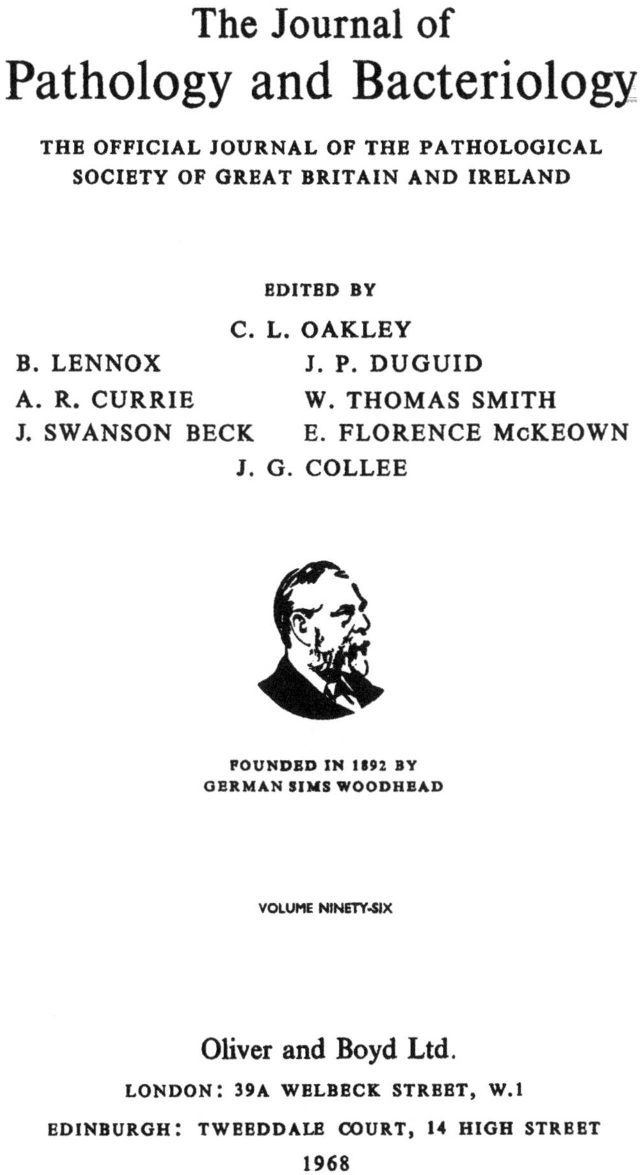

The Journal of
Pathology and Bacteriology

THE OFFICIAL JOURNAL OF THE PATHOLOGICAL
SOCIETY OF GREAT BRITAIN AND IRELAND

EDITED BY

C. L. OAKLEY

B. LENNOX J. P. DUGUID
A. R. CURRIE W. THOMAS SMITH
J. SWANSON BECK E. FLORENCE McKEOWN

J. G. COLLEE

FOUNDED IN 1892 BY
GERMAN SIMS WOODHEAD

VOLUME NINETY-SIX

Oliver and Boyd Ltd.
LONDON: 39A WELBECK STREET, W.1
EDINBURGH: TWEEDDALE COURT, 14 HIGH STREET
1968

Figure 8.6 A Front covers of (A) the last issue of the *Journal of Pathology and Bacteriology* and (B) the first issue of the *Journal of Pathology*.

was overseen by C. L. Oakley, who initially edited both Journals. He continued as editor of the *Journal of Pathology* until 1973, being succeeded by W. Spector (Fig. 8.7), who was editor until his untimely death in 1982. Several significant events took place around this time. The Committee Minutes of 1981 make mention that the *Investigative and Cell Pathology* journal was to change its name to *Diagnostic Histopathology* and become a Society journal. The death of Spector in early 1982 precipitated a special meeting of the officers, at which D. Willoughby was appointed acting editor. The Minutes for that year also record some of the problems with the publisher, including loss of copy, publication of volumes in the wrong order, failure to use corrected page proofs, a large backlog and long delays in publication. Later in 1982, the decision was taken to change the

The
Journal of Pathology

AN OFFICIAL JOURNAL OF THE PATHOLOGICAL SOCIETY OF GREAT BRITAIN AND IRELAND

EDITED BY
C. L. OAKLEY
J. P. DUGUID W. THOMAS SMITH
J. SWANSON BECK E. FLORENCE McKEOWN
J. G. COLLEE

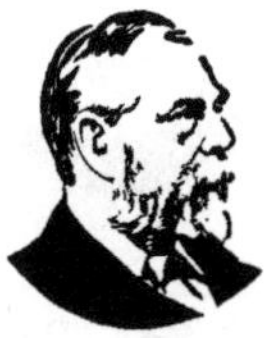

GERMAN SIMS WOODHEAD
Founder of The Journal of Pathology and Bacteriology

VOLUME NINETY-SEVEN

Oliver and Boyd Ltd.
EDINBURGH: TWEEDDALE COURT, 14 HIGH STREET
1969

Figure 8.6 B (*Continued*)

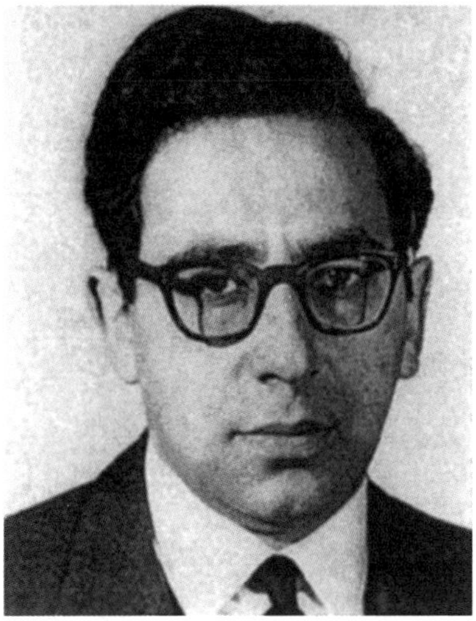

Figure 8.7 W. Spector, Editor 1974–1982.

publisher from Longmans to John Wiley and Sons and to merge it with *Diagnostic Histopathology*. Dennis Wright (Fig 8.8) was appointed the new editor. These decisions were ratified in 1983 and the publisher changed from January 1984 (Walker, 2006). As an aside, the Journal came to be published by Longman's as a result of Oliver and Boyd becoming a division of that publishing house in 1970: this change can be gleaned from the front covers of the Journal issues, which alter to reflect this fact in January 1970.

The Journal went from strength to strength throughout the 1980s and into the early 1990s when it celebrated its centenary, which was marked by an editorial (Wright, 1994). In the same year, the editorship passed to Peter Toner (Fig. 8.9), during whose term of office the transition to electronic publication began to have a significant effect on the Journal. In addition, the publication of Annual

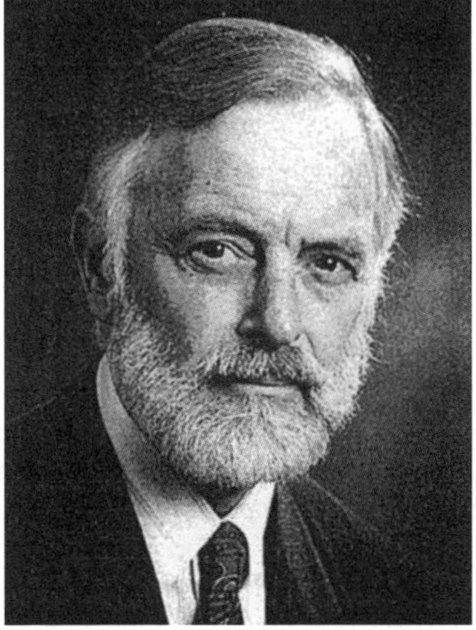

Figure 8.8 D. H. Wright, Editor 1983–1994.

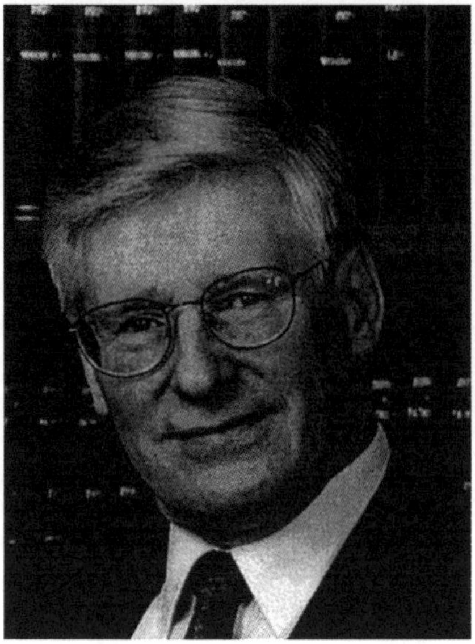

Figure 8.9 P. G. Toner, Editor 1994–2002.

Review Issues was instigated (Toner, 1998), the first of these dealing with Molecular and Cellular Themes in Cancer Research and appearing in January 1999. This development has been highly successful, producing high quality contributions to the review literature that have the significant added benefit of being good for the impact factor, of which more later!

THE NEW MILLENNIUM

In 2000, the Journal appeared on the worldwide web, through Wiley Interscience, with electronic versions of all papers back to 1997 appearing as pdf files (Toner and Reece, 2000a). This was supplemented later the same year by introduction of the EarlyView service, whereby papers that are ready for publication but are waiting in the queue to appear in a paper issue are published online (Toner and Reece, 2000b). Importantly, these papers are visible to the clinical and scientific communities through electronic search engines and are indexed through the PubMed system.

The meeting of the Journal editorial board in 2000 was a landmark event. The structure of this meeting was a departure from the traditional approach, allowing more time for 'brainstorming' and discussion. As a result, a new editorial structure was developed and several significant changes were made to the running of the Journal. Six associate editors (Fred Bosman, Peter Hall, James Kirkpatrick, Richard Poulsom, Rosemary Walker and me) were appointed. The post of managing editor was created and it was agreed that this individual would be based in the London offices of the Society, rather than in the offices of the editor. Jeremy Theobald was appointed to this post in October 2001 and I took up office as editor in January 2002 (Fig. 8.10). During this time, John Wiley and Sons had been developing the Manuscript Central online manuscript tracking system for use with several of their journals. The Belfast office of the *Journal of Pathology* piloted the system during 2001 and it went 'live' in February 2002 (Toner and Herrington, 2002).

Manuscript Central has been extremely successful. It has allowed the online processing of all manuscripts, with easy and effective communication between the associate editors, assistant editor, authors and reviewers, who are distributed all over the world. This has led to an ever-increasing database of reviewers, a large proportion of whom are now based in countries other than the UK,

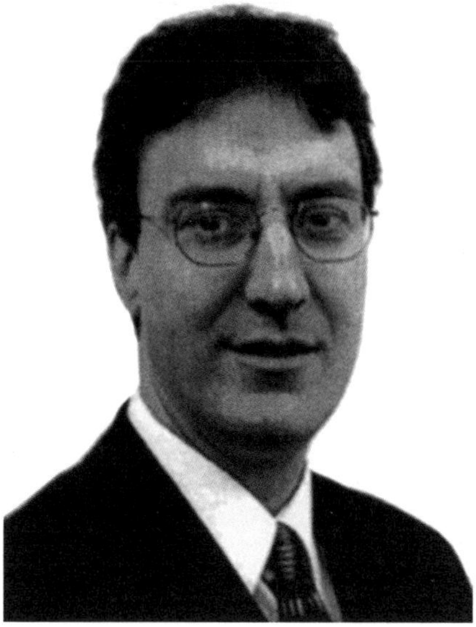

Figure 8.10 C. S. Herrington, Editor 2002–current.

with an increasing number from North America, Japan, Australia and many other countries. The authorship and global impact of the Journal are also broadening. For example, in June 2003 we published a paper from China describing the clinical pathology of SARS (Ding *et al.*, 2003): this attracted considerable media attention, particularly from the Far East and Australasia, and led to submission and subsequent publication of further influential papers on this infectious disease. Similarly, in July 2004 the Journal was mentioned on the front page of *The Times* newspaper as a result of publication of a paper describing the prevalence of prion proteins in archival tonsillar and appendiceal tissues (Hilton *et al.*, 2004). There is no doubt that the development of electronic publishing, and the wider effects of the web, played major roles in these successes.

Another major development took place in 2005. As a result of a gargantuan effort by John Wiley and Sons, the entire archive of the *Journal of Pathology* (*and Bacteriology*) was published online. This is available via the Journal website at http://www3.interscience.wiley.com/cgi-bin/jhome/1130, is fully searchable and provides electronic access to pdf files of all papers published in the Journal from its foundation in 1893. The archive is fascinating. It is now possible to search for, download, print and read any paper published in the Journal, including seminal works by many distinguished investigators. It also allows analysis of how the Journal has changed throughout its history. For example, changes in the volume of published copy can be gleaned from the data contained in the archive (Fig. 8.11). Note that the effects of the two World Wars are evident, as is the decline in copy in the 1970s (said to be related to poor performance of the then publishers, Longmans), with a rebound increase to deal with the backlog when the publisher changed in 1984. The effect of the introduction of Annual Review Issues is also clearly visible.

THE FUTURE

So what of the future? As Peter Toner and I remarked in 2002, 'nothing stands still in the world of publishing'! Our impact factor currently stands at 5.33; we are ranked second in pathology (first for immediacy index) and are closing the gap on the *American Journal of Pathology* (Fig. 8.12). Although impact factor is not everything, it is an important parameter by which we are judged.

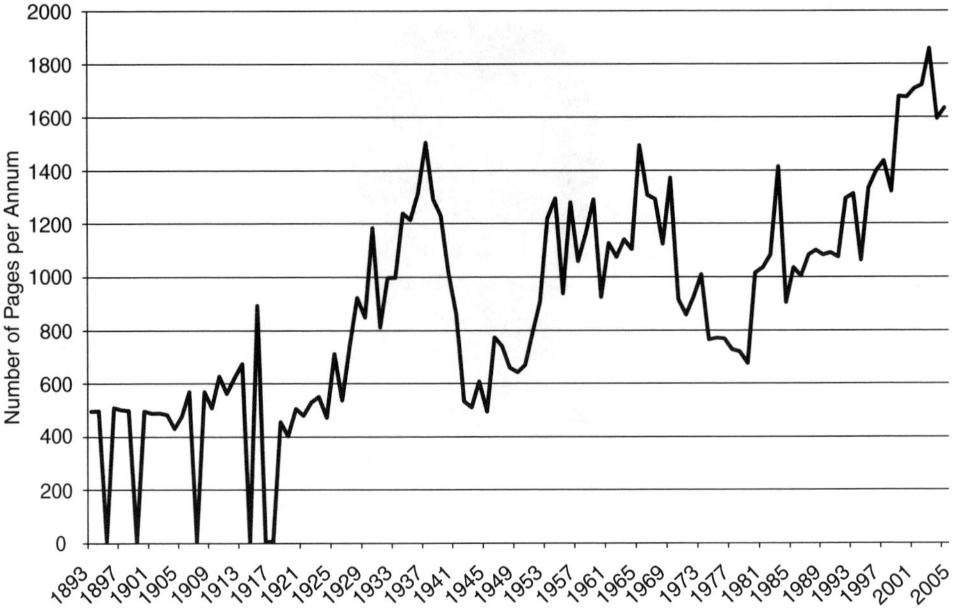

Figure 8.11 The number of pages published per annum from 1893 to 2005. No issues were published in some calendar years early in the Journal's history but volumes at this time were often dated across two years, e.g. 1913–1914. Note the slow recovery in copy after both World Wars, with a remarkable peak in the intervening period. The trough in the 1970s may be related to the problems with the publisher at that time. The increase due to the introduction of Annual Review Issues in 1999 is also visible.

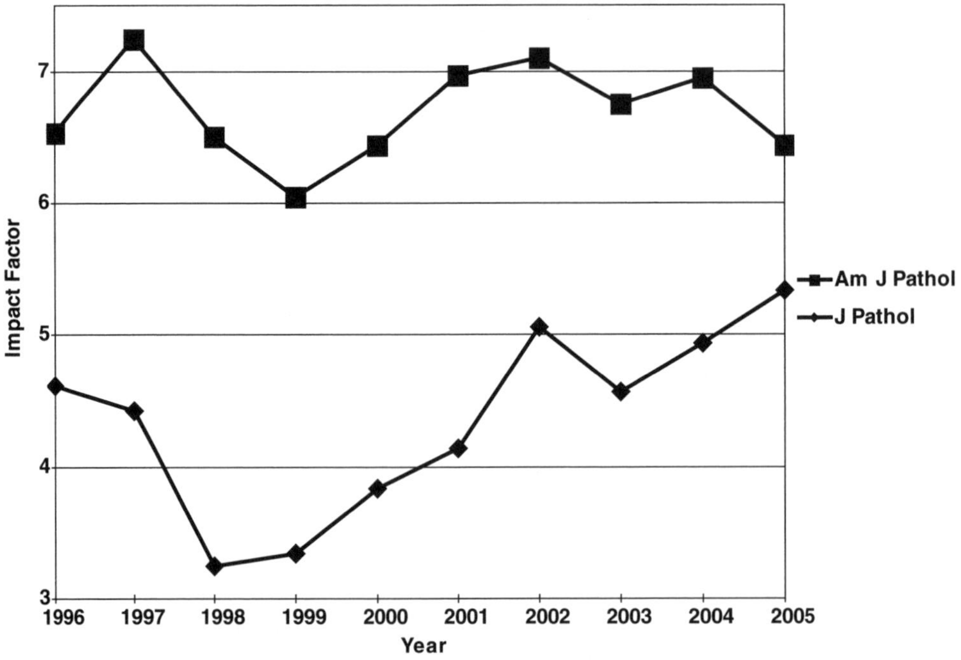

Figure 8.12 Trends in impact factor for the *Journal of Pathology* and its main competitor the *American Journal of Pathology* (1996–2005).

Plans for the future must therefore take it, as well as other considerations, into account. At a recent meeting of the editorial board, we discussed how we can improve the quality of the Journal still further, or 'raise the bar' as it was put. This requires careful thought but increasing our profile in other parts of the world, particularly China and the USA, is an important part of our plans. There is no doubt that the Annual Review Issues have been hugely successful and appropriate management of these, with timely publication, is crucial. Open Access publishing is a challenge that faces the Journal, the Society and the publisher. The appearance and expansion of specific journals that employ the 'author pays', rather than the 'subscriber pays', model, together with the adoption by some journals of various approaches to providing 'free' content to readers, has the potential to damage the fiscal health of the Journal, with potential knock-on effects on both the publisher and the Society. As you can imagine, we are watching the development of this publishing model very closely, both in the UK and abroad. Although the concept of providing journal content free to all who want to read it is laudable, the practical implementation of such a policy is more difficult to envisage unless there are major alterations to how research, particularly the publication of research data, is funded. Naturally, the editors of the *Journal of Pathology*, the officers of the Society and the publishers will be keeping a close eye on developments to ensure that the Journal does not suffer from any changes in corporate or government policy.

FINAL THOUGHTS

The *Journal of Pathology* (*and Bacteriology*) has an illustrious history. Compiling this short account made this clear to me and also demonstrated that many of the issues faced by my predecessors are still relevant today. The Journal is in good shape. We are holding our own in an increasingly global market but we cannot be complacent. Through continued quality improvements we aspire to improve our position still further and, with the help of authors, reviewers, editors and publishers, not to mention the Society, we will endeavour to do so.

Acknowledgements

I would like to thank all those who have contributed to the running and production of the Journal since its inception. This includes the Journal's founder and the succession of editors, assistant editors and now associate editors, not forgetting the members of the editorial board, the authors, the reviewers and, of course, the publishers, John Wiley and Sons, who have supported the Journal unfailingly for many years. Finally, as you can see from the above account, the Journal is inextricably linked with The Pathological Society of Great Britain and Ireland and I thank the Society officers, committee, administrators and members for their continued support. Specific thanks go to the current Secretary of the Society, Peter Hall, for sharing his findings from the Committee Minutes with me, and to Jeremy Theobald (managing editor) and Louise Ryan (assistant editor) for their constant support. I also thank Jeremy for providing Fig. 8.11, which was initially included in the publisher's report for 2005.

REFERENCES

Dible, J. H. (1957) A history of The Pathological Society of Great Britain and Ireland. *J. Pathol. Bacteriol.* **73(Suppl)**: 1–35.

Ding, Y., Wang, H., Shen, H., Li, Z., Geng, J., Han, H., *et al.* (2003) The clinical pathology of severe acute respiratory syndrome (SARS): a report from China. *J. Pathol.* **200**: 282–289.

Duerden, B. I. and Collee, J. G. (2006) Microbiology and The Pathological Society. In *Centenary of The Pathological Society of Great Britain and Ireland* (eds P. A. Hall and N. A. Wright). Wiley: Chichester.

Editorial (1908) *J. Pathol. Bacteriol.* **12**: xi.

Hilton, D. A., Ghani, A. C., Conyers, L., Edwards, P., McCardle, L., Ritchie, D., *et al.* (2004) Prevalence of lymphoreticular prion protein accumulation in UK tissue samples. *J. Pathol.* **203**: 733–739.

Lendrum, A. C. (1981) *75th Anniversary Tribute to The Pathological Society of Great Britain and Ireland*, Dundee.

Metchnikoff, E. (1893) On aqueous humour, micro-organisms, and immunity. *J. Pathol. Bacteriol.* **1**: 13–20.

Sims-Woodhead, G. (1893) Introduction. *J. Pathol. Bacteriol.* **1**: i–ii.

Toner, P. G. (1998) Editorial – The Annual Review Issue. *J. Pathol.* **186**: 339.

Toner, P. G. and Herrington, C. S. (2002) A new editorial system for the Journal of Pathology. *J. Pathol.* **196**: 249–251.

Toner, P. G. and Reece, D. (2000a) Into 2000: The Journal of Pathology on the web. *J. Pathol.* **190**: 1–2.

Toner, P. G. and Reece, D. (2000b) The Journal of Pathology publishes faster on EarlyView. *J. Pathol.* **191**: 111.

Virchow, R. (1893) Transformation and descent. *J. Pathol. Bacteriol.* **1**: 1–12.

Walker, F. (2006) The 1980s: People, Events and Meetings. In *The Centenary of The Pathological Society of Great Britain and Ireland* (eds P. A. Hall and N. A. Wright). Wiley: Chichester.

Wright, D. H. (1986) Jubilee volume: Journal of Pathology (G. S. Woodhead). *J. Pathol.* **150**: 1–4.

Wright, D. H. (1994) 100 years of the Journal of Pathology. *J. Pathol.* **172**: i–iii.

Wright was right

Stromal reactions to tumour cells had captured my interest in the early 1970s. I devised an elegant (well, I thought so) *in vitro* assay to measure the fibroblast growth-stimulating effect of dialysed human tumour extracts. I assessed this by tritiated thymidine uptake in serum-deprived (G0) fibroblast cultures. I expected to find a positive correlation with the degree of stromal desmoplasia and eventually discover the growth factor. After presenting this to The Pathological Society audience, the memorable question came from Dr Nicholas Wright. 'How can you be so certain that the uptake of tritiated thymidine is a measure of fibroblast proliferation rather than DNA repair?' he asked. 'A good question' I replied, and then blathered. That alternative explanation had never crossed my mind. I learnt two lessons from this. First, avoid surrogates (tritiated thymidine uptake) for what is directly measurable (more cells). Second, don't be seduced into believing that trendy sophisticated techniques make the work more 'scientific'.

James Underwood

Stay single

When slide projectors were the norm, those who wanted to make the greatest impression used dual projection. While few could compare with Julia Polak's vivacious manner, many sought to emulate her wide-screen visual extravaganzas. My one and only foray into using dual projection was when I presented the results of a study of non-A non-B (as it was then called) hepatitis in haemophiliacs. The key message was this: despite initial liver biopsies showing low-grade 'chronic persistent' hepatitis, repeat biopsies in these patients showed progressive disease with a high risk of cirrhosis. Within the first minute of my presentation, the bulb went in one of the dual projectors! I quickly adapted what I was going to say, and tried to remember the prompts that would have appeared on the now blank half of the screen. If I had stuck with single projection, the risk of technical failure would have been halved and the slide carrier could have been moved to the functioning projector. I have never witnessed dual PowerPoint projection. But I have seen plenty of irritating animation. Remember: it's the message, not the medium, that matters.

James Underwood

9 The Waxing and Waning of Academic Pathology: A Personal View

Nicholas A. Wright

INTRODUCTION

Let us start with a definition of terms. What is academic pathology? Ah, 'there's the rub' as they used to say. Because on what people have understood by the term 'academic pathology' whole careers have been decided, departments withered on the vine and the discipline itself placed in severe jeopardy. Overstated? Alarmist? Wait and see.

The life of a clinical academic working in pathology is usually said to be *tripartite* – research, teaching and practice – with different individuals having strengths in each sphere and thus doing more of one and less of the others. So far, so good. But what sort of research? Now we are down to the wire. From my own perspective, some time in the 1950s – it may indeed have been before that – a great divide opened in the ranks of British academic pathologists, arranging the profession into two major groupings: in the first group were the *academic surgical pathologists*, who based their research on the clinical material that came their way. So, what is this academic surgical pathology? It is difficult to define and some very eminent colleagues of ours would claim that it does not exist as a discipline – but I believe strongly that it does. It is the use of morphological and usually histological observational methods to define new clinicopathological entities and refine old ones, to identify and develop prognostic indices, to correlate treatments with its effects, to support clinical trials by correct histopathological diagnosis and classification, to accurately classify diseased tissues for tissue banks and microarrays and, most recently, to support mouse genetics through the phenotyping of transgenic and knockout animals. Techniques may include histochemistry, immunohistochemistry and/or *in situ* hybridisation, expression profiling and sophisticated three-dimensional reconstruction but, make no mistake, this research is based centrally and unequivocally in *morphology* – our core technique. Surgical pathology is frequently derided, often not appreciated at all and, most disgracefully of all, not thought to be internationally competitive with other disciplines within the context of the Research Assessment Exercise (RAE). In the 1950s and 1960s cardinal examples of such individuals were Herbert Spencer, Basil Morson, John Azzopardi and Harold Fox, and as the century advanced we saw the likes of Roddy MacSween, Peter Scheuer, Chris Elston, Chris Fletcher, Thomas Krauz, Ian Ellis, Mike Wells, David Slater and Neil Shepherd emerge to make their contribution.

And then there were the experimental or investigative academic pathologists – those who believed that only the study of basic pathological processes, often in non-human systems, was the way to advance the discipline. For many of these the future lay in non-morphological methods, in well-planned animal experiments and in the new developments in cell and tissue culture. Early examples can be found in the work of Cameron, Florey, Heppleston, Spector, Willoughby and Harris, and latterly Chambers, Pignatelli, Lemoine, Hall and Wynford-Thomas, who have embraced modern cell and molecular biology and made them work in solving problems in pathobiology and pathogenesis.

So what, you might say. Indeed, it would have been all sweetness and light had the two philosophies lived in peaceful coexistence and mutual support, but they did not. I have heard Professors of Pathology – dyed in the wool, London-shrunk, copper-bottomed, out and out experimentalists – refer to research in surgical pathology as 'muck-raking' (A. G. Heppleston, ca. 1969, in my presence) and its protagonists as 'the hacks', (C. Lumsden, ca. 1968), and even one who was seemingly proud to be the 'only Professor of Pathology (In the country? In the world?) who has never performed an autopsy' (H. Harris, ca. 1978, in my presence). Nor has the invective been all one way: anyone who has visited Australia will have heard the scorn reserved by the surgical pathologists for their 'academic colleagues' (here, for academic, read experimental) and, closer to home, many has been the vituperative comment directed at the basic end of the spectrum by the clinical pathologists.

Why should this be? What is the cause of this mutual antipathy? Pass. My own personal view, for what it is worth, is that the Pharisees of the experimental method regard the quintessentially morphological approach of the surgical pathologist as being somehow intellectually inferior. On the other hand, the disdain felt by some surgical pathologists for basic pathological research might be based on the feeling that it is impractical, arcane and recondite, and thus of very limited interest to them.

A moment's reflection will show that both groups are absolutely wrong. The thoughtful investigative pathologist will quickly appreciate that it is surgical pathology that presents the problems that are really worth working on: what defines the differences in invasiveness or metastatic potential seen so often between different tumours? What is the cause of the metaplasia seen diagnostically in Barrett's oesophagus? Which cells are responsible for the ductular reaction in the liver? How are the multiple urothelial tumours in the bladder related to each other? And when the surgical pathologist stains for Her2, defines a cytokeratin phenotype or assesses the proliferative status of a melanocytic lesion with Ki67 or mcm2, he/she uses the fruit of a great deal of basic science. You can, I am sure, think of many more examples from both spheres of endeavour.

But what has this to do with the development of academic pathology over the last 45 years, I hear you ask. A great deal, and dire. I suppose that up to the very early 1990s it was possible to run a University Department as a *spectrum*: at one end there were the star investigative pathologists with high grant income and graduate students, whereas at the other were the academic surgical pathologists, deriving their research material from the routine service and their referral practice. Somewhere in the middle were some who, although good surgical pathologists, also had a reasonable, or in some cases considerable, basic or translational research presence. Everyone did some teaching. So, at the end of the year, all activities – the research, the practice and the teaching – were covered. I know, you see, because this was the way I ran the Hammersmith Department for nigh on 17 years, and there is no doubt, at least my mind, that it worked there, as I am sure in other places. The whole was greater than the sum of the parts, and pathology flourished.

Then, in the 1960s universities were expanding and Heads of Departments were actually being *offered* positions rather than having them taken away. I recall my first professor, a certain A.G. Heppleston, actually *refusing to accept* another lecturer, presumably on space grounds. Can you imagine that happening today? So the number of positions in academic pathology rose, and new medical schools were established in those days with proper departments of pathology,[1] such as Southampton, to be populated with the likes of Dennis Wright and Peter Isaacson, and Leicester, with first Eric Walker and then Ian Lauder and Rosemary Walker. Then there

[1] I was incensed by a piece in acpNews reporting a debate entitled 'Medical students do not need to be taught the pathological basis of disease', held at one of these new medical schools – the Peninsula – and fired off arguably the most vituperative article I have ever written, full of personal invective against the (named) proposers of the motion. To my surprise, it was accepted and can be found in acpNews, Autumn 2003.

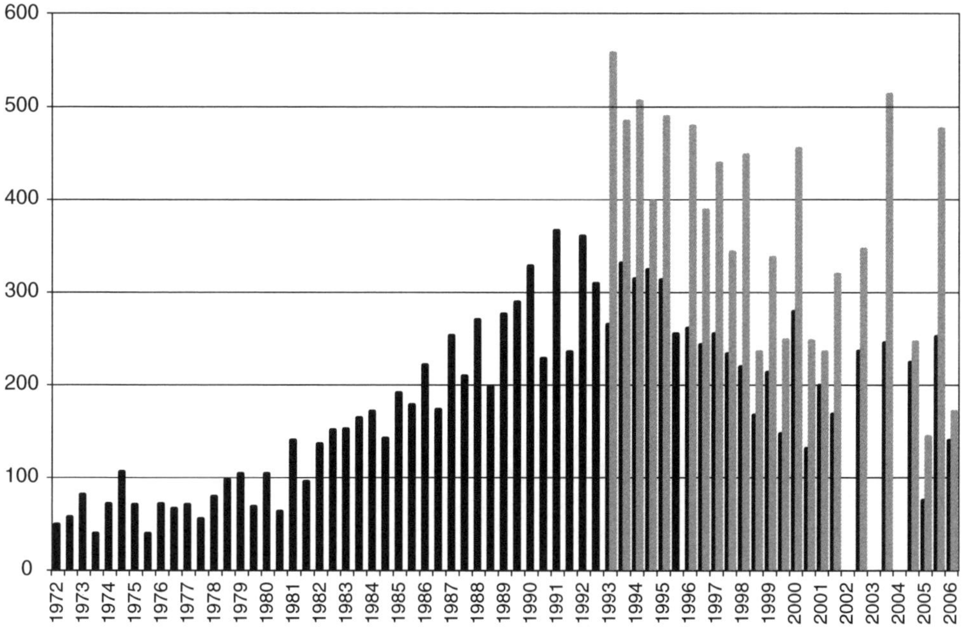

Figure 9.1 The number of abstracts received (black bars) and the number of registrants (grey) attending Pathological Society meetings from 1972 to 2006 (compiled by Professor Peter Hall). Note that prior to 1993 registration data are not available.

were the new techniques for studying disease, at the ultrastructural level, for measuring cell proliferation and cell death, and then the impact of the ability to localise proteins (see Chapter 15) and then mRNA species in tissue sections. Then came the explosion in cell and molecular biology, and by the late 1980s academic pathology in this country was really booming. The investigative pathologists were driving forward the development of these methods and the academic surgical pathologists were applying these advances to practical problems. And in those days pathology did indeed wax: I know that such metrics are not to everyone's taste, but Fig. 9.1 shows the number of abstracts presented at the Society's meetings from 1972 to the present day. When I joined the Society, meetings were small; I remember a meeting in Aberdeen with some 70 participants, most of whom gave papers. Using this metric for the number of abstracts presented at Pathological Society meetings over the years, it can be seen that in the 1970s (and indeed in preceding decades) meetings of the Society were small, with about 50–60 presentations per meeting. But then the number of abstracts rose steadily, reaching a peak in the early 1990s, possibly the Society's heyday. I can well recall a winter meeting at the Hammersmith Hospital in the early 1990s when I was reliably informed that there were nearly 800 registrants on one of the days.

But the dark clouds were even now gathering over academic pathology. Since then we have seen a decline, so much so that in 1999 the Society voted to stop the winter meeting because it was felt that there was insufficient material to be presented, with the result that, bizarrely, the summer meeting became the main meeting of the Society.[2] Now these data are of course open to different interpretations, but it is very clear that, judged by activity, research in academic pathology was now waning. The dark clouds I spoke of had now brought rain.

[2] I recall being told by Professor J. O'D. McGee in 1977, on my arrival in Oxford, that 'the Winter Meeting was for science, but the Summer Meeting was mainly a social occasion'.

THE RESEARCH ASSESSMENT EXERCISE AND ITS EFFECTS

In the latter years of the Thatcher era, a clamour arose that universities should be accountable for the vast (!) amounts of money they received, and should in some way be able to measure the efficacy of their outputs. Thus was born the QAA inspections, which 'measured' how good we were at teaching our students. Fortunately, there were no financial penalties for poor performance. However, in the early 1990s we began, with some trepidation, to prepare for the Research Assessment Exercise (RAE). New terms arose, such as grant expenditure/FTE[3] and impact factors of journals and citation indices of papers,[4] matters that academic pathologists of both persuasions had hitherto been oblivious to. And so we moved blindly into the first RAE. It now became important for *individual* senior members of staff to become 'RAE returnable' – each had to have grant income, preferably from a research council, to be supervising research students and to publish in high impact journals. And who suffered? The answer is, both groups, but the academic surgical pathologists suffered much, much worse because effective surgical pathology research does not require much in the way of grant income. Most surgical pathologists worked with junior medical staff, or at most a clinical fellow, and a few supervised PhD students. And where do they publish?: in the *American Journal of Surgical Pathology*, in *Histopathology* or *Human Pathology*, which is hardly comparable to *Nature*, *Cell* or the *Journal of Clinical Investigation* in which *some* of their experimental colleagues published. And it has done them little good to be part of a large team doing good clinical research, even when publishing in good journals, as many have done.[5] But by no means all the experimentalists did well: in recent years the surrogate metric for a 5* (the highest score) has been an average of £150K/FTE expenditure and two graduate students per year. Few academic pathologists could reach those dizzy heights. Consequently, with a few notable exceptions, university departments of pathology began to score badly. Unlike the QAA, the RAE has a financial sting in its tail, and the score, multiplied by the unit of resource, equals your research

[3] Grant expenditure/FTE (full-time equivalent of staff) has become an important metric in the RAE – in the last two assessments there seemed to be a linear relationship between grant expenditure/FTE and unit score in the RAE.

[4] Despite protestations that impact factors and citation indices are not used in the RAE, the author can vouch for their use in the 1996 RAE.

[5] In the 2001 RAE it was proposed that surgical pathology contributions to multi-author papers should automatically be graded 3a (a low score and unfunded by the High Education Funding Council). This was successfully resisted but it reflects the view of surgical pathology by some in these circles (Professor Simon Herrington told me this). It is thus very clear that surgical pathology research has been poorly regarded in successive RAEs. It is very difficult to understand from whence such a demeaning view has arisen; a moment's reflection will immediately reveal how critical a pure morphological observation actually is – we would not treat a melanoma without first assessing the Breslow thickness of the Clarke level, probably with serial section analysis of the sentinel node biopsy, nor a breast cancer patient without axillary node sampling or clearance and fairly exhaustive histological analysis. There have been recent British contributions where histopathological observations have been central, and where international interest and appreciation are manifest; space obviously precludes an exhaustive analysis of all fields where our research has made a significant impact, but I am sure you can add your own examples from your own field if I chose two or three examples that immediately come to mind. So what examples of British surgical pathology would I grade as 5*? I suppose that few would now issue a report on a breast cancer specimen without at least some mention or consideration of the Nottingham Prognostic Index (NPI), which has made a major impact internationally. Combining a measurement of the diameter of the tumour with an assessment of the tumour grade made using defined criteria with knowledge of the number of axillary nodes involved, the NPI is used internationally in clinical assessment, management, prediction and in obtaining comparative data in clinical trials. This is the definition of 5* research; I have yet to see Nottingham's pathology flagged as such. A second example would be that the resection margins of rectal carcinomas define the local recurrence rate. This is very much a multicentre effort, in which Basingstoke and Leeds figure largely. I have heard American surgeons at the 2004 Digestive Diseases Week agree that this was among the most prominent observations that defined clinical practice in this field in the last 10 years – if this is not again the definition of internationally competitive research, then what is? There are of course British observations that have attracted some credit among our peers – the recognition of complex sclerosing lesions in the breast, the adenoma/carcinoma sequence and the resultant molecular pathology, and MALT and the MALTomas – but there are others that remain totally unrecognised.

income from the Funding Council for the next few years. Poorly scoring medical schools lost money, and the brunt of the fallout hit the poorly performing departments. Senior lecturers with clinical interests moved into the National Health Service – some voluntarily, others forcibly. Clinical lectureships were either lost or changed into non-clinical lectureships or senior lectureships to provide positions for scientists who were RAE returnable, which is not a bad thing in itself but from the viewpoint of academic pathology it is disastrous. Most importantly, it was more or less the end of the road for those academic surgical pathologists hoping to be appointed to established chairs of pathology in this country. But our loss has been America's gain – we have watched while some of our best surgical pathologists have been enticed across the pond, because of their inability to land such a chair, to positions in the USA where, as surgical pathologists (an American term really), they are appropriately venerated and revered.

Just as academic surgical pathologists have felt the pressure of the RAE and the need to win grants in strong competition, investigative pathologists have felt under pressure from the demands of the National Health Service (NHS), have been unable to cope with the tripartite role and have departed into a career of research and teaching only or even into the NHS itself. An example from Kings: 'the last proper academic pathologist appointed as senior lecturer was Dr Vasi Sundaresan in 1997; he promptly buried himself within experimental pathology (which was always physically, and in reality administratively, separate from histopathology) and worked on lung cancer and neuronal developmental biology. He faced the classic dilemma of wanting to hold onto a clinical contract whilst realising that working six sessions a week for the hospital would wreck significant research activity. In reality he did about 1.5 sessions of diagnostic work (between 06.30 and 08.00 on some mornings), which did not sit well with purely diagnostic colleagues as the cancer networks got organised, and in 2004 he finally gave up to work full-time elsewhere in the NHS. There were no hard feelings on the part of St Thomas's Hospital, only contempt from Sunderesan at the lousy management structures of the medical school. When Sebastian Lucas approached the new Guy's, King's and St Thomas's Dean about appointing a new senior lecturer to replace him (intended as tongue in cheek), the answer was a straight 'No' ' (S. Lucas, personal communication).

And what have we done about this? Not a lot. There was a time when I thought I detected a cadre of academic pathologists who were widely respected for their diagnostic acumen but who also led a team of clinical academics and scientists doing internationally competitive research: individuals such as Peter Isaacson and Dillwyn Williams. This, I thought, was the way forward. I was probably wrong. We simply have not produced enough individuals with the happy knack of bestriding the two branches of our profession successfully. In addition, as Peter Hall pointed out,[6] we also have not produced enough good experimentalists to win programme grant support in a highly competitive environment. And where are the surgical pathologists now? Mainly in the NHS out of the way of the RAE, some with honorary chairs (if they are lucky at the local university, or in some cases further afield).[7] The Society has, with the help of the Private Patients Plan (PPP) and the College, established a few clinician scientist positions in pathology, but transparently not enough. The Society's Centenary will hopefully provide a new impetus to this!

And so academic pathology positions have been lost, and people have now begun to notice.[8] The Council of Heads of Medical Schools recently wrote to the Royal College of Pathologists to enlist its help in reversing this trend. The Trent Regional Committee of the College was trenchant in its criticism: 'We found it risible that the Council of the Heads of Medical Schools should look

[6] In his talk 'Academic Pathology – a Way Forward', delivered to the Academic Forum at the winter meeting of the Society in January 2006.

[7] Professor Neil Shepherd, working in Gloucester, is a Professor (now a Visiting Professor) at the University of Cranfield.

[8] In 2005 the Council of Heads of Medical Schools Report on Academic Staff Numbers drew attention to the loss of positions in histopathology.

to the College for action over the decimation of academic pathology while it was the heads of medical schools themselves who had wilfully closed 40% of academic pathology posts in a single year and closed 81% of lectureships in pathology since 2000'. I can really see their point but I can also (well I would, wouldn't I) see it from the viewpoint of the hard-pressed Dean of Medicine with a deficit budget, desperately casting about to increase the School's score in the next RAE or else see the School go even deeper into the financial mire.

There have been other explanations for the waning of academic pathology, and the examinations of the Royal College of Pathologists has been an old chestnut in this respect. 'Young people were being forced to learn innumerable facts, and to concentrate on the examinations over a five or six year period – to the exclusion of anything else – during what is supposed to be their most formative years when they should be laying the foundations of a research career' was the cry from one side. 'The examination has driven up standards of diagnostic pathology in this country' came the counter from the other side. And so it went on, with Professor Dennis Wright having many a fight with his opponents, whom he christened, a trifle ungraciously I thought, the 'backwoodsmen'. In fact the Association of Professors of Pathology, in perhaps its only effective political action, decided to run a number of candidates for the College Council with the express policy of changing the examination system to a single exam to be taken after three years of training. In this they succeeded, only to see the 'backwoodsmen' subsequently flood the Council and re-apply for a further tough exit examination at 5 years – perhaps the worst of all worlds. But I have always been ambivalent about the effect of the examination on academic aspirations; believing, as I do, that academic pathologists should at least endeavour to have a foot planted firmly in both experimental and surgical pathology, I can see nothing really wrong in taking the Part 1 examination, then getting a fellowship to do a PhD and then returning to take Part 2 and obtain a CSST or CST – as it will be called in the future. That is what I did, and I think it behoved me well, actually.

The academic expansion of the 1960s was matched in the 1980s and 1990s by a crisis in recruitment, largely brought about by ourselves (well, some of us). Alarmed at the apparently large number of senior registrars seeking consultant appointments, our College and the Department of Health actually *froze* recruitment into our discipline for 18 months – an unmitigated disaster for pathology, which then saw recruitment plummet even when the ban was lifted. The reasons for this are complex and have been discussed elsewhere (see Chapters 12 and 13), and the trend is only now being reversed with the establishment of the SHO Schools. But even with the recruitment of more individuals into pathology, we are not seeing many naturally follow an academic interest: the Society is now having to make a special effort to interest juniors in an academic career. Why then is the situation compounded by an apparent decline in research interest among junior pathologists? Apart from saying the obvious – that this is a position seen in most, if not all, other clinical academic disciplines in this country – there are probably several reasons: lack of local academic leadership and encouragement; knowledge that consultant appointment within 5 years of starting training is standard (the issue of the shortage of pathologists); lack of money to take time out for research; clinical lectureships being stopped, or made it impossible to appoint, through the simple rule that appointees would have a substantial opus already to be presented for the RAE (S. Lucas, personal communication).

Because this is a personal piece, I can give you another view. There has been much comment on the lack of exposure of medical and dental students to pathology in the undergraduate curriculum, so that, unlike in other disciplines, students do not know what pathologists do. This has been argued effectively and evocatively elsewhere (see Chapter 12) but there may be another reason why recruitment into the pathology disciplines has fallen so precipitously since the admissions procedure of 1984. About 15% of students make up their minds to do pathology *before* they apply to medical school – I know I did. When asked why I wanted to read medicine, I told the interviewers and they appeared entirely unfazed. These days they would probably call for security, such is the concentration on 'aptitude', 'communication skills' and 'empathy': we could well be selecting against those individuals who regard medicine as merely a first scientific degree.

RECENT EVENTS

The impact of the Alder Hey and Bristol episodes on recruitment in pathology and on the incidence of autopsies has been discussed frequently but their effects on research and teaching have received less attention. In the days when the Retained Organ Commission was sitting, I can recall distinguished surgical pathologists being literally terrified of the consequences of sending out sections for a slide seminar, and several who almost broke down under the strain. And the impact on tissue-based research has been really quite dreadful. The inclusion of surgically acquired tissues within the Human Tissue Act was an issue that the Society fought long and hard against. Despite the Retained Organ Commission assuring us, on multiple occasions, that these tissues were not on their agenda, they appeared as part of the Act and no amount of lobbying on our or anyone else's part could get them off the statute book. Initially they needed to be consented for research *and* teaching (the latter prior to any diagnosis – whatever that was supposed to mean). At least we were able to get the teaching and training for research off the consent agenda, with a great deal of help from our friends, some of them noble. Interestingly, the Scots, as in so many things, were wiser, exempting surgically acquired tissues from the legislation; whether this will result in a move over the border by disenfranchised tissue researchers is a matter for the future.

As I write, nobody is yet clear how the Human Tissue Act is going to work, but we will definitely see the licensing of all tissue banks, the need to consent all tissue (including blood and cerebrospinal fluid) and the need to get ethical approval for even the smallest tissue-based project that in any way will count as research. This might be as innocuous, for example, as looking for male cells in the archived biopsies of female patients who have received a bone marrow transplant: for this, one currently has to fill in an entire COREC form (over 60 pages long) and wait at least 60 days before you can actually cut the sections. There is no doubt that researchers in this country generally, and especially in pathology, feel ground down by the sheer bureaucratic burden of prosecuting research, and wonder if it is worth the candle. It is interesting to note that a recent consultation document from the Department of Health seeks to reduce this bureaucratic burden, which is especially piquant when you think who created all this bureaucracy in the first place.[9]

Finally, and somewhat at the risk of being labelled a dinosaur, there is the attack on professionalism in this country to consider: we have seen the introduction of the new consultant contract, at huge expense, which in my view has done a great deal to expedite this loss. We used to be paid a fair amount to do a job that was, by its nature, open-ended: now we have slavishly accepted a deal that actually measures what we do and pays us accordingly. From the professional viewpoint, I consider this a debasing step. However, when I expressed this view at a recent College Council meeting I was subjected to considerable abuse – this is how far we have come. Of course, I am sure that many of us, especially in universities, carry on much as before, but it is the principle underlying the contract to which I object. It leads to a certain mind set: I well remember feeling close to despair when, at a recent meeting held to consider the Society's strategy over the next few years, I heard a young woman describe how she set up her period in research with funding and a project, but on reflection pulled out of it because 'she would lose her banding' and any way, during this proposed period, a consultant position in her area that she had had her eye on would become vacant. If her research mattered so little to her, what is the point anyway, I reasoned. Before becoming maudlin and bemoaning the death of idealism, I had to remind myself that it was I who was probably being unreasonable and expecting more from her than she was prepared to give. But it upset me, nonetheless.

[9] 'Best Research for Best Health', Department of Health, 2005.

THE SCOTTISH CONNECTION

It is difficult to dissociate the happenings in the last few years without to some extent discussing the men and women who contributed to this process: in this book there are several chapters that deal with people and happenings in relation to the Society, but where have our leaders come from over this period? Well, first things first – there is no reasonable doubt that from the 1950s and well into the 1970s the era was dominated by what has been called the 'Scottish Mafia' or even more specifically as the 'Glasgow Mafia', although other Scottish cities might also claim that title. A number of people who were appointed to the Aberdeen Department by Alastair Currie subsequently went on to be appointed to chairs of pathology elsewhere in the UK (John Beck, Dundee; Colin Bird, Leeds and Edinburgh; Eric Walker, Leicester and Aberdeen; Andrew Wylie, Edinburgh and Cambridge). But it has to be emphasised that the Scottish hegemony held considerable sway not only in Scotland, where you would *a priori* expect them to dominate, but also in England: Anderson in Liverpool, Bird in Leeds, Crane in Sheffield, Curran in St Thomas's, McGee in Oxford, Walker in Leicester, Wylie in Cambridge, Munro Neville at the Institute of Cancer Research, Wilson Horne in Newcastle and Levison at Guy's. Together with their indigenous Scottish brethren – Currie, MacSween, Goudie *et al.*, who are always active in the Society – it is probably true to say that they dominated the academic scene in the period leading upto the 1980s.

That is not to say that other departments were not active in producing professors: from Birmingham came Donald Heath, chair in Liverpool, Douglas Brewer, chair in morbid anatomy in Birmingham; Walter Smith, chair in neuropathology in Birmingham. Dennis Wright joined the department and later was appointed from Uganda to the foundation chair of pathology in Southampton in the early 1970s, and of course Lyn Jones held the chair in Birmingham for many years. But it is clear that the Scottish mafia held sway and I have often wondered why this should be so. Did, or do, Scots have a special talent for pathology, or does the subject hold a special attraction for Scots? Could it be that the shade of Robert Muir still held influence? I well recall being told of the 'red carpet' treatment meted out to promising undergraduates in Glasgow if they selected pathology as a career (A. J. Watson, personal communication). Certainly, having been trained by a product of the Glasgow School of Pathology, I can vouch for their high standards and critical thinking, but times were changing. In more recent years we have seen a decline in the export of pathologists to departments south of the border, and even the accession of a Sassenach, Barry Gusterson, to that Holy of Holies – the chair in Glasgow. Apart from what might be called the Hammersmith/ICRF axis, which sent Evans to St Mary's, Foster to Liverpool, Hall to St Thomas's, Dundee and Belfast, Krausz to Chicago, Pignatelli to Bristol, Ilyas to Nottingham, El-Lalani to Birmingham and Stamp to Hammersmith itself, no one department has dominated in the manner in which Glasgow did. Where will our leaders be trained in the next centennium? Who will take up the banner?

So the face of pathology has changed. In London we have seen massive mergers and the example of Guy's, King's and Thomas's, which became the United Medical and Dental School, is most instructive (S. Lucas, personal communication):

> 'Tighe resigned in a huff and left early in Sept 1990 (too much hospital and district administration and too little practical pathology mainly) and, oddly, a replacement professor was appointed (Hall) although the UMDS already had one in Levison. Hall left for what appeared to be a better offer in Dundee in 1993. Levison was then the single UMDS professor, took a good look at the difficult people at St Thomas' Hospital (McKee, Fletcher etc) and was attracted back home to Dundee in 1995. A long hiatus followed and Sebastian Lucas was appointed. This was actually bizarre, since there was an excellent local personal chair pathologist *in situ* (Fletcher), but three times he was rejected by the appointments committee, once with no appointment and twice in favour of outsiders (Hall, Lucas). Such was local politics! More bizarre was the fact that Lucas had strong backing from the Experimental Pathology Professor, Frank Walsh, even though anyone with open eyes would know that Lucas had no basic science research leanings

whatsoever, and little ability to stimulate such activity in others. In 1997, Whimster died whilst lecturing at Kings College London and there was no question of re-appointing a pathologist professor to Kings College Hospital, even though 'Guys, Kings and Thomas' had not yet happened. So from three to one professor in 4 years'.

And other parts of the country have faced similar problems: the period of most rapid and profound change was during the 1990s. The tension between the increasing pressure of service commitments and the drive to improve research quality and productivity led to the creation of NHS consultant posts to work alongside the clinical academic consultants. The headship of the histopathology service, historically an *ex officio* role of the academic head of department, became a rotational position open to NHS and academic consultants. The number of clinical lecturer posts was cut, although Sheffield is one of the few academic centres to have been able to retain as many as two!

In others we have seen appointments of non-pathologists to chairs of pathology, e.g. in Bristol when Tom Hewer retired (who was not only a general pathologist of the old school who carried full clinical responsibilities, but also an expert botanist; he was also a keen Comparative Pathologist and was extremely interested in the results of the autopsies on animals that died at the Bristol Zoo) he was succeeded by Professor Sir Michael Anthony Epstein. Professor Epstein is well-known as one of the discoverers of the Epstein-Barr virus and was succeeded in 1981 by Ian Silver, a Professor of Comparative or Veterinary Pathology. Although there is no room for doubt about the quality of Epstein as a scientist, I have yet to be persuaded that such appointments really do anything for our discipline: chairs of pathology should really be about developing our subject and providing role models for young people starting out in our subject, the scope of which I have defined above. Talented as such individuals are, I would argue emphatically that chairs of pathology are not appropriate for them.

However, more than one Professor of Pathology has asked me about their future and their role in the future academic firmament. Consider Sebastian Lucas: 'from being the leader within the Pathology Division of the old medical school, there is no such now, and he is a member of the Division of Immunobiology solely on the basis of an interest in HIV and other infectious diseases. He will not be included in the next RAE, because the medical school only wants 5 and 5* persons on its books. The reason why he has survived without transfer to the Trust, along with all (*sic*) the other clinical pathology professors in the medical school hospitals, is simple: the chair that he inherited from Levison is funded 80/20 by the NHS and the medical school. Because he does sufficient teaching to occupy the 20%, it is not worth the fuss (the medical school has handled the transfers with staggering cack-handedness and it is surprising that so many good people stay on into Trust positions). When he retires in 2012, he will not be replaced in the same mould. The gold-inscribed board listing Lecturers and Professors of Pathology at St Thomas's has some space under his name, but it is unlikely that a molecular biologist would want his or her name associated with the other names above. What is the role of a Professor of Pathology in modern times and how can he/she survive in the RAE climate of 'money is all'? The answers are, respectively, important and with considerable difficulty! Either by single-mindedly ploughing a field that is brilliant in output despite the odds (e.g. Isaacson); or by being less research interested but developing a special interest that makes him locally and nationally important in pathology governance. We do have a leadership role for our peers and trainees nationally, and the destruction of the old system is diminishing this.' (S. Lucas, personal communication).

ENVOI

Well, I can hear you saying, what a desperate situation! What is he doing writing this stuff and not out there doing something about it? I think there is a need for a sense of perspective. These are troublesome times for academic medicine, and we are not alone, In the 'craft specialties' in particular, where there is the expectation that a high level of practical competence has to be combined with internationally competitive research, as in academic surgery, we have suffered. There has to be a remedy for this somewhere. Moreover, we tend to compare ourselves now with the situation in the 1980s, when academic pathology was really motoring: what I hope this piece has set in perspective is that this was not always so. We have seen the waxing and waning of our subject and we can debate, as I have above, the reasons for this, but a visit to one of the Society's meetings does show, quite unequivocally in my view, that pathology research of the highest quality is being presented. I would concede that there is not enough of it: so what must be done? What we have to find now is a recipe for resurgence that is consistent with the new rules of the game. How can we re-establish an environment where both investigative and surgical pathology can regenerate in this country?

Of course, it is really a simply matter: we have to attract the right people and train them properly in the right environment. We need to nurture and support them but there are several barriers to this simple solution. Firstly, we have to get the career structure right. The recent Walport proposals,[10] which really codify the path that a number of successful researchers have taken in recent years, but supported with (hopefully) acceptance and financial backing, will help considerably. I sincerely hope that the by-word will be 'flexibility', which will mean that those intent on pursuing an academic career will not meet with obstructionism in realising the level of their professional expertise: that is not to plead for a lapse in standards, but a more flexible approach to meeting those standards in a more specialised field. Then there is the nature of our subject. I would argue that there are a growing number of younger investigators in British academic pathology who are competing at the right level, and we need to encourage these and develop more of them; on the principle of like breeds like, these are the people we look to be the role models for the next generation and to found the next dynasty of academic pathologists in this country, and they must not shrink from this responsibility. At the same time, it is absolutely imperative that we support and underpin academic surgical pathology in this country and bring it back where it belongs – into university departments. This will be far from easy – the barriers have been pointed out above; we could start by trying to heal the breach between investigative and surgical pathology, and a good place to start is to recognise our mutual interdependence. We have to make surgical pathology recognised again as a legitimate academic pursuit of the highest order – the case is easily made but, as I have made clear, remains unrecognised. This rehabilitation must start from within – we ourselves have to recognise its importance and unashamedly proselytise to those outside. There are many avenues in which we can do this, and we should start now.

I hope it is also clear that the environment for conducting clinical research in this country is becoming more and more hostile: everywhere one looks there are barriers and more are erected by the year, much of it rabbinical in its complexity. We have let this happen to ourselves and now we have to reverse the trend. We now need leaders in all branches of our profession who are prepared to stand up and be counted and to say that enough is enough: the bureaucracy surrounding research has to be simplified and in some areas disappear. The Pathological Society should be an advocate of this and act as a catalyst for this broad view of pathology.

Finally, there is a case for remembering that, as Oliver Lacon remarked, 'we are not keepers of a sacred flame; we have to adapt'.[11] To some extent this is true and academic groupings may indeed change: we may see the demise of the traditional Department of Pathology, as has happened

[10] In March 2005 a report was produced by the academic subcommittee of Modernising Medical Careers (MMC) and the UK Clinical Research Collaboration (UKCRC), providing recommendations for the future training of medically and dentally qualified academic staff. The subcommittee is chaired by Dr Mark Walport, Director of the Wellcome Trust, and has become known anecdotally as the 'Walport' report. The aim of the report is to set out clear training pathways for those doctors and dentists wishing to pursue an academic career. The recommendations in the report are supported by £2.5 million from the Department of Health as part of their commitment to establishing integrated academic training programmes for academic clinicians of the future.

[11] Smiley's People' by John Le Carre, Hodder and Stoughton, 1980.

in several medical schools, but this should not be a matter for despair. What we must hold to is our firm belief that pathology is the foundation of medicine, that change in structure caused by disease and their cellular and molecular basis is arguably the most important field in medical research now and for the foreseeable future; and those who prosecute it, be they developmental biologists, neuroscientists, mouse geneticists or whatever, are really, whether they like it or not, thinking and working as pathologists. We simply have to make people recognise this, harness this effort and bring pathology back to centre stage, where it really belongs.

Fetal or foetal?

I had the great privilege of working for a year with Sam Freedman, the Canadian co-discoverer of CEA. We shared sabbaticals at the Chester Beatty Research Institute with Munro Neville and Tom Symington. Sam was keen for us to seek a substance in fetal lymphoid tissues that might be re-expressed in lymphomas and lymphocytic leukaemias, and having similar utility to that of CEA. We soon identified a candidate substance in splenic tissue harbouring lymphoma and we set about its characterisation. Eventually we realised that we had rediscovered fetal globin using immunological methods. It was expressed in the extramedullary haemopoietic tissue sometimes accompanying splenic infitration by lymphoma.

After my presentation to The Pathological Society, Professor Bernard Lennox (1914–1997) challenged my use of 'foetal'. I had avoided 'fetal', believing that it was an Americanised spelling (as with 'tumor'). However, Professor Lennox suggested correctly that it should be 'fetal', derived from the Latin *fetus*. There was no time left to discuss the pathological aspects of my paper! I discovered only on reading Lennox's obituary (*British Medical Journal* 1997;**315**:432) that he was the principal medical consultant to the *Oxford English Dictionary*.

James Underwood

The origins of Finnan Haddie

It was the summer meeting in Aberdeen, at a Civic Reception, hosted by the Provost at City Hall. Surprisingly, it was a glorious evening. The Provost was a man of such imposing stature as to rival Munro Neville, but about as useful for the purposes of conversation as a sea cucumber. So boring was he that the Officers of the Society were deputed to keep him company one by one, in rotation. It was my turn, and as the Program Secretary I followed Munro. I wished him a good evening, which he countered with a mere nod. Silence. I frantically casted about for a conversational gambit. Finally I had one – I had studied a local map on the plane coming up. Quoth I: 'You're very lucky having the seaside village of Findon so close to Aberdeen'. Raised eyebrows as the Provost growled 'And why might that be, young man' (I was younger then). 'Well', said I, 'Because of the Finnan Haddie that comes from there'. (My senior colleague Alec Watson had told me this many years before). 'Och no', was the crushing response. 'A Finnan Haddie is a special type of haddock. It has nothing to do with Findon'. 'Oh,' I said, very taken aback, 'I'm sure you're right'.

You may have noticed, but Englishmen have a way of saying these words which mean the very opposite, and this attribute had obviously kicked in without my realising it. The Provost glowered at me, and looking over my shoulder, called out to one of his colleagues – aldermen – or whatever they are called north of the border. 'Angus. Tell the young man here the origin of the term "Finnan Haddie".' Of course he had to answer 'Why, because they originally came from Findon, quite close to here'. Oh my God, I thought. Sure enough, the Provost was now exceedingly exercised, called over another colleague, and interrogated him, with the same result. I was now becoming quite agitated, since the Provost was showing every sign of losing his temper, and heads were beginning to turn. But then the lovely Dr Boyd, a very senior member of the Society from Glasgow came across to my rescue, and pointedly asked me in a loud voice. 'Professor Wright, what appears to be the problem here'. 'The Provost and I were ruminating on the origins of the term "Finnan Haddie",' I replied, weakly. 'It's well known,' said the formidable Dr Boyd, in the same very loud voice that reverberated across the room. 'It's because they came from Findon. I'm very surprised, Provost, that you did not know this, it being so close to Aberdeen'. As they used to say in Punch, 'collapse of stout party'.

But this was not the end of this affair. The following Tuesday, I received a letter. It was from Dr Boyd, enclosing a photocopy of a page from a Scottish Dictionary of Phrases, which gave chapter and verse about the Finnan Haddie. I noted, initially with consternation, and then with growing admiration, that the letter and enclosure had been copied to the Provost of the City of Aberdeen. How this was received I know not – but it increased my respect for that generation of Scottish pathologists, before whom, if you spoke at all, you had to be entirely sure of your ground and of your references. I have not forgotten this lesson.

Nicholas Wright

The value of stygian darkness

The meeting of The Pathological Society that remains most vividly in my memory is the first one that I ever attended in July 1959. This was shortly after I had come to Britain and started to apply the, then fairly new, technique of immunofluorescence to vascular lesions. The session at which I was to give my presentation was well attended, most notably by Professor Dorothy Russell from the London. I thought her terrifying, an impression that was reinforced by her savaging the presentation and its presenters that immediately preceded mine. In those days the degree of immunofluorescence obtainable was much inferior to what developed subsequently and, in order that my preparations would be clearly visible, I gave my paper in stygian darkness. The fact that the members of the audience, instead of the transparencies, were invisible, did wonders for my confidence and enabled me to give a blush-free presentation.

Neville Woolf

A gentleman pathologist

An anecdote has emerged from my foggy old brain! It illustrates the image that pathologists' had of themselves over 50 years ago. The occasion was a Path Soc meeting in the early 1950s to which I went as a very junior trainee at the invitation of my chief, Professor Robert Scarff, the Director of the Bland-Sutton Institute of Pathology at the Middlesex Hospital. Scarff was a dour, down to earth character with a dry sense of humour. On this occasion I recall him pointing out the figure of Professor Hewer of Bristol who was very formally attired in wing collar and tie, black jacket, striped trousers and highly polished shoes. Scarff said 'Ah, there is Professor Hewer, a gentleman Pathologist, the only one!'

Basil Morson

10 Microbiology and The Pathological Society

Brian I. Duerden and J. Gerald Collee

INTRODUCTION

For its first 75 years The Pathological Society encompassed the broad church of pathology and microbiology (primarily bacteriology) as interrelated and mutually supportive disciplines. The Society's meetings addressed both of these in a single programme and the *Journal of Pathology and Bacteriology* reflected this unity of purpose. The accounts of H. Dible (Chapter 2) and A.C. Lendrum (Chapter 3) provide good records of the combined fortunes of pathology and bacteriology up to the 75th Anniversary of the Society. Here we attempt to trace the changes that drove our disciplines along separate lines in the later decades of the 20th century and into the new millennium.

The last quarter of the 20th century saw increasing divergences in the academic activities and service provisions of the two disciplines. The first major result for the Society was the separation of the *Journal of Pathology and Bacteriology* into its two component subject areas as the *Journal of Pathology* and the *Journal of Medical Microbiology*. The meetings themselves also divided the subject matter with parallel sessions on histopathology and morbid anatomy and microbiology, although continued and often very successful attempts were made to provide cross-disciplinary sessions that emphasised the scientific unity of pathology. Nevertheless, by the end of the century the academic and professional bases of the disciplines had diverged to such an extent that a broad pathology-based society was no longer the most appropriate forum for microbiology. An amicable separation was therefore agreed, with the microbiology section of the Society moving into the newly created clinical microbiology group of the Society for General Microbiology (SGM). At the same time, the responsibility for and ownership of the *Journal of Medical Microbiology* was also transferred to the SGM.

Three themes are inextricably linked in the story of microbiology and The Pathological Society during this period: (i) the changing pattern of microbiology as a scientific and clinical discipline; (ii) the creation of new societies and associations and the exponential growth in scientific conferences and symposia; and (iii) the increasing volume and specialisation of medical and scientific publications.

THE SUBJECT AND PRACTICE OF MICROBIOLOGY

The Society's recognition of medical microbiology as an independent and expanding discipline with the launch of the *Journal of Medical Microbiology* in 1968 coincided with a period of political (and medical) disregard for the continued threat of infection and infectious diseases. Infection was conquered; antibiotics and vaccines had controlled infectious diseases. This misguided view had serious consequences for medical microbiology as a profession, for its academic base and for patient care in developed and developing countries. There was an ever-increasing disparity

Table 10.1 Examples of 'new' infections described since 1975

HIV/AIDS
Hepatitis C, E
HTLV
HHV6, 7, 8
Lassa, Ebola viruses
Nipah, Hendra viruses
Hantavirus (SN)
Avian influenza
SARS
Legionella spp.
Campylobacter spp.
Clostridium difficile
Helicobacter pylori
Escherichia coli O157 (VTEC)
Vibrio cholerae O139
Cryptosporidium parvum
Chlamydia trachomatis
vCJD

between what was happening within microbiology and how it was perceived elsewhere in medicine, particularly by those responsible for the policy and management of health services. Modern medical advances focused particularly on cancer treatment and heart disease. The increased life expectancy, huge advances in cancer treatment by radiotherapy and chemotherapy (with the inevitable immunosuppression and risk of infection), ever more complex surgery in the fields of cardiac, orthopaedic and neurosurgery and the increasing numbers of patients living far longer with chronic illnesses all created a population at greater risk of infection; but the infections were considered a nuisance rather than a priority. At the same time, medical microbiology and infection control were moving apace. There was new technology as the genomics revolution took hold, new antibiotics (and new resistance mechanisms), new societies, new journals, new guidelines for dealing with infection and a succession of new diseases. Examples of the new infections that have been recognised since 1975 are shown in Table 10.1. However, increasingly infection and infection control were deemed to be the province of the microbiologists and infection control specialists rather than the mainstream of medicine. During the 1980s and 1990s there were increasing clinical problems with healthcare-associated infections (methicillin-resistant *Staphylococcus aureus*, antibiotic-associated diarrhoea and colitis due to *Clostridium difficile*, opportunist infections with *Acinetobacter* spp., explosive outbreaks of norovirus diarrhoea, etc.), increasing antimicrobial resistance (and fewer new antibiotics to combat these infections) and threats of new pandemics of influenza and other infectious diseases. These increased the need for microbiology and microbiologists, but the profile of infection specialists and the supply of microbiologists were decreasing. Within medicine in the UK there were fewer training posts for microbiologists, and on the academic front the profile of medical microbiology became much reduced. There was less impact on medical students and their training, and the successive research assessment exercises led further to a dislocation of the academic and service interface as they focused more on basic science research than on applied aspects of infection diagnosis, treatment and control.

By the 1960s it had become clear that the research bases of bacteriology and virology were pulling microbiology away from its traditional links with histopathology and were developing rapidly as separate scientific pursuits, supported and contested by the burgeoning disciplines of immunology, molecular biology and microbial genetics. We also had to take account of advances in mycology, protozoology and helminthology. Within this, microbiology had to adapt to rapidly developing approaches to nucleic acid interactions and genetic engineering in all its many forms, from phage-mediated genetic exchange to antibiotic resistance transfer by conjugation. While we adopted genome sequence analysis for taxonomic and virulence investigations, we were also adapting to major technical advances in diagnostic laboratory work. Similarly, histopathology was contending with huge advances in immunology, clinical chemistry and haematology, in which new concepts of molecular interactions from cytokines to pathophysiological cascade systems became the order of the day.

The whole genomics revolution in medical science grew out of microbiological science (Judson, 1996) but this had mixed effects on medical microbiology. In some areas, academic medical microbiology disappeared as a recognisable entity, subsumed into 'molecular medicine,' whereas, sadly, clinical microbiology was often slow to embrace the new technology and remained firmly entrenched in diagnostic methods that traced their direct lineage from the work of Pasteur, Koch and their colleagues in the 19th century. Although there were rapid advances in our understanding of the pathophysiology of infectious diseases and the genetics of virulence, especially in virology, applied research and development work in important public health areas such as microbial epidemiology and infection control did not attract major research funding, weakening the clinical microbiology research base. Senior academic posts were not being refilled; indeed, in the 1980s, Professor Kevin McCarthy (chairing the Association of Professors of Medical Microbiology) declared that professors of medical microbiology were an endangered species. Moreover, changes were occurring in undergraduate medical education as it moved from a subject-based, taught curriculum, with pathology and medical microbiology strongly represented as the scientific bases of medical practice. Integrated, system-based curricula with a strong emphasis on self-directed and problem-based learning became fashionable. This further weakened the academic base of medical microbiology and reduced the visibility of the subject as a potential medical career (see Chapter 12).

Towards the end of the 20th century the tide began to turn again. Major hospital outbreaks of salmonellosis (Wakefield) and legionellosis (Stafford) in the UK generated public enquiries and the subsequent appointment of Consultants for Communicable Disease Control in all districts (the old Medical Officers of Health had been abolished in 1974). The inexorable spread of HIV/AIDS, the resurgence of tuberculosis, cholera and dengue and the continued presence of malaria focused international attention on infectious diseases. Then the recognition of healthcare-associated infections as a major challenge (and cost) to healthcare services in developed as well as developing countries attracted fierce attention from politicians, the press and media and Departments of Health and health service managers. In the first few years of the 21st century infection was once again a healthcare priority and lessons of the previous 150 years (hand hygiene, asepsis and cleanliness) were having to be re-learned against a background of modern medical technology. The need for an understanding of the microbial world with training in infection control for all healthcare professionals and the importance of applied research and development were again recognised. Microbiologists, perhaps now better referred to as Infection Specialists, are once again obliged to accept the challenge and seize the opportunity to deliver their expertise to help reduce the impact of infection on the population's health. The pressing problem is that their numbers and resources have been badly depleted at a time when they are urgently needed.

SCIENTIFIC MEETINGS AND TRAINING IN PATHOLOGY

For the first 60 years of its existence The Pathological Society had played a leading role in training and career development for pathologists, including microbiologists. However, by the early 1960s there was a groundswell for change within the Society's ranks, and not least in connection with the need for recognition of our new sub-disciplines and the requirement for an examination system that would guide our training as our interests and their applications at academic and clinical levels diverged. The history of events that led to the foundation of the (Royal) College of Pathologists and the provision of a structure that served these needs is well documented by Goddard (2005) and in Chapter 11. Despite much debate and fierce protest from some members, the electorate of The Pathological Society in 1960–1961 were narrowly in favour of the founding of a College and supported the appointment of provisional officers, with Sir Roy Cameron as President in 1962. The first examinations were held in 1964 and our changed circumstances were set. Our continuing commitments to education and training became the province of the College, but with important input from many Society members.

During the same period it became clear that joint programmes with a major histopathology component were not attractive to either research or clinical microbiologists. The Society recognised this by breaking its long tradition of the unity of pathology to provide parallel programmes for pathology and microbiology, with some joint sessions of mutual interest. They were pioneered by R.E.O. Williams as Meetings Secretary, who did sterling work to edit microbiological contributions for publication in the new *Journal of Medical Microbiology*. However, this did not stem the flow of microbiologists away from the Society's meetings during the 1970s. As clinical microbiological interest focused on the problems of antimicrobial resistance and hospital infection, new societies such as the British Society for Antimicrobial Chemotherapy and the Hospital Infection Society were founded and their meetings became major focal points for medical microbiologists. In the 1980s the Association of Medical Microbiologists was formed to provide a professional forum for microbiology, and The Pathological Society meetings were no longer in the mainstream of professional interest for microbiologists. Attendance at the microbiology sessions reached a nadir in the late 1970s when a large coffee table seemed a more appropriate meeting venue than a small lecture theatre. A decision had to be made – either to disband the microbiology section or to make a determined effort to reinvigorate it. The remaining enthusiasts chose the latter route and the first action was to appoint a separate Microbiology Meetings Secretary to re-launch the meetings programme and to look for joint activities with other microbiology societies.

Under the successive guidance of Charles Easmon, Mary Cooke, Rosamund Williams and Curtis Gemmell, each supported by a small but enthusiastic Microbiology Subcommittee, this worked well and the reinvigorated microbiology programme continued for another 20 years. Meetings were well attended, especially the winter meetings in London. There were high quality and very successful symposia on Gram-negative sepsis, anaerobes, meningococcal disease, sexually transmitted infections, mycobacteriology and others that balanced academic research with clinical aspects of microbiology and the epidemiology of infection. However, as the 20th century neared its close, it was clear that medical microbiologists would not regard the Society as a major outlet for their activities. The Society for General Microbiology was the major academic and professional society for (mostly) non-medical microbiology but had raised its profile in the traditional Pathological Society area of microbial pathogenesis. At the same time, the professional societies that represented clinical microbiology and infectious diseases were pooling their resources to create an annual national meeting under the banner of the Federation of Infection Societies. Although not one of the original founding group, the microbiology section of the Society was very pleased to become a partner in the Federation. The microbiology section also gave strong support to the creation of a new clinical microbiology group to complement the existing microbial pathogenicity group at the SGM and, after due negotiations between the two societies, after 95 years The Pathological Society's microbiology section wound up its activities in 2002 and transferred allegiance to the SGM, along with its 'seat' in the Federation.

THE *JOURNAL OF MEDICAL MICROBIOLOGY*

The difficulties encountered in maintaining microbiological interest in the Society's meetings contrasted with the success and growth of the Society's microbiology journal. By the late 1960s it was clear that researchers wished to publish their work in journals specifically focused on their own subject (except for the higher echelons of *Nature* and the *Lancet*). The senior microbiological members of the Society were increasingly aware that scientists were demanding recognition of the many emerging sub-disciplines within the subject and were setting up successful independent journals to meet the demand. Despite his personal commitment to the joint journal, C.L. Oakley presided over the separation of the twins and the launch of their independent lives as the *Journal of Medical Microbiology* and the *Journal of Pathology*, initially acting as Editor-in-Chief of both. Under his dynamic and uncompromising leadership, the first editorial team, comprising S.D Elek, R. Blowers, J.P. Duguid, M.T. Parker, H. Stern and J.G. Collee, were very conscious of their responsibility for this break with tradition. The new journal was immediately successful and flourished under the successive editorships of Oakley, Elek, Collee and then B.I. Duerden. The journal developed an eclectic style of editorial management that created a strong 'collegiate' team ethos among its editors. For the first 20 years there was no traditional Editor-in-Chief. There was a Chairman of the Board, appointed by the Society's committee, but other senior editors took individual responsibility for running the reception and registry office and the rejection and rehabilitation office. In a novel but pivotal role, the sureditor was responsible for taking all accepted papers through to publication; he (they were all male) edited every paper, sorted out tables and figures, liaised with the publishers and printers, arranged the circulation and collation of proofs and did the contents make-up. Robert Blowers fine-tuned this role from 1977 and then handed it on to Brian Duerden in 1982. Proofreading was an essential quality assurance procedure for the journal. Not only were proofs sent to the authors and read line by line by the sureditor, but also to the original assigned editor and a third editor as 'collateral proofreader'. This gave the journal an enviable record of minimal corrigendum notices and served as a mutual education exercise for the editors.

The *Journal of Medical Microbiology* editors inherited from Oakley and his predecessors an unshakeable commitment to sustaining the quality, clarity and accuracy of scientific English. Many authors were amazed at the painstaking editorial work performed on their manuscripts but most were profoundly grateful for the improved clarity of their papers and their 'free tutorials' on scientific writing. Editorial colleagues and authors alike were indebted to Tom Parker and James Duguid for their sterling contributions in setting our standards of industry and care. From the Journal's inception, the editors felt a responsibility to authors to get worthwhile science into print even when initially poor presentation seemed to obscure the interesting science, especially when the author's first language was not English. This was why the rejection editor always had rehabilitation as an equal (and more time-consuming) part of the role.

When Duerden succeeded Blowers as the senior editor, the journal was still a quarterly publication with about 55 papers per year, perhaps a reflection of the less frenetic research environment of the time. By the 1980s, more papers were being submitted and there was an ever-increasing demand for faster review and publication. Under the guidance of Collee and Duerden, and ably supported by David Old and other senior colleagues, the journal expanded to first six and then eight issues per year, and reached the goal of monthly publication in 1988. Through the 1990s the editorial office at Chepstow and the meetings venue at Tintern became the *Journal's* nerve centre and spiritual home, with Marjorie Duerden working impressively to meet the heavy demands of increasing submissions and shorter turnaround times. To meet the demands of the modern readership and broaden the educational appeal, editorials, review articles, a technical note and a correspondence section were added to the essential core element of original reports of microbiological research.

A notable birthday was celebrated in 1993 with the Silver Jubilee of the *Journal of Medical Microbiology*. A memorable symposium that provided modern updates on the topics covered in the first issue (*Haemophilus influenzae*, *Bordetella pertussis*, *Escherichia coli* in farm animals, staphylococcal virulence, and listeriosis) was equally memorable as a microbiological event for those editors who were also members of the Pathological Society committee. Of 27 committee members and guests who attended the committee dinner 36 hours before the symposium, 21 became acutely ill with enteritis clinically characteristic of infection with norovirus (small round virus of Norwark type). The incident was a point source outbreak, probably linked to contaminated shellfish, with the onset occurring between 36 and 48 hours after the meal; symptoms of vomiting, diarrhoea, headache, fever, rigors and muscular aches ranged from moderate to incapacitating and two committee members were admitted to hospital. J.G.C. (who had not been at the dinner) shouldered the burden of chairing the whole symposium while the co-chairman (B.I.D.) was confined to his hotel room.

The growth of interest in medical microbiology research and education was further emphasised when the then publishers of the journal, Churchill Livingstone, launched a sister journal, *Reviews in Medical Microbiology*, with support from the Society and under the initial editorship of Rosamund Williams. However, the publishers and the Society soon parted company (the publishers believing that medical microbiology would be itself divided and subsumed in a combination of molecular medicine and clinical infectious diseases) and both journals came within the Chapman and Hall and subsequently the Lippincott Williams and Wilkins stable. At the start of the new millennium, as the Society's microbiology section moved closer to the SGM, it was recognised that the most appropriate publishing home would now be the publishing arm of the SGM. With this move, Ian Poxton took over the senior editorship with an enlarged editorial team now backed by a well-integrated professional publishing office. This move also secured electronic (in addition to continued hard copy) publication of the journal, which had been a priority for the editors, if not the publishers, for several years. The transfer of the Journal's ownership was a very generous 'dowry' from The Pathological Society to help launch the new clinical microbiology activities of the SGM and maintain the essence of continuity. The benefits of this change have been immediately evident in further increases in submissions and a higher profile in the microbiological community, with a notable increase in the Journal's impact factor.

FINALE

Microbiology has had a strong tradition in The Pathological Society. Our personal views are reflected in these individual comments:

> 'Early in my bacteriological career, I learned that The Pathological Society and its network was of enormous importance in our discipline. The Society set demanding standards in relation to professional competence, in the delivery of papers at meetings and at all stages of published work. It was, in effect, the labour exchange at which promising recruits for senior appointments were discreetly assessed. Our seniors were very regular attenders at all the Society's meetings and we were well aware of their interest in all that was on display. These were testing times and the experience was at once daunting and stimulating.
>
> The *Journal of Pathology and Bacteriology* occupied a central position in all of this. To publish in its pages was indeed a significant achievement. Authors quickly became aware of the meticulous refereeing and checking of manuscripts under editors who were very jealous of the reputation of such a medical scientific publication. When I joined the editorial team, I was deeply impressed with the wealth of talent and experience around me – a daunting challenge to a new recruit. I was profoundly grateful for all the help and advice that were generously given. These were important influences to guide me when it was my turn to be more senior and to guide the next generation of editors.' (J.G.C.)

> 'When I joined the Edinburgh Department of Bacteriology as a very young lecturer, J.G.C. immediately suggested I join The Pathological Society. My first individual paper was published in the *Journal of Medical Microbiology* and my first public presentation was at a Pathological

Society meeting – still a nerve-wracking experience. When I needed to move to widen my experience, it was through The Pathological Society and its then General Secretary, Michael McEntegart, who was very keen to offer me a post in his Sheffield department. I was then thrilled to be invited to join the *Journal of Medical Microbiology* editorial board in 1976 and it has been one of my proudest achievements to have subedited the journal for 20 years on behalf of The Pathological Society and to see it progressing so strongly with the transfer to the SGM under Ian Poxton.' (B.I.D.)

Microbiology has had to go its separate way but it owes much to its union with The Pathological Society over the last 100 years. Loyalties and pressures have changed and the new millennium presents new challenges and significant differences in our approaches to academic appointments, teaching, research, funding, training, recruitment and laboratory practice. There are equally demanding problems in providing effective microbiology services to our hospitals and to family and community doctors, and in maintaining proper links with the public health and health protection services. It is not surprising that these and other duties and obligations are pulling medical microbiologists in many different directions. Accordingly, academic and clinical microbiologists and epidemiologists and clinicians concerned with infectious disease must maintain contact with each other if we are to maintain the remarkably productive links that have advanced our discipline so well. Equally, in our continuing elucidation and understanding of the pathophysiology of human disease involving microbial systems, it is crucial that pathologists and microbiologists continue to nurture an essential partnership that has served the development of medical science so significantly in the past. It must be even more jealously guarded and valued as we face the challenges of the years ahead.

REFERENCES

Goddard, P.F. (2005) History of the College, Part 2. *Bull. R. Coll. Pathol.* **131**: 72–75.

Judson, H.F. (1996) *The Eight Days of Creation*. CSHL Press: Cold Spring Harbor, New York.

Trial by Senior Member

I gave my first ever public presentation to The Pathological Society at the Winter meeting in 1968; the paper was entitled 'The cellular reaction in choriocarcinoma'. It was, without doubt, the most terrifying experience of my professional life! There were two main reasons for this. In the first place, I asked a 'friend' to help me prepare the talk but he suggested that a more senior colleague would be more appropriate. Unfortunately this was a deeply unpleasant man who espoused the 'ritual humiliation' method of rehearsal and who very nearly convinced me that my results were fraudulent. The second reason was the 'Trial by Senior Member' that one endured at Path Soc in those days; all sessions were plenary and it was a truly daunting experience to be faced by serried ranks of eminent Professors, who, it was rumoured, could destroy a blossoming career with a single carefully worded question. In the end I was very lucky because the speaker before me was foolhardy enough to read her paper rather than give it from memory. When it was my turn the 'feeding frenzy' was over, appetites were sated and I was given a relatively easy time. My abiding memory of the day is actually a happy one because at the end of the session Professor Bill Robertson, whom I had never met before, made a point of taking me to one side and making kind remarks about my paper. So I survived both ordeals and giving lectures has never been quite so harrowing since!

Christopher Elston

Sense-of-humour failure?

It was a Cambridge January PathSoc meeting and very cold in Trinity Hall, where we were staying. Extra blankets and overcoats on the bed, with ice inside the windows. Late Friday afternoon, the domestic staff noticed that smoke was billowing from one the rooms. The fire brigade was called and arrived immediately. On entering the smoke-filled room, they encountered a desperate scene. The then Dr Phil Quirke had apparently been rehearsing his talk, and had left his slide projector on (imagine, carting a slide projector all the way from Leeds – talk about insecurity!) and this machine had overheated and caught fire. The room was a mess, and all Dr Quirke's clothes were utterly ruined. On his return to get changed for the evening dinner, Dr Quirke was confronted with the spectacle of all his belongings destroyed. Undaunted, he managed, in true PathSoc spirit, to borrow sufficient clothing to make a more-or-less respectable appearance at the dinner. But there was a slight, but perceptible, sense-of-humour failure, when I announced during my after-dinner speech that the fire had been caused by 'one of Dr Quirke's sex aids starting without him'. I remember telling the members, when the derisive laughter had died down, that 'Quirke was a man of few words, but he had just given me the benefit of two of them'.

Nicholas Wright

What's the fuss?

My first good (only?) presentation was in Dublin 1986 when I gave an oral presentation on AIDS in Uganda (hot stuff for the time), and nearly broke down whilst thinking and talking about the appalling statistics and mortality. Of course, it has got much worse since then in resource-poor countries. Mike Wells asked what I wore to protect myself during autopsy procedures on such patients, and I replied 'gloves', wondering (as I still do) what the fuss over risk was all about.

Sebastian Lucas

Reconnaissance is key

At Edinburgh 1993, I had a talk on paediatric AIDS all lined up for dual projection. Luckily I observed a very senior member of the Society giving an invited lecture and making a complete hash of the dual projection system. On inspecting the podium lectern, it transpired that the buttons were on asymmetric holders, at different heights on the podium, with the left button commanding the right projector and vice versa. I changed my talk to single projection!

Sebastian Lucas

The early Pleistocene

I remember giving a paper with Bob Curran in a forward row. At that time his grave demeanor and *basso profund* struck terror into the hearts of many juniors. He approached me after the talk and said 'I was going to ask a question' – at this stage I was nervous – 'but it was all very clear' – at which stage I was surprised, but by then he had gone. It will probably strike current Lecturers (if any are left) that it was absurd to be scared of the Professoriat but I speak of the early Pleistocene.

Colin Berry

11 A Short History of the Royal College of Pathologists

James C. E. Underwood[1]

ORIGINS OF THE MEDICAL ROYAL COLLEGES

Medical Royal Colleges have their roots in the early 16th century. The forerunner of the Royal College of Surgeons of Edinburgh, the oldest medical Royal College, was established in 1505 to regulate the barber surgeons. At that time, there were barbers who cut through hair and barber surgeons who, presumably with intent, incised skin and did other invasive procedures. Operative surgery was limited in anatomical extent by the absence of anaesthesia, but harm could result from even the most superficial procedures undertaken by untrained practitioners. Thus, the aim was to regulate clinical practice through a process of training and credentialling. This enduring principle was set out in the Seal of Cause granted in July 1505 by the Town Council of Edinburgh to the barber surgeons:

> '... that no manner of person occupy or practise any points of our said craft of surgery ... unless he be worthy and expert in all points belonging to the said craft, diligently and expertly examined and admitted by the Maisters of the said craft and that he know Anatomy and the nature and complexion of every member of the human body ... for every man ocht to know the nature and substance of everything that he works or else he is negligent.'

Surgery was in the vanguard of professional regulation through colleges because there was no other credentialling mechanism. Unlike physicians, who had to undergo a course of university education, surgeons learnt their craft through apprenticeship. The inclusion of surgery as part of the medical profession was completed through the Medical Act of 1858 and the establishment of the General Medical Council as the regulatory body for all doctors – physicians *and* surgeons.

The inception of Edinburgh's surgical college led, in the ensuing centuries, to the founding of colleges of surgeons and of physicians elsewhere. Thus, in England at the beginning of the 19th century there were just two medical Royal Colleges: the Royal College of Surgeons of England and the Royal College of Physicians of London. With increasing specialisation, some constituencies argued for creation of their own colleges separate from the ancient institutions. The first to secede was obstetrics and gynaecology, which delivered itself from the womb of the Royal College of Surgeons of England about 75 years ago. Other specialty-based colleges were established during the remainder of the 20th century: Royal Colleges of Radiologists, of Anaesthetists, of Psychiatrists, of Ophthalmologists, of Paediatrics and Child Health and of Pathologists.

EMERGENCE OF A COLLEGE OF PATHOLOGISTS

Although the word 'pathology' became widely used in medicine only as late as the 19th century, its principles nourished the early concepts underpinning Hippocratic medicine – medicine based

[1] Professor Sir James Underwood was President of the Royal College of Pathologists from 2002 to 2005.

on evidence and observation rather than on myth and superstition. Pathology was practised initially by physicians and surgeons, but its complexity and workload volume grew to the extent that it matured into a specialty in its own right. Its practitioners aspired to the same status, or higher, as that enjoyed by other consultants (Foster, 1982). Gradually, the Royal College of Physicians of London (RCP) came to be regarded as the appropriate body to represent pathology specialists.

In 1948, the RCP convened a Standing Committee on Pathology with the principal task of drafting recommendations for training and assessment, based on proposals from the Association of Clinical Pathologists (ACP) (Cunningham, 1992; Goddard, 2005). This led in 1951 to the Conjoint Diploma in Clinical Pathology ('conjoint' because it was a diploma of the Royal Colleges of Physicians of London and of Surgeons of England). However, trainee pathologists regarded this Diploma as having a status inferior to that of the MRCP standard to which they aspired. They feared that this would eventually brand them as 'sub-consultants'.

In his address in 1952 to the ACP, 'Does the pathologist need a faculty?', W.H. MacMenemey argued that pathology specialists should be credentialled with MRCP or FRCS, or another qualification with the same status. He did not favour a separate college. However, at its meeting in Exeter in 1953, the ACP debated and supported the motion that 'this meeting would welcome the institution of a college or faculty of pathologists'. To make progress towards this objective, the Association set up a committee under the chairmanship of Professor G. Hadfield. The most influential submission to the Hadfield Committee came in 1954 from five Sheffield pathologists – Eddie Blackburn, John Colquhoun, John Edwards, Arthur Jordan and Cecil Paine. The 'Sheffield memorandum' argued clearly and cogently for the establishment of a separate body (faculty or college); pathologists, they declared, should 'have their own house and be masters in it'.

The ACP's growing enthusiasm for a college contrasted with the neutrality, almost indifference, shown by The Pathological Society of Great Britain and Ireland. The Society declined to be represented on the Hadfield Committee, although it did accept observer status. The Society was not opposed to the formation of a college; its attitude stemmed from a belief that it was a purely scientific society and that it should distance itself from political issues (the proposal to form a college being regarded as such).

Hadfield's Committee reported in 1955, but without any decisive recommendation. Undoubtedly, the Committee realised that founding a new college would be no easy task and that the case for such a bold step would have to be very compelling. The Committee did, however, recognise the need to strengthen the training of pathologists and to have some means of satisfying consultant appointment committees that candidates were sufficiently competent to take on unsupervised responsibilities. Acting on the Hadfield Committee's findings, the ACP then voted against the formation of a college or faculty and reopened discussions with the RCP to set up a more acceptable pathology qualification, perhaps based on the MRCP. The MRCP offered by the Royal College of Physicians of Edinburgh was particularly favoured because it could be obtained after having sat a pathology component.

Unrest developed in the ranks of the ACP. In 1958, four branches persuaded its Council that the formation of a college should be considered afresh. A working party was established, chaired by Professor George Cunningham, and within a few months it issued proposals for a college and set out the procedure to be followed for its foundation. But there was still significant dissent. In his presidential address to the ACP in October 1958, W.H. MacMenemey (1958) summarised the arguments for and against a college of pathologists, and declared his personal opposition. However, a ballot of ACP members revealed a majority (69%) in favour of a college, so much so that they declared they would give it financial backing. The ACP's Council decided in 1959 that there was now sufficient support for the founding of a college, and The Pathological Society was approached for its view. Unfortunately, The Pathological Society's committee remained unenthusiastic, even though it declined to ballot its members and be guided by their views. Nevertheless, the Society allowed the ACP to conduct a ballot; this revealed only a small majority in favour and just 20% supported the financial proposals.

Concurrently, the Royal College of Physicians (London) revived its Pathology Committee, no doubt worried by the prospect of the secession of pathologists, and proposed a faculty within the College in which pathologists would have control of their discipline and run their own MRCP-equivalent examination.

Thus, in 1959, there were three options on the table:

1. Remain embedded within the general membership of the RCP.
2. Establish a Faculty of Pathologists within the RCP.
3. Set up a separate College of Pathologists.

The profession of pathology was now so strongly motivated to establish its own collegiate organisation that the first option was unsustainable; it was no longer seriously contemplated. Professor Cunningham was appointed chairman of a 'Ways and Means' committee to consider the remaining options. Cunningham's new committee reported in 1960 and, influenced by it, the ACP's Council resolved to pursue serious negotiations with the RCP, with a view to forming a faculty. (This was despite Cunningham's personal enthusiasm for an independent college.) Obviously, the RCP would need to be convinced that a majority of pathologists favoured a faculty, so voting papers were despatched with an explanatory booklet setting out the options. This watershed in the evolving professional representation of pathologists was the theme of Professor D. F. Cappel's ACP presidential address on 'Pathology at the crossroads' (Cappell, 1960).

The ballot process was heavily criticised and caused much dissent, but slightly more favoured (49.5%) than opposed (41.8%) an independent college. The ballot cannily gave voters the opportunity to reaffirm their faith in democracy by asking if they would support whichever option enjoyed greater support; 66% did so. So, substantial disagreement remained, but it was the younger pathologists who were most committed to a college. It was, after all, *their* future.

To pave the way to a College of Pathologists, the Council of the ACP set up a Joint Advisory Committee and invited representatives of The Pathological Society to serve on it. The Society's committee remained opposed to the idea, but it agreed to ballot the membership (even though many had already voted as ACP members); 52% supported the formation of a college. Guided by this albeit marginal majority, The Pathological Society's committee nominated five representatives, led by J. W. Howie, to sit on the Joint Advisory Committee. It reported in December 1961, proposing that the College of Pathologists be established with an entrance fee of £50. Consultants (including those in academic posts) and those becoming consultants within the next three years would be eligible for Founder Membership.

Thus, the College of Pathologists was formed. Its first meeting was held on 21 June 1962 at the London School of Tropical Medicine and Hygiene. Officers were appointed, and Professor Sir Roy Cameron, FRS, was installed as the first President. Examinations for membership began in 1964. The College of Pathologists was granted its Royal Charter in 1970 with Her Majesty Queen Elizabeth II as its patron.

The Royal College of Pathologists now has approximately 8000 members, most of whom work in pathology services and institutions in the UK. Through its Joint Committee on Higher Pathology Training, the College has responsibility for training curricula and assessments in histopathology, medical microbiology and chemical pathology. Curricula for the other pathology specialties, such as haematology and immunology, are administered through the Joint Committee for Higher Medical Training.

THE COLLEGE'S HEADQUARTERS

The Royal College of Pathologists is not a building. The College is its membership. But it does have a headquarters from which its many functions are delivered.

After a rather nomadic existence in its early years, 2 Carlton House Terrace in central London became the College's headquarters, with the Cancer Research Campaign (now Cancer Research UK) as joint tenants. Carlton House Terrace dates from the 1820s and is the work of John Nash (1752–1835) and Decimus Burton (1800–1881). This fine building is in the Crown Estate and is Grade 1 listed on account of its architectural importance. In 1941 it was gutted by an enemy bomb and it remained open to the sky until the late 1960s, when the lease was acquired on exceptionally favourable terms (due, no doubt, to the state of the building) through the generosity of Sir Michael Sobell, who died in 1993 at the age of 100 years. He is commemorated by a plaque in the College's foyer.

A major refurbishment, generously supported by a donation from The Pathological Society, was undertaken in the early 1990s. The next phase is a £3.5 million project to create an education centre in the lower ground floor (formerly known as 'the basement'), vacated a few years ago by Cancer Research UK which has now consolidated its activities elsewhere. This will include space for a public exhibition, part of the College's campaign to improve the public appreciation of pathology and its practitioners.

THE ACADEMY OF MEDICAL ROYAL COLLEGES

The growing number of medical Royal Colleges led to the need for a single voice that could speak for all on common issues. The first step in this direction led to the Standing Joint Committee of three major colleges (Physicians, Surgeons and Obstetricians & Gynaecologists). As new colleges formed, there was need for a fresh approach to cooperative working. Thus emerged in England, in 1974, the Conference of Royal Colleges and Faculties, mirroring one already established in Scotland and superceding the Standing Joint Committee. The Royal College of Pathologists was represented on the Conference.

In the early 1990s, the need for even stronger collegiate unison in British medicine became increasingly clear. The belief that the Conference could be administered by the college, of which its chairman was President, became unsustainable. So, in 1993, the Conference established its own office and staff, now located in the premises of the Royal Society of Medicine. Membership was extended to include presidents of the medical Royal colleges in the Republic of Ireland. In 1996, the Conference became the Academy of Medical Royal Colleges and was granted charitable status.

LINKS WITH THE PATHOLOGICAL SOCIETY OF GREAT BRITAIN AND IRELAND

The links between the College and The Pathological Society are not limited to sharing the same building. Histopathologists who have served as Presidents and other officers of the College have often been active members of The Pathological Society and contributed to the close working relationship between the two organisations. Recent evidence of this partnership includes well-attended annual meetings for trainees called 'Meet the Academics', subsequently emulated by haematologists in partnership with the British Society for Haematology.

The Pathological Society has been a generous contributor to the refurbishment of the College building and to academic aspects of the College's mission. In partnership with the Health

Foundation, The Pathological Society has contributed significantly to Clinician Scientist Fellowships administered by the College.

In contrast to the neutrality and indifference of The Pathological Society in the decades leading to the College's formation, it is now rightfully engaged in advising on the College's policies and strategies. For example, The Pathological Society is represented on the College's Specialty Advisory Committee for Histopathology.

ROUTES TO MEMBERSHIP OF THE COLLEGE

Among the original motives behind the founding of the College was the desire to have examinable standards for entry to the professional body of pathologists. The examination for membership has been in two parts probably since its inception. The first, taken after an initial period of training, assessed whether the trainee was suitable for higher professional training, eventually leading to eligibility for the final part of the examination. The final membership examination was proclaimed as an 'exit' examination, in contrast to the examinations of other colleges that tended to mark fitness to begin specialist training.

The timing of these examinations has provoked occasional controversy. During the 1980s, some senior academic (i.e. professorial) members of Council argued that trainees were obsessed with the examinations and that their interest in research was being stifled. This led to tinkering with the examination schedules, but many (including the author) believed – and continue to do so – that the research productivity of trainees has more to do with factors such as their intrinsic motivation, the academic milieu in which they work and the degree of competition for consultant posts (a publication-rich CV being advantageous).

The notion of the final examination as an 'exit' from training, hallmarking eligibility for consultant appointment, disappeared in the mid-1990s with the formation of the General Medical Council's specialist register and entry to it by the award of a Certificate of Completion of Specialist Training (CCST) from the Specialist Training Authority of the Medical Royal Colleges. In 2005, the authority to award the Certificate of Completion of Training (replacing the CCST, but equivalent in standard to it) passed to the Postgraduate Medical Education and Training Board, a statutory body on which the College is represented through the Academy of Medical Royal Colleges.

Membership of the College can also be achieved through the submission of published works, but this is not intended for those who wish to practice clinical pathology. Indeed, for medical graduates, MRCPath by this route confers no eligibility for CCT and entry to the specialist register. The publications route is popular with clinical scientists, particularly those working in highly specialised areas for which the broad and shallower scope of the examinations is inappropriate.

The third route to membership is by invitation of Council. With strengthening of the rigour of the process, this enables overseas-trained pathology consultants to be brought within the ambit of the College and its standards. With increasing movement of medical personnel within the European Union, many more consultant posts are being filled by doctors who have not achieved MRCPath by examination and entered the specialist register with that credential.

COALESCENCE AND CLEAVAGE

During the 1990s, the Royal College of Pathologists experienced two movements that would have had profound effects: the formation of a faculty of biomedical science and the separation of anatomical pathology (i.e. histopathology) from clinical pathology (haematology, chemical pathology, medical microbiology, etc). Neither movement developed sufficient momentum to change the structure of the College, but both merit brief attention.

The now infamous 'think tank' was set up by the College and the Institute of Biomedical Science (IBMS) to consider:

1. The creation of a single source of professional standards of practice.
2. The creation of a single institution for defining and assessing professional competence.
3. The creation, as a single conduit, of professional communication with other organisations, with the media and with Government.

The group was chaired by Professor John Lilleyman, who subsequently (1999–2002) became President of the College. Although the 'think tank' did not go as far as specifically proposing a faculty for biomedical scientists within the College, it was a logical extrapolation of its recommendations. When the general direction of travel was discussed with College Council, for many it was a step too far, although most shared the wish to work harmoniously and as closely as possible with the IBMS. The 'think tank' was dissolved, but in 2000 the Pathology Alliance was formed from its remnants, comprising representatives of the College, the IBMS and the Association of Clinical Scientists. However, the Alliance failed to realise its intended purposes – sovereignty remaining with the parent bodies – and it was replaced in 2005 by a concordat between its member organisations committing the signatories to work collaboratively on issues such as workforce, health and safety and quality assurance. Successful manifestations of what is achievable include conjoint (College and IBMS) initiatives on cervical cytology reporting and on specimen dissection and sampling.

Coalescence and cleavage characterise the life cycle of many organisations: colleges form; faculties develop within them and then secede to form separate colleges; realisation that strength lies in unity brings them closer together in a new federation; etc. So it was that, in the late 1990s, the organ retention 'scandal' in the UK led a small number (I think) of histopathologists to argue that their specialty would be represented better (i.e. defended) either by a body other than the Royal College of Pathologists or by a separate entity, such as a faculty, within it. This new grouping would be less distracted by issues affecting other pathology specialties. Although this never matured into a specific proposal, the episode highlighted the need for the College to pay attention to and support, with as much equanimity as possible, each of its constituent specialties. Ultimately, the College's overall handling of the organ retention issue drew praise from many quarters. The new legislation affects all pathology specialties and creates a further nexus between them. The Human Tissue Act 2004 (Scotland has separate legislation) applies to all bodily material containing cells, whether they be a few leucocytes in a wound swab in the custody of a medical microbiologist or the heart of a dead child removed by a histopathologist.

My own view is that what unites the pathology specialties is far greater than that which distinguishes them. Pathology in all its guises is the foundation of modern medicine.

THE COLLEGE'S DESTINY

Medical Royal Colleges cannot take their existence or authority for granted. Most of England's livery companies, such as the Worshipful Companies of the City of London, have long since lost their original standard-setting and training roles; many still thrive, but only as charitable bodies retaining their splendid premises. A similar destiny might befall the medical Royal Colleges if it was not for their resilience and adaptability. When the government first consulted on its proposals for reforming the governance of postgraduate medical training, eventually leading to the inception of the Postgraduate Medical Education and Training Board as a statutory body, many saw it as a threat to the colleges. However, by constructive engagement in the process, medical Royal Colleges have secured their continuing future in the landscape of specialist training.

Collegiate destiny is dependent on three factors:

1. Relevance: Are the College's functions needed? Could they be fulfilled by another body?
2. Effectiveness: Does the College deliver what it promises? Does it 'add value'?
3. Awareness: Does the College recognise the needs of patients and the public? And is it visible to them?

I regard the last of these as being supremely important. Medicine is changing rapidly from being profession-centred to patient-centred. Patients are becoming much more savvy about their diseases, diagnoses and treatments. The public now has ready access to medical information sources and often goes to see their doctor with a folder stuffed with printouts from Google searches.

In these early years of the 21st century the Royal College of Pathologists has become a much more patient-centred organisation. It has a thriving and influential Lay Advisory Committee with representation on numerous other committees, including Council. This befits the College's status as a charity, conferred because its primary concern is not the welfare of its members but that of patients. Pathology is the science behind their cure.

Acknowledgements

This account of the Royal College of Pathologists, particularly its origins, relies extensively on relevant chapters in W. D. Foster's *Pathology as a Profession in Great Britain and the Early History of the Royal College of Pathologists*, Professor George Cunningham's *The History of British Pathology* and on his papers donated to the College as described in two articles in the *Bulletin of the Royal College of Pathologists* by Dr Peter Goddard, the College's Librarian. I acknowledge these sources.

REFERENCES

Cappell, D.F. (1960) Pathology at the crossroads. *Lancet* **2**: 863.

Cunningham, G.J. (1992) *The History of British Pathology* (ed. G.K. McGowan). White Tree Books: Bristol.

Foster, W.D. (1982) *Pathology as a Profession in Great Britain and the Early History of the Royal College of Pathologists*. Royal College of Pathologists: London.

Goddard, P.F. (2005) The archive papers of Professor George John Cunningham. *Bull. R. Coll. Pathol.* Part 1: **130**: 54–57; Part 2: **131**: 72–75.

MacMenemey, W.H. (1958) The future of the pathologist in medicine. *Lancet* **2**: 841.

Get your adjectives right, you wee Sassenach

1986 at the London Hospital was my presenting debut at The Pathological Society. One of several fascinating X-ray analysis projects, courtesy of David Levison and Peter Crocker, had come to fruition at Barts. We had noticed that all adult Peyer's patches had funny black granular pigment in histiocytes towards their basal aspect. Curiously analysis had shown that this pigment contained aluminium, silicon and titanium. We postulated that these inorganic metallic elements derived from either food, especially vegetables, or toothpaste. We even dared to suggest that this study substantiated the toothpaste theories of the genesis of Crohn's disease.

So nervously I stood up before the great and good of the Society. My great mistake was, as ever, adjectival and I dared to use the term 'geographic' to describe the notable distribution of this pigment in the human body. Now one of the legions of Scottish Professors of Pathology, who always sat at one end of the front row of the lecture theatre, soon rebuked me with the canny words 'I think you mean anatomical and not geographic.' I clearly thought little of this man's observations, as, according to another eminent Scottish Professor of Pathology, soon to be our President, I made no retort whatsoever but merely turned my back to him and faced the opposite side of the lecture theatre. How was I to know that he was the Editor of one of our best known Medical Dictionaries? Ouch.

Neil Shepherd

Distilling disappointment

Belfast 1991, the first time The Pathological Society had met in the province for aeons. Professor Peter Toner, now my colleague in rural Gloucestershire, had organised a stunning meeting academically and socially but there was just one detail that had been overlooked..........

The Society Dinner was a marvellous affair in the City Hall but I have to admit to imbibing a little too much wine and you can blame Nigel Kirkham (whisky in the Europa Hotel) for Messrs Hall, Shepherd and Warren staggering down the Malone Road at 3 in the morning eating chips. The problem came the next day on the Conference Tour. The boys were a bit worse for wear but were still keen to see the Giant's Causeway and the renowned Bushmills' Distillery, although partaking of the latter's products was not foremost in their minds. The Giant's Causeway was magnificent and the whistling wind and roaring sea did wonders for sore heads. The problem came with the Distillery. It was closed...........

Neil Shepherd

12 The Changing Role of Pathology in the Undergraduate Curriculum

Paola Domizio

INTRODUCTION

In November 1906, Hubert Maitland Turnbull, a founder member of The Pathological Society, was appointed Director of the Institute of Pathology at the London Hospital. He recalls in his memoirs that shortly after taking up the post 'I realised how greatly handicapped my students were by having no knowledge... of what for instance a solid lung or fibrotic liver was like or even understanding pathological terms' (Turnbull, 1953). He goes on to describe how '... we persuaded the College Board that pathology in its most elementary form should be added to the introductory course' (Turnbull, 1953). A century later, Turnbull's words strike a familiar chord with pathology teachers nationwide. The difference between then and now is that it is no longer so easy to persuade the 'Board' that pathology teaching should be increased.

In the last 100 years, the role of pathology in the undergraduate curriculum has turned full circle – from being a supporting act, to playing a major role, to being a bit-part player once again. In this chapter I will give an overview of how pathology teaching has changed in the 20th century in the context of the overall development of medical education. I will also discuss the possible impact of modern medical curricula on recruitment in pathology and try to predict what the future holds for pathology teaching and its teachers.

THE GOALS OF PATHOLOGY TEACHING

Pathology bridges the gap between basic sciences and clinical medicine, so a proper understanding of pathological processes is vitally important for medical practice. This tenet is as true today as it was in Turnbull's time. The main goals of undergraduate pathology teaching have always been to provide a language or framework for the description of disease and to provide students with knowledge of the functional and structural changes in disease so that clinical signs and symptoms can be understood and interpreted.

The question 'should medical students be taught pathology?' has provoked much debate in the pathology popular literature. Arguments for and against the motion that 'Doctors don't need to know about the pathological basis of disease' have been vociferously argued (Jackson *et al.*, 2003; Wright 2003). The proponents maintain that 'medicine comprises more than a science and that more attention must be given to the humanist elements of medical practice and medical education' and that 'greater understanding of the pathological basis of disease has not contributed substantially to improved morbidity and mortality rates'. Opponents, on the other hand, respond that proper communication with colleagues and patients depends on a proper understanding of pathological language, that evidence-based practice depends on the scientific basis of medicine and that many advances in public health have been based on understanding of the underlying pathology of a disease.

There is little doubt that most pathologists would oppose the motion, but what about the 'consumers', the doctors of the future? It is interesting that a first-year student at one of the new medical schools has placed himself firmly in the opponents' camp (Jackson *et al.*, 2003), arguing that it is unethical for doctors to treat diseases that they have not been properly taught about: 'Not understanding how these diseases arise, present and are treated would be a criminal flaw. Ignorance is no defence.' Good communication skills are a *sine qua non* for tomorrow's doctors, but they must also have a sufficient knowledge base to communicate about.

PATHOLOGY TEACHING IN THE 20TH CENTURY

Information on pathology teaching prior to the 1980s comes solely from archival material, because the literature contains virtually no publications on teaching and learning in pathology before this time. The archives at St Bartholomew's and the Royal London Hospitals are a rich source of information on this particular subject and I have used them extensively to put together the description of early pathology teaching at their associated medical schools that follows. Other medical schools would have had their own approach to pathology teaching, and there would undoubtedly have been differences in course content and structure, but there is no reason to suppose that the progression of pathology teaching was significantly different from that at the Medical College of St Bartholomew's Hospital (Barts) and the London Hospital Medical College (LHMC).

The Early Years

At the end of the 19th century medical students at Barts and the LHMC were taught precious little pathology and what little teaching there was tended to be haphazard and disorganised. This was not surprising because the widely held view at the time was that 'morbid anatomy was defunct: Virchow had exhausted the subject' (Russell and Innes, 1956). By the start of the 20th century, the importance of applying science to medicine had begun to gain acceptance. The successes of bacteriology in diagnosing and controlling the spread of disease gave reformers a persuasive argument for placing greater emphasis on science in the medical curriculum, contradicting the prevalent view at the time that medicine was an 'empirical art' (Waddington, 2003a).

The real revolution in pathology teaching began in the early 1900s when, spurred on by increasing understanding of disease mechanisms, pathology began to be accepted as a specialty in its own right. Before Turnbull's appointment at the LHMC in 1906, surgeons gave the lectures in surgical pathology and also examined the specimens removed at surgery. At Barts, too, the surgeon Sir James Paget had 'held students captive with his lectures on surgical pathology' (Waddington, 2003b). Visiting physicians carried out the hospital autopsies and demonstrated their findings to medical students on an ad hoc basis. Turnbull soon realised not only the importance of having high-quality pathology teaching in the medical curriculum, but also the added value of pathologists actually carrying out the teaching themselves.

The Age of Reform

Turnbull's reform of the LHMC pathology course started in 1907. His first step was to introduce daily post-mortem demonstrations to clinical medical students, which he carried out himself for many years. Students were expected to attend these demonstrations whenever possible (Fig. 12.1) and were also encouraged to conduct autopsies themselves (London Hospital Medical College, 1936). There was certainly no lack of autopsies for the student to practice on, e.g. there were 3486 in 1938 (Turnbull, 1953).

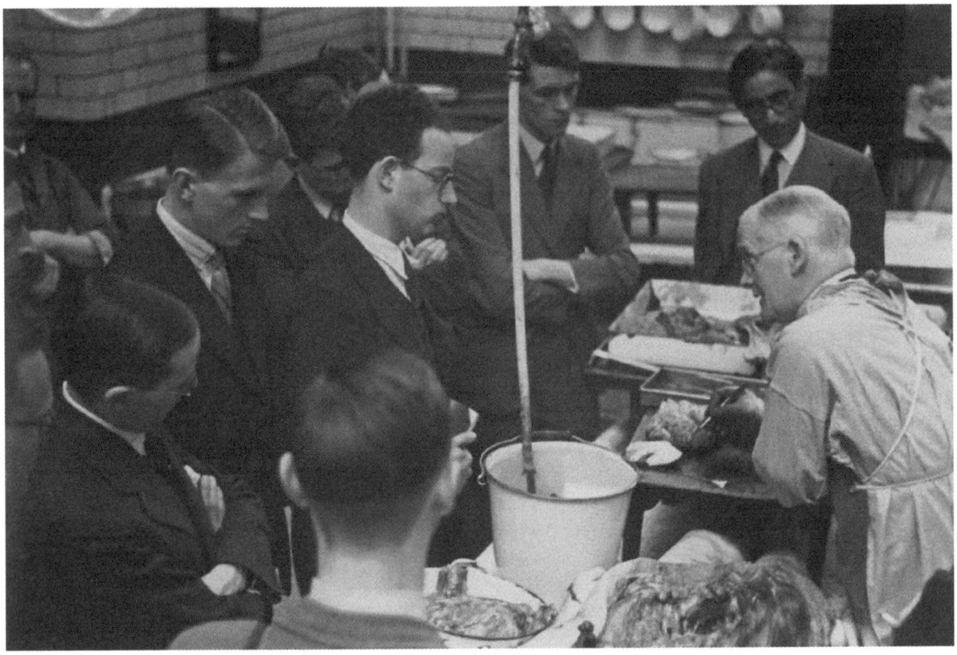

Figure 12.1 Turnbull demonstrating an autopsy, ca. 1930.

In 1909 Turnbull began a course of Directors' Lectures on the subject of 'special morbid anatomy and histology', supplemented by macroscopic and microscopic preparations to illustrate the conditions discussed. At first a single hour-long lecture was given once a week, increasing to twice a week to accommodate growing demand. The aim of the lectures was to 'treat individual organs and tissues in succession and introduce relevant general pathology as it occurred in the series' (Turnbull, 1953). Attendance at these lectures was voluntary and open to students of all years. Despite the fact that this was a new course whose importance may not have been immediately obvious to the students, its popularity grew rapidly. In typically meticulous manner, Turnbull kept an attendance sheet for all his lectures, and was able to demonstrate a steadily increasing number of students attending the lectures in the first few years.

Turnbull's style of teaching mirrored that of his own pathology teacher at Oxford, Professor Gotch, from whom he had learned meticulous attention to detail. Before the lecture started he would copy a list of headings onto a blackboard in order to jog his own memory and to help the audience follow the lecture – the forerunner of the modern-day lecture handout. Turnbull was a great believer in studying histology and pathology together and so 'made coloured diagrams of the histology of organs and other illustrations for the lectures, often enlarged pictures of actual microscopic fields, which I suspended from lattice of transverse laths behind the lectern' (Fig. 12.2) (Turnbull, 1953). Another blackboard was free for Turnbull to draw on with coloured chalks during the lecture.

Rather than use an 'epidiascope and lantern slides' to supplement his lectures, Turnbull preferred to lay out macroscopic specimens and glass slides under a microscope, which could be examined by students before or after the lecture (Fig. 12.3). Notes on the patient, their disease, and arrows to draw attention to particular points of interest accompanied the slides and specimens (Fig. 12.4). Turnbull's justification for what he himself called 'these somewhat antiquated methods' was that 'actual study of a section with a microscope is obviously better than a sight of it upon a screen' (Turnbull, 1953).

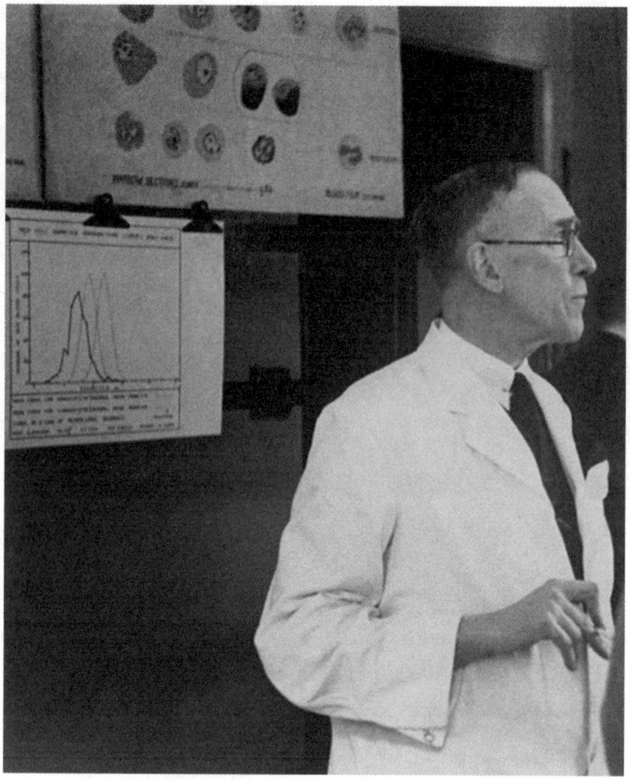

Figure 12.2 Turnbull lecturing, ca. 1925.

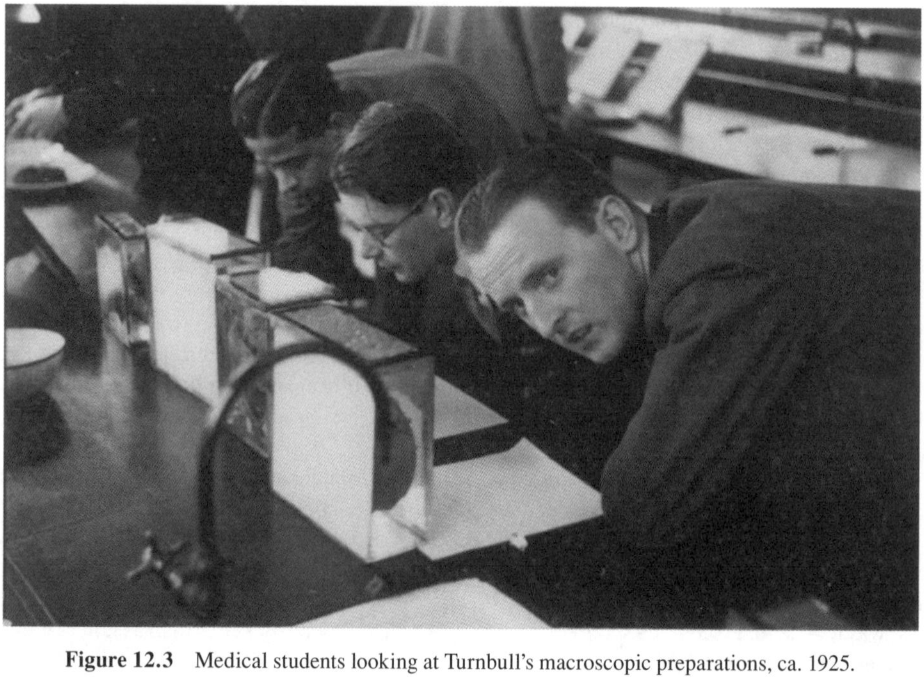

Figure 12.3 Medical students looking at Turnbull's macroscopic preparations, ca. 1925.

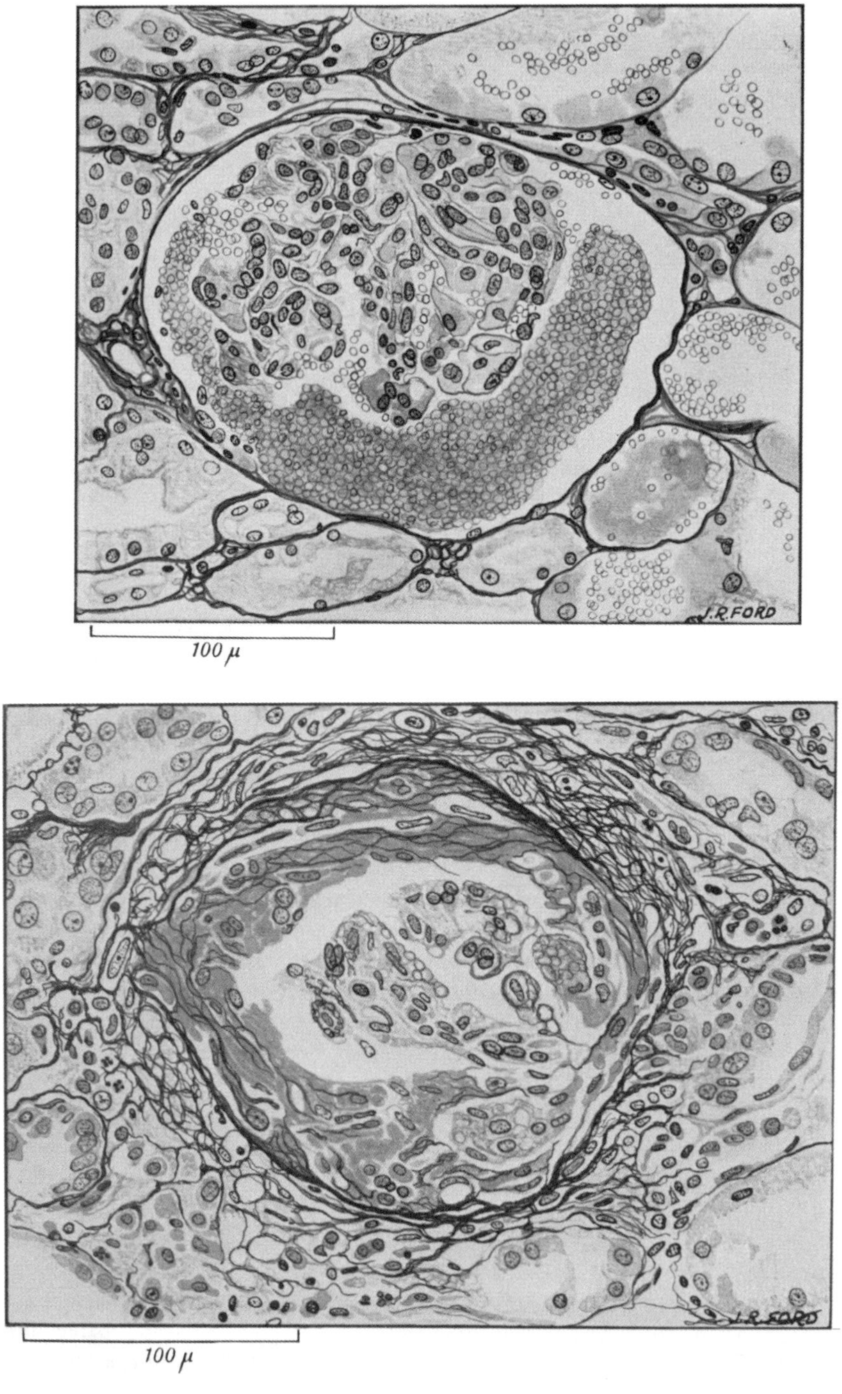

Figure 12.4 Turnbull's meticulous drawings of a diseased renal glomerulus. All his lectures and demonstrations were similarly illustrated.

There was no official feedback given to teachers in those days, but there is little doubt that Turnbull's lectures were well received. Clark-Kennedy, a future Dean of the LHMC, wrote of Turnbull's teaching 'the least intelligent of us perceived the truth which pervaded his lectures and the wealth of personal knowledge this contained' (Ellis, 1986a). Turnbull's scholarly authority and passion for his subject made him a highly effective role model, as demonstrated by the large number of his pupils who went on to be pathologists themselves, including Donald Hunter and Dorothy Russell.

In 1926, Donald Hunter became curator of the pathology museum at the LHMC and, together with Tumbull, completely reorganised the museum, discarding many older specimens and replacing them with new ones, rewriting the old museum catalogue at the same time. During the 1930s, pathology museums were in their heyday and remained so for the next few decades. Nearly all teaching hospitals had a pathology museum of some sort and the specimens therein were used widely during teaching. At the LHMC, the newly stocked museum became an important learning resource for medical students, and, benefiting from the 'imaginative and energetic care' of Donald Hunter, was said to 'augment all teaching' (Ellis, 1986a).

Pathology Teaching in the Clinical Course

At the LHMC, pathology teaching in the second and third clinical years was expanded in 1911 to include a compulsory three-month course devoted entirely to pathology. The first six days were spent learning staining techniques, ranging from haematoxylin and eosin to Schmorl's stain, and the remainder of the three months combined lectures in pathological histology (given by the Senior Assistant Director) with 'clerking in the post-mortem room, and with microbiology, chemical pathology and haematology in the clinical laboratory' (Turnbull, 1953). Interestingly, the course also included visits to the local Fever Hospital to receive instructions on fevers, and visits to the local asylum for instruction in 'lunacy' (London Hospital Medical College, 1936).

The introductory course in pathology that Tumbull had been so keen on when he was first appointed did not actually get off the ground until 1925. Until then, students entering their clinical years were given an introductory course in medicine and surgery in which they were taught 'percussion, other physical signs, how to examine medical and surgical patients and write clinical histories and notes' (Turnbull, 1953). The new introductory pathology course aimed to give early exposure to pathology and to 'establish not only a process of thought but also a basis of factual knowledge which should enable the student to learn more readily and think more independently during his first clinical year' (Turnbull, 1953). The course lasted for one month and was taught by the Junior Assistant Director. The students were given one hour's lecture every weekday on topics in general pathology, supplemented by examination of macroscopic specimens, 'especially those of which they would be taught the clinical signs, such as consolidation of the lung or valvular diseases of the heart' (Turnbull, 1953). Three afternoons a week were spent in the post-mortem room and other times were divided between the clinical laboratory and the wards. Through this course, students were encouraged to appreciate the pathological basis of clinical symptoms and signs, clinicopathological correlation and the importance of pathology to clinical medicine.

At Barts, a new scheme of pathological clerkships was adopted in 1912, mainly at the insistence of William Girling Ball, who had recently been appointed senior demonstrator in pathology. This scheme was greatly aided by the construction of a new pathology block with separate diagnostic and teaching laboratories. Before 1912, students working in the pathology department had been unsupervised and their work had often been 'unreliable'. Under Girling Ball's scheme, students were placed under the supervision of the demonstrator (pathologist) on duty in the hope that they would receive training in 'direct reference to individual patients'. As a result, 'clinical teaching was reorganised and a system of practical lectures and demonstrations introduced with clinical practice in mind' (Waddington, 2003c).

Despite the introduction of this scheme, the pressure on students at Barts to gain the widest possible clinical experience meant that pathology tended to be overlooked. By 1927 it was recognised that pathology had been inadequately taught with 'new classes added here and there whenever necessity arose' (Waddington, 2003d). To resolve this, pathology teaching was restructured, the teaching staff enlarged and more demonstrations organised. By 1931 a three-month full-time pathology course had been introduced into the final clinical year, similar to that already in place at the LHMC, thus preventing pathology teaching from being diluted.

The Influence of Flexner and Haldane

At about the time that Turnbull was transforming pathology teaching at the LHMC, several reports on medical education were sending shock waves through the medical establishments on both sides of the Atlantic. In 1910, Abraham Flexner published a scathing report on behalf of the Carnegie Foundation for the Advancement of Teaching on the standard of medical education in the USA and Canada (Flexner, 1910). Two years later, he published a similar report on medical education in Europe (Flexner, 1912). Flexner's reports triggered much-needed reforms in the standards, organisation and curricula of North American medical schools, which until then had operated more for profit than for education. With respect to the curriculum, Flexner advocated strong emphasis on biomedical sciences, to meet society's expectations that medical care be more scientifically based. He also proposed that clinical training should follow the model of clerkships introduced at Johns Hopkins by the renowned clinician and teacher William Osler.

In 1913, the Royal Commission on University Education in London, established years previously and chaired by Lord Haldane, published its findings (Haldane, 1913). Like Flexner, Haldane stressed the need to raise the level of science in the medical curriculum and called for the strengthening of traditional scientific departments (Haldane, 2005). Osler too, on a visit to the UK in 1911, had noted the 'glaring defects in provision of teaching of laboratory based medicine' and pleaded for 'more funding to support hospitals' scientific work' (Osler, 1911).

The effects of the Flexner and Haldane reports were felt worldwide. Turnbull and Girling Ball's attempts to increase pathology teaching were taking place at the very same time that there was rising momentum for greater scientific content in the medical curriculum. Consequently, they found no great obstacle to achieving their aims.

THE PERI- AND POST-WAR YEARS

The idea of a National Health Service had first been proposed by the Dawson Committee of 1920 (Dawson, 1920) but it was not until 1941 that the government announced plans for a post-war state hospital service. In 1942, the Goodenough Committee was established to look at the organisation of medical schools, their facilities for clinical training and research and their relationship to hospital services. The report, published in 1944 (Goodenough, 1944), recognised that doctors of the future would need to be able to think and reason things out for themselves and acquire even greater command of the scientific method. In essence, they would need education as well as training. This was the first time that such an approach had been proposed, and the authors realised the difficulties it might pose – after all, education encourages students to question what they are told while training requires students to do what they are told without question. The Goodenough report was published in the midst of the Second World War, and as a result its far-sighted recommendations went largely unnoticed. It was, however, to have substantial influence on medical education in later years.

By the time of Turnbull's retirement from the LHMC in 1946, pathology was an important part of the medical curriculum. Turnbull's successor as Director of the Institute of Pathology was Dorothy Russell, by then a distinguished neuropathologist. She continued to give the Directors'

Lectures in the same style and manner that Turnbull had. Her teaching was said to be 'less inspiring' than Turnbull's but certainly not less detailed – indeed, students felt that if they copied a full cycle of Russell's lectures from the blackboard they would have 'an entire textbook' (Ellis, 1986c). The compulsory pathology courses in the clinical years had also been continued after Russell's appointment, so that post-war medical students undoubtedly had significant exposure to pathology teaching.

A New Health Service for All

With the creation of the National Health Service in 1948, however, the environment in which medical students were taught began to change (Ellis, 1986b). Poor patients, who had previously been in receipt of charity and had been grateful for their care, were now entitled to expect the best treatment available free of charge. Duties such as surgical 'dressing', which were previously carried out by students, now had to be performed by qualified staff. Teachers, many of whom had previously been unpaid, now received a salary from the medical school, but teaching was becoming less of a priority against the new commitment to healthcare. Medical science was rapidly gathering pace. Not only were new drugs being licensed, but surgical sub-specialties were developing, obstetric services were improving and general practice was gaining influence. Consequently, the content of the clinical course changed repeatedly as new subjects were added and others were removed.

Throughout the 1950s, debate took place about the type of doctors the medical curriculum was producing. Reformers stressed the importance of an integrated approach that took account of the whole patient. The notion that a five-year undergraduate education could no longer hope to produce a complete doctor, as had been suggested in the Goodenough report, was accepted and the concept of a basic medical education as preparation for vocational training gained ground. Encouraged by a greater emphasis on social medicine arising from the birth of the NHS, a greater need was identified for training in a non-hospital environment, particularly in general practice.

With regard to pathology teaching at this time, the Professor of Pathology at Barts, John Blacklock, together with his colleague Alfred Stansfeld, argued for pathology lectures to be correlated with teaching in medicine and surgery. This did not happen until 1951, when yet another revised scheme was adopted and the amount of pathology in the clinical course was increased. The rationale behind this was to make students familiar with 'more complex tests which they might be expected to ask for and interpret' after they had qualified (Waddington, 2003e).

By the time Dorothy Russell retired from the LHMC in 1960, the practice started by Turnbull of teaching histology and pathology together had been discontinued. Instead, histology was taught alongside anatomy by anatomists in the preclinical course alone, emphasising the perceived scientific nature of these subjects. Lectures were given in both anatomy and histology but practical teaching was also provided. In anatomy, students worked in small groups dissecting a cadaver, whereas in histology each student had their own microscope, which they used to study the structure of tissues in detail.

Pathology was still prominent in the clinical course but the methods of teaching were beginning to change. The lectures and formal demonstrations so beloved of the old-school pathologists were giving way to small-group teaching. The LHMC prospectus from 1965 states: 'After his first clinical firm the student joins the clinicopathological course, which is designed so that pathology and clinical work are taught in close relation to one another; in this way the effect of disease on the structure and function of the various organs in the body may be illustrated... patients are demonstrated by individual students to their colleagues; teaching takes the form of discussion of the student's findings and conclusions' (London Hospital Medical College, 1965). This approach was the forerunner of modern-day integrated teaching. Pathology museums continued to be an important learning resource and the daily autopsy demonstrations remained popular with the students.

THE PRE-MODERN YEARS

The 1960s saw attitudes to education shift. Traditional divisions between the humanities and the sciences were starting to be questioned and the notion that medical graduates should have a wider educational experience, as had first been proposed by the Goodenough report, was increasingly promoted.

The Todd Report

In 1968 the Report of the Royal Commission on Medical Education, headed by Lord Todd (Todd, 1968), was published. This report proposed a five-year undergraduate course consisting of three years of basic medical sciences and two years of clinical work. The most radical proposal was that the preclinical course should be flexible and modular with students studying subjects of their choice in greater depth. In this aspect, Todd was the first to suggest that the undergraduate curriculum should include selected study modules. It also recommended that general pathology, which it termed a 'paraclinical' subject, should be included in the compulsory part of the preclinical course. To achieve these changes, the report called for the reduction of curriculum time devoted to traditional subjects such as anatomy, and the adoption of new teaching methods with less emphasis on didactic teaching. The report also saw continuing education as vital for medical graduates, to equip them 'with an understanding of medicine as an evolving science and art, and to provide the basis for future vocational training'. In this respect, the Todd report was confirming a shift in emphasis from a primarily vocational to an essentially educational course.

A Changing Curriculum

Throughout the 1970s, the preclinical–clinical divide continued but there began to be more emphasis on the humanities as applied to medicine – sociology, psychology, statistics and community medicine. Despite this, students (who had only recently been included in the debate on medical education) still perceived the preclinical teaching as boring and unrelated to medicine. There was no doubt that teaching concentrated on rote learning with assessment geared towards compartmentalisation of knowledge (Waddington, 2003f).

Pathology teaching at this time remained fairly 'traditional' at both Barts and the LHMC, with the bulk of the teaching occurring in dedicated blocks in the clinical years. Both lectures and small-group tutorials were given and daily autopsy demonstrations continued. The stand-alone pathology exam was a formidable hurdle and a potent driver for learning pathology.

The curriculum was under strain, however. New subjects had been introduced into both the preclinical and clinical courses without a sufficient reduction in existing subjects, so that students felt under increasing pressure. Curriculum overload was not a new concept; indeed, as early as 1876 Thomas Huxley had stated that 'the burden we place on a medical student is far too heavy... a system of medical education that is actually calculated to obstruct the acquisition of knowledge and to heavily favour the crammer and grinder is a disgrace' (Huxley, 1876) but it now became the stimulus behind major curriculum reform.

THE MODERN YEARS

Although 'medical educationalists' had been around for many years – indeed Turnbull and Russell were considered by their students to be enthusiastic and highly effective educationalists – it was not until the 1980s that medical education really began to be accepted as a specialty in its own right and departments of medical education were created in most medical schools.

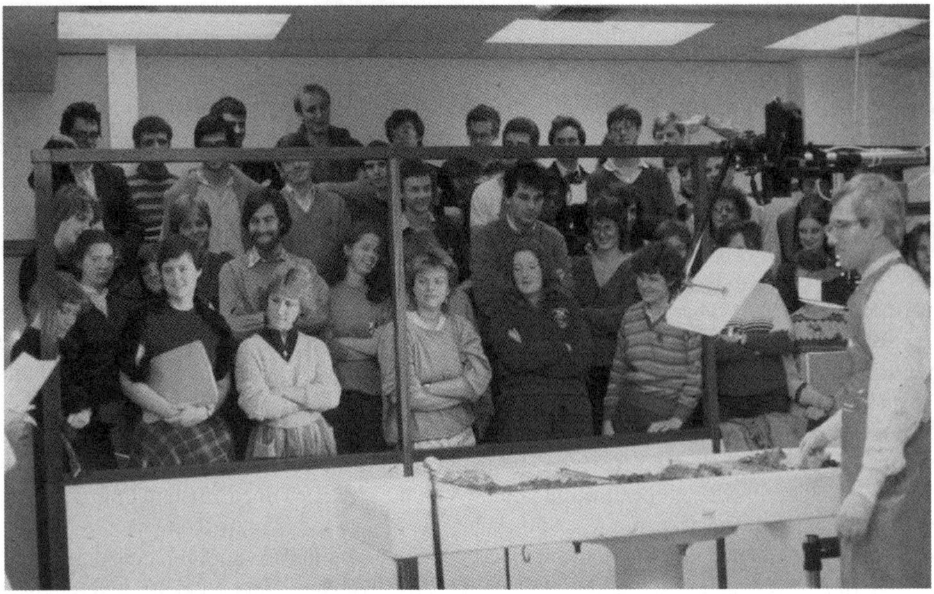

Figure 12.5 An autopsy demonstration, ca. 1980. David Levison is the pathologist.

Students were now being actively encouraged to participate in their own learning. The principles behind medical education, following on from the Todd report of 1968, were now not only to teach the fundamentals of medicine but also to encourage students to think and lay down the foundations of lifelong learning. New methods were required to enable students to develop critical reasoning and apply the knowledge they had learned. Self-directed learning (SDL) and problem-based learning (PBL), the latter developed in North America and The Netherlands, gained popularity.

The Turning Tide

By the late 1980s, significant change had taken place. In many medical schools, to counteract the criticism that preclinical teaching had little clinical relevance, the traditional preclinical course had been abandoned in favour of a systems-based approach. Emphasis on lectures was reduced, seminar-based work and small-group teaching was increasingly used and SDL became a key part of teaching practice. Despite this change in philosophy, individual departments were still reluctant to give up teaching time and there remained a feeling that the curriculum required an unrealistic degree of completeness.

Pathology teaching began to change to reflect these new ideas. In some medical schools, pathologists became involved in teaching histology, often alongside pathology to highlight its clinical relevance. Overall, however, pathology was looked upon as a fact-based science and so in most medical schools the pathology teaching time was cut. Instead, SDL packages were developed to supplement the pathology course content. Autopsy demonstrations, which had been so popular with generations of medical students, were becoming irregular and less well attended. The reasons for the decline in autopsy numbers are well documented and beyond the scope of this chapter, but there is little doubt that the impact was to reduce students' exposure to macroscopic pathology and clinicopathological correlation. Pathology museums were still functioning in most medical schools but their relevance to the new style of undergraduate course was beginning to be questioned and funding to maintain them was in short supply.

Tomorrow's Doctors

In 1991, the General Medical Council began a major review of medical education that culminated in1993 with the publication of *Tomorrow's Doctors* (General Medical Council, 1993). The drivers behind this review were numerous. Firstly, the preceding years had brought significant changes in patterns of disease and in the way that healthcare was organised. Secondly, the public now had a heightened expectation of doctors, which had led to a change in the doctor–patient relationship. Increasingly, doctors were being faced with difficult ethical and moral issues without sufficient instruction in how to manage these problems. Thirdly, despite the repeated recognition that curriculum overload was detrimental to medical education, not enough had been done to reduce the burden of factual information on students.

Tomorrow's Doctors sought to 'promote an approach to medical education... which differs substantially from that of the traditional curriculum' and to 'provide recommendations for a course which will produce graduates whose fitness to practice as pre-registration house officers is better assured' (General Medical Council, 1993). In 2003, the guidelines were updated to 'put the principles set out in Good Medical Practice at the centre of undergraduate education' and to 'identify the knowledge, skills, attitudes and behaviour expected of new graduates' (General Medical Council, 2003).

The main recommendations of *Tomorrow's Doctors* were that the medical curriculum should be organised around a core of essential knowledge and skills, augmented by a series of options (or selected study modules) that allowed students to study areas of particular interest to them in depth. The core curriculum should be integrated, with loss of the traditional divide between preclinical and clinical years and systems-based rather than discipline-based. The course should emphasise clinical, communication and practical skills and should instil into the student the professional attitudes of mind and behaviour befitting of a doctor and expected by the public. More emphasis should be put on the teaching of public health, ethics and law, and more of the curriculum should be taught in the community. Self-directed learning and critical evaluation should be encouraged, thereby preparing the student for life-long learning. In all areas of the curriculum, the burden of factual information on medical students should be substantially reduced.

Tomorrow's Doctors was to cause a seismic shift in the objectives of the undergraduate medical curriculum, away from the scientific,basis of medicine – a sound knowledge of which had been repeatedly advocated since Flexner's report of 1910 – towards patient-centred doctors, who had better communication and practical skills but whose knowledge of the basic medical sciences was inevitably much reduced. The effects on pathology teaching were profound.

The Effects of *Tomorrow's Doctors* on Pathology Teaching

In 2001, Professor Sir James Underwood carried out a survey on pathology teaching on behalf of The Pathological Society and presented the findings at a meeting on the future of academic pathology (Pathological Society, 2001); see also Appendix (11). This survey showed that in the preceding decade 10 of 19 medical schools in the UK (53%) reported a reduction in pathology teaching time, with only one medical school reporting an increase. Despite the fact that this study was not peer-reviewed, it does suggest, along with anecdotal evidence from individual lead teachers in pathology, that there has been a real reduction in pathology teaching time since the publication of *Tomorrow's Doctors*.

The aspects of pathology teaching that have suffered most from this reduction no doubt vary from school to school, but it would seem that the axe has fallen most heavily on histology and general pathology (personal observation). These two subjects were traditionally considered to be basic medical sciences and so were drastically cut in efforts to reduce factual overload. Systemic pathology has fared somewhat better, but even so, teaching on the morphological changes in disease is often neglected in favour of epidemiology and public health issues.

The teaching of pathology in blocks to 'avoid fragmentation' has all but disappeared, as has the traditional practice of teaching general pathology in the first two years and systemic pathology in the clinical years. Instead, pathology teaching is integrated throughout the course. A consequence of this is that in many medical schools 'pathology' is no longer a recognised subject. The multidisciplinary approach to teaching and learning is reflected in the modern-day integrated assessments, and the pathology exam, once a tough hurdle, is a thing of the past. In effect, pathology, which in Turnbull's time was as important as medicine or surgery, is no longer felt to be a core subject, although most medical schools will offer selected study modules in pathology to students who wish to study it in greater depth.

It is in teaching methods, however, that perhaps the biggest changes have been seen. The emphasis in medical education has switched from teaching to learning, which means that most of the curriculum is now student-centred rather than teacher-centred. Didactic instruction and tutor-led tutorials have given way in varying degree to SDL and PBL, and pathology tutors have been converted to PBL facilitators. Students no longer attend practical classes or look down microscopes, instead computer-assisted teaching has mushroomed and web-based learning is now the norm.

The organ retention affairs at Bristol and Alder Hey had several deleterious effects on pathology teaching. Firstly, the closure of pathology museums, which were already under threat by lack of funding, was hastened. Secondly, the number of consented autopsies, which had been in decline for some time, fell even further so that autopsy demonstrations have now become exceedingly rare. Consequently, the opportunities for today's medical students to observe real-life macroscopic pathology have virtually disappeared. Instead, partly through choice but largely through necessity, this aspect of pathology teaching has been devolved to computer-based learning packages.

The undergraduate medical curriculum has thus evolved from being teacher-centred to student-centred, from discipline-based to integrated core and options-based and from passive acquisition of knowledge imparted by real teachers to active problem-based learning with reliance on computers. Pathology learning has changed from seeing pots in pathology museums and real organs at autopsy to looking at images on CDs and websites: from daily contact with pathologists, to irregular interaction with anonymous computer screens. Both models have their good and bad points. Modernists maintain that the current curriculum better prepares students for modern medical practice whereas traditionalists complain that 'the baby was thrown out with the bathwater'. The challenge for medical educationalists of the future is to strike a balance between best practice and achievability.

THE IMPACT OF CHANGING CURRICULA ON RECRUITMENT IN PATHOLOGY

The changes in medical education outlined above have evolved over a number of decades, although the pace of change has undoubtedly accelerated in the last 15 years. During that time, the number of consultant vacancies in all the pathology specialties has risen substantially, resulting in a significant recruitment crisis. In histopathology particularly, the rise in vacancies has been rapid and spectacular, from 4 in 1992 to 219 in 2004 (figures supplied by the Royal College of Pathologists). This huge increase in vacancies is partly explained by early retirements, but until recently it has not been known whether it was also accounted for by a fall in the number of medical graduates entering pathology.

A recent study looking at the career choices of medical graduates showed that the number of newly qualified doctors selecting pathology as their first choice of career halved between 1983 and 1993 and has remained static ever since (Lambert *et al.*, 2006). The reasons behind this worrying trend were not specifically sought by the study, but there was evidence that 'experience of the subject as a student' and the influence of 'a particular teacher or department' are more important in encouraging students and junior doctors to enter pathology than they are for other medical careers. Although the impact of *Tomorrow's Doctors* cannot *per se* explain the substantial drop in pathology as a career choice, there is no doubt that the current medical curriculum, in which pathology is low profile and there is virtually no exposure to charismatic pathologists acting as role models, will do nothing to remedy the situation.

THE FUTURE FOR PATHOLOGY TEACHERS

Despite recommendations for proper government funding of medical schools going back to the Goodenough report of 1944, continued funding cuts in higher education in the last few decades have meant that medical schools have struggled to maintain sufficient staffing levels to sustain the major curricular changes adopted. In particular, the savage funding cuts instigated by the last Research Assessment Exercise (RAE) have hit academic pathologists particularly hard. Whole departments have disappeared, with individuals retiring early or being re-badged as NHS consultants. Those who have survived the cuts have had the strongest research output but, not surprisingly, their enthusiasm for undergraduate teaching is sometimes poor.

A recent survey by the Council of Heads of Medical Schools (CHMS) has highlighted the dramatic fall in the number of clinical academics in pathology (Council of Heads of Medical Schools and Council of Heads and Deans of Dental Schools, 2005). Between 2003 and 2004 there has been a 40% drop in total number of academic pathologists, and there are now only 45% of the numbers that there were in 2000. The situation with clinical lecturers in pathology is even worse. Numbers have dropped by 64% since 2003 and now stand at only 19% of their 2000 numbers. These figures are the worst for any of the medical specialties and prompted the CHMS to state in their commentary on the survey that 'a shortage of academic pathologists at all levels will compromise medical training as well as the UK's medical research capacity'.

The widespread dearth of academic pathologists has left pathology teaching in crisis, particularly as NHS consultants have been reluctant to take on the teaching mantle due to their own burgeoning workload and generally low morale. The result is that in several medical schools pathology is no longer taught by pathologists – whatever pathology remains in the curriculum is incorporated into PBL scenarios and is supervised by PBL tutors. The argument that in PBL-based curricula students should 'learn' and not 'be taught' could be used to justify the rejection of teaching by all but the most committed pathologists. There is little doubt, however, that students prefer to be taught (or supervised) by experts in the subjects they are learning. So, in the ideal world, pathologists should 'teach' pathology, just as surgeons should 'teach' surgery and psychiatrists should 'teach' psychiatry.

At the same time as the number of academics is falling, the number of medical students is continually increasing – by 40% since 2000, buoyed by the opening of four new medical schools. More students need more teachers, particularly in PBL-based curricula where the small-group nature of the teaching means that the teacher:student ratio is necessarily high.

But where will the teachers needed come from? The practice long-held by most 'traditional' universities of appointing academics on the basis of research profile and then expecting delivery of a significant teaching workload is no longer acceptable. It is being increasingly recognised that many of the skills required for research and teaching are different: good researchers do not necessarily make good teachers, and vice versa. The rapidly diminishing number of research academics is under greater pressure than ever, driven by the financial impact of the RAE, to obtain grant funding and publish papers in high-impact journals. This is particularly true of research-active pathologists, who, due to the 'unsexy' nature of much of their research, often have to work very hard to secure high-profile grants. Is it any wonder, therefore, that teaching comes low in their list of priorities? Until now, universities have not had to face financial consequences as a result of teaching quality assessments, but this may well change in the future as students switch from 'learners' to 'consumers' following the introduction of tuition fees. If this does happen, it is likely that good teachers will bring funding to universities, in the same way that good researchers currently do.

It is high time, therefore, for universities to recognise that these two academic pathways are fundamentally different, and to appoint not just high-profile researchers but also specialist teachers. Such a policy would allow committed teachers the time and resources to develop not only their courses but also their own careers, in the hope that they will eventually be recognised and promoted on the basis of their teaching portfolio alone. The effect on the pathology specialties, suffering as they are from chronic staff shortages and an ever-increasing clinical workload, would be dramatic.

PATHOLOGY TEACHING IN THE NEXT 100 YEARS

There is no doubt that the main objective of pathology teachers in the 21st century must be to raise the profile of pathology teaching in the undergraduate curriculum back to somewhere near its former level. This needs to be done not only to equip modern medical graduates with an understanding of disease mechanisms, but also to stimulate interest in pathology as a career. In order to do so, however, several issues need to be tackled. Firstly, the loss of pathology from modern curricula must be corrected, and, secondly, the pathology teaching workload must be adequately managed.

There is no doubt that managing the teaching workload will be a particularly difficult challenge for pathologists in the future and that novel solutions will need to be found. Given the savage loss of academic pathologists, unless the trend is reversed it will be impossible for universities to deliver pathology teaching without the help of NHS colleagues. Academic and NHS pathologists will need to work together to agree a model for delivering teaching. This might involve negotiation of job plans at a departmental level with protected time for teaching. Development of formulae for calculating the time required for teaching and its preparation will be particularly important, as will identifying and obtaining appropriate funding. Other ways of spreading the load include involvement of non-consultant staff in teaching, such as trainees, clinical scientists, postgraduate students or retired pathologists.

Raising the profile of pathology teaching depends on active involvement by pathologists in curriculum design and planning at a local level. As well as inclusion in the core curriculum, ways of incorporating pathology include offering selected study modules and clinical attachments or research projects in individual departments. Using multidisciplinary team meetings as an opportunity for teaching is another example of how pathologists can be actively involved in teaching without the need for substantial additional resources. Intercalated degrees in pathology are an important way of exposing interested students to pathology and, in the author's experience, provide a strong stimulus for eventual choice of pathology as a career.

The Pathological Society has been active in trying to re-invigorate pathology teaching. An Education subcommittee has been formed, chaired by the author, to tackle educational issues. This includes development of a database of e-resources, including images, tutorials and other computer-based teaching materials for use by hard-pressed pathology teachers nationwide. A joint project is ongoing with the Royal College of Pathologists to develop a realistic core curriculum in pathology. More importance will be given during Pathological Society meetings to research and innovation in medical education. Grants from the Open Scheme have been awarded for educational projects, one successful example being for the modernisation of the Crane Pathology Museum at the University of Sheffield (Bury and Burton, 2005). The existence of funds for supporting students in intercalated degrees in pathology will be advertised more widely and available funds may be increased. A student essay prize on a topical pathology title will be offered annually.

Through these initiatives, it is hoped to stimulate medical students' interest in pathology over the next 100 years!

CONCLUSIONS

Major reforms in medical education have led to a shift away from didactic discipline-based teaching with 'factual overload' towards integrated, systems-based education with an emphasis on SDL. Rightly or wrongly, pathology tends to be perceived as a fact-based science, and so has suffered the same fate as many of the basic science subjects in having teaching time drastically cut. From the position in Turnbull and Russell's time of pathology underpinning much of the medical curriculum, there is concern nowadays that pathology is disappearing from undergraduate curricula, especially those that are centred on PBL.

The problems facing pathology teaching and pathology teachers mirror those of most other medical disciplines, namely a lack of time and money, and competing pressures from many other sources. Academic pathology is in particular danger of extinction, however, so the questions must be asked: who will teach medical students pathology in the future and who will be the role models from whom the future generations of pathologists will come?

Teaching is a task that requires enthusiasm and time, but one that, if done properly, is greatly rewarding. If pathology teachers of the future can restore the profile of their subject there is hope that newly qualified doctors will understand the mechanisms of disease, use laboratories properly and be stimulated to become pathologists themselves. If not, there is the danger of producing doctors who cannot explain disease to their patients, who abuse laboratories and who have no interest in pursuing pathology as a career, leading to a slow and possibly irreversible decline in pathology as a medical profession.

REFERENCES

Bury, J. and Burton, J. (2005) *Modernisation of the WAJ Crane Museum of Pathology*. Report on work funded through the 'Open' scheme of The Pathological Society, 2003–2005. Pathological Society: London.

Council of Heads of Medical Schools and Council of Heads and Deans of Dental Schools (2005) *Clinical Academic Staffing Levels in UK Medical and Dental Schools: data update 2004*.

Dawson, B. (1920) *Interim Report on the Future Provision of Medical and Allied Services*. HMSO: London.

Ellis, J. (1986a) *The London Hospital Medical College 1785–1985. The Story of England's First Medical School*. London Hospital Medical Club: London, p. 77.

Ellis, J. (1986b) *The London Hospital Medical College 1785–1985. The Story of England's First Medical School*. London Hospital Medical Club: London, pp. 101–102.

Ellis, J. (1986c) *The London Hospital Medical College 1785–1985. The Story of England's First Medical School*. London Hospital Medical Club: London, p. 116.

Flexner, A. (1910) *Medical Education in the United States and Canada: A Report to the Carnegie Foundation for the Advancement of Teaching*. Carnegie Foundation: New York.

Flexner, A. (1912) *Medical Education in Europe: A Report to the Carnegie Foundation for the Advancement of Teaching*. Carnegie Foundation: New York.

General Medical Council (1993) *Tomorrow's Doctors: Recommendations on Undergraduate Medical Education*. GMC: London.

General Medical Council (2003) *Tomorrow's Doctors*. GMC: London.

Goodenough, W. (1944) *Report of Inter-Departmental Committee on Medical Schools*. HMSO: London.

Haldane, R. B. (1913) *Royal Comission on University Education in London*. Royal Commission: London.

Huxley, T. H. (1876) Lecture delivered at the opening of Johns Hopkins University, Baltimore.

Jackson, M., Arnott, B., Benbow, E. W., Marshall, R. and Maude, P. (2003) Doctors don't need to know about the pathological basis of disease. *ACP News* **Spring**: 33–39.

Lambert, T. W., Goldacre, M. J., Turner, G., Domizio, P. and du-Boulay, C. (2006) Career choices for pathology: national surveys of graduates of 1974–2002 from UK medical schools. *J. Pathol.* **208**: 446–452.

London Hospital Medical College (1936) *Prospectus.*

London Hospital Medical College (1965) *Prospectus.*

Osler, W. (1911) On the hospital unit in university work. *Northumb.Durham Med. J.* **18**: 178–189.

Pathological Society (2001) *Future of Academic Pathology.* Report of the residential meeting held at the Bellhouse Hotel, Beaconsfield, 28th–30th March 2001.

Russell, D. S. and Innes, J. R. M. (1956) In Memoriam. Hubert Maitland Turnbull 1875–1955. *J. Pathol. Bacteriol.* **LXXI**: 535–543.

Todd, A. (1968) *Report of the Royal Commission on Medical Education.* HMSO: London.

Turnbull, H. M. (1953) Autobiographical notes (unpublished work) .. Royal London Hospital Archives PP/TUR.

Waddington, K. (2003a) Medical Education at St Bartholomew's Hospital 1123–1995. The Boydell Press: Woodbridge, p. 123.

Waddington, K. (2003b) Medical Education at St Bartholomew's Hospital 1123–1995. The Boydell Press: Woodbridge, p. 136.

Waddington, K. (2003c) Medical Education at St Bartholomew's Hospital 1123–1995. The Boydell Press: Woodbridge, pp. 157–158.

Waddington, K. (2003d) Medical Education at St Bartholomew's Hospital 1123–1995. The Boydell Press: Woodbridge, p. 199.

Waddington, K. (2003e) Medical Education at St Bartholomew's Hospital 1123–1995. The Boydell Press: Woodbridge, pp. 326–327.

Waddington, K. (2003f) Medical Education at St Bartholomew's Hospital 1123–1995. The Boydell Press: Woodbridge, pp. 380–381.

Wright, N. A. (2003) Doctors don't need to know about the pathological basis of disease? Absolute cobblers! *ACP News* **Summer**: 10–12.

13 The Changing Nature of Training in Pathology

Patrick J. Gallagher

In almost every medical school in the world the teaching of pathology to undergraduates is supported by qualified staff and appreciated by students. Most members of a pathology department accept this role, usually with considerable enthusiasm. Other chapters in this celebratory book have chronicled the rise and fall in this activity over the last century. The training of pathologists is a related but different function of pathology departments. Although the development of undergraduate education programmes has been discussed repeatedly in papers and book chapters (Foster, 1961; Rolleston, 1961; Long, 1965), there are few records of exactly how pathologists became pathologists as our specialty emerged.

THE FIRST BRITISH PATHOLOGISTS

At the time The Pathological Society was formed, Sir William Osler held the Chair of Medicine in Oxford. The earliest surviving membership lists of The Pathological Society are from 1947 so we can only assume that he was a founder member! His enthusiasm for pathology was legendary. Like so many physicians and surgeons of his day, he had held an appointment as a pathologist during his training. Osler is said to have travelled widely to many hospitals in the UK. He always asked to see the clinical laboratory and is said to have expressed his displeasure if it was inadequate or absent (Cunningham, 1992). It is likely that microbiological and serological investigations were the bulk of the work of these laboratories. In the first 40 years of the last century pathologists emerged as specialists. We know that by 1939 there were 85 so-called pathologists in Britain (Table 13.1) and can probably assume that there was one in most large hospitals. Exactly how they trained was uncertain but they probably learned by a system of apprenticeship. Most had either completed the Membership of the Royal College of Physicians or had an MD degree by thesis (Foster, 1982). In 1947 a subcommittee of the Association of Clinical Pathologists recommended five years of post-registration experience with a minimum of three years of laboratory training (Cunningham, 1992) How these doctors spent their day, how they interacted with their colleagues and how much they earned in relative terms is uncertain. Nevertheless between 1940 and 1960 the number of practising pathologists increased by almost tenfold (Table 13.1) and this subsequently provided the impetus for the formation of our College. Training posts involved a rotation between microbiology, haematology and so-called morbid anatomy. At this time the Departments of Chemical Pathology were less well developed and some were staffed only by scientific graduates (Lathe, 1971). Hospital post-mortems were as much a part of a day's work as surgical pathology cut-ups and reporting. Consultant vacancies at this time were limited and a proportion of senior registrars emigrated. On appointment, many histopathologists also undertook haematology. At this time few, if any, surgeons or gynaecologists reported their own surgical pathology. In her book *The History of Pathology in Texas*, Marilyn Baker recalled that it was in 1939 that the last surgeon reported on his own specimens (Baker, 1966).

Table 13.1 Consultant numbers in England and Wales (adapted from Foster, 1982)

	1939	1960
Physicians	500	2280
Surgeons	1100	2040
Gynaecologists	170	450
Pathologists	85	725

THE EARLY INFLUENCE OF THE COLLEGE

In his account of the early history of the Royal College of Pathologists, Foster (1982) comments on the development of the examination structure and notes that:

> 'in undertaking to set an examination the college felt also that it must set some responsibility for the education of trainee pathologists.
>
> The Academic Affairs Committee was in no doubt that the proper training of recruits to pathology was more important than any form of the examination....evidence presented made it clear that certain establishments, including some teaching hospitals, did not provide adequate rotational training.'

A leading article in *The Lancet* in 1966 was entitled 'Training of pathologists'. Although anonymous, it was clearly written by someone with close connections with our College. The article specifically describes the periods of training that are desirable in particular sub-specialties. There are some comments that ring true today: 'trainees should not be sought by heads of laboratories to act as assistants because they cannot secure established posts for more senior staff'. The article ends with a plea that the College of Pathologists should 'not exclude those eccentrics whose unorthodox progress may do it honour'.

Until 1971 the Primary examination required candidates to take a moderately demanding practical examination in two disciplines as well as a somewhat challenging multiple-choice question in all aspects of clinical pathology. At that time there were comparatively few departments that offered a well-planned and integrated training programme. The vast majority of the trainees were UK graduates. Training usually included substantial periods of on-call duty as a resident pathologist, cross-matching blood and performing simple emergency investigations. The educational value of this potentially gruelling duty was limited. Those who survived the experience acquired a life-long familiarity with the laboratory bench. Even the most sophisticated new molecular technique cannot be more demanding than cross-matching 40 units of blood in the middle of the night.

Training in the 1970s and 1980s was largely the preserve of Teaching Hospital laboratories. Rotational training positions, such as the Senior Registrars who rotated between St. Thomas's and Portsmouth and Southampton and Poole, were exceptional but very successful. Trainees generally gained District General Hospital experience by acting as locum consultants. Senior Registrars were encouraged to report independently, which is a very different situation to the current system of graded reporting schedules. Generally an MD or PhD thesis was a requirement for a Teaching Hospital position. This was usually performed 'on the job' rather than as a dedicated research fellow.

In the September 1979 issue of *Human Pathology*, five distinguished American academic pathologists (Conn *et al.*, 1979) addressed the training issues that would be required to produce pathologists for the 1980s and 1990s. Many of the assertions in this article ring true today.

'We have no shortage of people willing to tinker with the medical education system. Pathologists must develop more effective ways of attracting medical students into the field. Pathology must maintain diversity in its training programme to meet the diverse needs in our field.'

However, during the 1970s and 1980s the training of pathologists experienced relatively few changes. Numbers expanded only slowly and most training was performed in teaching hospitals. Senior trainees were a mixture of clinical lecturers and senior registrars, and most of the training departments had a strong academic lead. Few, if any, trainees spent time abroad. Consultant vacancies generally matched the supply of successful examination candidates. The number of overseas graduates obtaining UK consultant positions increased slowly but significantly. All regions provided MRCPath teaching programmes and the Royal College, the British Division of the International Academy of Pathology and the Association of Clinical Pathologists supplemented these with short courses that were attended by a mixture of consultants and trainees. A proportion of younger pathologists attended Pathology Society meetings but they were regarded as of marginal benefit in terms of preparing for the final examination. In retrospect this was a period of extended calm before the storm that descended on histopathology in the 1990s.

Nowadays it is hard to imagine 30 UK graduates applying for each and every District General Hospital vacancy. However, this was the case for several very anxious years in the 1990s. Pathology immediately became less popular than it always will be. New consultant positions were created but sometimes in tandem with a reduction in trainee positions. By the end of the decade the situation was exactly reversed. There were insufficient applicants for the growing number of vacancies advertised.

In terms of mechanisms of postgraduate training, the 1990s was a decade of introspection and perhaps stagnation. Although this may have been true also of North American training programmes, matters were very different in Europe. Surgical pathology was blossoming in many different European centres. European meetings were attracting large numbers of young pathologists. Traditionally these pathologists were not restrained by an examination system (Rinsler, 1977) and were clearly applying themselves to clinical and research work with enthusiasm.

THE PRESENT AND THE FUTURE

At the opening of the new century British histopathologists were both demoralised and overworked. Economic upturn raised the possibility of many new consultant appointments but there were insufficient trained pathologists in the pipeline. In addition, there was a paucity of applicants for Senior House Officer positions. In part this was a result of the poor public profile of pathology, but prolonged lack of innovation in recruitment and training methods may also have played a role. Three doctors from different backgrounds addressed this particular problem: Phil Quirke, a Professor of Pathology at Leeds; Julia Moore, anaesthetist working in Medical Manpower at the Department of Health; and Professor Mike Richards, the National Director of Cancer Services. It was clear that advances in cancer diagnosis could not be implemented without a ready supply of trained histopathologists, so their solution was to establish and fund training schools for first-year histopathologists. The ethos was that these doctors would be treated humanely and taught enthusiastically. Training was to be in cohorts of up to eight 'new starters' and trainees would come together for periods of block teaching. The immediate impression was that the project was successful and training schools have now been established throughout England (Gallagher *et al.*, 2003; Giles *et al.*, 2005). A total of 100 first-year trainees were recruited in a national selection process in 2005 and dispersed among 12 schools. Training schools work in clusters in order to deliver teaching more effectively. For example the 40 doctors working in London and the South of

Table 13.2 Current issues in the training of histopathologists

Concerns
There are insufficient UK/EU-trained applicants for first-year training positions
Although most positions attract a salary supplement, some do not. We are in direct competition with General Practice training posts, which do have supplements.
Despite reassurances to the contrary, there is a suspicion that there will be insufficient consultant posts for the 100 or so trainees that are recruited each year in England
Failure rates and lack of standardisation in the final MRCPath examination concern trainees.
Some centres have lack of access to, or limited numbers of, autopsies
Achievements
e-Learning and recruitment has been successfully introduced
All trainees have high-quality microscopes
Seamless ('run through') training is under development
Cultural diversity is an integral feature of training centres
Increasing numbers of recently recruited trainees are expressing an interest in an MD/PhD degree

England spent their first full week in August in Bristol. The teaching laboratories of the university are especially well equipped for microscopy and ideal for an introductory week.

Histopathology will be one of the first specialties to adopt the pattern of seamless or 'run through' training that will be introduced as part of the Department of Health's programme of Modernising Medical Careers. This is a somewhat dubious honour and at the time of writing we are unsure how trainee histopathologists will move from year to year. Trainees are concerned that salary supplements may soon be reduced or removed. A new method of assessing first-year trainees has been developed, which is hopefully more of a test of aptitude than basic knowledge. Remarkably there was a very close relationship between performance in this test at the end of the first year and the scores achieved in the interview process a year previously.

We hope and believe that the worst is past. Training in histopathology has a new profile and has benefited from substantial funding from the Department of Health. Improving recruitment of UK/EU graduates into histopathology is now the major challenge. (Table 13.2). The 2005 round of appointments attracted over 500 applicants but less than 15% were UK/EU graduates. In a recent survey 89% of final-year Cardiff medical students gave a lack of patient contact as the major disincentive to choosing pathology as a career (Howarth, Syred and Douglas-Jones, 2005). This has been confirmed by each of the first-year trainees who have left training programmes to date. It is unlikely that histopathologists will ever have substantial patient contact but in the recruitment rounds we emphasise the enhanced clinical role of pathologists in the new Cancer initiatives. Other comments in the Welsh study were that histopathology is 'too academic' (35%), has a poor public and professional profile (20%) and involves autopsy practice (19%). The autopsy examination is now a stand-alone part of the final MRCPath examination and it is likely that autopsy-free training will shortly be introduced. A website has been developed to provide information about training and recruitment (www.nhshistopathology.com) and there is an e-learning resource (www.pathnet.org.uk) (Naik *et al.*, 2005). British pathology has a debt of gratitude to the many overseas graduates working as NHS consultants. A so-called Intensive Training and Assessment Programme has been developed to fast-track experienced overseas graduates into second-year positions (Bharucha *et al.*, 2005). Each large department in England has a breadth of cultural diversity that could not have been imagined even 10 years ago (Fig. 13.1).

THE FUTURE ROLE OF THE PATHOLOGICAL SOCIETY

How will the trainee pathologists of today be practising when The Pathological Society celebrates its 125th Anniversary? How will molecular pathology have developed and how will it interface

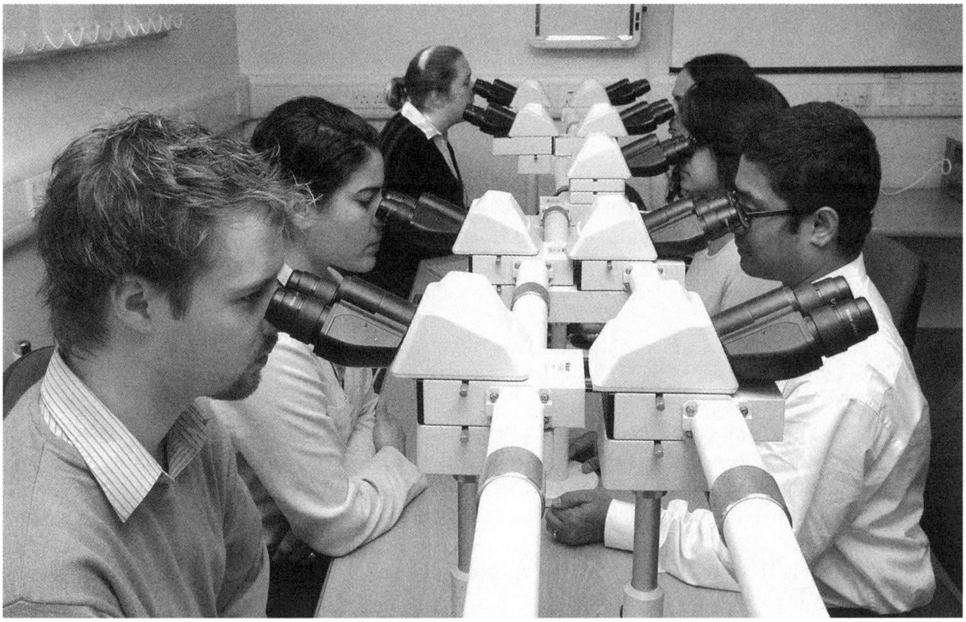

Figure 13.1 Learning histopathology in 2005. Note the excellent modern microscope and the cultural diversity of both senior and junior histopathologists.

with diagnostic surgical pathology? Will pathology still exist in District General Hospitals or will large groups of sub-specialists work from tertiary hospitals, communicating with distant sites with electronic efficiency that we can only imagine at present. Will pathology be restored to the undergraduate curriculum and will recruitment to our specialty be enhanced as a result?

A more relevant question is how will our Society have influenced the training and continuing education of young pathologists? The investment that has been provided to establish Histopathology Training Schools is aimed to deliver specialists who will serve the needs of the National Health Service by diagnosing disease. The Pathological Society mission is 'understanding disease', which is a wider role than pure diagnosis. It is probably fair to say that the input that our Society has had in the training of pathologists has been insufficient. This is recognised and is set to change. A trainees committee has been formed and each meeting will include days or half-days for presentations by, or the teaching of, trainees. Trainee membership is rising and is available for a nominal sum until Consultancy. It is important that trainers are recognised and supported by The Pathological Society, especially if they are not regular attenders at Pathology Society meetings. It is clear from many of the contributions to this volume that The Pathological Society is approaching its Centennial with pride but with a degree of concern about its future. Any effort or resource that the Society puts into the education of young colleagues will be time and money well spent.

Acknowledgements

I thank my teachers, Professors Austin Gresham and John Tighe, for information on their own experiences as trainees.

REFERENCES

Anonymous (1966) Training of pathologists. *Lancet* **2**: 93.

Baker, M.M. (1996) *The History of Pathology in Texas*. Texas Society of Pathology: Austin: TX.

Bharucha, H., Coles, C., Foria, V., Gallagher, P.J. and Mountford, B. (2005) The intensive training and assessment scheme in histopathology. *Hosp. Med.* **66**: 566–568.

Conn, R.B., Anderson, R.E., Benson, E.S., Hill, R.B. and Straumfjord, J.V. (1979) Training pathologists for the 1980s and 1990s. *Hum. Pathol.* **10**: 493–495.

Cunningham, G.J. (1992) *The History of British Pathology.* White Tree Books, Redcliffe Press: Bristol.

Foster, W.D. (1961) *A Short History of Clinical Pathology.* Livingstone: Edinburgh.

Foster, W.D. (1982) *Pathology as a Profession in Great Britain and the Early History of the Royal College of Pathologists.* Royal College of Pathologists: London.

Gallagher, P.J., Dixon, M.F., Heard, S., Moore, J.K. and West, K.P. (2003) An initiative to reform senior house officer training in histopathology. *Hosp. Med.* **64**: 302–305.

Giles, T., Griffin, N., Leonard, N. and McGregor, A. (2005) Histopathology training schools 4 years on. *Hosp. Med.* **66**: 560–562.

Howarth, S.M., Syred, K.S. and Douglas-Jones, A. (2005) Histopathology in the foundation two (F2) year. Will it work? *J. Pathol.* **207**: Suppl. 42A.

Lathe, G.H. (1971) Training of pathologists. *Lancet* **1**: 909.

Long, E.R. (1965) *A History of Pathology.* Dover Publications: New York.

Naik, P., Rashbas, J., Bennett, M., Cossins, S. and Griffin, N.R. (2005) IT innovation in histopathology recruitment, training and research. *Hosp. Med.* **66**: 563–565.

Rinsler, M.G. (1977) Training of pathologists in countries belonging to the European Economic Community. *J. Clin. Pathol.* **30**: 788–799.

Rolleston, H. (1961) The early history of the teaching of: I. Human Anatomy in London; II. Morbid Anatomy and Pathology in Great Britain. *Ann. Med. Hist.* **1**: 203–238.

14 The Changing Work Patterns of Pathology

Chris W. Elston, Alastair D. Burt and Neil A. Shepherd

INTRODUCTION

The history of British pathology can be traced back to the 18th century when the best clinicians, such as the Hunter brothers, William and John, began to perform autopsies on their patients and to collect their autopsy and biopsy specimens into museums. The first half of the 19th century saw the introduction of microscopy and the setting up of laboratories, staffed initially by part-time clinicians. Later in the century some full-time appointments were made and Chairs of Pathology were established in major cities; most were in morbid anatomy, with some in bacteriology. However, in comparison with Continental Europe, the recognition of clinical pathology (which included diagnostic histopathology) as an independent discipline in the UK was delayed until the second decade of the 20th century. Furthermore, although Pathology Departments were present in most Medical Schools, there were very few in non-teaching hospitals (Cunningham, 1992). Pathology tests were, therefore, available to only a very small number of privileged patients. Today, 100 years on, all clinicians and their patients have access to high-quality diagnostic histopathology services, including the latest molecular and genetic techniques. It is pertinent to this celebration of the centenary of The Pathological Society that this review gives an account of the profound changes that have taken place in the provision of these services and their impact on workload in diagnostic histopathology. For balance we have divided the century into two 50-year periods, 1906–1956 and 1957–2006.

THE FIRST 50 YEARS (1906–1956)

Background

Before the question of workload patterns can be discussed it is important to describe the nature of Pathology Services in this period. Pathology in Medical Schools was based in Departments of Morbid Anatomy, which were mainly concerned with teaching medical students (largely from autopsies) and carrying out basic pathophysiological research. However, in the early period after the First World War many had little involvement in patient care and some influential academics, such as Boycott at University College, London, even believed that the carrying out of 'blood tests' was more the preserve of clinicians than pathologists (Cunningham, 1992). Bacteriology was established as a discipline in its own right but the emerging field of clinical pathology, encompassing histopathology, chemical pathology, haematology and immunology, was in its infancy and many of the duties that are now accepted as the preserve of pathologists were carried out by clinicians. The next 20 or 30 years saw the gradual establishment of Pathology Departments in the larger District General Hospitals. These were usually general departments covering all disciplines and headed by a single-handed pathologist whose main interest was morbid anatomy and histology. According to Cunningham (1992), the proper pattern for a modern Pathology Department was established in 1934 by Kettle at the newly founded British Postgraduate Medical School at the Hammersmith Hospital, London. He divided his department into sections that operated independently under a sub-departmental head, covering morbid anatomy, bacteriology, chemical patho-logy and haematology. During the Second World War clinical pathology developed more rapidly, largely under the auspices of the Emergency Medical Service. Under this scheme the establishment of laboratories in London and throughout the provinces formed the basis of the pathological services that came into being when the National Health Service was introduced in 1948.

Workload

It is difficult at this distance to give an accurate account of the typical workload of a pathologist in those early days. Apart from overseeing the technical aspects of all the disciplines, he or she would have had a substantial autopsy practice, including work for HM Coroner, although many of the latter cases were being performed by general practitioners and even hospital-based clinicians. Diagnostic (or surgical) pathology usually occupied less time and the majority of specimens were derived from major surgical procedures such as gastrectomy, colectomy, hysterectomy and mastectomy; the main purpose of histological examination of these specimens was simply to confirm the clinical diagnosis. Biopsy specimens would have been restricted to easily accessible sites such as skin, endometrial curettings and those to which a rigid 'scope' could be applied, such as recto-sigmoid, larynx, oesophagus and bronchi. Liver biopsies could only be obtained during procedures such as exploratory laparotomy and were nearly always performed to investigate discrete lesions found incidentally at this time, rather than as part of a general diagnostic work-up.

In most cases diagnosis was based on examination of a small number of blocks from the specimens, stained with conventional haematoxylin and eosin (H&E). Special stains such as van Gieson, periodic acid–Schiff and Congo Red were used sparingly. Histopathology reports were largely descriptive and contained little prognostic or predictive information.

There was little or no direct involvement in patient management and no concept of multidisciplinary team working. Perhaps the closest that the pathologist came to participation in the decision-making process was in the performance of intra-operative frozen sections. Despite the fact that the freezing microtome was introduced in the latter part of the 19th century and was advocated for examination of tissues at operation (Senn, 1895; Gal, 2001), it was not until 1905 that it became accepted as a routine procedure (Wilson, 1905). According to Haagensen (1986) this technique was first suggested for breast disease by the gynaecologist Thomas Cullen at Johns Hopkins, Baltimore, USA in 1900. At this time Halsted, the renowned breast surgeon, was still dependent on clinical diagnosis alone to select patients for radical mastectomy and about 10% were operated on unnecessarily for benign disease. One of Halsted's assistants, Bloodgood, learnt how to perform frozen sections and solved the problem (Bloodgood, 1914). The equipment was rather basic and it was not possible to produce thin sections of the quality obtained by a modern cryostat; nevertheless, by 1938 Breuer reported an overall accuracy of 88.9%, with no false-positive results, although in general the false-positive rate was about 1–2% (Breuer, 1938). Frozen sections were carried out most frequently on samples from breast (30%), lymph node (15%), gastrointestinal tract (10%) and lung/thorax (10%). In most cases the procedure was carried out to confirm a clinical diagnosis of malignancy before proceeding to therapeutic surgery, whereas in others an unexpected mass or nodule might be sampled to exclude metastatic disease.

We noted above that, in some general hospitals, pathology testing was carried out by clinicians. This usually applied to autopsies and such 'blood tests' as were available, but in some hospitals clinicians also ran Diagnostic Histopathology Departments. For example, at St Bartholomew's Hospital, London, it was traditional for the gynaecologists to report on their own specimens and this practice even continued until the 1970s. The same can be said for dermatopathology. Even today many clinical dermatologists are expert histopathologists, particularly in the assessment of inflammatory diseases of the skin.

THE SECOND 50 YEARS (1957–2006)

Background

In general the practice of diagnostic histopathology differed little in the first decade of this period from the previous 20 or 30 years. There was still a relatively large autopsy workload, the case mix in diagnostic histopathology was unaltered and intra-operative frozen section was practised widely as a precursor to major surgery. Indeed, the basic technology of histopathology has not changed significantly during the whole of the century since the foundation of The Pathological Society. The majority of specimens are still fixed in formalin and embedded in paraffin wax, sections are still cut on microtomes, H&E is the routine first-line stain and light microscopy is the main means of arriving at a diagnosis.

In 1963, when one of us (C.W.E) was about to embark on his career in histopathology, it was perceived as outmoded and only marginally relevant to patient management; some predicted that the discipline would disappear altogether, to be replaced by more sophisticated techniques such as the automated multichannel analysers being developed in clinical chemistry laboratories. How wrong the doubters were can be seen very simply in the steady and significant rise in overall workload in this second 50-year period in one District General Hospital, which can be regarded as representative for the whole discipline (Fig. 14.1). Yet few, if any, could have envisaged the profound changes that would occur in our discipline in the last 40 years, greater than at any time in the history of histopathology. This renaissance has been due to a number of different but interconnected factors, but the key to its continuing importance, even in the modern 'molecular' age, is the imperative to establish an accurate tissue diagnosis before treatment is started. Most of the factors

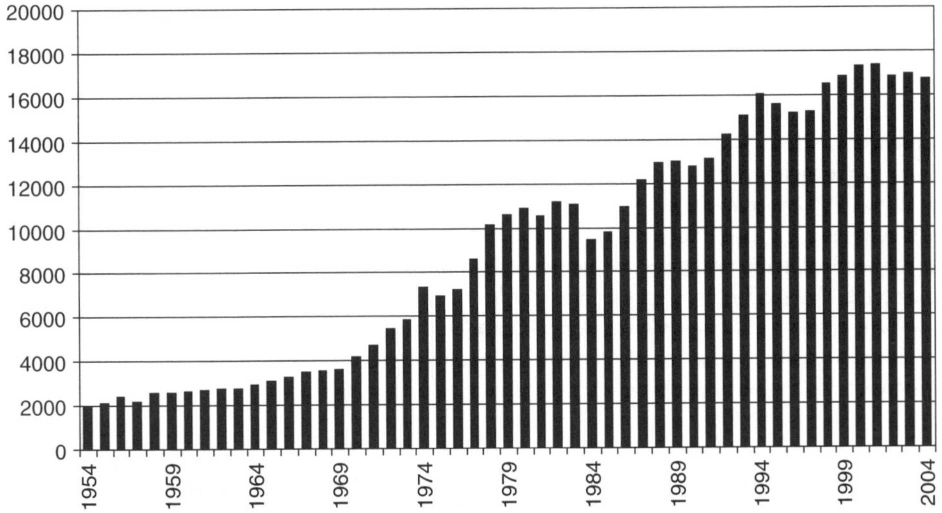

Figure 14.1 Cumulative histopathology workload figures for the 50-year period 1954–2004 at the Gloucestershire Royal Hospital. Although demonstrating a relatively consistent rise, there are two notable dips. The first, in 1984–1985, is an artefact because of a change in the way the specimens were counted. The second, in 1995–1996, was the result of the pathologists' proactivity, with the prohibition of routine antral biopsies for the diagnosis of helicobacter infection.

that have driven the changes in our discipline are clinically related and due to improvements in our understanding and treatment of the major diseases, such as cancer, whereas some, such as the development of immunohistochemistry (Taylor and Kledzik, 1981; Gatter, 1989), are intrinsic to the discipline itself. There are two broad clinical areas in which histopathology has become increasingly influential: pre- or non-operative diagnosis; and prognostication and prediction of disease outcomes. We will discuss the general implications of these changes but in order to illustrate their impact on workload patterns we will give examples from our own sub-specialties.

Pre- or Non-operative Diagnosis

General considerations

There have been huge improvements in biopsy techniques in the last 50 years. A major advance was the introduction of percutaneous needle biopsy, which enabled the investigation of solid internal organs not previously accessible without exploratory surgery. The first such needle, the Vim-Silverman, was initially introduced to improve the preoperative diagnosis of cancers (Silverman, 1938) but was also used for liver biopsy. A similar needle was devised for renal biopsy by Iversen and Brun (1951). The Vim-Silverman needle was subsequently superseded by the Menghini needle (Menghini, 1958), which was safer and easier to use than the Vim-Silverman, produced sufficient tissue to support techniques such as histochemistry in addition to light microscopy and gave less crush artefact. Following its success in liver biopsy (see also below), the Menghini needle was subsequently applied to other areas such as renal, prostate and lung biopsy. Even greater improvements were heralded by the development of disposable needle-core-cutting devices such as the 'Tru-Cut' needle (Rake *et al.*, 1969; Vitums, 1972) and, more recently, automated spring-loaded biopsy guns (e.g. the Bard Magnum and the Manan Pro-mag). Allied to high-resolution ultrasound guidance and, where necessary, 'long throw' needles, most organs in the body, including para-aortic or mediastinal lymph nodes, are now accessible to needle biopsy. The other major advance has been the invention of flexible fibre-optic endoscopic devices in the early 1970s (Kirsner, 1998; Cotton and Williams, 2003), which are not only much safer than rigid endoscopes but permit far more extensive sampling, especially in the gastrointestinal tract (see below).

In parallel with these improvements in biopsy technique, conventional light microscopy has been complemented by refinements in ancillary diagnostic methods: histochemistry, which retains considerable importance in the evaluation of liver, renal and gastrointestinal biopsies; electron microscopy, which is a central component of renal biopsy assessment; and immunohistology, which has revolutionised the accuracy of differential diagnosis in tumour pathology.

These developments have, of course, contributed to the steady and significant rise in workload referred to above; for example, at the Nottingham City Hospital biopsy specimens have nearly doubled in the last 10 years and now account for 40% of the overall workload (Table 14.1). They have also led to the establishment of pre-non-operative Multidisciplinary Team Meetings (MDTM), which is another significant call on a pathologist's time. There is a general consensus that team-working in cancer management is good for the patient and in particular should lead to consistency of therapeutic approaches with, it is hoped, enhanced quality of care. What is less

Table 14.1 Comparison of biopsy and resection specimens at Nottingham City Hospital in 1994–1995 and 2004–2005

Year	Biopsies	Resection	Total	Biopsy percentage
94/95	4306	13 508	17 814	24%
04/05	7749	12 296	20 045	40%

clear is whether the MDTMs are a cost-effective way of achieving such team-working. There was a very lively debate about this at the Summer 2005 Newcastle Pathology Meeting.

Breast disease

Although fine-needle aspiration cytology (FNAC) became popular throughout Europe as an alternative to frozen section in the diagnosis of breast lesions (Franzen and Zajiceck, 1968), it was used only sparingly in the UK. Instead, a variety of needles that produced a histological sample were developed, the most successful of which was the manual 'Tru-Cut' (Roberts *et al.*, 1975; Elston *et al.*, 1978). Use of this technique enabled a definite preoperative diagnosis of carcinoma in 75% of cases. This resulted in a substantial reduction in the number of 'open-ended' frozen sections, many of which, it should be noted, revealed benign disease only. Operation lists became more efficient and there was more productive use of pathologist's time. 'Tru-Cut' biopsy was less successful in the diagnosis of benign lesions; for example, a definite diagnosis was only possible in 50% of fibroadenomas. Nevertheless, a significant reduction in unnecessary excision biopsies for benign disease was achieved.

About a decade later the introduction of mammography as both a diagnostic and a screening procedure led to the need to sample smaller palpable and impalpable lesions. More precise targeting was provided by high-resolution ultrasound guidance. Paradoxically, the 'Tru-Cut' needle was unsuitable in this setting, for technical reasons, and this led to a resurgence in interest in FNAC.

In many centres, for the next 10–15 years FNAC was the main diagnostic technique, so that in the Nottingham City Hospital, for example, the annual total of breast FNAC specimens rose to approximately 2500. The Standard of Care for the pre- or non-operative assessment of breast lesions became the Triple Approach, based on clinical examination, imaging (mammography and/or ultrasound) and FNAC (Dixon *et al.*, 1984; Hermansen *et al.*, 1987). The preoperative diagnosis rate for invasive carcinoma was approximately 90%, but that for ductal carcinoma *in situ* (DCIS) was only 75–80% due to the difficulty in obtaining representative samples from small areas of mammographically suspicious microcalcifications. This problem was solved in the 1990s by the introduction of automated spring-loaded needle core biopsy (NCB) and more recently vacuum-assisted mammotomy (VAM). These developments eventually led to the replacement of FNAC by NCB in most UK breast units. Audit for the Nottingham Breast Screening Service shows that even for screen-detected breast carcinoma a preoperative diagnosis rate of close to 100% can be achieved (Table 14.2). Definite positive diagnosis of benign lesions such as fibroadenomas is also possible in the majority of cases, thus reducing the need for excision biopsy. This approach has resulted in an annual workload of, on average, 2000 NCBs, about a third of which require multiple levels for the assessment of microcalcifications or suspicious epithelial proliferations (11 109 biopsies January 2000–November 2005).

The use of immunohistology in NCB has increased dramatically in the last 10–15 years for both diagnostic and therapeutic reasons. Diagnostically, for example, the use of a panel of epithelial immunostains can differentiate an infiltrate of carcinoma cells from an inflammatory process, or a metaplastic spindle cell carcinoma from a soft-tissue sarcoma. In terms of therapy there is an

Table 14.2 Audit of preoperative diagnosis of carcinomas in the Nottingham Breast Screening Service, 2003–2004

Type	Number of cases	Preoperative diagnosis
Invasive	156	156 (100%)
Ductal carcinoma *in situ*	34	33 (97%)
Total	190	189 (99.5%)

Table 14.3 Reporting categories for needle core biopsy of breast, recommended by the National Coordinating Committee for Breast Pathology

B1 – Unsatisfactory/normal tissue only
B2 – Benign
B3 – Uncertain malignant potential
B4 – Suspicious
B5 – Malignant

increasing demand from clinicians for assessment of hormone receptor status (aestrogen receptor and progesterone receptor) on core biopsy, particularly in elderly patients or those with locally advanced disease in whom primary hormone therapy is contemplated.

A further development in many Breast Units has been the introduction of synoptic rather than narrative reporting, based on the B1–B5 system (Table 14.3) recommended in the National Health Service Breast Screening Programme (Non-operative Diagnosis Subgroup of the National Coordinating Committee for Breast Pathology, 2005); this saves both pathologist and secretarial time, especially if applied electronically.

Liver disease

As noted above, the introduction of the Menghini needle helped put liver biopsy interpretation 'on the map'. This procedure provided tissue of sufficient quality to support light microscopic, histochemical and even ultrastructural studies. Newer core biopsy devices such as the 'Tru-Cut' biopsy and biopsy guns have refined the technique; this includes coating the needles with synthetic materials thought to contribute to better quality histology with reduced artefact (Fukuda and Inokuti, 2004). For most conditions percutaneous biopsy yields a satisfactory specimen. Ultrasound guidance can be particularly helpful in dealing with small focal lesions but is also increasingly applied to obtain samples in patients with diffuse disease. The development of biopsy via the transjugular approach has been particularly helpful in providing specimens from patients who are more unwell, e.g. those who have a bleeding diathesis or marked ascites (McAfee *et al.*, 1992). In many centres such specimens are now almost as impressive as those taken percutaneously using ultrasound.

In the early days liver biopsy was used primarily in the investigation of obstructive jaundice and suspected infections (including, in some parts of the world, diagnosis of disorders such as schistosomiasis). Biopsies are now much less commonly seen from patients with biliary obstruction because imaging procedures have improved and complications of biopsy are recognised to be greater in patients with obstruction than in other situations. The general approach to liver biopsy interpretation has not altered radically since the mid-1950s/early 1960s. For the majority of cases, routine H&E-stained sections together with a panel of simple histochemical stains is sufficient for a full histopathological diagnosis.

Immunohistochemistry has, arguably, played a lesser role in hepatopathology compared to many other areas, although it is of particular help in defining the nature of malignant tumours (primary versus secondary; hepatocellular versus cholangiocarcinoma). There are a number of commercially available reagents that can identify infective agents but much of the important clinical information in relation to hepatitis B and hepatitis C, for example, can best be obtained from serological/virological analysis. There is a growing interest in the application of proteomics and genomics on liver biopsy material but this remains an adjunct and is currently best regarded as being within the research domain rather than applied practice.

It is worth remembering that the procedure of liver biopsy carries a not insignificant morbidity and even mortality. Deaths from biopsies are said to occur in between 1 in 1000 to 1 in 10000 examinations; the procedure is therefore not to be undertaken lightly. A number of centres have sought to develop FNAC as an alternative to needle biopsy. Although there is little doubt that this can be a safe and effective approach in the diagnosis of mass lesions, it is not of any value in the investigation of common necro-inflammatory conditions or in the monitoring of post-transplant complications.

Throughout the latter half of the 20th century there was a continued rise in the use of liver biopsy; this was probably contributed to by the development of clinical hepatology as a distinct sub-specialty. There was an almost exponential rise in the number of biopsies undertaken following the identification of hepatitis C as an important human pathogen. Even the earliest studies of this very common condition showed that investigation of liver function tests did not provide any indication of the severity of the disease; as discussed below, liver biopsy interpretation has remained a cornerstone for assessing patients for therapy in this condition. The other stimulus for an increase in liver biopsy numbers, at least in the larger centres, has been the development of liver transplantation. Again, it became clear that clinicians could not rely on the common 'liver function tests' to monitor how the liver was faring postoperatively and in particular whether there was any rejection (Sebach and Samuel, 2004).

Since the late 1990s many departments, including the large tertiary centres with supra-regional liver units, have seen a plateau in the number of liver biopsy requests. In the transplant units there has been a decline in the interest and justification of protocol biopsies (in the past many patients would have an annual 'MOT' biopsy). Clinical algorithms have been drawn up for certain conditions that have obviated the need for biopsy diagnosis; clearly this is driven by the morbidity and even mortality referred to above. Such algorithms are not without their problems and frequently overlook the fact that the liver often harbours more than one pathological process! Biopsies are still regarded as the 'gold standard' for assessing the degree of fibrosis (see below) but a number of international groups have sought to identify surrogate markers that would again overcome the need for biopsy (Rosenberg *et al.*, 2004); although these are exciting developments they are yet an unproven clinical utility (Afdhal, 2004). Thus, we may see a slight decline in liver biopsy requests over the next decade or so but it is highly likely that this investigation will remain pivotal in clinical hepatology way beyond the retirement date of each of the authors of this chapter.

Gastrointestinal disease

The last 50 years have seen extraordinary changes in the practice of gastroenterology and, thereby, the practice of gastrointestinal pathology. As noted above, undoubtedly the major influence has been the dramatic improvement in endoscopy and the ability to reach areas of the gastrointestinal tract previously only accessible by intra-operative techniques. Flexible upper gastrointestinal endoscopy became more available to most practitioners in this country in the late 1970s and early 1980s. Furthermore, flexible sigmoidoscopy and colonoscopy also wrought dramatic changes in colorectal clinical practice. Not only have these techniques allowed excellent access for pathological diagnosis but they have also dramatically increased our understanding of the pathological processes at play, particularly in the oesophagus and the stomach.

Oesophagus

Although the oesophagus was reasonably accessible by rigid oesophagoscopy, there is no doubt that flexible endoscopy has rapidly increased our knowledge of oesophageal disease. The advent of such endoscopy, particularly with open access, allowing endoscopic and pathological assessment of many patients with reflux-type symptoms, has in part influenced the dramatic increase in the number of cases of Barrett's oesophagus now detected. Although there has been a true increase in the prevalence, the better recognition by clinicians of the disease, particularly the short segment variant, has also led to a significant rise in the number of cases detected histopathologically. At the same time, our understanding of the diagnosis of reflux disease has also changed pathological practice. It is clear that endoscopic techniques are much better at assessing the presence and degree of reflux-associated disease than pathology. There really can be no indication, now, for routine biopsies of reflux oesophagitis.

Stomach

Flexible endoscopy has greatly increased our knowledge of the pathology of gastritis and peptic ulcer disease. This particularly relates, of course, to Helicobacter infection. Before the discovery of this highly prevalent bacterial infection by the 2005 Nobel Laureates Marshall and Warren (Marshall and Warren, 1983), we had very limited understanding of the pathogenesis of gastritis and peptic ulceration. It rapidly became clear that Helicobacter infection has had a major influence on the epidemiology and pathogenesis of gastric peptic ulceration, duodenal peptic ulceration and on gastric carcinogenesis. Indeed the bacterium is now regarded as a type 1 carcinogen. When all three of us were medical students, we were taught that it was inconceivable that significant bacterial infection could survive the acidic environment of the stomach. We now know that the bacterium is uniquely able to withstand such an acidic environment and, indeed, is the chief cause of gastritis, peptic ulceration and gastric carcinoma in most countries.

Although there is no doubt that Helicobacter infection is the most common significant bacterial infection in the world and that it is so potent in the genesis of gastric cancer, we are seeing evidence of a decreasing prevalence of Helicobacter-associated gastritis, in the UK at least. This is probably mainly related to enhanced socio-economic circumstances. At the same time, the incidence of gastric carcinoma is falling and the disease is now relatively more common in the proximal stomach, compared to the antrum, the most prevalent site in former years. Because of a diminution in Helicobacter infection of the stomach, we have also seen a notable reduction in Helicobacter-associated peptic ulceration in both the stomach and the duodenum. Reactive gastritis, most usually due to drugs, is now the most common type of gastritis demonstrated in endoscopic specimens from the stomach in the UK.

Even in our professional lifetimes, we have been able to see these quite dramatic evolutionary changes, almost entirely related to the epidemiology of Helicobacter infection. There is now good evidence that the age of acquisition of Helicobacter infection, in a population as a whole, is a major determinant of the predominant gastro-duodenal pathological phenotypes in that population (Blaser, 1998). Furthermore, there is tantalizing evidence that the high prevalence of Helicobacter infection in the stomach protects that population from oesophageal disease, most notably reflux oesophagitis, Barrett's oesophagus and adenocarcinoma complicating the latter.

The last 50 years, especially the last 20 years, have seen a dramatic increase in our understanding of gastric pathology, particularly gastritis and peptic ulceration. However, although research by biopsy should of course continue, there is little evidence that the routine biopsy of the stomach, without an endoscopic lesion, can be justified, particularly with the pressure of work that UK pathologists face at this time. For instance, there is little evidence that the additional information provided by histopathological assessment of antral biopsies is of any use to individual patient management; microbiological and serological methodology, for the demonstration of Helicobacter, is now just as effective as histopathological assessment (Howat *et al.*, 2006). With the advent of open-access flexible endoscopy, there has been an ever-burgeoning biopsy practice and we would argue that pathologists should resist the routine biopsy. There also needs to be an intensive educational drive by pathologists to ensure that endoscopists understand the indications for histopathological assessment throughout the gastrointestinal tract.

Small bowel

The histopathological diagnosis of coeliac disease has undergone considerable change. Formerly, jejunal biopsy, usually performed by a Crosby capsule, was the method of choice for harvesting small-intestine mucosa. This technique, using radiological guidance, was prevalent, particularly in children, in the 1970s. Flexible endoscopy has now ensured that endoscopists are easily able to reach the duodenum and biopsies from its second and third parts are now preferred for the accurate diagnosis of coeliac disease. At the other end of the small intestine, colonoscopists reach the terminal ileum in more than 90% of procedures. Indeed, they can regularly intubate the terminal ileum and this allows pathological assessment of terminal ileal disease, particularly, of course, in Crohn's disease. Even newer techniques, such as capsule enteroscopy, are not yet sufficiently developed to allow such capsules to take biopsies but one might envisage that, in the future, biopsies from areas of the small intestine at present wholly inaccessible may be possible.

Colorectum

It is, once again, flexible endoscopy that has dramatically influenced the practice of diagnostic histopathology in colorectal disease in the last few decades. This particularly relates to the assessment and differential diagnosis of chronic inflammatory bowel disease, but open-access colonoscopy has also influenced our understanding of carcinogenesis in the large intestine. Furthermore, colorectal cancer screening will be instituted, in the UK, in 2006 and this will have a major influence on workload patterns in histopathology departments. There are tentative proposals for medical staff to undertake the histopathological assessment of polyps generated from the Colorectal Cancer Screening Programme.

Prognostication and Prediction of Disease Outcome

General considerations

At the beginning of this 50-year period the treatment options for many diseases were relatively limited. In the field of cancer, for example, surgical excision with or without postoperative irradiation was the standard procedure for operable tumours whereas palliative radiotherapy was given in inoperable cases. Cytotoxic therapy was being introduced for the leukaemias and some lymphomas but was not used for solid tumours. The main role of the histopathologist was to confirm the diagnosis of malignancy but there was little input to therapeutic decision-making. Although correlations between histopathological features and prognosis were well established, they were disregarded by clinicians. Gradually, however, new therapeutic regimes emerged as surgical techniques became more precise, radiation therapy better targeted and more effective cytotoxic therapy was developed.

Instead of a standard regime for all those with a particular tumour, it was recognised that patients should be stratified so that each individual receives appropriate therapy. As a result, histopathological assessment has assumed greater importance, specimens are examined more extensively, reports have become more detailed and minimum data sets have been established for all tumour sites. These changes have all contributed to an increased workload not only numerically but particularly in the complexity of the process. Another important consequence has been the inexorable move, especially in large departments, towards sub-specialisation, with pathologists restricting their reporting to one or two organ systems.

Breast disease

Until the last 10–20 years the treatment of all breast lesions, benign or malignant, was predominantly surgical. For invasive breast carcinoma the standard treatment was mastectomy, either simple or radical, with axillary clearance and/or postoperative irradiation to the axilla. Histopathology reports were mainly descriptive and the only prognostic information supplied (or required) was lymph node stage, even in clinical trials of cytotoxic therapy. The resurgence of interest in other prognostic factors began with the demonstration that an index based on a combination of factors (histological grade, lymph node stage and tumour size) gave a more accurate prediction of survival (Haybittle *et al.*, 1982). The relevance to the stratification of patients for adjuvant systemic therapy of such an index is now established, as is its validation in other centres (Clark, 1992; Galea *et al.*, 1992; Blamey, 1996; Balslev *et al.*, 1994).

Assessment of oestrogen receptor status by immunohistology is now performed routinely on formalin-fixed paraffin-embedded material (Snead *et al.*, 1993). Oestrogen receptor status is accepted as a reliable means of predicting response to hormone therapy (Barnes and Millis, 1995) and is part of the minimum data set in most Breast Units. The novel drug trastuzumab, a recombinant humanised monoclonal antibody directed against the epidermal growth factor receptor 2 (HER2), previously used only in advanced cases, has now been shown to be effective as an adjuvant therapy in early breast cancer (Romond *et al.*, 2005). Approximately 15% of breast cancers are HER2 positive, but it is envisaged that testing will be carried out on patients in the very near future – a further and expensive addition to the pathology workload. Earlier presentation, partly as a result of mammographic detection, has led to an increasing demand for conservation surgery; approximately 40% of patients now choose this option. This, in turn, has emphasised the need for more thorough pathological assessment of excision specimens and the importance of clear margins (Gage *et al.*, 1996).

Although a weak prognostic factor compared with grade, histological type is of importance in our understanding of the biological aspects of breast cancer. For example, the association between the medullary and medullary-like phenotype with BRCA-1 gene mutation carrier status provides interesting insights into genetic and hereditary aspects of the disease (Lakhani *et al.*, 1998). The critical role of these and other prognostic factors in patient management has become established in a comparatively short space of time, certainly less than 20 years. They are incorporated in the Royal College of Pathologists histopathology minimum data set and their inclusion in the standard breast histopathology report is now mandatory (Guidelines Working Group of the National Coordinating Committee for Breast Pathology, 2005). Their impact on workload is illustrated by comparing the average number of blocks from a mastectomy specimen ca. 1975 (6–10) with that for a mastectomy (15–20) and wide local excision (25–30) in 2005. Furthermore, in the personal experience of one of us (C.W.E), there is a considerable difference in the time taken to report such resection specimens: an average of 15–20 min in 1975 compared with 45–60 min in 2005. To this must be added the time spent in attending therapeutic MDTMs.

Liver disease

Liver biopsies are used for grading and staging much more in the field of necro-inflammatory disease and for the monitoring of rejection than in neoplastic disease. Although there are grading systems described for hepatocellular carcinoma – the most common malignant liver tumour – overall survival for all grades is pretty appalling and assessment on needle biopsy has not been helpful in prognostication. Indeed, current European protocols have indicated that biopsy of suspected hepatocellular carcinoma should not be performed using any form of needle because of the risk of dissemination of tumour along the needle track (Scholmerich and Schacherer, 2004).

It is principally in the field of viral liver disease in which assessment of severity has been of most value. The various treatment modalities that have been developed for dealing with hepatitis C virus are expensive, associated with significant side-effects and certainly not 100% effective. As a consequence it has been extremely important to develop systems that stratify patients for therapeutic intervention. Over the past 20 years or so there have been a number of scoring systems developed to assess the histological severity of chronic hepatitis.

For many years the most widely used was the Knodell Score, which was developed by Kamal Ishak and colleagues at the Armed Forces Institute of Pathology. In essence this uses numeric scores for a number of different parameters of necro-inflammation and fibrosis, and these are summated to give an overall histological activity index. In the 1990s it became apparent that it would be important to separate out the assessment of necro-inflammation (grade) from the degree of fibrosis (stage). Furthermore, there is no good biological justification for summating the numeric scores for each of the different assessed features. The modified HAI described by Ishak and colleagues is thus a profile of features, although inevitably many of our clinical colleagues do the summation themselves! Some have argued that we would have been more sensible applying letters rather than numbers to the system, avoiding the misuse of statistics.

Liver pathologists have, however, been concerned with the important issue of sampling (Scheuer, 2003). There are now several well-conducted studies that have demonstrated that unless the biopsy is greater than 2 cm the reliability of grading and staging is substantially reduced. Furthermore, there have been numerous studies looking at inter- and intra-observer variation of such semi-quantitative scores. Some of these have demonstrated a quite appalling lack of consistency, particularly across observers, but, more reassuringly, in individual centres where there has been training of the observers as a group (what Professor Valeer Desmet refers to as 'tuning the violins') the Kappa values are very much better. More recently, similar grading and staging systems have been used increasingly in the assessment of fatty liver disease. In particular they are likely to be applied quite widely to the assessment of non-alcoholic fatty liver disease as new therapies become available to treat this common condition (Brunt *et al.*, 2004).

Gastrointestinal disease

Accurate prognostication of cancer started with the meticulous pathological studies of Dukes and his staging system for colorectal cancer (Dukes, 1932; Dukes and Bussey, 1958). In the early 1920s, Dukes first demonstrated that accurate pathological assessment of the spread of colorectal cancer had a profound influence on prognosis. His studies, performed at St Mark's Hospital in London, were based on accurate macroscopic pathological assessment and, in fact, depended relatively little on microscopic assessment. Certainly in the 1970s and 1980s the importance of such macroscopic assessment was somewhat disregarded and we believe that this was a major influence in the overall poor quality of colorectal cancer assessment in pathology departments in the UK (Morson, 1981; Shepherd and Quirke, 1997). Only more recently, with the advent of initiatives by the Royal College of Surgeons and then the Royal College of Pathologists, and the introduction of reporting proformas and minimum data sets, has the quality of colorectal cancer reporting improved in routine pathological practice.

It was perhaps the success of the Dukes classification, which effectively only assesses penetration of the bowel wall and local lymph node involvement, that accounts for the dearth of accurate research on parameters that are now regarded to be of supreme importance in colorectal cancer prognostication. A dramatic change undoubtedly occurred in the early 1980s with the recognition of the importance of surgical complete mesorectal excision (Heald *et al.*, 1982; Heald and Ryall, 1986). It was Quirke who championed the importance of pathological assessment of this margin and the influence of margin involvement on local recurrence and prognosis (Quirke *et al.*, 1986). Such assessment of margin involvement, and the techniques that accompanied it, is now applied also to colonic cancer and oesophageal cancer.

The same initiatives have occurred in the assessment of oesophageal and gastric cancer. In the last 50 years there has been a dramatic change in the prevalence of these two diseases, with less gastric cancer and much more adenocarcinoma of the oesophagus, the latter related to reflux disease and Barrett's oesophagus. Pathological practice, of course, reflects surgical practice but we have seen a large increase in resections for oesophageal adenocarcinoma and a notable decrease in resections for oesophageal squamous cell carcinoma and gastric adenocarcinoma. The quality of pathological assessment has been improved, particularly in oesophageal cancer resection specimens, with the recognition of the importance of circumferential margin involvement and lymph node involvement.

As with breast cancer, there is no doubt that the accurate assessment of these gastrointestinal cancer resection specimens has had an important influence on the workload of the pathologists. Accurate and diligent assessment of these specimens now takes at least one hour, whereas formerly the macroscopic assessment was often detailed to a junior member of staff or alternatively took a very little time. There has also been the advent of the cancer MDTMs; these have had a significant influence on the pathologist's workload. Most pathologists appreciate the importance of such meetings because they allow accurate analysis of the needs of individual cancer patients in terms of appropriate investigations, surgery, oncological treatment, palliative care and overall prognosis.

SUMMARY

In the last 100 years diagnostic histopathology has developed from a largely passive discipline to one that is proactive and at the forefront of modern patient management. The most dramatic changes have taken place in the last two to three decades due to a combination of improved therapeutic options and well-constructed clinicopathological research. As a result, our discipline has more relevance today than at any time in the past century. The most striking changes have been the growth of pre- and non-operative diagnosis and the provision of factors that are prognostic and predictive of disease outcome. Establishment of a tissue diagnosis is still the 'gold standard' for all cancers and many other diseases. As a result, there has been a steady year-on-year rise both in the overall number of specimens examined and in the complexity of pathology reports.

There is another example where the proactivity of diagnostic pathologists is important. Formerly, the passivity of the specialty was such that pathologists had no influence on which specimens were to be submitted for pathology and thus we accepted all samples sent to us. The first changes occurred nearly 30 years ago when Fox (1978) first argued that the routine examination of placentas from live births was unproductive. Nowadays, most notably in the gastrointestinal tract, pathologists are even more involved in influencing the type of specimens they receive (Fig. 14.1) (Howat *et al.*, 2006). Perhaps the best example of this is antral biopsies for the diagnosis of Helicobacter infection. There is no doubt that other much simpler methodologies are easier to perform and cheaper, and we strongly believe that there can be no indication for the routine diagnosis of Helicobacter infection by histopathology. There is an argument that non-malignant disease has lagged behind in developing quality standards utilising minimum data sets, although these do exist in some areas. For both tumour and non-tumour pathology it is essential that we continually assess the evidence base for items that are considered minimum data. This is a stated objective of the Royal College of Pathologists but there are some who believe that at least a proportion of existing minimum data sets contain, from a clinical perspective, redundant information.

It would be injudicious to attempt to predict the long-term future of diagnostic histopathology but in the short to medium term we believe that light microscopy will still retain its importance, complemented by data from evolving molecular and biological techniques.

REFERENCES

Afdhal, N.H. (2004) Biopsy or biomarkers: is there a gold standard for diagnosis of liver fibrosis? *Clin. Chem.* **50**: 1299–1300.

Balslev, I., Axelsson, C.K., Zedelev, K., *et al.* (1994) The Nottingham Prognostic Index applied to 9149 patients from the studies of the Danish Breast Cancer Cooperative Group (BDCG). *Breast Cancer Res. Treat.* **32**: 281–290.

Barnes, D.M., and Millis, R.R. (1995) Oestrogen receptors: the history, the relevance and the methods of evaluation. *Progress in Pathology* (eds N. Kirkham and N.R. Lemoine), vol. 2. Churchill Livingstone: Edinburgh, pp. 89–114.

Blamey, R.W. (1996) The design and clinical use of the Nottingham Prognostic Index in breast cancer. *Breast* **5**: 156–157.

Blaser, M.J. (1998) *Helicobacter pylori* and gastric diseases. *BMJ* **316**: 1507–1510.

Bloodgood, J.C. (1914) Diagnosis and treatment of borderline pathological lesions. *Surg. Gynecol. Obstet.* **8**: 19–34.

Breuer, M.J. (1938) Frozen section at operation. *Am. J. Clin. Pathol.* **8**: 153–169.

Brunt, E.M., Neuschwander-Tetri, B.A., Oliver, D., *et al.* (2004) Non-alcoholic steatohepatitis: histologic features and clinical correlations with 30 blinded biopsy specimen. *Hum. Pathol.* **35**: 1070–1082.

Clark, G.M. (1992) Integrating prognostic factors. *Breast Cancer Res. Treat.* **22**: 187–191.

Cotton, P.B., and Williams, C.B. (2003) *Practical Gastrointestinal Endoscopy* (5th edn). Blackwell Science: Oxford.

Cunningham, G.J. (1992) *The History of British Pathology* (ed. G. Kemp McGowan). White Trees Books: Bristol.

Dixon, J.M., Anderson, T.J., Lamb, J., *et al.* (1984) Fine needle aspiration cytology, in relationships to clinical examination and mammography in the diagnosis of a solid breast mass. *Br. J. Surg.* **71**: 593–596.

Dukes, C.E. (1932) The classification of cancer of the rectum. *J. Pathol. Bacteriol.* **35**: 323–332.

Dukes, C.E. and Bussey, H.J.R. (1958) The spread of rectal cancer and its effect on prognosis. *Br. J. Cancer* **12**: 1016–1023.

Elston, C.W., Cotton, R.E., Davies, C.J. and Blamey, R.W. (1978) A comparison of the use of the 'Tru-Cut' needle and fine needle aspiration cytology in the pre-operative diagnosis of carcinoma of the breast. *Histopathology* **2**: 239–254.

Fox, H. (1978) Pathology of the placenta, vol. 7. *Major Problems in Pathology* (ed. J. L. Bennington). W.B. Saunders: Philadelphia, PA.

Franzen, S. and Zajiceck, J. (1968) Aspiration biopsy in the diagnosis of palpable lesions of the breast: critical review of 3479 consecutive biopsies. *Acta Radiol. Ther. Phys. Biol.* **7**: 241–262.

Fukuda, H. and Inokuti, Y. (2004) Aspiration biopsy using new ceramic-coated stainless steel puncture needle. *J. Biomed. Mater. Res.* **71**: 392–397.

Gage, I., Schnitt, S.J., Nixon, A.J., *et al.* (1996) Pathologic margin involvement and the risk of recurrence in patients treated with breast-conserving therapy. *Cancer* **78**: 1921–1928.

Gal, A.A. (2001) In search of the origins of modern pathology. *Adv. Anat. Pathol.* **1**: 1–13.

Galea, M.H., Blamey, R.W., Elston, C.W. and Ellis, I.O. (1992) The Nottingham Prognostic Index in primary breast cancer. *Breast Cancer Res. Treat.* **22**: 207–219.

Gatter, K.C. (1989) Diagnostic immunocytochemistry: achievements and challenges (CL Oakley Lecture, 1989). *J. Pathol.* **159**: 183–190.

Guidelines Working Group of the National Coordinating Committee for Breast Pathology (2005) *Pathology Reporting of Breast Disease*, NHSBSP Publication No. 58.

Haagersen, C.D. (1986) Biopsy and local cision of breast tumours. In *Diseases of the Breast* (ed. C.D. Haagersen). W.B. Saunders: Philadelphia, PA, pp. 615–624.

Haybittle, J.L., Blamey, R.W., Elston, C.W., *et al.* (1982) A prognostic index in primary breast cancer. *Br. J. Cancer* **45**: 361–366.

Heald, R.J., Husband, E.M. and Ryall, R.D.H. (1982) The mesorectum in rectal cancer surgery – the clue to pelvic recurrence. *Br. J. Surg.* **69**: 613–616.

Heald, R.J. and Ryall, R.D.H. (1986) Recurrence and survival after total mesorectal excision for rectal cancer. *Lancet* **i**: 1479–1482.

Hermansen, C., Poulsen, H., Jensen, J., *et al.* (1987) Diagnostic reliability of combined physical examination, mammography and fine needle puncture ('triple-test') in breast tumors. A prospective study. *Cancer* **60**: 1866–1871.

Howat, A., Boyd, K., Jeffrey, M., *et al.* (2006) *Histopathology/Cytopathology of Limited or No Clinical Value* (2nd edn). Royal College of Pathologists: London.

Iversen, P. and Brun, C. (1951) Aspiration biopsy of kidney. *Am. J. Med.* **11**: 324–330.

Kirsner, J.B. (1998) The origin of 20th century discoveries transforming clinical gastroenterology. *Am. J. Gastroenterol.* **93**: 862–871.

Lakhani, S.R., Jacquemier, J., Sloane, J.P., *et al.* (1998) Multifactorial analysis of differences between sporadic breast cancers and cancers involving BRCA1 and BRCA2 mutations. *J. Natl. Cancer Inst.* **90**: 1138–1145.

Marshall, B.J., and Warren, J.R. (1983) Unidentified curved bacilli in the stomach of patients with gastritis and peptic ulceration. *Lancet* **1**: 1311–1315.

McAfee, J.H., Keeffe, E.B., Lee, R.G. and Rosch, J. (1992) Transjugular liver biopsy. *Hepatology* **15**: 726–732.

Menghini, G. (1958) One second needle biopsy of the liver. *Gastroenterology* **35**: 190–199.

Morson, B.C. (1981) Histopathology reporting in large-bowel cancer. *BMJ* **283**: 1493–1494.

Non-operative Diagnosis Subgroup of the National Coordinating Committee for Breast Pathology (2001) *Guidelines for Non-operative Diagnostic Procedures in Breast Cancer Screening*, NHSBSP Publication No. 50.

Quirke, P., Dixon, M.F., Durdey, P. and Williams, N.S. (1986) Local recurrence of rectal adenocarcinoma due to inadequate surgical resection. Histopathological study of lateral tumour spread and surgical excision. *Lancet* **ii**: 996–999.

Rake, M.O., Murray-Lyon, I.M., Ansell, I.D. and Williams, R. (1969) Improved liver-biopsy needle. *Lancet* **ii**: 1283–1284.

Roberts, J.G., Preece, P.E., Bolton, P.M., Baum, M. and Hughes, L.E. (1975) The 'Tru–Cut' biopsy in breast cancer'. *Clin. Oncol.* **1**: 297–303.

Romond, E.H., Perez, E.A., Bryant, J. *et al.* (2005) Trastuzumab plus adjuvant chemotherapy for operable HER2-positive breast cancer. *N. Eng. J. Med.* **353**: 1673–1684.

Rosenberg, W.M., Voelker, M., Thiel, R., *et al.* (2004) Serum markers detect the presence of liver fibrosis: a cohort study. *Gastroenterology* **127**: 1704–1713.

Scheuer, P.J. (2003) Liver biopsy size matters in chronic hepatitis: bigger is better. *Hepatology* **38**: 1356–1358.

Scholmerich, J. and Schacherer, D. (2004) Diagnostic biopsy for hepatocellular carcinoma in cirrhosis: useful, necessary, diagnostic, or academic sport? *Gut* **53**: 1224–1226.

Sebach, M. and Samuel, D. (2004) Place of the liver biopsy in liver transplantation. *J. Hepatol.* **41**: 897–901.

Senn, N. (1895) *The Pathological and Surgical Treatment of Tumors.* W.B. Saunders: Philadelphia, PA, p. 107.

Shepherd, N.A. and Quirke, P. (1997) Reporting colorectal cancer: are we failing the patient? *J. Clin. Pathol.* **50**: 266–267.

Silverman, I. (1938) A new biopsy needle. *Am. J. Surg.* **40**: 671–672.

Snead, D.J.R., Bell, J.A., Dixon, A.R., *et al.* (1993) Methodology of immunohistochemical detection of oestrogen receptor in human breast carcinoma in formalin fixed paraffin embedded tissue: a comparison with frozen section morphology. *Histopathology* **23**: 233–238.

Taylor, C.R. and Kledzik, G. (1981) Immunohistologic techniques in surgical pathology – a spectrum of 'new' special stains. *Hum. Pathol.* **12**: 590–596.

Vitums, V.C. (1972) Percutaneous biopsy of the lung with a new disposable needle. *Chest* **62**: 717–719.

Wilson, L.B. (1905) A method for the rapid preparation of fresh tissues for the microscope. *J. Am. Med. Assoc.* **45**: 1737.

15 The Antibody Revolution: How 'Immuno' Changed Pathology

Elizabeth Soilleux and Kevin C. Gatter

"You are young still, pathologist", the old professor said,
"And your slides aren't just purple and pink,
They have staining in brown, of both nuclei and membranes,
Pray, is this a good thing, do you think?"

Rather dramatically adapted from 'Father William' by Lewis Carroll.

INTRODUCTION

What we Mean by the Antibody Revolution

In the early 1980s one of our senior consultants in Oxford was asked to review a case of head and neck lymphoma that had been misdiagnosed as carcinoma. He could not find the H&E because this was out with us 'young thrusters' alongside the frozen section immunostains. An immediate letter was sent to the ENT consultant with copies to all and sundry. The gist was 'I don't mind these young chaps playing around in the lab, but when they get in the way of my diagnostic practice I really do draw the line'. He was actually a kindly old stager and we (David Mason and K. C. G.) portrayed him as such in a cartoon illustrating an early review of ours on the diagnostic value of immunohistochemistry (Fig. 15.1) (Mason and Gatter, 1987).

The whole thing seems ludicrous now. There is no pathologist in this country, or possibly the world, who does not use some immunocytochemistry regularly for diagnosis. You would certainly be up before 'his lordship' if you made wrong diagnoses through resistance to incorporate antibodies. That is probably not true for any other technique in histopathology and is one way of introducing this as a revolution. It has completely and permanently changed our routine practice.

Another way of assessing the revolution is to look at the impact of immunocytochemistry on the laboratory workload. In 1980 in Oxford this was, to all intents and purposes, zero. By 1992 it had moved to form nearly 3% of our workload, whereas now it is almost 15%. In 2004 we produced 24 798 immunostained glass slides against an overall output of 166 332 slides for all purposes. Four boxes of glass slides with 50 slides to a box weighs 1 kg which means that we imported 124 kg of glass into the department just to perform immunostains. Multiplied around the country and to other developed nations the 'immuno' revolution is, if nothing else, a significant contributor to road transport use.

When was the Revolution?

We stated previously (Mason and Gatter, 1987) that although there were forays into immunocytochemical methods in the 1960s the game as we know it today started in 1974 with the work of Taylor and Burns demonstrating immunoglobulin in plasma cells in paraffin sections (Taylor and

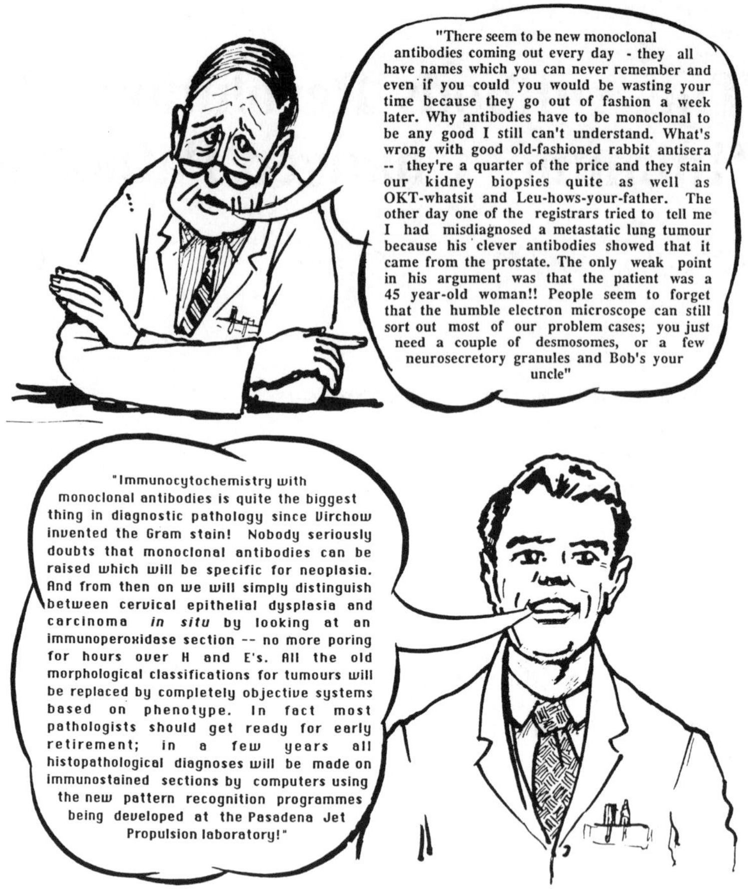
"There seem to be new monoclonal antibodies coming out every day - they all have names which you can never remember and even if you could you would be wasting your time because they go out of fashion a week later. Why antibodies have to be monoclonal to be any good I still can't understand. What's wrong with good old-fashioned rabbit antisera -- they're a quarter of the price and they stain our kidney biopsies quite as well as OKT-whatsit and Leu-hows-your-father. The other day one of the registrars tried to tell me I had misdiagnosed a metastatic lung tumour because his clever antibodies showed that it came from the prostate. The only weak point in his argument was that the patient was a 45 year-old woman!! People seem to forget that the humble electron microscope can still sort out most of our problem cases; you just need a couple of desmosomes, or a few neurosecretory granules and Bob's your uncle"
"Immunocytochemistry with monoclonal antibodies is quite the biggest thing in diagnostic pathology since Virchow invented the Gram stain! Nobody seriously doubts that monoclonal antibodies can be raised which will be specific for neoplasia. And from then on we will simply distinguish between cervical epithelial dysplasia and carcinoma *in situ* by looking at an immunoperoxidase section -- no more poring for hours over H and E's. All the old morphological classifications for tumours will be replaced by completely objective systems based on phenotype. In fact most pathologists should get ready for early retirement; in a few years all histopathological diagnoses will be made on immunostained sections by computers using the new pattern recognition programmes being developed at the Pasadena Jet Propulsion laboratory!"

Figure 15.1 Cartoon showing how we thought of the situation in histopathology with regard to immunocytochemistry in 1987, reproduced from a previous review (Mason and Gatter, 1987).

Burns, 1974). This was soon confirmed by a number of laboratories but remained largely a laboratory oddity due to the lack of markers of real diagnostic value other than light chains. In addition, the techniques used at the time were relatively insensitive so antigen detection was a variable and unreliable endeavour. Indeed, as a number of workers have stated, it was lucky that Taylor and Burns chose immunoglobulin for their experiments because it is so abundant in plasma cells that it allows easy detection.

Enhanced Methods

The next significant advance made in the introduction of diagnostic immunocytochemistry was the discovery that proteolytic digestion of paraffin sections considerably enhanced both the intensity and reliability of antigen detection (Huang *et al.*, 1976; Reading, 1977; Mepham *et al.*, 1979). Of course this early example of importing kitchen technology into laboratory science has been supplemented by many others, most notably recent methods using microwave ovens and pressure cooking in a variety of different pH buffers (Leong *et al.*, 2003) – if only we had thought to do it the other way round and we would have beaten a certain well-known chef to best restaurant in the world and become millionaires!

The Repertoire of Reagents

With all of these wonderful technical advances in the 1970s, why did it take so long for immunocytochemistry to become a standard technique in routine diagnosis? The answer is simple in retrospect. There were just no useful antibodies. This hurdle was solved immediately when pathologists realised that the invention of monoclonal antibodies by Kohler and Milstein (Kohler and Milstein, 1975) enabled a continuous production of new markers for evaluation. At first many of these needed frozen sections to detect their antigens, but as antigen retrieval methods improved and further antibodies were produced, an extensive range of diagnostic markers emerged.

One measure of this progress is to look at the work of the various conferences set up to characterise and classify monoclonal antibodies against human leucocyte differentiation antigens. These are the so-called CD conferences from which the CD numbers used mainly in haematopathology have come. CD stands for 'Cluster of Differentiation' and represents an internationally agreed system for classifying antigens and their respective monoclonal antibodies. A CD group is a cluster of antibodies recognising the same antigen. Where there is a series of related genes giving rise to antigenic variants, the CD groups have been subdivided, e.g. CD1 a, b, c or CD11 a and b. These groupings are defined at International Workshops on Human Leucocyte Differentiation Antigens. The first of these was held in Paris in 1982, when 15 CD groups were defined. To date there have been eight workshops and the number of clusters has increased to 247. Although this seems a large number it is nothing compared to the thousands of antibodies, each with their own 'laboratory' names, that have been allocated to the clusters. Interested readers can discover more about the CD system from the relevant workshop reports or about many of the antibodies from a number of antibody companies that have information fact sheets available, e.g. R&D Systems, DAKO or Visionbiosystems – all of these have websites and in addition there are many antibody search and review sites available on the web.

The anti-CD antibodies are of course only the tip of the immunocytochemical iceberg. The number of reagents against other markers of diagnostic usage, only some of which will be mentioned here, is now very extensive. To detail them all would take several times more space than is available for this review. An excellent starting point for the novice is the recent laboratory manual on diagnostic antibodies by Leong and colleagues (Leong *et al.*, 2003).

WHAT DO WE USE ANTIBODIES FOR?

Today a formidable range of antibodies, monoclonal and polyclonal, from a variety of animals and increasingly from gene expression libraries, is available to the pathologist. So what do we actually use them for? In our view there are three major areas of practical value at present. These are:

1. To make or confirm a diagnosis.
2. To provide prognostic information.
3. To determine treatment.

The remainder of this short overview will attempt to summarise these three areas, mainly in the form of tables, with some comments, specific and general, where we feel that they will be useful. In order to make the tables reasonably aesthetic, we have used frequent abbreviations, which may not be familiar to all readers. These abbreviations are explained in the footnotes to the tables, in order of appearance.

Table 15.1 Differentiating major tumour types

Class of neoplasm	Antibodies	Comments
Carcinoma	Cytokeratin, epithelial membrane antigen (EMA)	EMA is not epithelial-specific (vascular lesions, plasma cells, meningioma and some lymphomas (Theaker *et al.*, 1986; Gatter and Delsol, 2002). It has a particular use in some poorly differentiated carcinomas that express little or no cytokeratin, such as renal cancers (Langner *et al.*, 2004)
Sarcoma	Vimentin and markers of lineage (see Table 15.3)	Some overlap with carcinoma and melanoma, depending on the type of sarcoma (Fletcher *et al.*, 2002)
Melanoma	S100, melan-A (Mart-1), HMB-45, MITF, PNL2 (Rochaix *et al.*, 2003)	S100 is sensitive but not specific, so a combination of these markers is needed (Fletcher, 2000)
Lymphoma	CD45 and lineage markers (see Table 15.5 and 15.6)	Hodgkin lymphoma and myeloma are typically negative (Jaffe *et al.*, 2001)

To Make or Confirm a Diagnosis

The first area of diagnostic impact was in differentiating the major groups of malignant tumours when they were too poorly differentiated histologically (Gatter *et al.*, 1982, 1984; Warnke *et al.*, 1983). There was some grumbling at the time that we needed to do this because we, the new generation of pathologists, were not up to scratch morphologically. We countered this with a wicked little study that dug out cases of poorly differentiated tumours from the Oxford archives and showed that there was a 40% error rate in assigning these to their major tumour types (Hales *et al.*, 1989). Initially these studies were heavily biased towards the commoner and crucial distinction of carcinoma from lymphoma (Gatter *et al.*, 1985) but today, as shown in the tables below, the range of uses is much larger.

Table 15.1 shows a current plan of action for differentiating so-called anaplastic tumours. This has not changed much in the last ten years and most modern pathologists probably think much more of immunostaining for subdividing or classifying tumour types. Indeed, the act of classifying will usually give a robust assignation, e.g. a B-cell phenotype is a lymphoma. Nevertheless, the correct identification of a tumour's origin is crucial and the role of immunostaining in this should not be overlooked.

Table 15.2 is similar to Table 15.1 but deals with tumour types confronted less commonly as unknowns or anaplastic lesions. Nevertheless, a few poorly differentiated tumours are met in practice that fail to be categorised by the antibodies of Table 15.1 – they have no clinical or morphological clues or do not make sense clinically or morphologically. In these cases in adults the tumours in Table 15.2 are worth considering, and in children and adolescents those in Table 15.3. An obvious difference from Table 15.1 is the much greater number of antibodies recommended by various experts. This reflects the heterogeneity of many of these tumours, especially those of germ cell or paediatric type.

The phenotypes of paediatric tumours given in Table 15.3 are an amalgamation of several detailed reference works and should not be considered in any way definitive. Paediatric tumours that are classified only on immunophenotype are a peculiarly primitive group of tumours and great overlap in marker expression does exist (Kleihues and Cavenee, 2000; Jaffe *et al.*, 2001; Fletcher *et al.*, 2002, Mills *et al.*, 2004; Sebire *et al.*, 2005).

Table 15.2 Differentiating less common tumour types

Class of neoplasm	Antibodies giving positive immunostaining	Comments
Germ cell tumour	PLAP, AFP, HCG, CD30, CD117, CK	All of these markers appear on other tumour types (Mills *et al.*, 2004)
Mesothelioma	CK5/6, CK7, WT-1, calretinin, mesothelin, thrombomodulin, EMA, HBME-1	Expression of many of these antigens is variable (Fletcher, 2000; Mills *et al.*, 2004; Politi *et al.*, 2005)
Central nervous system (CNS) tumours	GFAP, neurofilaments, S100	CNS tumours show a wide range of different immunophenotypes (Kleihues and Cavenee, 2000)

PLAP, placental alkaline phosphatase; AFP, alpha fetoprotein; HCG, human chorionic gonadotrophin; CK, cytokeratin; WT-1, Wilon's tumour protein 1; EMA, epithelial membrane antigen; GFAP, glial fibrillary acidic protein.

Quite frequently poorly differentiated tumours are clearly of haematological origin, perhaps because of a distinctive morphology or after a first round of immunostaining. However, it may still be unclear what type of tumour one is dealing with. Before launching out on detailed immunophenotyping it may be sensible to undertake a further small study such as is illustrated in Table 15.4. Here it can be seen that with a limited range of markers it is usually possible to identify the major tumour group that one is dealing with, and then a more detailed classification can be undertaken (Jaffe *et al.*, 2001).

Tables 15.5 and 15.6 feature B-cell lymphomas classified into low and high grade. Strictly speaking the terms low and high grade for lymphomas were abolished by the WHO classification in 2002 (Jaffe *et al.*, 2001) but they have lingered on as pathologists have struggled to find a better term for their comparison and differential diagnosis. A few comments may be helpful. Cyclin D1 staining has revolutionised the recognition of the important entity of mantle cell lymphoma. Initially this was a difficult marker for routine laboratories but the introduction of new rabbit monoclonal antibodies has changed all of this. Most centres now use these but caution is needed when interpreting focal or weak staining. Some normal cells such as endothelium and macrophages express cyclin D1 and with enhanced staining techniques the rabbit antibodies are starting to show some weak positivity in other lymphoma types, especially follicular lymphomas. Follicular lymphomas are clearly different from the other tumours here but are easily confused with reactive lymph nodes. Here the key immunostains are CD10 and bcl2: CD10 positivity in interfollicular lymphocytes is diagnostic of follicular lymphoma, as is bcl2 positivity in their neoplastic germinal centres. Immunostain bcl2 does not appear in Table 15.5 because all of these tumours are positive. Sometimes nodular lymphocyte predominant Hodgkin lymphoma looks like follicular lymphoma but here the large abnormal cells, although bcl6 positive, are CD10 negative (Jaffe *et al.*, 2001; Gatter and Delsol, 2002).

At present the important differential to make among the high-grade B-cell lymphomas is to recognise Burkitt and lymphoblastic lymphoma. Burkitt lymphoma is the entity that usually causes most problems but if strict immunocytochemical criteria are applied then the diagnosis is usually pretty robust and consistent. If in doubt it is better to call it a diffuse large cell lymphoma. Lymphoblastic lymphoma is generally more obvious, especially in a younger patient, when one is thinking of this entity. Care should be exercised in older patients not to confuse mediastinal T lymphoblastic lymphoma with a thymoma (see Table 15.4).

Although they took some time to catch up with lymphomas, epithelial tumours now have a useful panel of markers for helping to assess their type and origin, as shown in Table 15.7 for

Table 15.3 Paediatric tumour differential diagnosis

Tumour/ antibody	Vimentin	Cytokeratin	EMA	NSE	Myogenin	Desmin	MyoD1	Muscle – specific actin	CD99	TdT	WT-1	NB84	NF
Neuroblastoma	−	−	−	+	−	−	−	−	−	−	−	+	+
Ewing's sarcoma/ PNET	+	−	−	−/+	−	−	−	−	+	−	−	−/+	−
Rhabdomyosarcoma	+	−	−	−	+	+	+	+	−	−	−	−	−
(Intra-abdominal) desmoplastic small round cell tumour	+	+	+	+	−	+	−	−	−	−	+	−	−
Congenital rhabdoid tumour	+	+	+	+	?	+/−	?	−	−/+	−	−	−	−
Lymphoblastic lymphoma	+	−	−	−	−	−	−	−	+	+	−	−	−
Synovial sarcoma	+	+	+	−	−	−	−	−	−/+	−	−	−	−
Wilm's tumour	+/−	+/−	−	−	−	−	−	−	−	−	+/−	−	−

PNET, peripheral neuroectodermal tumour.

Table 15.4 Haematological tumours

Haematolymphoid tumour	Immunostaining panel	Comments
B-Cell lymphoma	CD20, CD79a, Pax-5 (Torlakovic *et al.*, 2002)	Anti-CD20 antibody therapy may alter the staining in relapse
T-Cell lymphoma	CD3, CD2, CD5, CD7, CD4/8	Frequently have abnormal T-Cell antigen patterns
Hodgkin lymphoma	CD15, CD30, MUM-1 (Carbone *et al.*, 2002)	CD15 may be focal or absent
Myeloma	CD38, CD138, VS38c, kappa, lambda, CD79a, CD56, MUM-1	About a third of cases are also CD20+, which can be confusing
Histiocytic lymphoma	CD68, S100, CD1a, lysozyme	Covers a wide range of tumour types
Granulocytic sarcoma or other myeloid neoplasm	MPO, lysozyme, CD43	CD43 can cause confusion with T-cell lymphoma
Thymoma	CK (for epithelium) CD1a, TdT, CD99 (for lymphocytes) (Travis *et al.*, 2004)	Easily misdiagnosed as lymphoblastic lymphoma if the CK is overlooked

CK, cytokeratin; TdT, terminal deoxynucleotidyl transferase.

Table 15.5 Classification of low-grade B-cell lymphomas

Lymphoma type	IgM	IgD	CD5	CD10	CD23	CD43	bcl6	Cyclin D1
Chronic lymphocytic leukaemia	(+)	(+)	+	−	+	+	−	−
Lymphoplasmacytic lymphoma	+	−	−	−	−/+	−/+	−	−
Marginal zone lymphoma	+	−	−	−	−	+/−	−	−
Splenic marginal zone lymphoma	+	+	−	−	−	−	−	−
Follicular lymphoma	+	−/+	−	+	−/+	−	+	−
Mantle cell lymphoma	+	+/−	+	−	−	+	−	+

Table 15.6 Classification of high-grade B-cell lymphomas

Lymphoma type	CD5	CD10	CD23	Ki67	TdT	bcl2	Cyclin D1
Burkitt lymphoma	−	+	−	>95%	−	−	−
Diffuse large B cell	−/+	−/+	−	<90%	−	+/−	−
Mantle cell blastic type	+	−	−	<90%	−	+/−	+
CLL Richter's transformation	+	−	+	<90%	−	+/−	−
B lymphoblastic	+	+	−	<90%	+	−	−

TdT, terminal deoxynucleotidyl transferase; CLL, chronic lymphocytic leukaemia.

Table 15.7 The differentiation of epithelial tumours with cytokeratins 7 and 20

CK7+ CK20+	CK7+ CK20−	CK7− CK20−	CK7− CK20+
Transitional cell	Breast	Hepatocellular	Colorectal
Pancreatic mucinous	Non-small-cell lung	Renal cell	
Ovarian mucinous	Ovarian serous	Prostate	
	Mesothelioma	Squamous	
	Endometrial	Neuroendocrine	
	Pancreatic		
	Thyroid		

Table 15.8 The differentiation of epithelial tumours with other markers

Carcinoma	Cytokeratin, epithelial membrane antigen (EMA), keratin subtyping (see Table 15.7)
Thyroid	Thyroglobulin, TTF-1, calcitonin (medullary)
Prostate	Prostatic acid phosphatase or prostate – specific antigen
Breast	Oestrogen receptor, progesterone receptor, c-Erb B2
Lung	TTF-1
Liver	CK8, CK18, hep-par-1, AFP
Pancreas	Ca19.9
Endometrium/ovary	CA125
Neuroendocrine	NSE, pgp9.5, NCAM (CD56), synaptophysin, chromogranin A

TTF-1, thyroid transcription factor 1; NSE, neuron-specific enolase; NCAM, neural cell adhesion molecule.

cytokeratin subtyping (Chu and Weiss, 2002) and Table 15.8 for a range of other antigens (Mills *et al.*, 2004).

We could continue with many more tables of differential diagnoses but space dictates we call a halt. Just to show that not everything is tissue or tumour in pathology, we shall finish with renal disease, cytology and infection. Differentiating the different types of renal glomerular disease is a highly specialised area, but we hope that Table 15.9 gives a flavour of how immunostaining, still predominantly by immunofluorescence, may assist.

Differentiating mesothelioma from carcinoma in serous effusions has long been extremely difficult. Indeed, reactive mesothelial cells can also look very malignant at times so care is still needed in this differentiation. Nevertheless, the panel of markers available (shown in Table 15.10), which continues to grow, is of great assistance to cytologists today (Fletcher, 2000; Mills *et al.*, 2004; Politi *et al.*, 2005).

The number of infectious agents (whether viruses or bacteria) that can be identified in routine tissues continues to expand regularly. Table 15.11 outlines some of the commoner and more reliably identified agents in current practice.

Table 15.9 Immunostaining in renal disease with glomerular crescent formation

Diagnosis	Common immunofluorescent staining pattern
Antiglomerular basement membrane antibody disease (Goodpasture's Syndrome)	Linear GBM staining for IgG and C3 in majority, with fibrin/ fibrinogen in crescents
Immune complex crescentic glomerulonephritis related to infection	Coarse granular capillary wall staining with C3 +/− IgG, with fibrin/ fibrinogen in crescents
Immune complex crescentic glomerulonephritis related to lupus	Granular capillary wall and mesangial staining for C3, C1q (and C4), IgG, IgM and IgA, with fibrin/ fibrinogen in crescents
Pauci-immune necrotising glomerulonephritis (ANCA-related)	Negative immunofluorescence for complement and immunoglobulin in majority, with fibrin/ fibrinogen in crescents
IgA nephropathy/ Henich-Shönlein purpura	IgA and often C3 positive immunofluorescence, with fibrin/ fibrinogen in crescents

ANCA, anti-neutrophilic cytoplasmic antibody.

Table 15.10 Identification of malignant cells in serous effusion

Antibody/condition	Adenocarcinoma	Mesothelioma
EMA	+ cytoplasm and membrane	+ membrane
CEA	+ (usually)	−
B72.3	+	−
CK7	+ (variable)	+
CK20	+/−	−
LeuM1 (CD15)	+	−
MOC-31	+	−
CK5/6	−	+
Thrombomodulin	−	+
HBME-1	−	+
WT-1	−	+
Calretinin	−	+
Vimentin	−	+

EMA, epithelial membrane antigen; CK, cytokeratin; WT-1, Wilm's tumour protein 1.

To Predict Prognosis

Almost from the start as the early studies of tumour typing with antibodies were emerging, there was a dawn chorus from our clinicians of 'but does it tell us anything about prognosis?'. Sadly 25 years later immunostaining is still not a very reliable or helpful means of predicting prognosis. Nevertheless, there are a few tried and tested stains that have stood up to the unpredictability of human cancer. Some of these are summarised in Table 15.12.

For most other tumours, in spite of a huge amount of effort there just has not been enough data to substantiate any markers as truly meaningful for prognosis (Compton *et al.*, 2000; Compton, 2003; Altman and Riley, 2005). Three antigens p53, bcl2 and Ki67 are (and have been for some time) front-runners as generic markers of prognosis in many, if not all, tumours. There is evidence (though not conclusive) that positivity for p53 and a high proliferative index with Ki67 are associated with a more aggressive tumour and hence a poorer prognosis (Steele *et al.*, 1998; Brown and Gatter, 2002). Bcl2 is more problematic, with some tumours showing positivity in aggressive

Table 15.11 Infectious agents identifiable by immunohistochemistry

Infectious agent	Site
Helicobacter	Stomach
Polyoma	Urogenital tract (including positive immunostaining in urine cytology)
Herpes simplex virus	Epithelia: skin, orogenital, oesophagus
Cytomegalovirus	Endothelial cells and macrophages in many sites (especially immunosuppressed patients)
Hepatitis B virus	Liver
Human immunodeficiency virus p24	Lymphoid tissue
Epstein Barr virus	Lymphoid tissue, nasopharyngeal carcinoma
HHV-8	Human herpes virus 8, involved in the pathogenesis of Kaposi's sarcoma, primary effusion lymphoma and the plasma cell variant of Castleman's disease
Toxoplasma	Central nervous system, placenta

Table 15.12 Use of immunohistochemistry in the prediction of prognosis

Tumour type	Prognosis	
	Good	Bad
Breast	ER, PR	Her2
Colon	bcl2, beta-catenin	p53
Chronic Lymphocytic leukaemia		ZAP70, CD38
Anaplastic large cell lymphoma	Alk-1	
Diffuse large B-cell lymphoma	CD10, bcl6	p53, bcl2
Neuroblastoma	Trk-A	

ER, oestrogen receptor; PR, progesterone receptor; Alk-1, anaplastic lymphoma kinase 1.

tumours and others negativity. Many studies show complete conflict of results in the same tumour type. An example of this is diffuse large B-cell lymphoma. Here, a variety of studies have shown bcl2 to be either good or bad. It looks as though the resolution is that bcl2 is a poorer prognostic marker in non-germinal centre type tumours, which basically means, in antibody terms, when CD10 and bcl6 are negative (See Table 15.11) (Berglund *et al.*, 2005; Biasoli *et al.*, 2005).

To Determine Treatment

The most striking (and also in some cases expensive) change in immunocytochemical practice for pathologists has been the introduction of immunocytochemical testing as a precursor to the selection of therapy. This has been most dramatically demonstrated by the use of antibodies against the Her-2 oncogene on cases of breast cancer selected by immunostaining for a high level of expression of it on the tumour cells (Slamon *et al.*, 2001; Vogel *et al.*, 2002). There are now a number of other examples of immunohistochemical testing to determine or at least strongly guide treatment, as indicated in Table 15.13.

IN SUMMARY: THE PROS AND CONS OF THE ANTIBODY REVOLUTION

Pros

Any list of benefits or deficiencies in diagnostic immunocytochemistry must inevitably be subjective. Nevertheless, it seems to us that the following are definite benefits.

Table 15.13 The use of immunohistochemistry to determine treatment

Disease type	Relevant antibodies	Treatment
Breast cancer	ER, PR	Tamoxifen and analogues
Breast cancer	HER-2	Herceptin
Gastrointestinal stromal tumour	CD117	Imatinib mesylate/ STI571/ Glivec
B-Cell lymphoma	CD20	Rituximab
Chronic lymphocytic leukaemia	ZAP-70, CD38	Consideration of autologous stem cell transplantation
Infections	Identification of any infection agent (see Table 15.11)	Appropriate chemotherapy

1. Improved accuracy of diagnosis.
2. Increased reliability of diagnosis (fewer sleepless nights).
3. More objectivity in classification (e.g. lymphomas).
4. Preservation of morphology when stained (advantage over DNA technology).

Cons

1. Significant increase in laboratory workforce and consumables (see Introduction).
2. Increased temptation to ignore morphology, with consequent deskilling.
3. Increased delay in diagnosis, especially if repeating or ordering more immunostains.
4. Overlap of immunophenotypic profiles causes confusion ('tumours haven't read the textbooks' syndrome).
5. Now almost a legal requirement to do certain immunostains when they are possibly unnecessary, e.g. cyclin Dl on every lymphoma in case a mantle cell is missed.

CONCLUSION

Basically antibodies in the routine laboratory are here to stay. The public and governments are demanding the introduction of modern methods into diagnosis to prevent avoidable errors. Any costs will just need to be subsumed into our practice somehow. It is often suggested that the days of immunostaining in diagnosis are numbered. But will antibody technology ever be superseded by genomic methods, e.g. DNA microarray technology? We think probably not, because antibody technology is relatively cheap, very sensitive and now highly reliable. In addition, it can be readily automated. Finally, the thrust of modern biological research is moving the action towards proteins and not DNA or RNA, and that is exactly where immunostaining is targeted.

Antibodies are here to stay!

REFERENCES

Altman, D. G. and Riley, R. G. (2005) *Nat. Clin. Pract. Oncol.* **2**: 466–472.

Berglund, M., Thunberg, U., Amini, R. M., Book, M., Roos, G., Erlanson, M., *et al.* (2005) *Mod. Pathol.* **18**: 1113–1120.

Biasoli, I., Morais, J. C., Scheliga, A., Milito, C. B., Romano, S., Land, M., Pulcheri, W. and Spector, N. (2005) *Histopathology* **46**: 328–333.

Brown, D. C. and Gatter, K. C. (2002) *Histopathology* **40**: 2–11.

Carbone, A., Gloghini, A., Aldinucci, D., Gattei, V., Dalla-Favera, R. and Gaidano, G. (2002) *Br. J. Haematol.* **117**: 366–372.

Chu, P. G. and Weiss, L. M. (2002) *Histopathology* **40**: 403–439.

Compton, C. C. (2003) *Mod. Pathol.* **16**: 376–388.

Compton, C. C., Fielding, L. P., Burgart, L. J., Conley, B., Cooper, H. S., Hamilton, S. R., Hammond, *et al.* (2000) *Arch. Pathol. Lab. Med.* **124**: 979–994.

Fletcher, C. D. M. (2000) *Diagnostic Histopathology of Tumors.* Churchill Livingstone: New York.

Fletcher, C. D. M., Unni, K. K. and Mertens, F. (2002) *Pathology and Genetics of Tumours of Soft Tissue and Bone.* IARC Press: Lyon.

Gatter, K. C. and Delsol, G. (2002) *The Diagnosis of Lymphoproliferative Diseases.* Oxford University Press: Oxford.

Gatter, K. C., Abdulaziz, Z., Beverley, P., Corvalan, J. R., Ford, C., Lane, E. B., *et al.* (1982) *J. Clin. Pathol.* **35**: 1253–1267.

Gatter, K. C., Alcock, C., Heryet, A., Pulford, K. A., Heyderman, E., Taylor, P. J., Stein, H. and Mason, D. Y. (1984) *Am. J. Clin. Pathol.* **82**: 33–43.

Gatter, K. C., Alcock, C., Heryet, A. and Mason, D. Y. (1985) *Lancet* **1**: 1302–1305.

Hales, S. A., Gatter, K. C., Heryet, A. and Mason, D. Y. (1989) *Leuk. Lymph.* **1**: 59–63.

Huang, S. N., Minassian, H. and More, J. D. (1976) *Lab. Invest.* **35**: 383–390.

Jaffe, E. S., Harris, N. L., Stein, H. and Vardiman, J. W. (2001) *Pathology and Genetics of Tumours of Haematopoietic and Lymphoid Tissues.* IARC Press: Lyon.

Kleihues, P. and Cavenee, W. K. (2000) *Pathology and Genetics of Tumours of Nervous System.* IARC Press: Lyon.

Kohler, G. and Milstein, C. (1975) *Nature* **256**: 495–497.

Langner, C., Ratschek, M., Rehak, P., Schips, L. and Zigeuner, R. (2004) *Mod. Pathol.* **17**: 180–188.

Leong, A. S.-Y., Cooper, K. and Leong, F. J. W.-M. (2003) *Manual of Diagnostic Antibodies for Immunohistology.* Oxford University Press: Oxford.

Mason, D. Y. and Gatter, K. C. (1987) *J. Clin. Pathol.* **40**: 1042–1054.

Mepham, B. L., Frater, W. and Mitchell, B. S. (1979) *Histochem. J.* **11**: 345–357.

Mills, S. E., Carter, D., Greenson, J. K., Oberman, H. A., Reuter, V. E. and Stoler, M. H. (2004) *Sternberg's Diagnostic Surgical Pathology.* Lippincott Williams & Wilkins: Philadelphia, PA.

Politi, E., Kandaraki, C., Apostolopoulou, C., Kyritsi, T. and Koutselini, H. (2005) *Diagn. Cytopathol.* **32**: 151–155.

Reading, M. (1977) *J. Clin. Pathol.* **30**: 88–90.

Rochaix, P., Lacroix-Triki, M., Lamant, L., Pichereaux, C., Valmary, S., Puente, E., *et al.* (2003) *Mod. Pathol.* **16**: 481–490.

Sebire, N. J., Gibson, S., Rampling, D., Williams, S., Malone, M. and Ramsay, A. D. (2005) *Appl. Immunohistochem. Mol. Morphol.* **13**: 1–5.

Slamon, D. J., Leyland-Jones, B., Shak, S., Fuchs, H., Paton, V., Bajamonde, A., *et al.* (2001) *N. Engl. J. Med.* **344**: 783–792.

Steele, R. J., Thompson, A. M., Hall, P. A. and Lane, D. P. (1998) *Br. J. Surg.* **85**: 1460–1467.

Taylor, C. R. and Burns, J. (1974) *J. Clin. Pathol.* **27**: 14–20.

Theaker, J. M., Gatter, K. C., Esiri, M. M. and Fleming, K. A. (1986) *J. Clin. Pathol.* **39**: 435–439.

Torlakovic, E., Torlakovic, G., Nguyen, P. L., Brunning, R. D. and Delabie, J. (2002) *Am. J. Surg. Pathol.* **26**: 1343–1350.

Travis, W. D., Brambilla, E., Müller-Hermelink, H. K. and Harris, C. C. (2004) *Pathology and Genetics of Tumours of the Lung, Pleura, Thymus and Heart.* IARC Press: Lyon.

Vogel, C. L., Cobleigh, M. A., Tripathy, D., Gutheil, J. C., Harris, L. N., Fehrenbacher, L., *et al.* (2002) *J. Clin. Oncol.* **20**: 719–726.

Warnke, R. A., Gatter, K. C., Falini, B., Hildreth, P., Woolston, R. E., Pulford, K., *et al.* (1983) *N. Engl. J. Med.* **309**: 1275–1281.

16 The Changing Face of Neuropathology

Ingrid V. Allen

ORIGINS

1906 was an auspicious year to have been alive: it saw the birth of The Pathological Society of Great Britain and Ireland with obstetrician James Lorrain Smith and attendant midwife William Osler (Cushing, 1924). In that same year the Nobel prize for Physiology or Medicine was awarded jointly to Santiago Ramón y Cajal and Camillo Golgi for their separate studies on the nervous system, using similar techniques, but reaching very different conclusions. These two events, the one of national importance, the other of great international significance, are reflective of the genesis and nature of neuropathology as a subject, rooted in general pathology, but having seminal links with basic and clinical neuroscience. Given its complex origin, neuropathology has developed in a different way from other branches of pathology, and this is reflected in the practice of the subject throughout the 20th century and at the present time. If one takes Rudolf Virchow as an example of the influence of pathology on neuropathology, then we are indebted not only for the broad principles of cellular pathology, but also for specific concepts for which his terms, e.g. 'myelin' and 'neuroglia', have become part of the standard neuropathological vocabulary (Virchow, 1860).

However, it is to Cajal, often described as the father of neuroscience, that we owe the concept of the neuron as the basic unit of the nervous system (Cajal, 1906) and to Cajal and his disputatious but correct younger colleague, Pio del Rio-Hortega, that we now understand the nature and origin of the cells that make up the neuroglia (Cajal, 1909, 1911; Rio-Hortega, 1919). The great contribution of Rio-Hortega to our understanding of neuroglia must be recognised, but the incomplete descriptions of W.H. Robertson are worthy of note (Robertson, 1900; Penfield, 1932).

Anatomists and physiologists before the 20th century had established the phenomenon of cerebrospinal fluid secretion and circulation. It only remained for Paul Ehrlich, a nobel laureate two years after Cajal and Golgi, to establish the concept of the blood–brain barrier (Ehrlich, 1902), and the cardinal discoveries underpinning neuropathology were in place. How then did neuropathology emerge as a distinct discipline? The answer is: very differently in different parts of the world. For example, in Spain and Italy its origins lie in the neurohistological schools of Cajal and Golgi. In France, neuropathology was initially practiced by neurologists under the influence of Jean-Martin Charcot, Professor of Neurology at the Salpêtrière in Paris, who himself made many contributions to neuropathology, and with his friend and fellow neurologist Alfred Vulpian, established a systematic museum of anatomical pathology (Corvisier-Visy and Poirier, 1996). In Germany the main influence came from the German Research Institute for Psychiatry in Munich where Alois Alzheimer, Korbinian Brodmann, Bernhard von Gudden, Emil Kraepelin, Franz Nissl and Walther Spielmeyer, all psychiatrists as well as neuropathologists, made lasting contributions. Similarly in the rest of mainland Europe the links to neuroanatomy and histology were strong, but the practitioners were frequently neuropsychiatrists, of which Sigmund Freud is an example, a knowledgeable neurohistologist and Professor of Neuropathology in Vienna until he left for England in 1938.

ANGLOPHONE CONNECTIONS

In the English-speaking world neuropathology developed rather differently. Here the influence of neurology and neurosurgery is important; for example, in England, Hughlings Jackson, William Gowers, Victor Horsley and R.H. Clarke combined neurophysiological and pathological techniques to elucidate the functions and to understand diseases of the nervous system. The influence of neurosurgery was even stronger in the USA where Harvey Cushing, working with Percival Bailey, established the field of neuro-oncology, while again neurologists were the key influence in the Boston school (Richardson *et al.*, 1994). In Canada the influence of neurosurgery is also apparent, where neurosurgeon Wilder Penfield in 1934 realised his vision of a multidisciplinary institute for the study of neurology with the opening of the Montreal Neurological Institute. Throughout the English-speaking world the links of neuropathology with the parent subject of pathology have always been strong. The Institutes of Neurology and Psychiatry in London from the early days had departments of neuropathology, in many cases staffed by those trained in mainstream pathology. British academic departments of pathology, often because of clinical service commitments, usually had at least one member of staff who was an expert on the nervous system.

To summarise, neuropathology is fortunate in having a diverse background, with roots in pathology, anatomy, neurology, neurosurgery and psychiatry. One might facetiously represent the different origins by the use of the paraffin section (pathology!) versus the use of the celloidin section (neuroanatomy!).

The turbulence in Europe in the first half of the 20th century had at least one good effect in that it brought the different practices of neuropathology together. Neuropathologists trained in different ways and from different backgrounds, some of whom were forced to leave mainland Europe and move to Britain or America, began to work together, thus establishing the multidisciplinary framework that is so necessary at the present time. An early example of this blending of disciplines and of collaboration between workers trained in Germany and in Britain is seen in the work of Alfred Meyer and Elizabeth Beck. Both were refugees from Germany: Alfred Meyer trained in psychiatry and neuropathology, and Elizabeth Beck in neuroanatomical techniques. They worked together and with Turner McLardy made the definitive study of the anatomical effects of prefrontal leucotomy (Cavanagh, 2004). Alfred Meyer, while in Germany, had been influenced by the work of his friend Walther Spielmeyer, who among others in the German school of neuropathology considered that definite evidence of ischaemic cell change in the human brain was only apparent some 7 days after the hypoxic event. This view from the Munich school, propagated by Alfred Meyer at the Maudsley Hospital in London, awakened in the young James Brierley a lifelong devotion to the study of cerebral hypoxia. His innovative human and experimental studies, carried out with the cooperation of Alwyn Brown and Brian Meldrum, led to a complete revision of views as to the timescale of cellular changes in brain hypoxia, a conclusion that has profound implications for clinical practice (Graham *et al.*, 2005).

KEY FIGURES: GREENFIELD AND RUSSELL

Two figures stand out in the emergence of specialist neuropathology in 20th century Britain. Both remained part of the general family of pathology and contributed to The Pathological Society and to the Association of Clinical Pathologists, but both realised that the complexity of the nervous system, with the requirement for special techniques, necessitated specialisation. Godwin Greenfield (1884–1958) (Fig. 16.1) was for many years pathologist to the National Hospital, Queen Square, London. Described by William McMenemey in his admirable and full obituary (McMenemey and Walshe, 1959) as the architect of British neuropathology, he was very much the clinician's pathologist, remembering above all else that he gave a clinical service. His publications therefore

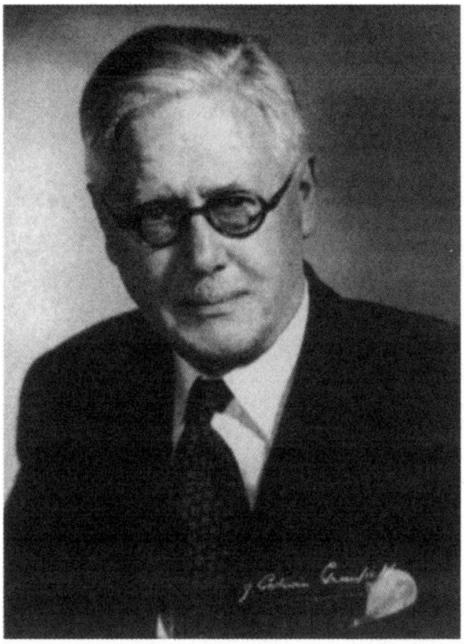

J.G. Greenfield, MD, FRCP, LLD
(1884–1958)

Figure 16.1 Godwin Greenfield.

are not in the field of experimental neuropathology, but include classical pathological descriptions that still stand, e.g. on measles encephalomyelitis (Greenfield, 1929), on late infantile metachromatic leucodystrophy (Brain and Greenfield, 1950) and on the spino-cerebellar degenerations (Greenfield, 1954).

The year 1950 has great significance for British neuropathology; it was in that year that Greenfield established, with 28 founder members, the Neuropathological club, later to be known from the same year in which the College of Pathologists was founded, i.e. 1962, as the British Neuropathological Society. By the year 2000 when the Society celebrated its 50th Anniversary there were more than 200 active members (Geddes, personal communication). Greenfield could not have foreseen how the formation of the club in 1950 would influence the yet to be formed College of Pathologists. By 1962 British neuropathologists were well organised and through the efforts of the honorary secretary of the Neuropathological Society, Marion Smith, and others, the College from the beginning recognised neuropathology as a sub-specialty with its own slanted examination, for which the present author had the honour to be the first candidate.

Dorothy Russell (1895–1983) (Fig. 16.2), Professor of Morbid Anatomy at the London Hospital Medical College from 1946 until 1960, like Greenfield did much to establish neuropathology as a specialty. Her training was in general histopathology, but the formation of a neurosurgical unit at the London Hospital, led by Hugh Cairns, encouraged Russell to take up neuropathology (Geddes, 1998). She worked with Frank Mallory, Wilder Penfield and Pio del Rio-Hortega and pioneered the use of tissue culture in the study of brain tumours. Her MRC monograph 'Observations on the Pathology of Hydrocephalus' is a classic that remains a key text for the condition. She is, however, remembered most for her contributions with Lucien Rubinstein to neuro-oncology. These included the identification of the so-called 'pinealoma' as a teratomatous lesion, and of 'microgliomas' as distinct from gliomas, now generally accepted as lymphomas.

She was the first woman to become head of a department of pathology in Britain, and her achievements contributed greatly to the advancement of women in British medicine (Rubinstein,

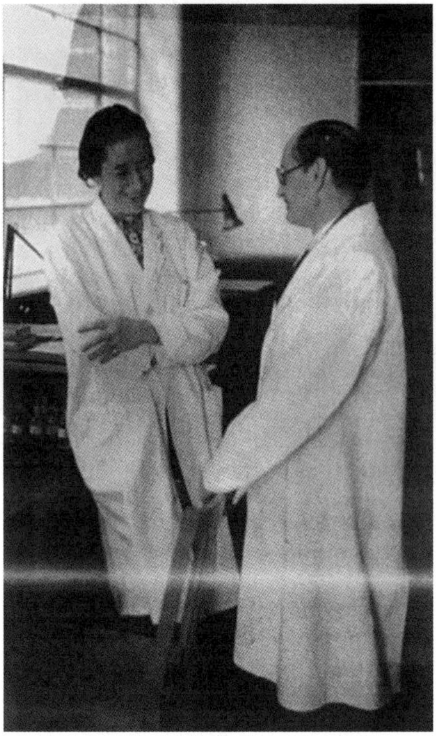

Figure 16.2 Dorothy Russell and Pio del Rio-Hortega, Oxford.

1984). The rarity of women in high academic positions at that time is perhaps typified by her soubriquet – she was always known as 'The Lady'. She was privately warm and caring, but publicly, possibly because of the vigour of her intellect, often described as intimidating (Geddes, 1998). She would probably be surprised today to see the predominance of women in British medical schools and their equal influence with their male colleagues in neuropathology. She received many honours in her lifetime and is remembered eponymously by a biannual lecture, sponsored by the journal *Neuropathology and Applied Neurobiology* and by the British Neuropathological Society.

The different development of pathology in Scotland, Wales, Ireland and the English provinces as compared with London, where historically pathology was not regarded as a separate subject (Foster, 1981), has in many ways been an advantage to British neuropathology. The first chair of pathology was established in Edinburgh in 1831, followed 50 years later by the second at Aberdeen. By the beginning of the 20th century, most medical schools outside London had chairs in pathology, thus providing job opportunities from which all branches of pathology benefited. With the advent of the National Health Service in 1948 and the establishment of regional centres for neurology, neurosurgery, neuroimaging and neuropathology, there were already well-trained neuropathologists to fill the new posts. These regional centres have provided a framework not only for the clinical service, but for teaching, training and research. Research contributions, experimental and clinical, from British neuropathology are therefore wide ranging in subject and from diverse geographical centres. In assessing British neuropathological research output, the value of the National Health Service in ensuring that cases are easily collected and are available for research must be acknowledged. It is invidious to be selective about achievements: sufficient to say that British researchers have contributed to all fields in neuropathology and the strength of

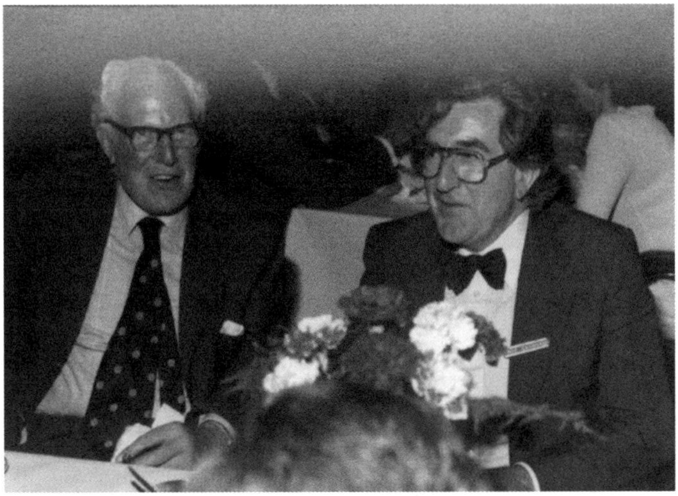

Figure 16.3 John Cavanagh and Harold Millar, Belfast, 1981.

the contributions is reflected in the ensuing publications. Until 1958 the only British textbook of neuropathology was that of Biggart (1936). This small book, described as 'a student's introduction', is elegantly written and displays clarity of thought. For many years it was used widely by pathologists and neurologists in training and ran into three editions. By 1958, however, knowledge had advanced to such a degree that a more detailed textbook was needed; this was provided by Greenfield and is now in its seventh edition (Graham and Lantos, 2002). The 1958 edition of Greenfield's 'Neuropathology' was complemented the following year by Russell and Rubinstein's 'Pathology of Tumours of the Nervous System', which was intended to be an accompanying volume and is now in its sixth edition (Bigner et al, 1998). Of even greater importance for the publication of research findings was the establishment of the journal *Neuropathology and Applied Neurobiology* in 1974, sponsored by the British Neuropathological Society. This initiative was the brainchild of John Cavanagh (Fig. 16.3), Director of the Medical Research Council Group in Applied Neurobiology at the Institute of Neurology in London. Cavanagh became the journal's first editor and it was he who set the high standards that have achieved the international reputation that the journal enjoys today.

CURRENT CHALLENGES

Given the excellence of the tradition of neuropathology in Britain, one must consider what endangers the specialty at the present time. Recruitment to the specialty has long been a problem. Undergraduates get little exposure to neuropathology in their formative years and the training is prolonged with increasing necessity of knowledge of cognate subjects such as neuroanatomy and neuroimaging. The rapid developments in the clinical neurosciences in the last few years, with input from genetics, molecular biology, neuroimaging and neuropharmacology, highlight the centrality of neuropathology in this spectrum of disciplines. Interpretation of results, whether in basic or applied neuroscience, requires precise phenotyping at the level of the whole person, the tissue and the cell. One can only hope that the intellectual excitement that comes from such an approach will continue to attract the very best graduates to neuropathology, be their training medical or scientific.

A further challenge is the wide range of pathological conditions in which neuropathologists providing a clinical service, often few in number in each centre, have to be proficient. Regional centres were initially established to support the broad spectrum of neurology and neurosurgery. Thus, most neuropathological laboratories process tissue from brain, spinal cord, peripheral nerve, striated muscle, the autonomic nervous system and pituitary. Some laboratories are also responsible for ophthalmic pathology and for cerebrospinal fluid cytology. The range of tissues is great, but the spectrum of diseases is even greater. Thus the practising neuropathologist must be conversant with infections, vascular disorders, inborn errors of metabolism, metabolic and toxic diseases, trauma, epilepsy, neurodegenerative diseases, demyelinating diseases, movement disorders, psychiatric disorders, peripheral nerve and muscle diseases and tumours affecting organs as different as the pituitary and the brain. Not only is the disease range wide, but the clinical age span extends from the perinatal period to old age. With the growth of sophisticated molecular techniques it is doubtful if all regional centres in Britain can retain total proficiency across the broad historical spectrum. Some networking of centres is desirable, and this may follow similar trends in neurology and neurosurgery. Opportunities from increased automation in histopathology generally have focused attention on the requirements for the specialist neuropathology service. Certainly nervous tissue requires special processing and staining, but the next few years will almost certainly see greater automation in histopathology, which should allow neuropathology staff to concentrate on specialist techniques, both classical and innovative. Furthermore, the use of telemedicine, with dynamic-imaging systems, will allow the acquisition of biopsies at one site but their reporting elsewhere at a centre of excellence (Walter *et al.*, 2000).

An even greater difficulty is the question of clinical research (Allen, 1996), yet the need has never been greater. For example, the application of the importance of accurate pathological description in the interpretation of gene and protein arrays is acknowledged. These techniques as applied to the nervous system are, at the present time, largely experimental but may soon be important in patient management. It is vital therefore that regional centres of neuropathology have sufficient staff to allow high-quality translational and clinical research to continue.

What then of the distant horizons? Most of the big questions in neuropathology have been posed many years ago but imperfectly answered, largely because of lack of suitable techniques. For example Virchow, writing in 1893, rather than posing a question, made the following statement that is still the subject of intense experimentation:

> 'every case of descent, in the sense in which Darwin uses the term, that is to say, every deviation from the type of the parent animal, must have its foundation on a pathological accident.'

Considering the tools available to Virchow in terms of microscopy and tissue stains, it is incredible how accurate have been the observations that he and others have made. There have been dramatic technical advances over the 100 years of neuropathology: the initial phase with beautiful and accurate drawings, but bound by the limitations of the light microscope and the available stains; the succeeding era of electron microscopy and enzyme histochemistry; the development of immunocytochemistry with specific antibodies; and *in situ* hybridisation with mRNA probes for cellular and pathogen gene expression. But how exciting the present era with laser capture of single cells, fluorescent *in situ* hybridisation, tissue, gene and protein arrays, and the developments in confocal microscopy and computational science that make these techniques at least semi-quantitative. The opportunities have never been greater.

Cajal in his *Advice for a Young Investigator* (1999) wrote:

> 'If we knew the entire chemical composition of living cells, results due to the application of a particular staining reagent could be deduced simply from biochemical principles. However, because we are so far from this position, those aspiring to discover new biological methods are forced to submit live tissues to the same blind tests resorted to by chemists for centuries in the hope of now and then finding some unforeseen combination of reactions or mixtures of elements.'

Neuropathologists today can test the veracity of Virchow's statement, using techniques and reagents that Cajal craved!

REFERENCES

Allen, I.V. (1996) The Clinician Scientist – an endangered species? *Ulster Med. J.* **65**: 61–67.

Biggart, J.H. (1936) *Pathology of the Nervous System – a Student's Introduction.* E. & S. Livingstone: Edinburgh.

Bigner, D.D., McLendon, R.E. and Bruner, J.M. (1998) *Russell and Rubinstein's Pathology of Tumors of the Nervous System.* Oxford University Press: Oxford.

Brain, W.R. and Greenfield, J.G. (1950) Late infantile metachromatic leucoencephalopathy, with primary degeneration of the interfascicular oligodendroglia. *Brain* **73**: 291–316.

Cajal, S.R. (1906) Nobel lecture. http://nobelprize.org/medicine/laureates/1906/index.html

Cajal, S.R. (1909, 1911) Histologie du Système Nerveux de l'Homme et des Vertébrés (trans. L. Azoulay). Maloine: Paris. Translated into English in 1995 as *Histology of the Nervous System of Man and Vertebrates* (trans. N. Swanson and L.W. Swanson). Oxford University Press: New York.

Cajal, S.R. (1999) *Advice for a Young Investigator* (trans. N. Swanson and L.W. Swanson). MIT Press: New York.

Cavanagh, J.B. (2004) Obituary – Elizabeth Beck (1907–2002): an appreciation. *Neuropathol. Appl. Neurobiol.* **30**: 193.

Corvisier-Visy, N. and Poirier, J. (1996) Neuropathology in France (19th–20th centuries). Semantic and institutional misadventures. *Arch. Anat. Cytol. Pathol.* **44**: 18–27.

Cushing, H. (first published 1924, republished 1940) *The Life of Sir William Osler.* Oxford University Press: Oxford, pp. 741–742.

Ehrlich, P. (1902) Über die Beziehungen von chemischer Constitution, Vertheilung, und pharmakologischer Wirkung. Reprinted and translated in 1906 in *Collected Studies in Immunity.* Wiley: New York, pp. 567–595.

Foster, W.D. (1981) *Pathology as a Profession in Great Britain and The Early History of the Royal College of Pathologists.* Royal College of Pathologists: London.

Geddes, J.F. (1998) Why do we remember Dorothy Russell?. *Neuropathol. Appl. Neurobiol.* **24**: 268–270.

Graham, D., Brown, A., Cavanagh, J. and Meldrum, B. (2005) Obituary – James Brunskill Brierley (1916–2004). *Neuropathol. Appl. Neurobiol.* **31**: 206–209.

Graham, D.I. and Lantos, P.L. (2002) *Greenfield's Neuropathology* (7th edn) Arnold: London.

Greenfield, J.G. (1929) The pathology of measles encephalomyelitis. *Brain* **52**: 171–195.

Greenfield, J.G. (1954) *The Spino-Cerebellar Degenerations.* Blackwell Scientific Publications: Oxford.

McMenemey, W.H. and Walshe, F.M.R. (1959) Obituary notices of deceased members – Joseph Godwin Greenfield. *J. Pathol. Bacteriol.* **78**: 577–592.

Penfield, W. (1932) *Cytology and Cellular Pathology of the Nervous System* (3 vols). Paul B. Hoeber: New York.

Richardson, E.P. Jr., Astrom, K.E. and Kleihues, P. (1994) The development of neuropathology at the Massachusetts General Hospital and Harvard Medical School. *Brain Pathol.* **4**: 181–188.

Rio-Hortega, P. del (1919) El tercer elemento de los centros nervios. I. La microglía en estado normal. II. Intervención de la microglía en los procesos patológicos (células en bastencito y cuerpos gránulo-adiposos). III. Naturaleza probable de la microglia. *Biol. Soc. Esp. Biol.* **9**: 69–129.

Robertson, W.F. (1900) A microscopic demonstration of the normal and pathological histology of mesoglia cells. *J. Ment. Sci.* **46**: 733–752.

Rubinstein, L.J. (1984) Obituary – Dorothy Stuart Russell. *J. Pathol.* **142**: iii–v.

Virchow, R. (1860) *Cellular Pathology as based upon Physiological and Pathological Histology.* John Churchill: London.

Virchow, R. (1893) Transformation and descent. *J. Pathol. Bacteriol.* **1**: 1–12.

Walter, G.F., Matthies, H.K., Brandis, A. and von Jan, U. (2000) Telemedicine of the future: teleneuropathology. *Technol. Health Care* **8**: 25–34.

17 Debate: Whither Haematoxylin and Eosin?

SETTING THE SCENE

The technical advances of the past 30 years and the burgeoning scope of molecular and genetic analyses have been predicted by some to be the harbingers of the demise of pathology as a diagnostic discipline. It has been suggested that the traditional heamotoxylin and eosin stained preparation interpreted and considered by a histopathologist using a light microscope will be replaced in short order by molecular analyses and perhaps by automated and robotic procedures.

At the beginning of the second century of The Pathological Society we have challenged a leading molecular pathologist to argue the case that *H&E will be replaced by 'chips'*. Nick Lemoine has advanced this thesis with his sub-heading *Microarrays are the way: adding value to precious tissue in the molecular era*. This proposition has been rebutted by Jason Hornick and Chris Fletcher from the more traditional camp of diagnostic (or surgical) pathologists. They have responded to the progressive molecular view with the response that *H&E will hold sway*! and the sub-heading of *The invaluable role of morphology in the molecular era*. The reader will have their own view and the future will indicate where the truth lies!

The Editors

H&E Will Be Replaced by 'Chips'

Microarrays Are the Way: Adding Value to Precious Tissue in the Molecular Era

Nick R. Lemoine

INTRODUCTION: MODERNISE OR DIE!

Since the founding father of the science of histopathology, François-Xavier Bichat, worked throughout his career without a microscope 200 years ago, perhaps we can consider the subsequent focus on cells and microscopy introduced by Rudolf Virchow to be but a passing phase in the evolution of the specialty. Maybe we can now at last join the molecular revolution and move on to a new era where pathologists become central rather than peripheral to patient management, and proactive rather than reactive to scientific and clinical developments.

Medicine is generally a conservative profession, and many believe histopathology to be among the most conservative of its specialties. This might hold some superficial attractions in the rapidly changing world of healthcare: investigative fashions may come and go but clinicians have continued to recognise the gold standard of '30 years of experience and an H&E' when it comes to diagnostics for treatment decisions. However, healthcare professionals – and perhaps more importantly, patients – are now more informed than ever about the potential for individualised therapy, and managers are examining more closely the cost–benefit issue of the laboratory services. If the right information cannot be delivered from a pathology service to make resource-critical decisions on a patient's treatment pathway, then the resource will be withdrawn and invested elsewhere. It is absolutely critical that pathologists are forewarned with the right intelligence and armed with the right tools as the molecular revolution sweeps through the practice of medicine.

It is crucial that molecular pathology is recognised and encouraged as a specialty if we are to contribute to progress. The shift in thinking represented by systems biology means that we must have the expertise to analyse biological complexity and exploit it in predictive, preventive and personalised medicine. The profession must modernise or die.

APPLICABILITY IN CLINICAL PRACTICE

A criticism frequently levelled at the use of molecular approaches in the analysis of clinical material is that tissue handling, transport and storage all make a significant impact on gene and protein profiles independent of the disease process under study. Indeed, when healthy and malignant colon tissue samples were snap-frozen at various time points after colon resection, and gene and protein expression were determined by the two common platform technologies (Affymetrix microarray HG-U133A chips and surface-enhanced laser desorption/ionisation time-of-flight mass spectrometry (SELDI-ToF-MS), respectively) changes in profiles were already observed 5–8 min after colon resection (Spruessel *et al.*, 2004). Fifteen minutes after surgery, 10–15%

(and, after 30 min, 20%) of all detectable genes and proteins differed significantly from the baseline values. Studies such as this have meant that control of these variables has become mandatory to obtain reliable data in screening programmes for molecular targets and diagnostic molecular patterns.

However, many of the same criticisms over the handling and storage of tissue samples apply equally to technologies that the classical histopathogist now regards as part of his standard armentarium, such as immunohistochemistry. A long delay between cutting the sections and immunohistochemical staining can decrease the immunohistochemical reaction intensity, as revealed in a recent study of the influence of slide age on the results of IHC analyses for oestrogen receptor (ER), progesterone receptor (PR), cyclin D1, HER2 (HercepTest) and E-cadherin (Mirlacher *et al.*, 2004). The frequency of positivity on old sections (stored for 6 months at 4 °C) compared to freshly cut sections decreased from 65 to 46% for ER ($P < 0.0001$), from 33 to 18.5% for PR ($P < 0.0001$), from 16.3 to 9.6% for HER2 ($P = 0.0047$), from 45.1 to 37.7% for cyclin D1 ($P = 0.10$) and from 58.9 to 32.9% for E-cadherin ($P < 0.0001$). Hence both classical and molecular pathologists need to take care of their tissues if they are to have confidence in their outcomes.

More reassuringly, a recent study evaluated the validity of assessing gene expression in cervical tissues acquired in a clinical setting, investigating whether standard procedures such as the application of acetic acid and/or Lugol's iodine, employed for the visualisation of colposcopically directed biopsies, altered patterns in oligonucleotide array analysis (Wang *et al.*, 2005). Microarray profiles were compared in tissues from six women, each with three adjacent samples removed from benign hysterectomy specimens and either immediately frozen or had acetic acid only or both acetic acid and Lugol's iodine applied. They found that standard precolposcopic procedures do not substantially affect the overall gene expression patterns in the normal cervix.

As clinical practice moves ever further towards minimally invasive diagnostic procedures, it is important to note that it is feasible to generate gene expression profiles from both fine-needle aspirates and core needle biopsies that yield (from breast cancers, for instance) an average of 1–2 μg of total RNA (Assersohn *et al.*, 2002; Ellis *et al.*, 2002; Sotiriou *et al.*, 2002; Pusztai *et al.*, 2003; Symmans *et al.*, 2003). The rate of successful profiling is around 70–80% with both biopsy methods, and the gene expression profiles obtained from matching fine-needle aspirates and core needle biopsies of the same tumour are similar (Symmans *et al.*, 2003). At least one commercial laboratory in the USA already offers comprehensive gene expression profiling of formalin-fixed, paraffin-embedded human cancer tissues, although currently for research purposes only (US Laboratories, Irvine, CA).

MOLECULAR DIAGNOSIS OF TUMOURS OF UNKNOWN PRIMARY SITE

Although classical histopathology is well equipped to make the diagnosis of malignancies in their primary site or typical metastatic locations, it is less powerful for the identification of tumours of unknown primary site and because such cases make up perhaps 5% of new cancer presentations (Briasoulis and Pavlidis, 1997) this is a significant limitation to practice. These neoplasms (often adenocarcinoma) represent a clinically diverse group, typically presenting with moderately to poorly differentiated tumours involving multiple organs, including liver, bone, lung, lymph nodes, pleura and brain (Le Chevalier *et al.*, 1988). Such a diagnosis may be a potential source of financial frustration for the patient because in the USA Medicare and many private insurers will not pay their drug costs because the diagnosis of 'unknown primary site' is not listed in the indications for various drugs in the United States Pharmacopeia Dispensing Information (Reynolds, 1998). Tumours of unknown primary site also cause much clinical frustration, because patients with such disease represent a disproportionate fraction of cancer deaths due to their poor median survival, which is typically a matter of months (Abbruzzese *et al.*, 1995). This is unsatisfactory in today's world because treatments are becoming increasingly specific, with approaches varying significantly depending on the cellular origin (and molecular subtype) of the cancer. With recent advances in chemotherapy, specific regimens have led to improvements in survival and quality of life even for tumour types that traditionally have been regarded as relatively chemoresistant, such as pancreatic and non-small-cell lung cancers.

Gene expression profiling could be an important tool to identify the site of origin of these malignancies, and indeed several studies have shown that it is possible to identify correctly metastatic tumours from known primary carcinoma using this approach (Ramaswamy *et al.*, 2001; Su *et al.*, 2001; Bloom *et al.*, 2004), although until recently no study had benchmarked the efficacy of such tests for predicting the site of origin of tumours against clinical diagnostic variables. Now a highly accurate multiclass classifier designed for clinical application to tumours of unknown primary has been reported (Tothill *et al.*, 2005). A large and comprehensive data set of gene expression was obtained from microarray analysis of 229 tumour samples, representing 14 common sites of origin in the differential diagnosis of tumours of unknown primary site. A single cDNA microarray platform was used to profile 229 primary and metastatic tumours representing 14 tumour types and multiple histological subtypes (which addresses the confounding issue of molecular heterogeneity of specific tumour classes). This data set was subsequently used for training and validation of a support vector machine (SVM) classifier that demonstrated 89% accuracy using a 13-class model.

Of course an objection raised to the application of expression profiling in clinical practice is that microarray analysis typically requires as a substrate fresh-frozen tissue harvested and stored in pristine condition. However, a number of studies have shown that accurate classification of multiple cancer types can be made using a reduced number of genes – hundreds rather than thousands (Su *et al.*, 2001; Giordano *et al.*, 2001; Shedden *et al.*, 2003; Bloom *et al.*, 2004). Hence a classification could be achieved using cheaper, faster and more robust platforms for quantifying gene expression, such as quantitative polymerase chain reaction (PCR), and already several studies have demonstrated that expression analysis from fixed material using quantitative PCR is perfectly feasible (Specht *et al.*, 2001; Abrahamsen *et al.*, 2003; Cronin *et al.*, 2004). Generating low-density quantitative-PCR arrays or using multiplex reactions therefore offers an attractive alternative to standard high-density microarrays for eventual clinical application in a conventional pathology laboratory using formalin-fixed, paraffin-embedded material. Tothill and colleagues selected 79 optimal gene markers and achieved the translation of a five-class classifier to a quantitative-PCR low-density array, allowing the assay of both fresh-frozen and formalin-fixed, paraffin-embedded tissue. Data generated using both quantitative PCR and microarray were subsequently used to train and validate a cross-platform support vector machine model with high prediction accuracy, and on prospective application to a test series the classifiers were capable of making high-confidence predictions in 11 of 13 cases of tumour of unknown primary site. Importantly, Tothill *et al.* emphasise that it is likely that there will be cost savings from the application of such a molecular genomics test because it will enable more directed clinical evaluation of patients. The average cost for diagnostic evaluation of patients with a tumour of unknown primary site at a major US cancer centre was estimated at $18 000 when a large series was considered (Schapira and Jarrett, 1995), whereas a test similar to that described here is likely to cost under $1000 (Tothill *et al.*, 2005).

BIOLOGICAL INSIGHT INTO CONTROVERSIAL TUMOUR ENTITIES

There are some areas of oncology where classical light microscopy has probably gone as far as it is ever likely to go and the classification of sarcomas is a good example (as even the protagonists for the survival of the H&E might concede). For instance, the malignant fibrous histiocytoma was for some decades regarded as the most common soft-tissue sarcoma of adult life, but almost from its first description in the early 1960s controversy has raged over its histogenesis and its validity as a clinicopathological entity (indeed the latest World Health Organization classification no longer includes malignant fibrous histiocytoma as a distinct diagnostic category but rather as subtypes of an undifferentiated pleomorphic sarcoma). Similar, if less incandescent, arguments break out over other entities in the sarcoma spectrum and some order needs to be established for clinical practice to advance.

Perhaps because it is such a fertile hunting ground for those determined to classify objectively on grounds other than individual, subjective opinion on morphology, microarray technology has been applied extensively in the analysis of sarcomas (Allander *et al.*, 2001; Nielsen *et al.*, 2002; Segal *et al.*, 2003). Some of the most interesting reports have described expression profiles associated with poor clinical outcome in leiomyosarcoma (Lee *et al.*, 2004) and Ewing's sarcoma (Ohali *et al.*, 2004), and novel biomarkers in dermatofibrosarcoma protuberans (West *et al.*, 2004) and clear cell sarcoma (Schaefer *et al.*, 2004). Recently, a comprehensive study examined 181 tumors representing 16 classes of human bone and soft-tissue sarcomas on a 12 601-feature cDNA microarray (Baird *et al.*, 2005). A set of 2766 probes differentially expressed across this sample panel clearly delineated the various tumour classes. Many genes previously associated with specific tumour types were among those most highly weighted (for example: the muscle markers *MYLK, CNN1* and *ACTG2* in leiomyosarcoma; *KIT* in gastrointestinal stromal tumours; *SSX1* in synovial sarcoma; and *PDGFB* in dermatofibrosarcoma protuberans), but each group was also associated with a highly informative list of other associated genes, including numerous genes not previously associated with sarcoma.

The group of tumours pathologically classified as malignant fibrous histiocytomas proved to be a rather complex group at the molecular level. On unsupervised clustering of the microarray data, the majority of malignant fibrous histiocytoma tumours co-clustered with the more poorly differentiated tumours, forming a large branch that included dedifferentiated and pleomorphic liposarcomas, malignant peripheral nerve sheath tumours and the sarcomas that are not otherwise specified. Interestingly, the most closely adjacent branch on the unsupervised clustering dendrogram contained the leiomyosarcomas.

Unsupervised hierarchical cluster analysis of the malignant fibrous histiocytoma tumors identified two groups of nearly equal proportions. The group of genes associated with the first group carried a muscle profile with the genes *myosin X, sarcoglycan ß* and *tenascin C* among the ten genes, with the most significant differences in expression. In contrast, the second group of tumours was characterized by a cluster of immune regulatory genes, with *HEM1, MX1, DAP10, PLCG2* and *FOLR3* constituting the five most highly weighted genes. The distinction of malignant fibrous histiocytoma with myogenic differentiation versus inflammatory characteristics could prove clinically significant. Certainly it is known that the presence of myogenic differentiation in malignant fibrous histiocytoma and undifferentiated sarcomas correlates with a poor prognosis (Fletcher *et al.*, 2001), although the prevalence of such differentiation is approximately 30% on classical histological criteria rather than 50% on molecular profiling. Quite what the significance is of the inflammatory signature needs more investigation, because classical histopathologists recognise an inflammatory-type malignant fibrous histiocytoma only rarely. However, an inflammatory profile is correlated with good prognosis in other malignancies (Lotze and Rees, 2004), such as colorectal cancer with microsatellite instability (Banerjea *et al.*, 2004) and follicular lymphoma (Fujii *et al.*, 2005), which is considered in more detail below.

A really significant advantage that large-scale molecular analysis such as this offers over simple histopathological descriptions is the facility for other investigators to mine the data and build their own hypotheses to test in other clinical series or model systems. The complete raw data from the study are available through the Gene Expression Omnibus (GEO) data repository (GEO accession number GSE2553) and the expression profiles of the 7788 probes of highest quality from the gene expression array can be viewed at http://watson.nhgri.nih.gov/sarcoma/. Similar facilities now exist for many different tumour panels, and the future entry of clinical trial series will increase the value of such resources.

LYMPHOMA – THE EXEMPLAR OF MOLECULAR PROGNOSTICATION

Follicular lymphoma is a disease with marked clinical heterogeneity in which some patients undergo rapid transformation to aggressive lymphoma and die, whereas others survive for years with indolent disease. Reliable prognostic markers have not been established to guide therapy and it is well recognised that pathological grading is highly subjective and the clinically based International Prognostic Index identifies relatively few high-risk patients (Decaudin *et al.*, 1999). Significantly, it was in this disease that expression profiling had its first high-profile successes in prognostication (Dave *et al.*, 2004; Glas *et al.*, 2005), and highlighted the critical impact of the cytokine milieu in the lymphoma microenvironment (Fujii *et al.*, 2005).

More recently, follicular lymphoma has been the exemplar for the identification of biologically relevant differences in protein expression using reverse-phase protein microarrays (Gulmann *et al.*, 2005). By using reverse-phase protein microarrays and antibodies to proteins in the intrinsic apoptotic pathway, it was shown that high ratios of Bcl-2/Bak and Bcl-2/Bax were associated with early death from disease, with differences in median survival times of 7.3 years ($P = 0.0085$) and 3.8 years ($P = 0.018$), respectively. Such data are powerful arguments to incorporate proteomic endpoints in clinical trial protocols to validate fully their clinical utility.

A CLASSIC EXAMPLE: DUKES' STAGING ONLY TAKES US PART OF THE WAY – MOLECULAR PROFILING IS NEEDED TO COMPLETE THE JOURNEY

One of the best examples of how classical histopathology can be exploited to guide clinical practice is Dukes' staging of colorectal cancer, which has long been the gold standard for prognostication and treatment decisions. However, considerable variability exists in the long-term survival of patients within each class. Notably, around 50% of Dukes' C patients will have disease recurrence and die as a result of their disease after surgery with curative intent, whereas the other half are surgically cured, and it has not been possible by histopathological means to distinguish between these two subgroups of patients. The advent of routine adjuvant treatment for these patients over the last decade has significantly improved the survival of 10–20% of these patients, but at the cost of overtreating those who are already surgically cured. Hence, although classical histopathology has served us well, it has reached the limit of its power in this group and more sophisticated stratification is needed.

A recent study used high-density oligonucleotide microarray analysis to identify profiles of expression in tumours from Dukes' C patients who had surgery as the only form of treatment (Arango *et al.*, 2005). A total of 218 genes showed a significant difference in expression in tumours from patients with good and bad outcomes. Microarray-based expression profiling outperformed other genetic markers previously investigated, such as *TP53* and *K-RAS* status or allelic imbalance in chromosome 18q. One of the genes with the most significantly reduced expression in tumours from patients with bad prognosis compared with tumours from good-prognosis patients was the RAS homologue gene *RHOA*. Using immunohistochemistry and a tissue microarray, the level of expression of *RHOA* was assessed in an independent set of 137 formalin-fixed, paraffin-embedded tumour samples from Dukes' C patients. Patients with low RHOA levels in the tumour had significantly worse overall ($P = 0.03$) and disease-free ($P = 0.01$) survival compared with patients whose tumours had high *RHOA* protein levels. Interestingly, shorter survival of patients with low *RHOA* tumour protein levels could also be observed in those patients who received 5-fluorouracil–based adjuvant chemotherapy. Therefore, *RHOA* could be used to identify a subset of patients with a higher probability of recurrence and for whom a more aggressive treatment may be justified. Although adjuvant treatment with 5-fluorouracil has become the standard treatment of Dukes' C colorectal cancer, effective alternatives exist in irinotecan and oxaliplatin. Reduced *RHOA* levels could therefore identify a group of patients who could benefit from combined treatment with 5-fluorouracil and CPT-11 and/or oxaliplatin.

TREATMENT INDIVIDUALISATION BY MOLECULAR PROFILING

Two subgroups of patients do not get any benefit from adjuvant chemotherapy: the first one comprises patients who are already cured by locoregional treatment alone (as exemplified in the Dukes' C group reviewed above), and the second one is represented by patients who do not profit from adjuvant chemotherapy because of resistance to the regimens employed. There are two ways in which we can improve the cost–benefit issue of this treatment strategy: one is to improve the sensitivity of prognostic factors to be able to select a specific group with a good signature that does not need adjuvant treatment; the second is to identify predictive factors that may help us to select the optimal therapeutic strategy or the optimal regimen or drug for individual patients.

When chemotherapy is administered preoperatively to women with breast cancer, a complete and partial response rate assessed clinically exceeding 70% is achieved with many regimens. However, a lower percentage ranging from about 5% to 38% of patients achieve tumour eradication when response is assessed by careful pathological examination of the surgical specimen after chemotherapy (Bonadonna *et al.*, 1998; Fisher *et al.*, 1998; Smith *et al.*, 2002; Kaufmann *et al.*, 2003). Several studies have shown that, together with nodal status at surgery, pathological complete response is the most significant independent variable associated with the likelihood of benefit as measured by disease-free and overall survival. In principle, diagnostic tests that predict, before administration of neoadjuvant therapy, which patients are going to experience Pathological complete response will identify patients who are likely to benefit from treatment and will also identify individuals with low or no likelihood of benefit, sparing them the toxicity of an inactive treatment and allowing earlier application of alternative approaches. Successful prediction of a durable benefit of chemotherapy using routinely obtained fixed tumour tissue would make possible and widely applicable the tailoring of toxic chemotherapy to individual patients. The identification of a predictive multivariate marker from microarray expression data involves three main steps: invariant genes must be filtered from the data set to prevent noise obscuring true biological associations, and the remaining genes of interest are ranked by their strength of association with the outcome; a model is identified that can predict outcome using the gene expression values as input to a mathematical formula; and a prediction rule is defined that categorises the output from the model into clinically defined classes using cut-off points.

Expression of 250 candidate genes in tumour tissues from a total of 447 patients identified a 21-gene panel and a Recurrence Score (RS) algorithm. The RS was clinically validated to quantify the risk of distant recurrence in 668 women with ER-positive, node-negative breast tumours treated with adjuvant tamoxifen in a clinical trial conducted in the USA as the National Surgical Adjuvant Breast and Bowel Project (Paik *et al.*, 2004). The expression of 384 genes, including the RS panel of 21 genes, was similarly quantified in fixed diagnostic biopsy specimens of women with locally advanced breast cancer who were treated with chemotherapy before surgery (Gianni *et al.*, 2005). The 86 candidate genes that were significantly correlated with pathological complete response in this cohort of patients were then tested for their correlation with pathological complete response in a separate cohort of 82 patients treated with similar neoadjuvant chemotherapy whose tumour tissue was profiled by DNA microarrays. The predictive genes included three particularly prominent co-expression clusters. Pathological complete response correlated, as expected, with higher expression of genes regulating proliferation (e.g., *CDC20*, *E2F1*, *MYBL2* and *TOPO2A*) and lower expression of genes related to expression of the ER (e.g., *ER*, *PR*, *SCUBE2* and *GATA3*). The third cluster predicting pathological complete response comprised a group of upregulated genes associated with immune response (e.g., *MCP1*, *CD68*, *CTSB*, *CD18*, ILT-2, *CD3z*, *FasL* and *HLA.DPB1*) and hence it is possible that the pretreatment host response may enhance the ability of chemotherapy to eliminate cancer cells.

Validation of the recurrence score will require a randomised phase III study such as that being planned by the US Intergroup Program for the Assessment of Clinical Cancer Tests. A large randomised multinational trial (Microarray In Node-negative Disease may Avoid Chemo Therapy, MINDACT) will compare the information obtained with genomic profiling and the classical clinicopathological index (St Gallen classification); the objective is to allow women not to be treated with adjuvant chemotherapy if their genomic signature is 'good'. Another trial (EORTC 10994) is being conducted to investigate whether, in patients with p53-mutated tumours, neoadjuvant chemotherapy with docetaxel is more efficient than an anthracycline-containing regimen (a supplementary study will evaluate gene profiles in each group). This type of treatment response prediction may be more broadly applicable: expression profiling of pancreatic cancer cells with differential resistance to gemcitabine has revealed that analysis of as few as six genes (among which downregulated *TNFSF6* – also known as Fas ligand – *BNIP3* and *AKT* may be the most informative combination) may allow the development of an algorithm for stratification of patients before treatment (Akada *et al.*, 2005; Nakai *et al.*, 2005). This is now being tested as part of large-scale prospective clinical trials in which the construction of tissue microarrays is an integral component of protocol design.

An important outcome of the confirmatory trials will be to determine whether the new predictors of response are specific for particular chemotherapy regimens, or whether they predict response to any cytotoxic treatment. To be most useful clinically, a pharmacogenomic predictor would need to be regimen-specific and a portfolio of such predictors developed for assisting decision points in the treatment pathway of individual patients. Multigene predictors using prediction scores and machine-learning algorithms have several features distinct from traditional single (gene) markers. The number of genes (as well as the individual sequences) included in the prediction model can change over time as more data become available, allowing the introduction of a series of sequential predictors with increasing predictive accuracy. Different mathematical methods and alternative combinations of genes could yield a number of different predictors with similar performance. The profiling methods that will be used routinely in the clinic are not yet clear. Limited profiling using real-time reverse-transcription (RT)-PCR or small custom arrays that measure only the genes that contribute to a prognostic predictive signature are already commercially available (OncotypeDX®, Genomic Health, Inc, Redwood City CA; MammaPrint®, Agendia, Amsterdam, The Netherlands). Similar products for chemotherapy prediction could soon appear on the market soon after completion of the ongoing validation studies. External validation will entail the use of any molecular test in different laboratories to show that the methods are reproducible and widely applicable to tissue in routine clinical practice.

HAS MICROARRAY TECHNOLOGY IDENTIFIED A UNIVERSAL DEATH-FROM-CANCER SIGNATURE?

A highly provocative report has suggested recently that a 'death-from-cancer' gene expression signature may be identifiable in tumour biopsies at the time of presentation, and this represents dominance of a stem cell population in the malignancy (Glinsky, 2005; Glinsky *et al.*, 2005). The hypothesis is that activation in transformed cells of normal stem cells' self-renewal pathways might contribute to the survival of cancer stem cells and promote tumour progression. The gene expression pathway driven by the BMI-1 oncogene is essential for the self-renewal of haematopoietic and neural stem cells, and now it appears that it may be a critical determinant in cancer cell fate. A mouse/human comparative translational genomics approach was used to identify an 11-gene (*GBX2, KI67, CCNB1, BUB1, KNTC2, USP22, HCFC1, RNF2, ANK3, FGFR2, CES1*) signature that consistently displays a stem-cell-resembling (BMI-1-driven) expression profile in distant metastatic lesions, as revealed by the analysis of metastases and primary tumours from cancer patients. The 11-gene set comprises two groups: those in which elevated expression levels are associated with stem cell-ness and a poor prognosis (*Ki67, CCNB1, GBX2, BUB1, KNTC2, USP22* and *RNF2*, in descending order of strength of association), and those for which decreased expression levels are associated with stem cell-ness and a good prognosis (*CES1, FGFR2* and *ANK3*).

The prognostic power of the 11-gene signature was validated in several independent therapy-outcome sets of clinical samples obtained from 1153 cancer patients diagnosed with 11 different types of cancer, including five common epithelial malignancies (prostate, breast, lung, ovarian and bladder cancers) and five non-epithelial malignancies (lymphoma, mesothelioma, medulloblastoma, glioma and acute myeloid leukaemia). Kaplan-Meier analysis demonstrated that a stem cell-like expression profile of the 11-gene signature in primary tumours is a consistently powerful predictor of a short interval to disease recurrence, distant metastasis and death after therapy in cancer patients diagnosed with any of these distinct types of cancer. These data suggest the presence of a conserved BMI-1-driven pathway, which is similarly engaged in both normal stem cells and a highly malignant subset of human cancers diagnosed in a wide range of organs and uniformly exhibiting a marked propensity towards metastatic dissemination as well as a high probability of unfavourable therapy outcome. Other authors (Lahad *et al.*, 2005) have already replicated part of the analysis of the stem-cell-like phenotype association index (SPAI) in a lung cancer study that included survival data on 125 patients and microarray data from Affymetrix U95Av2 GeneChips, and so more universal application may be possible.

TISSUE MICROARRAYS: WHERE CLASSICAL HISTOPATHOLOGY HANDS THE BATON ON TO MOLECULAR PATHOLOGY

The validation required for translation of tissue biomarkers from the research laboratory to the clinical setting will depend on the combination of tissue microarray (TMA) technology with automated quantitative analysis. Tissue microarrays offer molecular information for both RNA and protein within the context of cellular morphology and tissue architecture. Using conventional histopathology slides, a study of 20 biomarkers in a 400-sample cohort would take weeks to assemble and months to process. Tissue microarrays allow processing of the biomarkers on serial sections of the array on the same day, and at a fraction of the cost. Classical histopathologists are clearly required for initial selection of representative areas for harvesting donor cores, but much of the remaining processing and analysis can be automated. The high-density format of TMAs allows variables such as antigen retrieval, temperature, washing time and reagent concentration to be standardised for the entire cohort, and combination with fully automated systems such as the Ventana Discovery platform (www.ventanadiscovery.com/) adds further quality control. A number of commercial software packages have been produced for the automated analysis of TMAs based on the optical density of chromagen-detected antigens, resulting in objective scores on a continuous scale. Some systems (e.g. Chromavision ACIS,® which combines both image acquisition and quantitative interpretation) achieve higher accuracy than microscopic analysis by classical histopathologists and better agreement with the standard FISH assay for the evaluation of HER-2/*neu* overexpression by chromagen-linked immunohistochemistry (Wang *et al.*, 2001). Similarly promising results have been reported for quantitative analysis of ER and p21 in tumours.

Immunofluorescence-based antigen detection has the well-established advantages of being more sensitive, more linear and having a wider dynamic range. An automated quantitative analysis system that measures protein expression in subcellular compartments on a continuous scale – including in arrayed specimens – has been validated for several biomarkers (Camp *et al.*, 2002). An alternative immunofluorescence technique using laser imaging has been shown to give a good correlation to well-studied biomarkers in colon cancer and can be applied to nucleic acid detection by mRNA *in situ* hybridisation (Jubb *et al.*, 2003). Using such technology, molecular definition of subcellular compartments beyond the range of classical histopathology is possible: fluorescence-based systems allow co-localisation with markers of specific subcellular compartments, such as the Golgi, mitochondria or endoplasmic reticulum, or even virtual compartments, such as components of signal transduction pathways.

Bioinformatics tools developed for the analysis of gene expression arrays are not suitable for TMA analysis, because the TMA data structure has absolute rather than relational values and missing data preclude the use of Euclidean distance algorithms. New methods that are specific to the problems of TMAs but include elements of microarray annotation and epidemiological analysis are now being developed. Advances in web-based browser systems that allow archiving and annotation of large sets of tissue microarray data (Kim *et al.*, 2005) will speed the process of validating individual or clustered markers while maintaining the quality assurance of pathological expertise.

CONCLUSION

So much is now possible in the molecular analysis of clinical material that it is important for pathologists to develop *modi operandi* that enhance their chances of survival in the evolving molecular world. Understanding the technology and embracing the informatics can be facilitated by specialist training. Adopting the new way of thinking encapsulated by systems biology should be mandatory, as should an open attitude to professional networks and the warehousing and mining of data (perhaps, controversially, including the biological data represented by tissue).

The future for molecular medicine is bright; it is up to us to ensure that pathology is part of it.

REFERENCES

Abbruzzese, J.L., Abbruzzese, M.C., Lenzi, R, Hess, K.R. and Raber, M.N. (1995) Analysis of a diagnostic strategy for patients with suspected tumors of unknown origin. *J. Clin. Oncol.* **13**: 2094–2103.

Abrahamsen, H.N., Steiniche, T., Nexo, E., Hamilton-Dutoit, S.J. and Sorensen, B.S. (2003) Towards quantitative mRNA analysis in paraffin-embedded tissues using real-time reverse transcriptase-polymerase chain reaction: a methodological study on lymph nodes from melanoma patients. *J. Mol. Diagn.* **5**: 34–41.

Akada, M., Crnogorac-Jurcevic, T., Lattimore, S., Mahon, P., Lopes, R., Sunamura, M., *et al.* (2005) Intrinsic chemoresistance to gemcitabine is associated with decreased expression of BNIP3 in pancreatic cancer. *Clin. Cancer Res.* **11**: 3094–3101.

Allander, S.V., Nupponen, N.N., Ringner, M., Hostetter, G., Maher, G.W., Goldberger, N., *et al.* (2001) Gastrointestinal stromal tumors with KIT mutations exhibit a remarkably homogeneous gene expression profile. *Cancer Res.* **61**: 8624–8628.

Arango, D., Laiho, P., Kokko, A., Alhopuro, P., Sammalkorpi, H., Salovaara, R., *et al.* (2005) Gene-expression profiling predicts recurrence in Dukes' C colorectal cancer. *Gastroenterology* **129**: 874–84.

Assersohn, L., Gangi, L., Zhao, Y., Dowsett, M., Simon, R., Powles, T.J. and Liu, E.T. (2002) The feasibility of using fine needle aspiration from primary breast cancers for cDNA microarray analyses. *Clin. Cancer Res.* **8**: 794–801.

Baird, K., Davis, S., Antonescu, C.R., Harper, U.L., Walker, R.L., Chen, Y., *et al.* (2005) Gene expression profiling of human sarcomas: insights into sarcoma biology. *Cancer Res.* **65**: 9226–9235.

Banerjea, A., Ahmed, S., Hands, R.E., Huang, F., Han, X., Shaw, P.M., *et al.* (2004) Colorectal cancers with microsatellite instability display mRNA expression signatures characteristic of increased immunogenicity. *Mol. Cancer* **3**: 21.

Bloom, G., Yang, I.V., Boulware, D., Kwong, K.Y., Coppola, D., Eschrich, S., *et al.* (2004) Multi-platform, multi-site, microarray-based human tumor classification. *Am. J. Pathol.* **164**: 9–16.

Bonadonna, G., Valagussa, P., Brambilla, C., Ferrari, L., Moliterni, A., Terenziani, M., *et al.* (1998) Primary chemotherapy in operable breast cancer: eight-year experience at the Milan Cancer Institute. *J. Clin. Oncol.* **16**: 93–100.

Briasoulis, E. and Pavlidis, N. (1997) Cancer of unknown primary origin. *Oncologist* **2**: 142–152.

Camp, R.L., Chung, GG and Rimm, D.L. (2002) Automated subcellular localization and quantification of protein expression in tissue microarrays. *Nat. Med.* **8**: 1323–1327.

Cronin, M., Pho, M., Dutta, D., Stephans, J.C., Shak, S., Kiefer, M.C., *et al.* (2004) Measurement of gene expression in archival paraffin-embedded tissues: development and performance of a 92-gene reverse transcriptase-polymerase chain reaction assay. *Am. J. Pathol.* **164**: 35–42.

Dave, S.S., Wright, G., Tan, B., Rosenwald, A., Gascoyne, R.D., Chan, W.C., *et al.* (2004) Prediction of survival in follicular lymphoma based on molecular features of tumor-infiltrating immune cells. *N. Engl. J. Med.* **351**: 2159–2169.

Decaudin, D., Lepage, E., Brousse, N., Brice, P., Harousseau, J.L., Belhadj, K., *et al.* (1999) Low-grade stage III-IV follicular lymphoma: multivariate analysis of prognostic factors in 484 patients – a study of the groupe d'Etude des lymphomes de l'Adulte. *J. Clin. Oncol.* **17**: 2499–2505.

Ellis, M., Davis, N., Coop, A., Liu, M., Schumaker, L., Lee, R.Y., *et al.* (2002) Development and validation of a method for using breast core needle biopsies for gene expression microarray analyses. *Clin. Cancer Res.* **8**: 1155–1166.

Fisher, B., Bryant, J., Wolmark, N., Mamounas, E., Brown, A., Fisher, E.R., *et al.* (1998) Effect of preoperative chemotherapy on the outcome of women with operable breast cancer. *J. Clin. Oncol.* **16**: 2672–2685.

Fletcher, C.D., Gustafson, P., Rydholm, A., Willen, H. and Akerman, M. (2001) Clinicopathologic re-evaluation of 100 malignant fibrous histiocytomas: prognostic relevance of subclassification. *J. Clin. Oncol.* **19**: 3045–3050.

Fujii, A., Oshima, K., Hamasaki, M., Utsunomiya, H., Okazaki, M., Kagami, Y., *et al.* (2005) Differential expression of cytokines, chemokines and their receptors in follicular lymphoma and reactive follicular hyperplasia: assessment by complementary DNA microarray. *Oncol. Rep.* **13**: 819–824.

Gianni, L., Zambetti, M., Clark, K., Baker, J., Cronin, M., Wu, J., *et al.* (2005) Gene expression profiles in paraffin-embedded core biopsy tissue predict response to chemotherapy in women with locally advanced breast cancer. *J. Clin. Oncol.* **23**: 7265–7277.

Giordano, T.J., Shedden, K.A., Schwartz, D.R., Kuick, R., Taylor, J.M., Lee, N., *et al.* (2001) Organ-specific molecular classification of primary lung, colon, and ovarian adenocarcinomas using gene expression profiles. *Am. J. Pathol.* **159**: 1231–1238.

Glas, A.M., Kersten, M.J., Delahaye, L.J., Witteveen, A.T., Kibbelaar, R.E., Velds, A., *et al.* (2005) Gene expression profiling in follicular lymphoma to assess clinical aggressiveness and to guide the choice of treatment. *Blood* **105**: 301–307.

Glinsky, G.V. (2005) Death-from-cancer signatures and stem cell contribution to metastatic cancer. *Cell Cycle* **4**: 1171–1175.

Glinsky, G.V., Berezovska, O. and Glinskii, A.B. (2005) Microarray analysis identifies a death-from-cancer signature predicting therapy failure in patients with multiple types of cancer. *J. Clin. Invest.* **115**: 1503–1521.

Gulmann, C., Espina, V., Petricoin, E., III, Longo, D.L., Santi, M., Knutsen, T., *et al.* (2005) Proteomic analysis of apoptotic pathways reveals prognostic factors in follicular lymphoma. *Clin. Cancer Res.* **11**: 5847–5855.

Jubb, A.M., Landon, T.H., Burwick, J., Pham, T.Q., Frantz, G.D., Cairns, B., *et al.* (2003) Quantitative analysis of colorectal tissue microarrays by immunofluorescence and *in situ* hybridization. *J. Pathol.* **200**: 577–588.

Kaufmann, M., von Minckwitz, G., Smith, R., Valero, V., Gianni, L., Eiermann, W., *et al.* (2003) International expert panel on the use of primary (preoperative) systemic treatment of operable breast cancer: review and recommendations. *J. Clin. Oncol.* **21**: 2600–2608.

Kim, R., Demichelis, F., Tang, J., Riva, A., Shen, R., Gibbs, D.F., *et al.* (2005) Internet-based profiler system as integrative framework to support translational research. *BMC Bioinformatics* **6**: 304.

Lahad, J.P., Mills, G.B. and Coombes, K.R. (2005) Stem cell-ness: a 'magic marker' for cancer. *J. Clin. Invest.* **115**: 1463–1467.

Le Chevalier, T., Cvitkovic, E., Caille, P., Harvey, J., Contesso, G., Spielmann, M., *et al.* (1988) Early metastatic cancer of unknown primary origin at presentation. A clinical study of 302 consecutive autopsied patients. *Arch. Intern. Med.* **148**: 2035–2039.

Lee, Y.F., John, M., Falconer, A., Edwards, S., Clark, J., Flohr, P., *et al.* (2004) A gene expression signature associated with metastatic outcome in human leiomyosarcomas. *Cancer Res.* **64**: 7201–7204.

Lotze, M.T. and Rees, R.C. (2004) Identifying biomarkers and surrogates of tumors (cancer biometrics): correlation with immunotherapies and immune cells. *Cancer Immunol. Immunother.* **53**: 256–261.

Mirlacher, M., Kasper, M., Storz, M., Knecht, Y., Durmuller, U., Simon, R., *et al.* (2004) Influence of slide aging on results of translational research studies using immunohistochemistry. *Mod. Pathol.* **17**: 1414–1420.

Nakai, Y., Otsuka, M., Hoshida, Y., Tada, M., Komatsu, Y., Kawabe, T., *et al.* (2005) Identifying genes with differential expression in gemcitabine-resistant pancreatic cancer cells using comprehensive transcriptome analysis. *Oncol. Rep.* **14**: 1263–1267.

Nielsen, T.O., West, R.B., Linn, S.C., Alter, O., Knowling, M.A., O'Connell, J.X., *et al.* (2002) Molecular characterisation of soft tissue tumours: a gene expression study. *Lancet* **359**: 1301–1307.

Ohali, A., Avigad, S., Zaizov, R., Ophir, R., Horn-Saban, S., Cohen, I.J., *et al.* (2004) Prediction of high risk Ewing's sarcoma by gene expression profiling. *Oncogene* **23**: 8997–9006.

Paik, S., Shak, S., Tang, G., Kim, C., Baker, J., Cronin, M., *et al.* (2004) A multigene assay to predict recurrence of tamoxifen-treated, node-negative breast cancer. *N. Engl. J. Med.* **351**: 2817–2826.

Pusztai, L., Ayers, M., Stec, J., Clark, E., Hess, K., Stivers, D., *et al.* (2003) Gene expression profiles obtained from fine-needle aspirations of breast cancer reliably identify routine prognostic markers and reveal large-scale molecular differences between estrogen-negative and estrogen-positive tumors. *Clin. Cancer Res.* **9**: 2406–2415.

Ramaswamy, S., Tamayo, P., Rifkin, R., Mukherjee, S., Yeang, C.H., Angelo, M., *et al.* (2001) Multiclass cancer diagnosis using tumor gene expression signatures. *Proc. Natl. Acad. Sci. USA* **98**: 15149–15154.

Reynolds, T. (1998) Patients with unknown primaries face unusual insurance problems. *J. Natl. Cancer Inst.* **90**: 269.

Schaefer, K.L., Brachwitz, K., Wai, D.H., Braun, Y., Diallo, R., Korsching, E., *et al.* (2004) Expression profiling of t(12;22) positive clear cell sarcoma of soft tissue cell lines reveals characteristic up-regulation of potential new marker genes including ERBB3. *Cancer Res.* **64**: 3395–3405.

Schapira, D.V. and Jarrett, A.R. (1995) The need to consider survival, outcome, and expense when evaluating and treating patients with unknown primary carcinoma. *Arch. Intern. Med.* **155**: 2050–2054.

Segal, N.H., Pavlidis, P., Antonescu, C.R., Maki, R.G., Noble, W.S., DeSantis, D., *et al.* (2003) Classification and subtype prediction of adult soft tissue sarcoma by functional genomics. *Am. J. Pathol.* **163**: 691–700.

Shedden, K.A., Taylor, J.M., Giordano, T.J., Kuick, R., Misek, D.E., Rennert, G., *et al.* (2003) Accurate molecular classification of human cancers based on gene expression using a simple classifier with a pathological tree-based framework. *Am. J. Pathol.* **163**: 1985–1995.

Smith, I.C., Heys, S.D., Hutcheon, A.W., Miller, I.D., Payne, S., Gilbert, F.J., *et al.* (2002) Neoadjuvant chemotherapy in breast cancer: significantly enhanced response with docetaxel. *J. Clin. Oncol.* **20**: 1456–1466.

Sotiriou, C., Powles, T.J., Dowsett, M., Jazaeri, A.A., Feldman, A.L., Assersohn, L., *et al.* (2002) Gene expression profiles derived from fine needle aspiration correlate with response to systemic chemotherapy in breast cancer. *Breast Cancer Res.* **4**: R3.

Specht, K., Richter, T., Muller, U., Walch, A., Werner, M., and Hofler, H. (2001) Quantitative gene expression analysis in microdissected archival formalin-fixed and paraffin-embedded tumor tissue. *Am. J. Pathol.* **158**: 419–429.

Spruessel, A., Steimann, G., Jung, M., Lee, S.A., Carr, T., Fentz, A.K., *et al.* (2004) Tissue ischemia time affects gene and protein expression patterns within minutes following surgical tumor excision. *Biotechniques* **36**: 1030–1037.

Su, A.I., Welsh, J.B., Sapinoso, L.M., Kern, S.G., Dimitrov, P., Lapp, H., *et al.* (2001) Molecular classification of human carcinomas by use of gene expression signatures. *Cancer Res.* **61**: 7388–7393.

Symmans, W.F., Ayers, M., Clark, E.A., Stec, J., Hess, K.R., Sneige, N., *et al.* (2003) Total RNA yield and microarray gene expression profiles from fine-needle aspiration biopsy and core-needle biopsy samples of breast carcinoma. *Cancer* **97**: 2960–2971.

Tothill, R.W., Kowalczyk, A., Rischin, D., Bousioutas, A., Haviv, I., van Laar, R.K., *et al.* (2005) An expression-based site of origin diagnostic method designed for clinical application to cancer of unknown origin. *Cancer Res.* **65**: 4031–4040.

Wang, S., Saboorian, M.H., Frenkel, E.P., Haley, B.B., Siddiqui, M.T., Gokaslan, S., *et al.* (2001) Assessment of HER-2/neu status in breast cancer. Automated Cellular Imaging System (ACIS)-assisted quantitation of immunohistochemical assay achieves high accuracy in comparison with fluorescence *in situ* hybridization assay as the standard. *Am. J. Clin. Pathol.* **116**: 495–503.

Wang, S.S., Dasgupta, A., Sherman, M.E., Walker, J.L., Gold, M.A., Zuna, R., *et al.* (2005) Towards improved biomarker studies of cervical neoplasia: effects of precolposcopic procedures on gene expression patterns. *Diagn. Mol. Pathol.* **14**: 59–64.

West, R.B., Harvell, J., Linn, S.C., Liu, C.L., Prapong, W., Hernandez-Boussard, T., *et al.* (2004) Apo D in soft tissue tumors: a novel marker for dermatofibrosarcoma protuberans. *Am. J. Surg. Pathol.* **28**: 1063–1069.

H&E Will Hold Sway

The Invaluable Role of Morphology in the Molecular Era

Jason L. Hornick and Christopher D.M. Fletcher

INTRODUCTION – THE DEATH OF MORPHOLOGY?

Despite remarkable (and rapid) advances in understanding the molecular genetic basis of human malignancies over the past several decades, recently coupled with the accumulation of vast and often overwhelmingly complex expression profiling data, traditional surgical pathology employing conventional haematoxylin and eosin (H&E)-stained slides remains the cornerstone of tumour classification and prognostication. It is indeed surprising how little these molecular developments have altered current clinical practice. This overview explores the ways in which ancillary molecular methodologies have already affected diagnostic histopathology, and emphasises the central role that 'old-school' light microscopic evaluation will continue to play in tumour diagnosis and in guiding emerging applications of molecular findings for prognostication and targeted therapeutics. Although conventional histopathological examination will also continue to dominate the evaluation of most other (non-neoplastic) diseases, because cancer classification and prognostication have been the most hotly debated areas in which molecular genetics might replace morphology, tumour pathology will be the focus of this discussion.

For decades, new biomedical scientific discoveries have led to increasingly frequent proclamations that H&E would soon be obsolete. Such pronouncements often criticise the lack of objectivity of the technique and praise an imminent 'scientific' tumour classification that will replace 'old-fashioned' surgical pathology. However, existing (and evolving) diagnostic categories, created in large part by meticulous attention to cytological and architectural findings, as well as careful correlation with clinical features and patient outcome, are (to employ an overused adjective!) 'robust' to say the least – a sea change in the diagnosis of cancer has yet to occur, despite the great advances in molecular genetics. Nonetheless, new techniques have refined the practice of surgical pathology and have added useful prognostic and therapeutic information in selected cases.

ROLE OF IMMUNOHISTOCHEMISTRY

Immunophenotypic evaluation is now the most widespread and routine ancillary approach to tumour classification (see Chapter 15 of this volume), which arguably plays its most prominent role in haematopathology. For example, in most centres, flow cytometric phenotyping is an integral part of the assessment of virtually all haematolymphoid malignancies. Similarly, in soft-tissue pathology, immunohistochemical findings also provide key support for the diagnosis of some of these rare tumour types. In perhaps its most widely used application outside of haematopathology and soft-tissue pathology, immunohistochemistry can help to suggest possible primary sites in many cases of metastatic carcinoma in which the primary site is clinically occult. In the uncommon cases of undifferentiated malignancies that show no specific morphological features to aid in classification, immunohistochemical evidence for a specific line of differentiation (e.g. carcinoma versus lymphoma) can be helpful to guide subsequent therapy. Immunohistochemistry has largely supplanted electron microscopy in this regard. In the case of pleomorphic ('MFH'-like) sarcomas, immunohistochemistry can help to support subclassification as leiomyosarcoma or rhabdomyosarcoma, which show significantly higher rates of metastasis than other pleomorphic sarcomas (Gaffney *et al.*, 1993; Fletcher *et al.*, 2001), such as dedifferentiated liposarcoma (McCormick *et al.*, 1994; Henricks *et al.*, 1997) or myxofibrosarcoma (Merck *et al.*, 1983; Mentzel *et al.*, 1996). Even in cases where subclassification is not possible, recent studies have suggested that myogenic differentiation *per se* (defined by immunohistochemistry) is a significant indicator of more aggressive behaviour in pleomorphic sarcomas (Fletcher *et al.*, 2001; Deyrup *et al.*, 2003; Massi *et al.*, 2004). This type of subclassification may in the future guide the development of specific or more intensive therapies exploiting these differences in clinical behaviour.

ROLE OF GENETICS

The earliest contribution that genetics made to tumour classification was the identification, nearly 50 years ago, of the Philadelphia chromosome (Nowell and Hungerford, 1960), resulting from the chromosomal translocation t(9;22) (Rowley, 1973), the defining feature of chronic myelogenous leukaemia (CML). Several decades later, this translocation was shown to result in the juxtaposition of *BCR* and *ABL* (Bartram *et al.*, 1983; Groffen *et al.*, 1984), the fusion transcript of which encodes a receptor tyrosine kinase, constitutive activation of which is believed to be the central pathogenetic event in CML (Shtivelman *et al.*, 1985). In the past decade, the first targeted therapy directed against a receptor tyrosine kinase, imatinib mesylate (Gleevec or Glivec), developed to inhibit the BCR–ABL fusion protein, has shown considerable clinical efficacy in CML (Druker *et al.*, 2001). This type of rational targeted molecular therapy has become a new model for the development of pharmacological reagents in oncology (see below).

Reciprocal chromosomal translocations and other karyotypic abnormalities are a recurring theme in haematological malignancies, including other myeloid disorders and lymphomas, the identification of which has, in most cases, confirmed existing diagnostic categories and occasionally has defined entities that were difficult to tease out. For example, mantle cell lymphoma is now recognised as a specific clinicopathological entity chiefly following identification of the t(11;14) chromosomal translocation, which results in fusion of the immunoglobulin heavy chain gene promoter to *BCL-1*, which drives overexpression of cyclin D1 (Williams *et al.*, 1990; Rosenberg *et al.*, 1991; Vandenberghe *et al.*, 1991). Since this discovery, an immunohistochemical assay for cyclin D1 has been developed and is now widely available (de Boer *et al.*, 1995; Swerdlow *et al.*, 1995; Zukerberg *et al.*, 1995), which can allow confirmation of the diagnosis of mantle cell lymphoma in the absence of cytogenetic (or other molecular) analysis. This paradigm, namely the development of simple immunohistochemical tests to demonstrate overexpression of proteins of pathogenetic importance, is widely applicable not only in the subclassification of tumours (numerous examples of which are already used clinically), but also will likely aid in prognostication and the identification of targets for specific cancer therapies (see below).

Cytogenetics is now an invaluable adjunct to the morphological classification and prognostic assessment of myeloid stem cell disorders. Specifically, defined chromosomal abnormalities predict outcome in myelodysplastic syndromes (Greenberg *et al.*, 1997), and cytogenetic findings are strong predictors of behaviour in acute myeloid leukaemias (AML) (Bloomfield *et al.*, 1998; Grimwade *et al.*, 1998; Slovak *et al.*, 2000). In fact, the presence of such recurrent chromosomal abnormalities has largely replaced the traditional morphological/histochemical FAB classification as being the more clinically meaningful distinguishing features among these leukaemias and this is reflected in the current World Health Organisation classification. Nonetheless, in the majority of cases, the traditional classification of AML subtypes correlates remarkably well with cytogenetics, underscoring the power of careful morphological assessment and validating pre-existing classification schemes.

There are also examples of chromosomal translocations that distinguish different prognostic groups among non-Hodgkin lymphomas that are not discernible by routine histological examination. For example, patients with anaplastic large-cell lymphoma showing translocations that result in rearrangement of the *ALK* gene (most frequently t(2;5)) have significantly better survival than those whose tumours lack such translocations. Moreover, immunohistochemical detection of the ALK protein serves as a clinically valuable surrogate for such translocations and has prognostic value (Shiota *et al.*, 1995; Falini *et al.*, 1999; Gascoyne *et al.*, 1999). As another example, in the case of gastric extranodal marginal zone B-cell lymphoma (MALT lymphoma), in which most patients experience sustained remission following eradication of *Helicobacter pylori* infection, the presence of the t(11;18) translocation correlates with resistance to *Helicobacter* eradication and a worse outcome (Alpen *et al.*, 2000; Liu *et al.*, 2001; Levy *et al.*, 2005).

Simple recurrent chromosomal translocations are also characteristic of some types of soft-tissue sarcomas, the presence of which, in the majority of cases, has served to validate existing morphological classification schemes rather than defining new entities. For example, the t(X;18) translocation resulting in the fusion of the *SYT* and *SSX1* or *SSX2* genes is found in essentially all cases of synovial sarcoma (Clark *et al.*, 1994; de Leeuw *et al.*, 1995), and translocations of *EWS* (most often t(11;22) involving *EWS* and *FLI1*) characterize the Ewing sarcoma/peripheral neuroectodermal tumour (PNET) family of tumours (Delattre *et al.*, 1992; Zucman *et al.*, 1992). These tumour types have sufficiently distinctive morphological and clinical features that the diagnosis can usually be based simply upon conventional H&E examination, supported by immunohistochemistry, and cytogenetic or molecular genetic analysis is generally reserved for cases with atypical histological or clinical features. However, recent clinical studies have suggested that the specific fusion types (or breakpoint sites) may alter the prognosis for patients with these sarcomas, but the results are contradictory. For instance, in synovial sarcoma, several studies have shown that tumours harbouring the *SYT–SSX1* gene fusion behave in a more aggressive fashion than those with the *SYT–SSX2* gene fusion (Kawai *et al.*, 1998; Nilsson *et al.*, 1999; Inagaki *et al.*, 2000; Panagopoulos *et al.*, 2001; Ladanyi *et al.*; 2002), but a recent large study found no survival difference between fusion types (Guillou *et al.*, 2004). Similar survival benefits for specific fusion sites have been suggested in Ewing sarcoma/PNET (Zoubek *et al.*, 1996; de Alava *et al.*, 1998; Ginsberg *et al.*, 1999) and alveolar rhabdomyosarcoma (Kelly *et al.*, 1997; Sorensen *et al.*, 2002), but the results of these studies are preliminary and also somewhat contradictory. Nonetheless, these types of molecular analyses may ultimately prove useful in adding prognostic information beyond that which is available from current histological and clinical parameters. It should be emphasised, however, that the apparent prognostic information gained from these expensive molecular tests (which can only be undertaken in specialised, usually academic, centres) is at best modest, and widespread application may not be a reasonable expectation nor cost-effective (Hahn and Fletcher, 2005).

In carcinomas, which constitute the overwhelming majority of human cancers, molecular genetics has had surprisingly little impact on tumour classification and prognostication. The conventional H&E-based assessment of tumour grade and the determination of tumour stage remain the most important predictors of outcome for carcinomas arising at most anatomic sites. One notable, but pretty much isolated, exception, which exemplifies an emerging role for molecular genetics, is in colorectal carcinomas (CRC). In these tumours, deficiencies in components of the mismatch repair (MMR) machinery correlate with improved survival (Sankila *et al.*, 1996; Gryfe *et al.*, 2000; Guidoboni *et al.*, 2001; Popat *et al.*, 2005), and, at the same time, decreased susceptibility to conventional 5-fluorouracil-based chemotherapy (Ribic *et al.*, 2003; Carethers *et al.*, 2004). As a consequence of MMR deficiency, these CRCs show high levels of microsatellite instability (MSI). Approximately 15% of all CRCs show MSI, most of which arise sporadically secondary to promoter methylation and transcriptional silencing of the *MLH1* gene (Herman *et al.*, 1998). In a relatively small proportion of tumours, MSI is caused by inherited mutations (most often in the *MSH2* or *MLH1* genes) (Peltomaki and Vasen, 1997), in patients with the hereditary non-polyposis colorectal carcinoma (HNPCC) syndrome. These patients also have an increased risk of developing carcinomas at other anatomic sites, most often the endometrium, renal pelvis, ureter and small bowel. Interestingly, there are some histological correlates to MMR deficiency. Specifically, right-sided mucinous CRCs and those showing poor differentiation and numerous tumour-infiltrating lymphocytes are more likely to show MSI (Jass *et al.*, 1998; Shashidharan *et al.*, 1999). However, although such features may suggest MSI, this correlation is not very strong. As described above in other tumour types, recent studies have shown that immunohistochemistry is a good surrogate for assessment of MSI (Marcus *et al.*, 1999; Chaves *et al.*, 2000; Lindor *et al.*, 2002; Shia *et al.*, 2005): loss of expression of either the MLH1 or MSH2 protein can serve as a good initial screening test, followed by polymerase chain reaction (PCR)-based assessment of microsatellite repeats to confirm MSI. Although MSI determination is not yet standard practice and is generally reserved for patients in whom there is a suspicion for HNPCC, it seems likely that this type of analysis, whether by immunohistochemistry or formal microsatellite testing, will in time be applied widely, given its significant prognostic and therapeutic implications.

GENE EXPRESSION PROFILING: CLINICAL APPLICATIONS?

Recently, there has been a remarkably rapid emergence of vast amounts of gene expression data for countless human tumours, mainly in attempts to identify genes or groups of genes, the expression of which correlates with either diagnosis or clinical outcome. Virtually all attempts at 'diagnostic' classification by this rather expensive route have done no more than validate long-standing (and much cheaper!) light microscopic classifications. Nevertheless, perhaps the best example thus far of the potential for this approach is in the case of the most common type of lymphoma, diffuse large B-cell lymphoma (DLBCL), which is clinically heterogeneous, with nearly half of the affected patients entering remission following combination chemotherapy, while the remainder die of progressive disease. Morphology alone cannot predict these differences in outcome. In 2000, a gene expression profiling study using DNA microarrays suggested two distinct subgroups of DLBCL, which have different expression patterns, that appeared to correlate remarkably well with outcome: a 'germinal centre B cell-like' group and an 'activated B cell-like' group (Alizadeh *et al.*, 2000). Patients in this study whose tumours showed the former expression profile had a significantly better overall survival than the latter. Because such a complex (and expensive) analysis is not currently feasible in routine clinical practice (and is unlikely to be so in the foreseeable future), expression array studies have in some cases stimulated follow-up studies utilising immunohistochemical analysis of the most promising markers that had been identified. Along these lines, several studies of DLBCL have attempted to recapitulate these data with a small group of tissue-based markers (Chang *et al.*, 2004; Hans *et al.*, 2004; Berglund *et al.*, 2005; Biasoli *et al.*, 2005). For example, detection of the 'germinal centre' markers CD10 and bcl-6 by immunohistochemistry appears to predict good outcome, whereas the 'activation' marker MUM1/IRF4 appears to correlate with poor outcome in patients with DLBCL (Chang *et al.*, 2004; Hans *et al.*, 2004). Although these studies are preliminary, they provide a model for the translation of gene expression profiling data to a much more widely applicable technology such as immunohistochemistry. It is critical that such immunohistochemical analyses of potential prognostic markers be performed rigorously in clinical trials to prove significance prior to introduction into the routine clinical arena.

In this regard, it is important to remember that the results of expression profiling studies are only as good as the initial diagnostic assignment of the tumour categories or subtypes being examined – invaluable annotation that can be provided only by a trained anatomic pathologist. For this reason, it is essential that a morphologist be directly involved in such studies to verify and specify diagnoses prior to analysis, not to mention confirm that the sample analysed is in fact lesional (and not adjacent non-neoplastic or necrotic tissue). Unfortunately, some high-profile expression microarray studies have not been appropriately meticulous; in fact, pathologists are frequently absent from such studies when they should be playing a central and critical role and such large-scale (and expensive) experiments run the significant risk of yielding data that are of dubious (if any) significance. At the same time, with few notable exceptions (such as those described above), there has generally been insufficient effort to validate the results of these molecular studies by tissue-based clinical trials using selected potentially prognostic markers, including critical multivariate analyses for comparison with conventional histological (and clinical) predictors of outcome. Again, this major gap in bridging bench-top research and clinical medicine stems in part from the lack of involvement in many such studies by histopathologists, who are uniquely qualified to assist in the development and evaluation of such tissue-based markers for appropriate translation to patient care.

TARGETED THERAPEUTICS

Another promising application of molecular genetics to cancer is the development of targeted therapeutics. One of the first examples of such a targeted therapy is trastuzumab (herceptin), a monoclonal antibody directed against the HER-2/neu oncoprotein in breast cancer. Approximately 30% of breast cancers show amplification (and consequent overexpression) of HER-2/neu, which not only serves as a therapeutic target but also correlates with poor prognosis (Slamon *et al.*, 1987, 1989). In most centres (and in most, but not all, cases), HER-2/neu testing is assessed by immunohistochemistry and light microscopy. Initial studies of patients with metastatic breast cancer overexpressing HER-2/neu showed a modest survival benefit with trastuzumab therapy (Baselga *et al.*, 1996; Cobleigh *et al.*, 1999), strengthened by the addition of chemotherapy (Slamon *et al.*, 2001), and very recent studies demonstrated a dramatic survival benefit for patients with early stage HER-2/neu-overexpressing breast cancers who were treated with adjuvant trastuzumab combined with chemotherapy following surgery (Piccart-Gebhart *et al.*, 2005; Romond *et al.*, 2005). In a second recent example of a targeted molecular therapy, a small subgroup of patients with non-small-cell lung cancer (NSCLC) respond dramatically to the epidermal growth factor receptor (EGFR) inhibitor gefitinib (Fukuoka *et al.*, 2003; Kris *et al.*, 2003). Very recently, activating mutations in *EGFR* were shown to predict gefitinib response (Lynch *et al.*, 2004; Paez *et al.*, 2004). Patients who respond to such therapy are also more likely to have adenocarcinomas (particularly those with a bronchioloalveolar component) (Miller *et al.*, 2004; Kim *et al.*, 2005; Yatabe *et al.*; 2005). Similarly, and as mentioned previously, the small-molecule tyrosine kinase inhibitor imatinib mesylate, directed against BCR–ABL, has clinical efficacy in CML (Druker *et al.*, 2001). This same drug is also effective in the treatment of metastatic gastrointestinal stromal tumours (GISTs) (Demetri *et al.*, 2002), due to its activity against the tyrosine kinase receptor *c*-kit (Heinrich *et al.*, 2000; Tuveson *et al.*, 2001), which is mutated in approximately 85% of GISTs (Hirota *et al.*, 1998), leading to constitutive kinase activity. Most of the remaining GISTs harbour analogous activating mutations in the tyrosine kinase platelet-derived growth factor receptor-alpha gene (*PDGFRA*) (Heinrich *et al.*, 2003b). Immunohistochemical detection of *c*-kit is invaluable to confirm the diagnosis of GIST, although a small subset of GISTs are *c*-kit-negative (Debiec-Rychter *et al.*, 2004; Medeiros *et al.*, 2004); most of these latter tumours have activating mutations in *PDGFRA*. Nonetheless, tyrosine kinase inhibitors such as imatinib may also be efficacious in some of these tumours by inhibiting PDGFRA. Interestingly, recent studies have indicated that the specific site of the *c-kit* or *PDGFRA* gene mutation in GISTs predicts the clinical response to imatinib (Heinrich *et al.*, 2003a; Corless *et al.*, 2005). The role of DNA sequence analysis for prognostication remains uncertain, however, because at present such an approach is time-consuming, expensive and not widely available. The imminent possibility of different targeted therapies, most effective against specific types of mutation, may well influence this situation.

LESS AND LESS TISSUE

Increasingly, radiology-guided core-needle biopsies and aspirations are replacing surgical (incisional) biopsies as alternative approaches to tumour sampling for diagnosis. Although such procedures may allow for decreased hospital stays and (arguably) less morbidity, the yield of diagnostic material is lower and, even if lesional tissue is obtained, the scant nature of the specimen may not allow for a specific (morphological) diagnosis. In this context, in at least some cases molecular genetics may provide useful and, at times, essential contributions to tumour classification. Appropriate examination of immunophenotype (e.g. using flow cytometry of a lymphoid neoplasm), detection of a fusion product of a chromosomal translocation (as described above, using fluorescence *in situ* hybridisation (FISH) or reverse-transcription PCR) and/or evaluation for an immunoglobulin or T-cell receptor gene rearrangement (to support clonality in the case of a low-grade lymphoproliferative disorder) may then lead to a specific diagnosis. However, even in this context, skilled morphological assessment is absolutely critical for guiding selection of the appropriate molecular investigation that should be undertaken.

CONCLUSION

In summary, light microscopic examination of tissue specimens by surgical pathologists will continue to remain central to tumour classification, at least for the foreseeable future. Without question, morphology remains the gold standard against which all newer technologies have to be validated and assessed. Expression profiling of tumours, instead of replacing conventional H&E-based morphological assessment, will likely aid in the identification of prognostic markers and targets for therapeutic intervention. Such an approach will likely require the development of immunohistochemical reagents for rapid and inexpensive assessment of protein overexpression in order for these discoveries to translate into routine clinical practice. In the future, it seems likely that a panel of markers will be evaluated in many human cancers as adjuncts to the standard prognostic parameters established by routine morphological assessment. The panel of markers investigated will, of course, be determined by the specific tumour type, as established by the surgical pathologist. Therapeutic targets can then be evaluated in a similar fashion. As we move into this new era of rational targeted molecular therapies, meticulous attention to precise tumour classification remains critical for the development of such therapies, and surgical pathology will undoubtedly continue to occupy a central role.

We should also remember that any new technologies must be both affordable and as widely available as possible to ensure maximum benefit for society, otherwise there will continue to be increasingly wide disparities in the distribution and quality of healthcare between the extremely wealthy and the remainder of society. Even now, 25 years after its introduction, immunohistochemistry is not used in many parts of the world because of its expense and a related lack of both technical training and interpretative expertise. If many of the world's healthcare systems cannot afford such established technology, it is difficult to justify the widespread dissemination of newer, much more expensive and technically challenging molecular diagnostic approaches to tumour classification and prognostication until broader and more basic needs are met.

REFERENCES

Alizadeh, A. A., Eisen, M. B., Davis, R. E., *et al.* (2000) Distinct types of diffuse large B-cell lymphoma identified by gene expression profiling. *Nature* **403**: 503–511.

Alpen, B., Neubauer, A., Dierlamm, J., *et al.* (2000) Translocation t(11;18) absent in early gastric marginal zone B-cell lymphoma of MALT type responding to eradication of Helicobacter pylori infection. *Blood* **95**: 4014–4015.

Bartram, C. R., de Klein, A., Hagemeijer, A., *et al.* (1983) Translocation of c-abl oncogene correlates with the presence of a Philadelphia chromosome in chronic myelocytic leukaemia. *Nature* **306**: 277–280.

Baselga, J., Tripathy, D., Mendelsohn, J., *et al.* (1996) Phase II study of weekly intravenous recombinant humanized anti-p185HER2 monoclonal antibody in patients with HER2/neu-overexpressing metastatic breast cancer. *J. Clin. Oncol.* **14**: 737–744.

Berglund, M., Thunberg, U., Amini, R. M., *et al.* (2005) Evaluation of immunophenotype in diffuse large B-cell lymphoma and its impact on prognosis. *Mod. Pathol.* **18**: 1113–1120.

Biasoli, I., Morais, J. C., Scheliga, A., *et al.* (2005) CD10 and Bcl-2 expression combined with the International Prognostic Index can identify subgroups of patients with diffuse large-cell lymphoma with very good or very poor prognoses. *Histopathology* **46**: 328–333.

Bloomfield, C. D., Lawrence, D., Byrd, J.C., *et al.* (1998) Frequency of prolonged remission duration after high-dose cytarabine intensification in acute myeloid leukemia varies by cytogenetic subtype. *Cancer Res.* **58**: 4173–4179.

Carethers, J. M., Smith, E. J., Behling, C. A., *et al.* (2004) Use of 5-fluorouracil and survival in patients with microsatellite-unstable colorectal cancer. *Gastroenterology* **126**: 394–401.

Chang, C. C., McClintock, S., Cleveland, R. P., *et al.* (2004) Immunohistochemical expression patterns of germinal center and activation B-cell markers correlate with prognosis in diffuse large B-cell lymphoma. *Am. J. Surg. Pathol.* **28**: 464–470.

Chaves, P., Cruz, C., Lage, P., *et al.* (2000) Immunohistochemical detection of mismatch repair gene proteins as a useful tool for the identification of colorectal carcinoma with the mutator phenotype. *J. Pathol.* **191**: 355–360.

Clark, J., Rocques, P. J., Crew, A. J., *et al.* (1994) Identification of novel genes, SYT and SSX, involved in the t(X;18)(p11.2;q11.2) translocation found in human synovial sarcoma. *Nat. Genet.* **7**: 502–508.

Cobleigh, M. A., Vogel, C. L., Tripathy, D., *et al.* (1999) Multinational study of the efficacy and safety of humanized anti-HER2 monoclonal antibody in women who have HER2-overexpressing metastatic breast cancer that has progressed after chemotherapy for metastatic disease. *J. Clin. Oncol.* **17**: 2639–2648.

Corless, C. L., Schroeder, A., Griffith, D., *et al.* (2005) PDGFRA mutations in gastrointestinal stromal tumours: frequency, spectrum and in vitro sensitivity to imatinib. *J. Clin. Oncol.* **23**: 5357–5364.

de Alava, E., Kawai, A., Healey, J. H., *et al.* (1998) EWS-FLI1 fusion transcript structure is an independent determinant of prognosis in Ewing's sarcoma. *J. Clin. Oncol.* **16**: 1248–1255.

de Boer, C. J., Schuuring, E., Dreef, E., *et al.* (1995) Cyclin D1 protein analysis in the diagnosis of mantle cell lymphoma. *Blood* **86**: 2715–2723.

de Leeuw, B., Balemans, M., Olde Weghuis, D., *et al.* (1995) Identification of two alternative fusion genes, SYT-SSX1 and SYT-SSX2, in t(X;18)(p11.2;q11.2)-positive synovial sarcomas. *Hum. Mol. Genet.* **4**: 1097–1099.

Debiec-Rychter, M., Wasag, B., Stul, M., *et al.* (2004) Gastrointestinal stromal tumours (GISTs) negative for KIT (CD117 antigen) immunoreactivity. *J. Pathol.* **202**: 430–438.

Delattre, O., Zucman, J., Plougastel, B., *et al.* (1992) Gene fusion with an ETS DNA-binding domain caused by chromosome translocation in human tumours. *Nature* **359**: 162–165.

Demetri, G. D., von Mehren, M., Blanke, C. D., *et al.* (2002) Efficacy and safety of imatinib mesylate in advanced gastrointestinal stromal tumours. *N. Engl. J. Med.* **347**: 472–480.

Deyrup, A. T., Haydon, R. C., Huo, D., *et al.* (2003) Myoid differentiation and prognosis in adult pleomorphic sarcomas of the extremity: an analysis of 92 cases. *Cancer* **98**: 805–813.

Druker, B. J., Talpaz, M., Resta, D. J., *et al.* (2001) Efficacy and safety of a specific inhibitor of the BCR-ABL tyrosine kinase in chronic myeloid leukemia. *N. Engl. J. Med.* **344**: 1031–1037.

Falini, B., Pileri, S., Zinzani, P. L., *et al.* (1999) ALK+ lymphoma: clinico-pathological findings and outcome. *Blood* **93**: 2697–2706.

Fletcher, C. D., Gustafson, P., Rydholm, A., *et al.* (2001) Clinicopathologic re-evaluation of 100 malignant fibrous histiocytomas: prognostic relevance of subclassification. *J. Clin. Oncol.* **19**: 3045–3050.

Fukuoka, M., Yano, S., Giaccone, G., *et al.* (2003) Multi-institutional randomized phase II trial of gefitinib for previously treated patients with advanced non-small-cell lung cancer (The IDEAL 1 Trial). *J. Clin. Oncol.* **21**: 2237–2246.

Gaffney, E. F., Dervan, P. A. and Fletcher, C. D. (1993) Pleomorphic rhabdomyosarcoma in adulthood. Analysis of 11 cases with definition of diagnostic criteria. *Am. J. Surg. Pathol.* **17**: 601–609.

Gascoyne, R. D., Aoun, P., Wu, D., *et al.* (1999) Prognostic significance of anaplastic lymphoma kinase (ALK) protein expression in adults with anaplastic large cell lymphoma. *Blood* **93**: 3913–3921.

Ginsberg, J. P., de Alava, E., Ladanyi, M., *et al.* (1999) EWS-FLI1 and EWS-ERG gene fusions are associated with similar clinical phenotypes in Ewing's sarcoma. *J. Clin. Oncol.* **17**: 1809–1814.

Greenberg, P., Cox, C., LeBeau, M. M., *et al.* (1997) International scoring system for evaluating prognosis in myelodysplastic syndromes. *Blood* **89**: 2079–2088.

Grimwade, D., Walker, H., Oliver, F., *et al.* (1998) The importance of diagnostic cytogenetics on outcome in AML: analysis of 1,612 patients entered into the MRC AML 10 trial. The Medical Research Council Adult and Children's Leukaemia Working Parties. *Blood* **92**: 2322–2333.

Groffen, J., Stephenson, J. R., Heisterkamp, N., *et al.* (1984) Philadelphia chromosomal breakpoints are clustered within a limited region, bcr, on chromosome 22. *Cell* **36**: 93–99.

Gryfe, R., Kim, H., Hsieh, E. T., *et al.* (2000) Tumor microsatellite instability and clinical outcome in young patients with colorectal cancer. *N. Engl. J. Med.* **342**: 69–77.

Guidoboni, M., Gafa, R., Viel, A., *et al.* (2001) Microsatellite instability and high content of activated cytotoxic lymphocytes identify colon cancer patients with a favorable prognosis. *Am. J. Pathol.* **159**: 297–304.

Guillou, L., Benhattar, J., Bonichon, F., *et al.* (2004) Histologic grade, but not SYT-SSX fusion type, is an important prognostic factor in patients with synovial sarcoma: a multicenter, retrospective analysis. *J. Clin. Oncol.* **22**: 4040–4050.

Hahn, H. P. and Fletcher, C. D. M. (2005) The role of cytogenetics and molecular genetics in soft tissue tumour diagnosis – a realistic appraisal. *Curr. Diagn. Pathol.* **11**: 361–370.

Hans, C. P., Weisenburger, D. D., Greiner, T. C., *et al.* (2004) Confirmation of the molecular classification of diffuse large B-cell lymphoma by immunohistochemistry using a tissue microarray. *Blood* **103**: 275–282.

Heinrich, M. C., Corless, C. L., Demetri, G. D., *et al.* (2003a) Kinase mutations and imatinib response in patients with metastatic gastrointestinal stromal tumour. *J. Clin. Oncol.* **21**: 4342–4349.

Heinrich, M. C., Corless, C. L., Duensing, A., *et al.* (2003b) PDGFRA activating mutations in gastrointestinal stromal tumours. *Science* **299**: 708–710.

Heinrich, M. C., Griffith, D. J., Druker, B. J., *et al.* (2000) Inhibition of c-kit receptor tyrosine kinase activity by STI 571, a selective tyrosine kinase inhibitor. *Blood* **96**: 925–932.

Henricks, W. H., Chu, Y. C., Goldblum, J. R, *et al.* (1997) Dedifferentiated liposarcoma: a clinicopathological analysis of 155 cases with a proposal for an expanded definition of dedifferentiation. *Am. J. Surg. Pathol.* **21**: 271–281.

Herman, J. G., Umar, A., Polyak, K., *et al.* (1998) Incidence and functional consequences of hMLH1 promoter hypermethylation in colorectal carcinoma. *Proc. Natl. Acad. Sci. USA* **95**: 6870–6875.

Hirota, S., Isozaki, K., Moriyama, Y., *et al.* (1998) Gain-of-function mutations of c-kit in human gastrointestinal stromal tumours. *Science* **279**: 577–580.

Inagaki, H., Nagasaka, T., Otsuka, T., *et al.* (2000) Association of SYT-SSX fusion types with proliferative activity and prognosis in synovial sarcoma. *Mod. Pathol.* **13**: 482–488.

Jass, J. R., Do, K. A., Simms, L. A., *et al.* (1998) Morphology of sporadic colorectal cancer with DNA replication errors. *Gut* **42**: 673–679.

Kawai, A., Woodruff, J., Healey, J. H., *et al.* (1998) SYT-SSX gene fusion as a determinant of morphology and prognosis in synovial sarcoma. *N. Engl. J. Med.* **338**: 153–160.

Kelly, K. M., Womer, R. B., Sorensen, P. H., *et al.* (1997) Common and variant gene fusions predict distinct clinical phenotypes in rhabdomyosarcoma. *J. Clin. Oncol.* **15**: 1831–1836.

Kim, K. S., Jeong, J. Y., Kim, Y. C., *et al.* (2005) Predictors of the response to gefitinib in refractory non-small cell lung cancer. *Clin. Cancer Res.* **11**: 2244–2251.

Kris, M. G., Natale, R. B., Herbst, R. S., *et al.* (2003) Efficacy of gefitinib, an inhibitor of the epidermal growth factor receptor tyrosine kinase, in symptomatic patients with non-small cell lung cancer: a randomized trial. *JAMA* **290**: 2149–2158.

Ladanyi, M., Antonescu, C. R., Leung, D. H., *et al.* (2002) Impact of SYT-SSX fusion type on the clinical behavior of synovial sarcoma: a multi-institutional retrospective study of 243 patients. *Cancer Res.* **62**: 135–140.

Levy, M., Copie-Bergman, C., Gameiro, C., *et al.* (2005) Prognostic value of translocation t(11;18) in tumoural response of low-grade gastric lymphoma of mucosa-associated lymphoid tissue type to oral chemotherapy. *J. Clin. Oncol.* **23**: 5061–5066.

Lindor, N. M., Burgart, L. J., Leontovich, O., *et al.* (2002) Immunohistochemistry versus microsatellite instability testing in phenotyping colorectal tumours. *J. Clin. Oncol.* **20**: 1043–1048.

Liu, H., Ruskon-Fourmestraux, A., Lavergne-Slove, A., *et al.* (2001) Resistance of t(11;18) positive gastric mucosa-associated lymphoid tissue lymphoma to Helicobacter pylori eradication therapy. *Lancet* **357**: 39–40.

Lynch, T. J., Bell, D. W., Sordella, R., *et al.* (2004) Activating mutations in the epidermal growth factor receptor underlying responsiveness of non-small-cell lung cancer to gefitinib. *N. Engl. J. Med.* **350**: 2129–2139.

Marcus, V. A., Madlensky, L., Gryfe, R., *et al.* (1999) Immunohistochemistry for hMLH1 and hMSH2: a practical test for DNA mismatch repair-deficient tumours. *Am. J. Surg. Pathol.* **23**: 1248–1255.

Massi, D., Beltrami, G., Capanna, R., *et al.* (2004) Histopathological re-classification of extremity plemorphic soft tissue sarcoma has clinical relevance. *Eur. J. Surg. Oncol.* **30**: 1131–1136.

McCormick, D., Mentzel, T., Beham, A., *et al.* (1994) Dedifferentiated liposarcoma. Clinicopathologic analysis of 32 cases suggesting a better prognostic subgroup among pleomorphic sarcomas. *Am. J. Surg. Pathol.* **18**: 1213–1223.

Medeiros, F., Corless, C. L., Duensing, A., *et al.* (2004) KIT-negative gastrointestinal stromal tumours: proof of concept and therapeutic implications. *Am. J. Surg. Pathol.* **28**: 889–894.

Mentzel, T., Calonje, E., Wadden, C., *et al.* (1996) Myxofibrosarcoma. Clinicopathologic analysis of 75 cases with emphasis on the low-grade variant. *Am. J. Surg. Pathol.* **20**: 391–405.

Merck, C., Angervall, L., Kindblom, L. G., *et al.* (1983) Myxofibrosarcoma. A malignant soft tissue tumour of fibroblastic-histiocytic origin. A clinicopathologic and prognostic study of 110 cases using multivariate analysis. *Acta Pathol. Microbiol. Immunol. Scand. Suppl.* **282**: 1–40.

Miller, V. A., Kris, M. G., Shah, N., *et al.* (2004) Bronchioloalveolar pathologic subtype and smoking history predict sensitivity to gefitinib in advanced non-small-cell lung cancer. *J. Clin. Oncol.* **22**: 1103–1109.

Nilsson, G., Skytting, B., Xie, Y., *et al.* (1999) The SYT-SSX1 variant of synovial sarcoma is associated with a high rate of tumour cell proliferation and poor clinical outcome. *Cancer Res.* **59**: 3180–3184.

Nowell, P. C. and Hungerford, D. A. (1960) A minute chromosome in human chronic granulocytic leukemia. *Science* **132**: 1497–1500.

Paez, J. G., Janne, P. A., Lee, J. C., *et al.* (2004) EGFR mutations in lung cancer: correlation with clinical response to gefitinib therapy. *Science* **304**: 1497–1500.

Panagopoulos, I., Mertens, F., Isaksson, M., *et al.* (2001) Clinical impact of molecular and cytogenetic findings in synovial sarcoma. *Genes Chromosomes Cancer* **31**: 362–372.

Peltomaki, P. and Vasen, H. F. (1997) Mutations predisposing to hereditary nonpolyposis colorectal cancer: database and results of a collaborative study. The International Collaborative Group on Hereditary Nonpolyposis Colorectal Cancer. *Gastroenterology* **113**: 1146–1158.

Piccart-Gebhart, M. J., Procter, M., Leyland-Jones, B., *et al.* (2005) Trastuzumab after adjuvant chemotherapy in HER2-positive breast cancer. *N. Engl. J. Med.* **353**: 1659–1672.

Popat, S., Hubner, R. and Houlston, R. S. (2005) Systematic review of microsatellite instability and colorectal cancer prognosis. *J. Clin. Oncol.* **23**: 609–618.

Ribic, C. M., Sargent, D. J., Moore, M. J., *et al.* (2003) Tumor microsatellite-instability status as a predictor of benefit from fluorouracil-based adjuvant chemotherapy for colon cancer. *N. Engl. J. Med.* **349**: 247–257.

Romond, E. H., Perez, E. A., Bryant, J., *et al.* (2005) Trastuzumab plus adjuvant chemotherapy for operable HER2-positive breast cancer. *N. Engl. J. Med.* **353**: 1673–1684.

Rosenberg, C. L., Wong, E., Petty, E. M., *et al.* (1991) PRAD1, a candidate BCL1 oncogene: mapping and expression in centrocytic lymphoma. *Proc. Natl. Acad. Sci. USA* **88**: 9638–9642.

Rowley, J. D. (1973) A new consistent chromosomal abnormality in chronic myelogenous leukaemia identified by quinacrine fluorescence and Giemsa staining. *Nature* **243**: 290–293.

Sankila, R., Aaltonen, L. A., Jarvinen, H. J., *et al.* (1996) Better survival rates in patients with MLH1-associated hereditary colorectal cancer. *Gastroenterology* **110**: 682–687.

Shashidharan, M., Smyrk, T., Lin, K. M., *et al.* (1999) Histologic comparison of hereditary nonpolyposis colorectal cancer associated with MSH2 and MLH1 and colorectal cancer from the general population. *Dis. Colon Rectum* **42**: 722–726.

Shia, J., Klimstra, D. S., Nafa, K., *et al.* (2005) Value of immunohistochemical detection of DNA mismatch repair proteins in predicting germline mutation in hereditary colorectal neoplasms. *Am. J. Surg. Pathol.* **29**: 96–104.

Shiota, M., Nakamura, S., Ichinohasama, R., *et al.* (1995) Anaplastic large cell lymphomas expressing the novel chimeric protein p80NPM/ALK: a distinct clinicopathologic entity. *Blood* **86**: 1954–1960.

Shtivelman, E., Lifshitz, B., Gale, R. P., *et al.* (1985) Fused transcript of abl and bcr genes in chronic myelogenous leukaemia. *Nature* **315**: 550–554.

Slamon, D. J., Clark, G. M., Wong, S. G., *et al.* (1987) Human breast cancer: correlation of relapse and survival with amplification of the HER-2/neu oncogene. *Science* **235**: 177–182.

Slamon, D. J., Godolphin, W., Jones, L. A., *et al.* (1989) Studies of the HER-2/neu proto-oncogene in human breast and ovarian cancer. *Science* **244**: 707–712.

Slamon, D. J., Leyland-Jones, B., Shak, S., *et al.* (2001) Use of chemotherapy plus a monoclonal antibody against HER2 for metastatic breast cancer that overexpresses HER2. *N. Engl. J. Med.* **344**: 783–792.

Slovak, M. L., Kopecky, K. J., Cassileth, P. A., *et al.* (2000) Karyotypic analysis predicts outcome of preremission and postremission therapy in adult acute myeloid leukemia: a Southwest Oncology Group/Eastern Cooperative Oncology Group Study. *Blood* **96**: 4075–4083.

Sorensen, P. H., Lynch, J. C., Qualman, S. J., *et al.* (2002) PAX3-FKHR and PAX7-FKHR gene fusions are prognostic indicators in alveolar rhabdomyosarcoma: a report from the children's oncology group. *J. Clin. Oncol.* **20**: 2672–2679.

Swerdlow, S. H., Yang, W. I., Zukerberg, L. R., *et al.* (1995) Expression of cyclin D1 protein in centrocytic/mantle cell lymphomas with and without rearrangement of the BCL1/cyclin D1 gene. *Hum. Pathol.* **26**: 999–1004.

Tuveson, D. A., Willis, N. A., Jacks, T., *et al.* (2001) STI571 inactivation of the gastrointestinal stromal tumour c-KIT oncoprotein: biological and clinical implications. *Oncogene* **20**: 5054–5058.

Vandenberghe, E., De Wolf-Peeters, C., van den Oord, J., *et al.* (1991) Translocation (11;14): a cytogenetic anomaly associated with B-cell lymphomas of non-follicle centre cell lineage. *J. Pathol.* **163**: 13–18.

Williams, M. E., Westermann, C. D. and Swerdlow, S. H. (1990) Genotypic characterization of centrocytic lymphoma: frequent rearrangement of the chromosome 11 bcl-1 locus. *Blood* **76**: 1387–1391.

Yatabe, Y., Kosaka, T., Takahashi, T., *et al.* (2005) EGFR mutation is specific for terminal respiratory unit type adenocarcinoma. *Am. J. Surg. Pathol.* **29**: 633–639.

Zoubek, A., Dockhorn-Dworniczak, B., Delattre, O., *et al.* (1996) Does expression of different EWS chimeric transcripts define clinically distinct risk groups of Ewing tumour patients?. *J. Clin. Oncol.* **14**: 1245–1251.

Zucman, J., Delattre, O., Desmaze, C., *et al.* (1992) Cloning and characterization of the Ewing's sarcoma and peripheral neuroepithelioma t(11;22) translocation breakpoints. *Genes Chromosomes Cancer* **5**: 271–277.

Zukerberg, L. R., Yang, W. I., Arnold, A., *et al.* (1995) Cyclin D1 expression in non-Hodgkin's lymphomas. Detection by immunohistochemistry. *Am. J. Clin. Pathol.* **103**: 756–760.

18 Pathology 2026: The Future of Laboratory Medicine and Academic Pathology

John J. O'Leary

Traverse: Into The Future

by Je' Free

What I say now may be elementary –
Once man unravels time and its mystery
We travel to the past by memory
Imagination's what our future will be

Delve in the theories of the human minds
It's heaven or hell or in between those lines
Push to one direction, a radical turn
We see this paradox a great concern

We have explored it almost endlessly –
How we can change the course of history
Kaleidoscopic the world seems to be
We need a mechanism to set us free...

INTRODUCTION

The future of laboratory medicine and academic pathology are inextricably linked. Predicting the future is considered by many to be a dangerous pursuit, not given to scientific validation, rather to conjecture. It is with the lines above echoing in my head that I write this chapter. Laboratory medicine in the past 30 years has achieved major advances, yet before attempting to predict the future for laboratory medicine and academic pathology in these islands, I think it is fitting for us to analyse where we as a discipline are now and how we are perceived by our medical/scientific colleagues, the public at large and our political and governmental masters.

In order to achieve this critical analysis, I will firstly carry out a SWOT (strengths, weaknesses, opportunities, threats) analysis of laboratory medicine and academic pathology in the year 2006.

Strengths of Laboratory Medicine and Academic Pathology as Assessed in 2006

We are fortunate to have a young vibrant scientific and medical staff in laboratory medicine who are highly motivated and committed to excellence, while sometimes working in difficult situations. There is a good standard of pathology practice in the UK and Ireland, with a major emphasis on diagnostic excellence, proficiency and accreditation. Greater numbers of clinical laboratories have now achieved accreditation and there is an expectation in the general public's mind that clinical laboratories are doing 'right by the patient', notwithstanding controversies over cytopathology screening in recent years.

Laboratory medicine still attracts bright medical and scientific graduates to work in the field, but this may not be sustainable in the future (see below).

The Royal College of Pathologists, the Association of Clinical Biochemists and Institute of Medical Laboratory Scientists (UK) and the Association of Medical Laboratory Scientists (Ireland) all operate successful and properly structured trainings schemes and provide further educational opportunities for members. The Pathological Society of Great Britain and Ireland, through their bi-yearly meetings and publication of the *Journal of Pathology*, acts as a strong advocate for academic pathology in these islands.

Greater research funding opportunities are now available to all pathology disciplines, and indeed young medical and scientific staff are encouraged to undertake research and pursue higher degrees as part of their professional development. Many pathology laboratories have now specifically set aside 'seed funding' to encourage staff to initiate research and to obtain preliminary research data in order to successfully compete for national/international research funding.

The biotechnology sector and reagent suppliers continue to seek the establishment of strategic research links with pathology laboratories in the UK and Ireland. Often this is pursued in an unstructured way with no specific operational guidelines for laboratories currently available. Specific R&D initiatives with third party companies are to be welcomed, because of the synergy that is achieved between basic science and the clinical laboratory. Access to future technology platforms, chemistries, etc. is to be welcomed, as this provides a vital spring board for innovation in our laboratories going into the future.

In general, laboratory scientists and physicians are not comfortable dealing with intellectual property rights (IPR) issues and discovery exploitation. This needs fundamental review by our college and professional bodies. The exploitation of discovery and protection of IPR are vital for the continuance of basic and translational research in our laboratories with/without the cooperation of external biotechnology interests. The informality of 'trying out a kit or testing reagents' for suppliers is no longer acceptable in a modern laboratory environment.

Weaknesses of Laboratory Medicine and Academic Pathology as Assessed in 2006

It is generally accepted that service demands are increasing year on year, with little strategic investment by health strategists and planners in pathology departments. Currently, there appears to be insufficient time for strategic thinking by laboratory scientists and physicians, with the emphasis largely on turn-around times and productivity, reflected in new contractual arrangements for medical practitioners in laboratories. Most of us complain about increasing workloads, but in the process do not pursue or indeed present the requisite analysis in order to overcome this difficulty. This problem requires fundamental analysis and correction. Most of us encounter inappropriate testing requests, duplication of requests and inappropriate use of direct laboratory testing facilities where point of care testing would adequately suffice.

Medical staffing shortages, particularly in histopathology, have highlighted problems with recruitment and maintenance of staff, which for that discipline in particular may have serious repercussions in the future.

Inadequate funding structures for laboratories are universally encountered by all of us. It is common to see pathology and radiology services in hospitals/trusts competing for 'residual' finance, even though specific service plans have been developed for the laboratory. We appear to be perceived as being peripheral, almost superfluous to general hospital activity. It is clear that our budget advocacy skills need significant sharpening if we are to compete with clinical disciplines in our hospitals/trusts. The development of directorate models has gone some way to addressing this, but has not cured the problem. Strategic *in silico* business modelling needs to be pursued by every laboratory medicine directorate in order to achieve the necessary recurrent income and capital investment stream to maintain activity and achieve strategic growth. Often, strategic growth is sacrificed on the altar of expediency, which we should not tolerate.

In recent years, laboratory infrastructure (premises and plant) has improved but there are still serious deficiencies. In Ireland, for example, capital depreciation analysis in not performed in public hospitals, which negates the normal capital depreciation cycle and makes it difficult for laboratories to achieve significant capital infrastructural resourcing.

The concept of tenure track promotion has not been embraced by British and Irish pathology. Although we encourage young scientific graduates to pursue research and achieve higher degrees, the non-reward system stymies significant career advancement in laboratory medicine for most of our bright, highly qualified scientists. We are all aware of the migratory tendencies to industry, etc. by such scientists, who represent a huge intellectual loss to laboratory medicine in the public sector. The politicians' mantra 'people are our greatest resource' is so true, particularly in laboratory medicine, but the people resource in laboratories is, I feel, often undervalued and poorly supported. Strategic tenure track programmes need to be developed for young science and medical graduates in laboratory medicine disciplines in order to retain and develop expertise in our disciplines.

The perception of pathology by the general public, particularly in wake of the recent organ retention controversy, is one of not understanding what pathology is, what pathologists/laboratory scientists do or indeed the relevance of pathology to modern medicine. I believe that in the past 20–30 years we, as laboratory medicine practitioners, have further re-enforced this idea of 'remoteness' from general hospital and community-based medicine because we have retreated to our laboratories and have not engaged with the general public to explain what laboratory medicine or to contextualise its role in modern medicine. Currently there are no substantive education outreach programmes in second-level education that critically examine career structure in laboratory medicine or indeed explore the world of laboratory medicine.

In the university sector, pathology-related subjects have been under pressure to be maintained in core curricula. Indeed, the traditional pathology department has disappeared from some of our medical schools and is on the edge of extinction in others. This has major implications for the future in our inability to attract good medical graduates to enter laboratory medicine disciplines. Without direct exposure to pathology subjects, to pathology laboratories and to pathologists and laboratory scientists, medical students will be unable to make informed decisions in relation to future careers in laboratory medicine.

How we view ourselves and how we are viewed by health administrators also constitutes a major weakness today. In general, pathologists and medical laboratory scientists are not good at marketing our skills base and tend to interact badly with the media. Health planners see laboratory medicine as low priority and constantly criticise us for not thinking strategically and in a business-like fashion. This is a valid criticism and one that needs addressing as we move forward into a more business- and strategy-focused healthcare sector.

Opportunities for Laboratory Medicine and Academic Pathology as Assessed in 2006

Enormous opportunities still exist for all laboratory medicine disciplines. Because our 'bread and butter' business is diagnostic testing, the whole area of diagnostic test/kit development and the impact of in vitro diagnostic (IVD) directives, etc. has brought into sharp focus the role of clinical and academic laboratories in diagnostic test development. Until now, test development and refinement has proceeded on an *ad hoc* basis, with clinical laboratories offering limited and non-contextualised testing for major reagent/kit manufacturers. There is now an absolute need for a standardised approach in this area with definition of IPR, discovery and the concept of added value being defined in any interaction between the laboratory and third part suppliers. To put it bluntly, kit and chemistry verification are central to successful technology platform development by industry, and laboratory medicine must see itself as a strategic partner in such a development.

The era of 'personalised medicine' offers enormous opportunities for laboratory medicine disciplines in the future, particularly in the area of devices, remote patient monitoring and custom-designed DNA, RNA and protein chips (see below).

New emerging technologies, including robotics, humanoid technology, lab-on-chip devices, nanodevices and patient 'smart' implants, will in the future offer unique opportunities for laboratories to develop new core business areas (discussed below).

The ability to form research networks within hospitals and universities and externally with industry offers a unique vehicle for laboratory medicine to achieve academic advancement. By placing laboratory medicine at the core of technology development in our hospital and medical schools, we will ensure a significant element of future-proofing for pathology. Strategically, pathology departments should even now be planning for future integration with the biotechnology sector through the development of 'bio-incubator units' in laboratories in order to develop translational cores in laboratory medicine.

The 1990s have seen unprecedented economic growth in the West. However, economies and economic growth usually follow cyclical trends: 'the boom bust cycle'. No-one knows for how much longer the 'boom cycle' will continue but it is certain that a decline will eventually supervene. Laboratory medicine is perceived as expensive by healthcare strategists and planners, with high staffing, capital and infrastructural costs, and consequently a sustained increase in base costs. It is clear that these costs, while sustainable in the current economic climate, are not sustainable in the long term. The lack of a unified and universally applied cost base analysis model for laboratory medicine disciplines again highlights the vulnerability in the current situation. Currently in Ireland a conversation has commenced in relation to the provision of laboratory medicine services in the Republic in order to achieve high economic cost benefit, controlled cost base and high quality service. Indeed, the provision of laboratory services in public hospitals is coming under increased scrutiny and how new models can be developed into the future is being assessed. The interaction between the public and private sectors has also received much attention and will become a dominant factor in relation to how laboratory medicine services are delivered in the future (see below).

Threats to Laboratory Medicine and Academic Pathology as Assessed in 2006

If we remain as we are and do not alter the way we are perceived, we risk marginalisation of laboratory medicine. We need to change disciplines or parts of disciplines in order to redefine who we are, what we are and what we do.

We need to develop a strategic out-reach education programme and identify a national figure who will serve as an advocate for laboratory medicine, its mission and its role. We need to target specifically second-level education in education programmes organised by the Royal College of Pathologists and/or professional bodies.

We need to redefine laboratory medicine and support the advancement of 'clinical pathology/laboratory medicine' akin to the US model, making the pathologist/laboratory scientist more accessible and visible to clinical colleagues and other healthcare workers. The laboratory needs to be redefined in terms of its role in the hospital, and the community as a centre of diagnostics that is important and pivotal to the needs of the patient.

We need specifically to address how pathology is taught in our medical schools and arrest the erosion of pathology teaching that is currently taking place.

We need to resist fragmentation of traditional laboratory medicine disciplines away from laboratories. Currently haematology and immunology, having significant clinical contact, are moving more towards becoming clinical medicine disciplines, which will further erode the cohesiveness of diagnostic and academic laboratory medicine.

LABORATORY MEDICINE AND ACADEMIC PATHOLOGY IN 2026

In 2026, laboratory medicine will be fundamentally different to practice in the year 2006. We will have come through a turbulent economic cycle of boom and bust and fundamental reviews of economic cost of healthcare provision will have taken place. The modern medicine environment will be organised on a hub and spoke motif: large supra-regional tertiary centres (hubs) and smaller local treatment centres (spokes). Laboratories will also be organised on a similar basis. Throughout the UK and Ireland, pathologists and laboratory scientists, in collaboration with venture capitalists, will have established limited liability companies in order to tender for laboratory services in their region. Variable success will have been achieved, with some companies facing liquidation or receivership. An extremely competitive market will exist, with two or three large private laboratory providers dominating and potentially controlling up to 35% of former public hospital laboratory practice. Significant benefits for the exchequer with reduced operating laboratory costs will be achieved. Significant investment in R&D by major private laboratory service providers will achieve strategic growth in the sector. Strategic alliances between large pharmaceutical companies and private laboratory service providers, to provide pharmacogenomic and metabologenomic biosensor diagnostic services in the home, will attract significant stock market interest and intensify debate in relation to artificial cell therapies for diabetes and hypertension.

The Environments in Which we will Work

The mix of public/private laboratories in the UK in 2026 will be around 35% private and 65% public, but it is anticipated that by 2030 the ratio will be almost equal. New laboratories will be built in green field sites adjacent to major routeways in the UK and in Ireland (see Fig. 18.1). The new laboratory facilities will offer state-of-the-art ergonomically designed modular laboratory units with high reliance on robotic and humanoid features. Modular 'all-contained' drop-down units will feature prominently in new laboratories, offering greater flexibility and expandability.

High dependence on robotics, automated specimen handling, automated specimen tracking and humanoid technology will greatly simplify the management and tracking of specimens within the laboratory. The hub laboratories will provide diagnostic services in the following areas:

- Cellular Sciences
- Blood Chemistry
- Clinical Microbiology and Infectious Disease
- Diagnostic Molecular Pathology
- Cytogenetics
- Devices and Microsystems
- Information technology

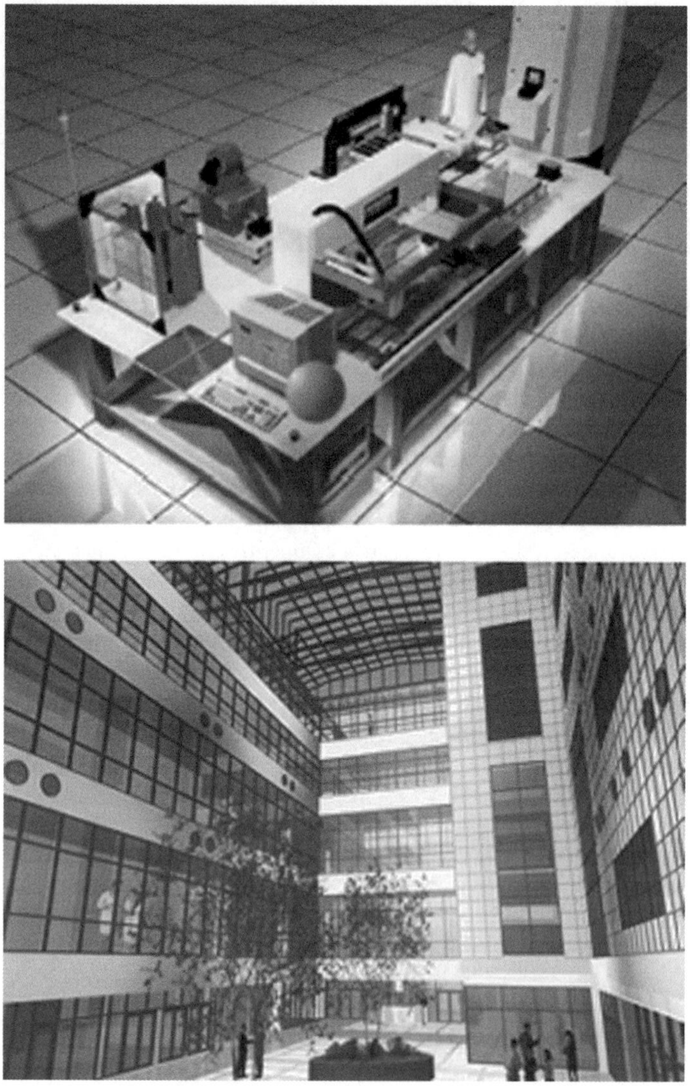

Figure 18.1 Interior and exterior of a modern laboratory in the year 2026, showing modular open laboratories built to high specification and ergonomically designed.

- Forensicogenomics
- Stem Cell Biology and Biobanking

Indeed the Royal College and Professional Associations will have ratified the above consolidated laboratory discipline list and will have issued strict guidelines in relation to professional qualifications and training in each unitary discipline for medical and scientific laboratory staff.

The introduction of advanced practitioner scientists, clinical diagnostic scientists, skills mix managers and audit managers within the laboratory environment will revolutionise how we, as practitioners of laboratory medicine, will deliver our service to the healthcare sector.

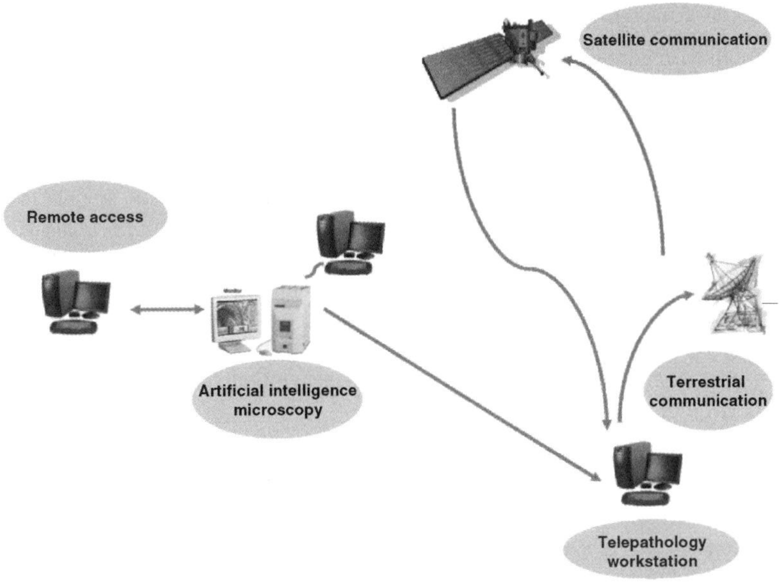

Figure 18.2 Reporting schema for cellular science in 2026, including use of artificial intelligence microscopy (AIM) and terrestrial and satellite communication.

Cellular Science

In 2026, the EUROPATH consortium, bringing together public and private laboratories throughout the European Union to develop vital sign technology (tele-medicine), will be a major focus for cellular science laboratories in the UK and Ireland. The schema will involve the use of satellite communication, remotely controlled microscopy, artificial intelligence microscopy (AIM), widespread high-speed hyper-band internet communication and telepathology workstation platforms remotely accessible from within and without the laboratory. In addition, an element of terrestrial communication will be involved in this new super-highway cellular science diagnostic service (see Fig. 18.2).

Within the UK and Ireland, telesynergy will be achieved between many hub laboratories in the areas of cellular science oncological pathology, with free exchange of digital imaging in real time between centres. The EUROPATH consortium will offer a virtual 'stat' reporting system that will allow instantaneous access to pathologists throughout the European Union. This new system will effectively allow 24-h, 7 days a week virtual pathology coverage in cellular science for European citizens and will herald a new era in global healthcare approaches.

The development of new artificial intelligence (AI) automated cytoscreening technology with automated robotic preparation will revolutionise how we practice cytopathology within cellular science laboratory medicine. Artificial intelligence rare cell event monitoring (RCEM) with protein tag labelling of abnormal cells will be in routine use, in parallel with lab-on-chip detection of human papilloma virus (HPV) genotypes using real-time PCR and nucleic acid base amplification chips. Greater than 95% of laboratories will offer a fully automated cytoscreening service as a primary screening tool. The advent of multivalent HPV vaccines will have a major impact on cervical cytology services throughout the European Union. The need for pre- and post-vaccination assessment using cervical cytology will increase dramatically the workloads in cytopathology laboratories. Non-gynaecological cytopathology will continue to grow significantly, with the greater use of molecular proteomic and metabolomic genetic assays on single- and group-cell aspirates.

The new era of nuclear magnetic resonance (NMR) microscopy will have arrived. This will allow cellular pathologists to look at patterns of cells in a tissue and facilitate examination of cells for the presence, absence or mutation of genes that control growth and function and will facilitate examination of specific markers of disease. The magnetic resonance microscope will allow, for the first time, non-invasive three-dimensional visualisation of single cells in living tissues. It will exquisitely allow cellular diagnostics and allow us to view intracellular and extracellular distribution of water and molecules within cells, it will be an important diagnostic adjunct in the assessment of artificial cell systems that will be used in disease treatment and molecular pharmacology. Nuclear magnetic resonance microscopy will allow the visualisation of contrast labels, substrates and materials, including monoclonal antibodies in normal tissues and organs and lesions derived therefrom, and will be a major breakthrough in cellular sciences. These new innovations will allow investigation of cellular metabolism in individual cells and tissues in real time (cellular metabolo-imaging). CytoNMR (cNMR) and newer generation technologies, including atomic sensitivity NMR, will lead to further advances in the assessment of individual cells and tissues at a subcellular/atomic level.

Blood Sciences

In 2026, the integration of haematology, transfusion medicine, biochemistry and immunology into a unified blood sciences discipline will have been achieved, largely reflecting the organisational infrastructure of modern laboratories based on open-design modular laboratories with high dependence on robotics and humanoid technology. Nanotechnology, bio-robots and microdevice detection systems (Microsystems) will be pervasive and will have revolutionised the analysis of bloods and blood-derived products in the laboratory. New specimen identification chips (SpecChip) will provide sample identification and incorporation of patient records within the sample cuvette and will revolutionise sample tracking within blood sciences.

The use of the personal profile chip (PPC) in haematology will be largely accepted and available for cardiovascular disease, autoimmune disease and detection of cancer signatures in peripheral blood. The majority of PPCs will be etched silicon wafers encompassing a number of biosensoring technologies, including mechanical, electrochemical, chemi-luminescence and optical. The PPC will be a semi-permanent implant, fully compatible with neighbouring tissues. The first generation of PPCs will read by passing a hand-held scanner device over the implant. It is anticipated that in the future PPCs will be read by remote telemetry. The PPC will be supplied with a memory bank of genetic and biochemical data that are directly related to major diseases and the disease from which the individual is known to be at risk from a pertinent family history. The PPC will be organised on the following basis: with a flow-through chamber for blood with channels, lanes and compartments in which cells are identified and sorted by size. In another chamber the sorted cells are analysed chemically and a third section of the chip will be used for drug delivery if required. Phenotypic monitoring gene chips (PMGCs), which have the capacity to analyse directly genes in cells and tissue *in vivo*, will be introduced.

The use of diagnostic nano-robots in blood sciences will be commonplace and will be particularly useful in the dynamic monitoring of diabetes, ischaemic heart disease, hypertension, the metabolic syndrome and inherited inborn errors of metabolism (see Devices section).

Clinical Microbiology and Infectious Disease

Clinical microbiology and infectious diseases will have undergone major innovation by the year 2026. Enhanced microbiological, virological and mycological susceptibility testing, advanced environmental monitoring, direct molecular microbiological epidemiology and organism strain identification with infectious disease tracking and population microgenomics will be pervasive. Microbiology and infectious disease will rely heavily on lab-on-chip devices, including automated DNA, RNA and protein/peptide extraction chips coupled to organism identification chips and sequencing chips giving real-time analysis of patient specimens. Hand-held microbiology detection devices will offer real-time dynamic monitoring of infectious diseases in the primary care setting, remotely monitored by laboratories. The development will bring increased workload for the devices and clinical microbiology/infectious disease sections of all our laboratories.

The rise in bioterrorism events throughout the world, particularly with recombinant viral and fungal pathogens, will focus increased attention in clinical microbiology and infectious disease departments in relation to the identification and monitoring of bioterrorism in the field and within the hospital environment. Newly developed bioterrorism hand-held devices for the top eight infectious pathogens worldwide will be available for monitoring efforts in this area.

Diagnostic Molecular Pathology

Diagnostic molecular pathology in 2026 will encompass the following sub-disciplines:

- Diagnostic genomics
- Transcriptomics
- Polysomics
- Proteomics
- Peptidomics
- Pharmacogenomics
- Metabalogenomics

The use of high-density 500 000 to 1 million SNP (short nucleotide polymorphism) diagnostic assays will be pervasive in laboratories. High-density cDNA array profiling of tumours will be commonplace. Custom-designed personalised SNP and cDNA and protein arrays will be available. High-density antibody and protein chip arrays will be used for the analysis of immune diseases and to assess the immune response to tumours in the context of therapy. Tumoural transcriptomics, polysomics and proteomics will form a substantial portion of diagnostic report formulation. As in blood sciences, patient-specific and disease monitoring chips will be widely available in order to monitor disease activity. Individual patient genome signature profiling will be commonplace, with the attendant ethical issues in relation to this type of screening. Individual laboratory and chip devices for specific disease monitoring will be available by custom design. The greater integration of metabalogenomics, proteomics and peptidomics will allow us to further stratify treatment responses in certain disease conditions. The integration of basic sciences and clinical diagnostic molecular pathology will further achieve academic advancement for the discipline of laboratory medicine. Molecular pathology will be highly reliant on the devices section of laboratories, particularly in the area of microsystems (lab-on-chip devices, microfluidics, nanotechnology, etc.).

Cytogenetics

Twenty-four-colour chromosome karyotyping/spectral analysis of tumours will be offered routinely in haematological malignancies and solid tumours. In addition there will be more widespread use of interphase cytogenetics, fine gene locus mapping and locus-specific sequencing of novel disease loci in patients with specific monitoring of locus-specific changes following treatment.

Devices and Microsystems

Electrochemical detection of infectious agents, gene mutations, specific gene transcripts and proteins will be possible through the use of devices that can be used in the primary healthcare setting. The PPC (see Blood Sciences section) will be in widespread use. The use of nanodevices and smart implants will be pervasive in the device sector of laboratory medicine. Laboratory medicine will work very closely with microsystem engineers, developing new surfaces for chip devices, chip milling formats, micropore systems, microfluidic systems and nano/picolitre technologies, in the design and formulation of lab-on-chip devices for use in hand-held formats, 'black-box' doctor's office format and in integrated laboratory chip devices.

Microelectromechanical systems (MEMS) will be developed to inoculate individual red cells as they travel through capillaries. The use of nanoparticles will be used to direct targets for specific cells or tissues. The ability of nanoparticles to seek out cells and identify specific molecules with the ability to report dynamically the presence or absence of molecules will act as an initiation point for treatment procedures and will feature prominently in diagnostic blood science departments.

Nano-encapsulation and nanorobot technology will facilitate the delivery of drugs to specific parts of the body by means of the use of magnetic fields. This is likely to boost therapeutic benefit while minimising side-effects on other parts of the body. The use of nanorobots in blood sciences will be dominant, particularly in the monitoring of haematological malignancy, anaemia, ischaemic heart disease, hypertension, diabetes and inborn errors of metabolism and the metabolic syndrome. The use of 'smart implants' will also offer endless potentials. These 'smart implants' consisting of nanosensors will have the ability to detect DNA sequences in the body, enabling simpler and more effective diagnosis. For example, implant devices could dispatch a signal to pump the release of a therapeutic agent, i.e. insulin in diabetic patients.

Smart medical implants including intelligent artificial chips may have the ability to detect and destroy bacteria, for use in molecular microbiology. These smart medical implants (MEMS) will contain sensors with the ability to identify microorganisms and then trigger the release of specific antibodies stored within the implant. Medical devices using biosensors and fuel cells will be in widespread use by 2026. One such approach in ischaemic heart disease could be where the implantable device would monitor the release of natural chemicals in ischaemic heart disease, such as troponins, which indicate that a heart attack is eminent. Another approach could use a subcutaneous biosensor implanted under the skin surface connected to a second device (an optical fibre) designed to be inserted into blood vessels near the heart. This second sensor could potentially couple to a cardiac pacemaker that may be required by the patient with ischaemic heart disease, thereby directly regulating the pacemaker device. This will result in a new discipline in clinical medicine (therapeutic nanodevices).

The use of microfluidic fuel cells will revolutionise the use of long-running medical implants. These miniature devices will provide long-term power for medical devices such as implants to detect glucose levels in diabetics. In general fuel cells require an ion conducting membrane or selective catalyst of the electrode to separate the fuel-containing fluids, which has proved problematic in relation to the development of smart devices implantable in patients. The use of microfluidics and taking advantage of how fuels flow in small channels (in that they do not mix) will mean that fuels can be separated without the use of membranes in such smart devices. Fuel cells will work in tandem to provide power under pulsating conditions that mimic blood flow in the normal body.

The use of the PPC, which is implanted under the skin, will allow instant access to a patient's record. This device will transmit a signal to a scanner that allows healthcare professionals to confirm a patient's identity and obtain detailed information from an accompanying database linked to that patient. The use of implantable radiofrequency identification (RFID) microchips will be widespread in the year 2026. These new devices will allow active real-time autonomous monitoring of many conditions, particularly those involved in metabolic control.

The introduction of humanoid technology into laboratories in 2026 will be finally realised. Currently several multinational corporations, including Honda, are developing humanoid technology for potential use in the laboratory context. Greater artificial intelligence capacity in these humanoid forms will greatly simplify laboratory workflow procedures in the future.

Information Technology

Information technology will feature very prominently in laboratories in the year 2026. The laboratory system of the future will:

- Focus on patients, enabling integration of community and hospital care and will increase the quality of care in patient outcomes through the integration of laboratory practice with the delivery of patient care.
- Deliver quality services that are responsive and sustainable.
- Use clinical outcomes as a primary measure of laboratory service efficacy.
- Coordinate the laboratory service delivery within health regions provincially and between hub and spoke laboratories.
- Employ various strategies, i.e. selected consolidation of testing, appropriate automations and standardisation (common laboratory information systems), to achieve cost effectiveness while attending to patient, clinician and systems needs.
- Employ information technology that facilitates the operation and management of the laboratory system and the delivery and management of healthcare.
- Utilise the systems approach to quality management issues and will foster the training, recruitment and retention of human resources within the laboratory system in order to pursue excellence.

Specialist scientists with degrees in information technology and laboratory medicine technology will be to the forefront in the development of information technology within our laboratories in 2026. They will have a pivotal role in relation to the interface between laboratories and their respective hospitals and between laboratories regionally and nationally.

Forensicogenomics

There will be widespread use of SNP genotyping high-density arrays for the forensic identification of persons, samples and the exclusion of perpetrators of crime. In addition, RNA and PPCs will be available for forensic identification. The recently published international Hap Map (HM) and subsequent updates and the combined DNA index system (CODIS) will be widely used in 2026. These maps and systems will facilitate a unified approach to the forensic identification of patients/perpetrators of crime. Forensicogenomics will be performed by selected laboratories within the hub and spoke motif of laboratory organisation. It is anticipated that forensic science services will be partially privatised in the future, which will require further standardisation of procedures and methodologies for participant laboratories providing forensicogenomic services.

Stem Cell Biology and Biobanking

Biobanking and stem cell biology will be extremely important components in laboratory medicine in the year 2026. Areas of development will include adult stem cell biology, tumour stem cell biology and somatic cell therapy. Stem cells will be selectively harvested and expanded for various therapies, including vehicles for gene therapy, and to genetically and cellularly engineer organs such as liver, pancreas or central nervous system cells to treat a myriad of diseases. Traditional blood banks and pathology departments will become cell banks or gene banks, where repositories of blood stem cells with attendant processing facilities will be available. Some of these processing facilities will involve changes to specific cell types that may need to be replaced or corrected, generated or expanded by adding appropriate genes and growth factors. Reconstituted blood cells and growing tissues, and organs and organoids reconstituted in three-dimensional matrixes, will become a reality.

Organ culture in 2026 will become a reality. The availability of bio-artificial livers, hearts, etc. using cell entrapment technology (CET) will have expanded enormously. Clearly developments in biobanking, stem cell biology, generation of organs/organoids and organ culture will involve other medical disciplines and will be increasingly interdisciplinary. The whole area of adult stem cell biology and embryonic stem biology will need careful ethical guidance and will require a significant input from medical laboratory physicians, scientists and ethicists in the future.

ACADEMIC PATHOLOGY IN MEDICAL SCHOOLS IN 2026

There will be widespread rationalisation of schools in the UK and the Republic of Ireland by 2026. In Ireland, I anticipate that four medical schools will provide medical, dental and paramedical education. It is anticipated that medical schools will be professional graduate schools much akin to the current US model. There will be an international network of medical schools throughout the European Union, with complete reorganisation of the current medical school complement. Medical schools will be required to support 300–400 graduate entrants per year, offering state-of-the-art facilities including virtual tele-medicine, nano-medicine and molecular medicine courses.

Academic pathology departments in medical schools in 2026 will largely have disappeared in the context of active expanding service departments. This appears a surprising statement but largely reflects the current decline of academic pathology departments in the UK and Irish medical schools unless we, as a discipline, fundamentally redefine ourselves in the future and seize the initiative and setout a bold agenda for academic pathology. One consequence of the current marginalisation of academic pathology in medical schools will be our inability to attract medically qualified graduates into laboratory medicine. I anticipate that there will be less medically qualified trainees available, particularly in the laboratory-based disciplines of cellular sciences, forensicogenomics, cytogenetics and molecular pathology. It is anticipated that the more clinically based disciplines such as haematology, immunology and clinical biochemistry will still be able to attract medically qualified trainees to their disciplines. With less medically trained trainees, this will bring about a fundamental realignment of how pathology diagnostic services are provided in laboratories. Today in 2006, the concept of consultant-led diagnostic services is foremost in all of our minds. However, the concept of medical-consultant-led diagnostic services in the year 2026 will not be sustainable if we are unable to attract medically qualified trainees. In this regard, I believe that there will be more consultant medical scientists, advanced medical science practitioners and skills mix managers within our laboratories who are not medically qualified.

The position of Professor of Pathology will largely have disappeared from medical schools in the year 2026. Individuals will still be called professors of a particular pathology discipline with individual chairs in divisions of clinical sciences or will have devolved very strategic areas of expertise, e.g. Professor of Pathology Microsystems, or Professor of Tumoural Protemics. Haematology, immunology and clinical biochemistry will continue to interface academically with clinical medicine disciplines. However, the cellular science disciplines of histopathology and cytopathology will largely remain laboratory based and will suffer from a lack of medical scientific graduate entrants into the discipline. However, molecular pathology and cytogenetics will be pivotal in terms of a laboratory/clinical medicine translational base and may offer growth opportunities within laboratory medicine going forward.

EDUCATION OF MEDICAL LABORATORY SCIENTISTS AND BIOCHEMISTS IN LABORATORY MEDICINE IN 2026

Strategic national centres of teaching and research excellence for medical scientists and clinical biochemists will in place by 2026. I anticipate that there will be formalised professional and academic MSc, PhD and DSc programmes for medical scientists and clinical biochemists who wish to avail themselves of this. There needs to be a diploma/membership of the Royal College of Pathologists for scientists who wish to pursue advanced practitioner status in their relevant pathology disciplines. In some disciplines such as cellular science (e.g. cytopathology) there will be an absolute need for specialised vocational MSc and PhD courses organised by laboratories with the support of local health agencies to further encourage, support and attract scientists into this discipline. Advanced practitioner courses and diplomas will have to be supported at this time. Indeed, the need for continuing professional development (CPD) will also require funding from source funders within our laboratories.

HOW DO WE MOVE FORWARD TO ACHIEVE EXCELLENCE IN 2026?

In the earlier part of this chapter I carried out a SWOT analysis of pathology in 2006. Although there are many strengths and many opportunities, there are significant weaknesses and threats in all disciplines within laboratory medicine. I believe that pathology needs to redefine itself as a unitary discipline and redefine its position within modern medicine, within society and within the world.

We need to develop greater advocacy skills for our disciplines and establish a European Pathology Forum to formulate strategies for education, research, service development and staff recruitment.

- We need to establish academic career advancement programmes, including tenure-track programmes for medical staff, medical trainees, medical laboratory scientists and biochemists.
- We need to encourage the formation of centres of research excellence in laboratory medicine based on the hub and spoke motif as outlined above.
- We need to establish pathology fellowship training programmes for medical and science trainees within laboratory medicine disciplines.
- In addition, we need to establish industrially supported MD, PhD and DSc studentships for medical and scientifically qualified graduates within laboratory medicine. This I believe is key in terms of achieving growth going forward for all laboratory disciplines in the greater family of laboratory medicine.

Laboratory medicine scientists and physicians need to be more proactive in spearheading service developments in pathology arising from the translational research they carry out and we need to properly address intellectual property rights and exploitation issues in relation to the fundamental basic science research that is currently being performed in laboratory medicine academic departments so that this is translated to the laboratory bench and exploited by the laboratories. Laboratories need to take a lead role in the biobanking, genome resource banking and national cancer genome survey initiatives that have recently been launched.

Most importantly, laboratory medicine needs to think like a business! We need to develop a pathology corporate strategy in our medical schools and hospitals to:

1. Attract external funding from the biotechnology sector (national and international agencies).
2. Establish international research and education networks.
3. Establish endowed studentships for MD, PhD, MSc and DSc students.
4. Establish endowed lectureships and professorships in laboratory medicine with significant support from biotechnology and industry partners.

Furthermore, we need to examine critically the role of private income generation and its potential use as seed capital funding for strategic academic, technological and scientific development within our laboratories. Pathology departments should now be establishing business translation incubator units (BTIUs), in collaboration with hospital institutions, universities and industrial/biotechnology partners. This is fundamental in relation to achieving growth within laboratory medicine. It allows significant technology transfer, access to 'blue sky' technology, access to innovative thought processing in relation to new chemistries and technology platforms that are currently being developed by the biotechnology sector. We need urgently to develop significant expertise in IPR in order to cope with the exploitation of discovery. Pathology disciplines should now start to provide essential core facilities for medical schools in order to regain the initiative and re-establish laboratory medicine/pathology as a fundamental discipline within medical schools. Such core facilities could include cDNA, CGH array facilities, tissue biobanks and laser capture microdissection, to mention just a few.

However, in the final analysis, laboratory medicine will only succeed based on its people resource. We need to create the pyramid effect in attracting and maintaining people of excellence in service and academic pathology. Mentoring programmes for medical and science graduates within laboratory medicine are extremely important in order to encourage the best, to retain the best and to ensure that the best seek academic advancement for themselves and their discipline. Only by employing this pyramid effect will we see strategic growth within laboratory medicine and protect a rich heritage that has been passed on to all of us.

SUGGESTED READING

Arney, K.R., Hopper, M.H., Tran, S.A., Ward, M.M. and Hanson, C.A. (2004) Quest for quality: department of laboratory medicine and pathology, Mayo Clinic. *Clin. Leadersh. Man. Rev.* **18**: 361–363.

Billings, P.R. and Brown, M.P. (2004) The future of clinical laboratory genomics. *MLO Med. Lab. Obs.* **36**: 8–10, 12–17.

Bountis, C. and Kay, J.D. (2002) An integrated knowledge management system for the clinical laboratories: an initial application of an architectural model. *Stud. Health Technol. Inf.* **90**: 562–567.

Brenner, B. (2003) Is the provision of laboratory results via the Internet acceptable to patients? A survey of private patients in a large, specialist gynaecology practice. *N. Z. Med. J.* **116**: U711.

Burke, M.D. (2000) Laboratory medicine in the 21st Century. *Am. J. Clin. Pathol.* **114**: 841–846.

Burnett, D., Blair, C., Haeney, M.R., Jeffcoate, S.L., Scott, K.W. and Williams, D.L. (2002) Clinical pathology accreditation: standards for the medical laboratory. *J. Clin. Pathol.* **55**: 729–733.

Campbell, D.A., Carmichael, J. and Chopra, R. (2004) Molecular pathology in oncology – the AstraZeneca perspective. *Pharmacogenomics* **5**: 1167–1173.

Davis, G.M., Lantis, K.L. and Finn, W.G. (2004) Laboratory hematology practice: present and future. *Cancer Treat. Res.* **121**: 167–179.

Finch, R., Hryniewicz, W. and Van Eldere, J. (2005) Report of working group 2: healthcare needs in the organisation and management of infection. *Clin. Microbiol. Infect.* **11**: 41–45.

Green, D.M. (2005) Improving health care and laboratory medicine: the past, present, and future of molecular diagnostics. *Proc. Bayl. Univ. Med. Cent.* **18**: 125–129.

Greinacher, A. and Warkentin, T.E. (2005) Transfusion medicine in the era of genomics and proteomics. *Transfus. Med. Rev.* **19**: 288–294.

Hallworth, M., Hyde, K., Cummings, A. and Peake, I. (2002) The future for clinical scientists in laboratory medicine. *Clin. Lab. Haematol.* **24**: 197–204.

Horvath, A.R. and Pewsner, D. (2004) Systematic reviews in laboratory medicine: principles, processes and practical considerations. *Clin. Chim. Acta* **342**: 23–39.

Kayser, K., Kayser, G., Radziszowski, D. and Oehmann, A. (1999–2004) From telepathology to virtual pathology institution: the new world of digital pathology. *Rom. J. Morphol. Embryol.* **45**: 3–9.

Koele, C. (2004) Building the lab workforce of the future. *MLO Med. Lab. Obs.* **36**: 28–29.

Kubik, T., Bogunia-Kubik, K. and Sugisaka, M. (2005) Nanotechnology on duty in medical applications. *Curr. Pharm. Biotechnol.* **6**: 17–33.

Lehmann, C. (2002) Management of point-of-care testing in home heath care. *Clin. Leadersh. Man. Rev.* **16**: 27–31.

Leong, F.J. and Leong, A.S. (2003) Digital imaging applications in anatomic pathology. *Adv. Anat. Pathol.* **10**: 88–95.

Narayanan, S. (2000) Technology and laboratory instrumentation in the next decade. *MLO Med. Lab. Obs.* **32**: 24–27, 30–31.

Plebani, M. (2005) Proteomics: the next revolution on laboratory medicine?. *Clin. Chim. Acta* **357**: 113–122.

Robertson, B.H. and Nicholson, J.K. (2005) New microbiology tools for public health and their implications. *Annu. Rev. Publ. Health* **26**: 281–302.

Valdes, R., Jr., Linder, M.W. and Jortani, S.A. (2003) What is next in pharamacogenomics? Translating it to clinical practice. *Pharmacogenomics* **4**: 499–505.

Weiss, R.L., Sundwall, D. and Matsen, J.M. (2002) Estimating the budgetary impact of setting the medicare clinical laboratory fee schedule at the national limitation amount. *Am. J. Clin. Pathol.* **117**: 691–695.

Wills, S. (2000) The 21st century laboratory: information technology and health care. *Clin. Leadersh. Man. Rev.* **14**: 289–291.

The sleeper down from Glasgow

In arranging the Winter meetings of the Society the committee showed scant, indeed no regard for Scottish traditions at Hogmanay (New Year's eve): the advent of New Year was always a cause for celebration, sometimes indeed (even frequently) more rumbustious than those for Christmas. It was traditional to 'first foot' neighbours and friends, to toast the New Year in uisge beatha (whisky) and the celebrations always ran into the first week of the New Year: indeed it was not uncommon to toast and wish friends a Happy New Year well into January. Winter meetings were not unknown to start on the 3rd of January and this was certainly an incursion on the traditional celebrations, as for that matter were meetings beginning on any date in the first week of the year.

The Glasgow contingent for the meetings was a large one combining the academic staffs at the Royal and Western Infirmaries – Professors, Senior Lecturers and Lecturers (and in the late 1960s the last group comprised 12). We travelled back and fore on British Rail sleepers: 2nd class, two berths per compartment with departures at both Glasgow and Euston being 23.50 hrs and a requirement to disembark no later than 08.00 hrs. Certainly on the outward journey there was much social intercourse and in keeping with time honoured custom drinks were exchanged; it is true to say that much whisky was consumed, but never to excess! The senior staff were generous but carefully abstemious; single malts were a specialty and in particular Talisker was the favourite – suited me well as part Sgiathanach (Skyeman): the juniors were sometimes experiencing their first single malt and there was the occasional mishap – one visiting trainee from East Africa found whisky to his liking and required some gentle care on arrival at Euston: there were occasional spillages and sometimes confusion reigned on trying to get back to one's own compartment only to find the sleeping car attendant had re-allocated what he presumed was a vacant bed/compartment.

On arrival at Euston we separated and made for our respective hotels: the Royal group favoured the Cora Hotel (Woburn Plate/Southampton Row) while the Western group were more up-market and enjoyed the luxury of the Bloomsbury hotels – the Ivanhoe and Kenilworth being favoured: additionally they reminded us of our Scottish literary heritage. However, when the meeting was at Oxford I recall the Royal group enjoying the luxury of the Randolph Hotel while we struggled furiously to keep warm in a stony, frigid, mediaeval College.

There was keen competitive rivalry between the two departments. Which one had the more papers accepted? Which ones were best presented? The 'Path Soc' meetings filled the juniors with fear and trepidation – serial ranks of Professors in the first few rows many of whom could spot a hair on the slide or a crack in the sections at a distance of 50 yards and this without spectacles; and woe betide any who read their script. The junior members from the Royal were apparently always advised to slip a Vitamin C tablet into their mouths just before beginning their delivery: it certainly avoided 'drying out', but on one occasion a now senior retired pathologist taking part in a telecast popped in a tablet without realising it was effervescent – the result was spectacular!

Socialising also took place in the course of the meeting, we discriminating Scots preferring the elegant a la carte cuisine of some Soho restaurants to the table d'hote of St Ermin's Hotel in the dingy surroundings of Victoria and where the dinner was wont to be held. On one such occasion the waiter asked for orders for the dessert and one of our group caused consternation when he demanded a 'pokey hat' (ice cream cone) and would not countenance refusal. It was our wont to continue some carousing on our return to the hotels in the evening. These were the days of last drinks at 22.00 hrs and one depended on the night porter getting us the necessary night cap. On one occasion 10 whiskies were ordered, and after a seemingly interminable wait a somewhat disgruntled porter eventually delivered. He was immediately asked for 10 more and again belatedly returned with but only 5 glasses and announced that the hotel had run out of whisky! A new venue was chosen for next year.

I have had various accounts of the following incident and can only vouch for the veracity of there having been a major shindig. Was it the Cora or the Randolph Hotel? Was the party in one of the Professors' rooms? Did the couple next door complain or did they join the festivities? In any event a shelf (or was it a wash-hand basin?) in the room was supporting a large collection of bottles and glasses when someone leaned heavily against it, detaching the shelf from the wall and releasing a cascade of bottles and drinks on the floor! The next morning when the incident was reported to the reception manager he re-assuringly remarked 'don't tell me the shelf has come away from the wall again'.

These are some of the printable fond memories of the sleeper trips and the winter meetings of the Path Soc, representing the usual extension of the Hogmanay celebrations for us Glaswegians. The recollections are now a little dim and the detailed accuracy less certain – whether due to amnesia close to the event or whether due to long-term memory impairment I am uncertain. The cameraderi engendered by these trips was unique and allowed the two departments to first foot each other and begin the year in good fellowship.

Roddy MacSween

I have not mentioned any names in the above, but I would acknowledge input from Professors Fred Lee and David Murray and Drs Peter Macfarlane and George Lindop

Appendices

Peter A. Hall, Roselyn A. Pitts and Julie Johnstone

APPENDIX 1: A CHRONOLOGICAL LIST OF PRESIDENTS

2000–2006	N.A. Wright
2006–2009	D.A. Levison (President elect 2005)

APPENDIX 2: A CHRONOLOGICAL LIST OF SECRETARIES,[1] GENERAL SECRETARIES AND CHAIRMAN

1906–1919	J. Ritchie and A.E. Boycott (Secretaries)
1920–1921	A.E. Boycott and H.R. Dean (Secretaries)
1922–1933	H.R. Dean and M.J. Stewart (Secretaries)
1934–1954	H.R. Dean and J.H. Dible (Secretaries)
1954–1958	J.H. Dible and A.W. Downie (Secretaries)
1959–1963	A.W. Downie and G.L. Montgomery (Secretaries)
1964–1965	R.E.O. Williams and G.L. Montgomery (Secretaries)
1966–1968	R.C. Curran and G.L. Montgomery (Secretaries)
1969–1977	B. Moore (General Secretary)
1977–1981	M.G. McEntegart (General Secretary)
1982–1992	R.B. Goudie (General Secretary)
1992–2000	F. Walker (General Secretary and Chairman)
2000–2003	M. Wells (General Secretary)
2003–date	P.A. Hall (General Secretary)

APPENDIX 3: A CHRONOLOGICAL LIST OF MEETINGS SECRETARIES

1966–1969	R.C. Curran
1970–1977	W.A.J. Crane
1978–1982	A.M. Neville
1982–1986	C.C. Bird
1987–1990	N.A. Wright
1991–1995	J.C.E. Underwood
1996–1999	M. Wells
1999–2002	C.S. Herrington
2002–date	M. Pignatelli

[1] Until the late 1960s the specific position of Meetings Secretary does not appear to have been distinguished and fell within the role of Secretary, of which two were elected (see Appendix 3).

In the period 1981–2000 there was a separate Meeting Secretary for Medical Microbiology

1981–1985	C.S.F. Easmon
1986–1990	E.M. Cooke
1991–1994	R.J. Williams
1995–2000	C.G. Gemmell

APPENDIX 4: A CHRONOLOGICAL LIST OF TREASURERS

1906–1912	C. Powell-White
1913–1922	J.C. Ledingham
1923	E. Emrys-Roberts (died in office)
1924–1927	E.E. Glynn
1928–1936	E.H. Kettle (died in office)
1937–1947	J. McIntosh (died in office)
1948–1965	R.W. Scarff
1966–1969	A.C. Thackary
1970–1981	W.G. Spector
1982–1993	A.M. Neville
1993–2003	D.A. Levison
2003–date	A.D. Burt

APPENDIX 5: A CHRONOLOGICAL LIST OF SOCIETY ADMINISTRATORS

1989–1999	Mrs J. Edwards
1999–2001	Mrs J. Edwards and Mrs R.A. Pitts (deputy)
2001–2003	Mrs R.A. Pitts and Miss J. Smith (deputy)
2003–date	Mrs R.A. Pitts and Ms J. Johnstone (deputy)

APPENDIX 6: A CHRONOLOGICAL LIST OF VENUES FOR MEETINGS SINCE 1980

1980	January	Oxford
	July	Manchester
1981	January	Middlesex Hospital Medical School, London
	July	Ninewell's Hospital Medical School, Dundee
1982	January	Cambridge
	July	Sheffield
1983	January	Birmingham
	July	Edinburgh
1984	January	RPMS, London
	May	Bergen, Norway (Joint Meeting with Norwegian and Dutch Pathological Societies)
	July	Leeds
1985	January	Northwick Park Hospital, London (the 150th Scientific Meeting)
	July	Cardiff
1986	January	The London Hospital Medical School, London
	July	Dublin

1987	January	Oxford
	July	Southampton
1988	January	St Bartholomew's Hospital Medical School, London
	July	Newcastle
1989	January	University College and Middlesex Hospital Medical School, London
	July	Aberdeen
1990	January	RPMS, Hammersmith Hospital, London
	July	Nottingham, Queen's Medical Centre
1991	January	Cambridge, Addenbrooke's Hospital
	July	Queen's University of Belfast
1992	January	Guy's and St Thomas's Hospital Medical School (note held at the RPMS, Hammersmith Hospital)
	July	Manchester (Joint Meeting with Dutch Pathological Society)
1993	January	St Mary's Hospital Medical School, London
	July	Edinburgh, held at Heriot-Watt University
1994	January	Royal London and St Bartholomew's (held at QE11 Conference Centre)
	July	Glasgow
1995	January	Nuffield Dept of Pathology, Oxford
	July	Amsterdam, Joint Meeting with Dutch Pathological Society
1996	January	King's College School of Medicine and Dentistry London (held at QE11 Conference Centre)
	July	Southampton
1997	January	Royal Free Hospital School of Medicine London (held at QE11 Conference Centre)
	July	Sheffield (joint meeting with Dutch Pathological Society)
1998	January	Charing Cross Hospital School of Medicine London (held at QE11 Conference Centre)
	July	Leicester
1999	January	Cambridge
	July	Ninewell's Hospital, Dundee
2000	January	St George's Hospital Medical School London (held at QE11 Conference Centre)
	July	Nottingham
2001	January	Maastricht (in association with Dutch Pathological Society)
	July	Liverpool (1st joint meeting with the British Division of the International Academy of Pathology)
2002	July	Dublin
2003	January	First Closed Study Group: Ploidy in Pathology
	July	Bristol (2nd Joint Meeting with the British Division of the International Academy of Pathology)
2004	January	Second Closed Study Group: Molecular Pathology and targeted therapy in cancer
	July	Amsterdam (joint meeting with the Dutch Pathological Society)
2005	January	Royal London and St Bartholomew's, London
	July	Newcastle (3rd Joint Meeting with the British Division of the International Academy of Pathology)
2006	January	Cambridge
	July	Centenary Meeting, Manchester

APPENDIX 7: THE OAKLEY LECTURERS

1979	Dr C.S.F. Easmon
1980	Dr B. Duerden
1981	Dr D.N. Slater
1982	Dr D.B. Lowrie
1983	Dr T.J. Chambers
1984	Dr J.E. Heckels
1985	Dr B.A. Gusterson
1986	Dr C.W. Penn
1987	Dr A.K. Foulis
1988	Dr S.G.B. Amyer
1989	Dr K.C. Gatter
1990	Dr S.P. Borriello
1991	Dr S. Fleming
1992	Dr R.C. Matthews
1993	Dr A.D. Burt
1994	Dr J. Ketley
1995	Dr N.R. Lemoine
1996	Dr T. Baldwin
1997	Dr C.S. Herrington
1998	Dr N. Woodford
1999	Dr J.J. O'Leary
2000	Dr G.I. Murray
2001	Dr M. Novelli
2002	Dr M.-Qu Du
2003	Not awarded
2004	Dr M. Ilyas
2005	Dr K. Oien
2006	Dr H. Grabsch

APPENDIX 8: THE DONIACH LECTURERS

2003	Professor Peter Isaacson
2004	Professor Julia Polak
2005	Professor Sir Dillwyn Williams
2006	Professor Munro Neville

APPENDIX 9: THE GOUDIE LECTURERS AND MEDALISTS

2005	Professor David Wynford-Thomas
2006	Professor Ian Hart

APPENDIX 10: A CHRONOLOGICAL LIST OF EDITORS OF THE *JOURNAL OF PATHOLOGY* (FORMERLY *JOURNAL OF PATHOLOGY AND BACTERIOLOGY*)

1892–1920	G. Sims Woodhead (founder)
1920–1922	J. Ritchie

1923–1933	A.E. Boycott
1934–1955	M.J. Stewart
1956–1971	C.L. Oakley
1971–1981	W.G. Spector (died in office)
1981–1992	D.H. Wright
1992–2002	P.G. Toner
2002–date	C.S. Herrington

APPENDIX 11: *FUTURE OF ACADEMIC PATHOLOGY*

Report of the Residential Meeting held at The Bellhouse Hotel, Beaconsfield, 28–30 March 2001

1. Introduction

1.1 There are many indicators that academic productivity in pathology in the UK is severely in decline: the reasons for this are manifold. However, it is difficult to understand because modern academic pathology underpins such a great deal of research. There is a need for accurate surgical pathological diagnosis in the context of clinical trials, in the classification of tissue banks (now so essential for the post-genomic era), the need for gene expression localisation in tissues and the burgeoning demand for phenotyping of transgenic and knockout mice, etc. In addition to this collaborative potential, pathologists are best placed to reap the benefits of translational research emanating from the enormous output from cell and molecular biology: before having as impact on therapy, these advances will benefit pathology, particularly in molecular diagnostics. Pathologists should be leading these programmes and, moreover, should be ideally placed to lead research groups looking at both basic and translational aspects of the pathogenesis of disease.

1.2 During the meeting, a number of areas were identified in an attempt to rectify this situation. In some cases these could be translated into discrete action points, with responsibilities. In some areas there was obviously further work needed before action could be taken and, finally, there were instances where the suggestions were rather nebulous and difficult to grasp in terms of specific actions, needing further consideration.

2. Research in pathology

2.1 It is fairly clear that, judged on a national level, research activity in pathology is in quite a desperate situation in terms of both quality and quantity. There is undoubtedly a problem in the recognition of pathologists as leaders in research: in many instances pathologists are viewed as mere 'facilitators' enabling other research group leaders to achieve their potential and appear well down in the authorship pecking order. This is notwithstanding the important observation that without such pathological collaboration, be it in the recognition of the phenotype of a knockout mouse and relating it to human disease, the detailed morphological analysis of an experimental or clinical procedure or the provision of accurately classified material from a tissue bank, such research cannot prosper. Nevertheless, within this environment, pathologists must assert ownership of their own ideas and fight for the right to be recognised.

At the same time, it is recognised that we are not producing sufficient numbers of research group leaders who, with programme grant level support, can pursue their own research questions from a pathology perspective. We stand accused of having limited horizons and being insufficiently innovative to attract programme support.

2.2 In general, two streams of research activity in pathology can be identified:
(i) research aimed at the elucidation of basic mechanisms of disease and the translation of these observations into the clinic and (ii) what might be termed 'academic surgical pathology'.

2.3 The training required to carry out effective research in these two spheres is different. The former requires the training of individuals who will be able to lead a research group of younger pathologists and doctoral and postdoctoral scientists. Research training for such a career would start with a clearly identified period of study leading to the award of a PhD. There was considerable discussion about the correct timing for this: either after the completion of the CCST or immediately after the SHO year, before specialist training is started. It was felt, without being prescriptive, that normally the best time was post-SHO, although it was recognised that by the time the CCST is completed there is a danger of techniques and concepts, etc. in the chosen field being out of date. However, it was felt that this was outweighed by the establishment of research experience and lines of thought at an early age. The need to ensure a smooth return to the NHS component of training was emphasised.

After completion of the CCST, this research career track should be continued with a period of postdoctoral study and in the case of medically qualified pathologists should be pursued in a Saville-type clinician scientist position, enabling the individual to have five or more years during which clinical work would be carried out but the majority of this time would be spent establishing the basis of a research career, with the usual provisos – mentoring, transferability, the achievement of consultant status (and salary), when appropriate, and the expectation of a career-post at senior lecturer level when this was completed.

In the past both of these avenues could be pursued via the clinical lecturer route. However, it was clear that the past decade has seen a dramatic reduction in the number of these positions, for several reasons, among them the need to contribute as a full-time equivalent (FTE) to the Research Assessment Exercise (RAE), problems in university funding, loss of the clinical epithet with conversion to non-clinical scientist posts, etc. It was felt very strongly that actions should be taken to rectify this position if at all possible.

2.4 In the case of academic surgical pathology, the training required may be quite different. Usually, individuals interested in this avenue would complete the examinations for Membership of the Royal College of Pathologists and then undertake a programme of training in a sub-specialty, such as gastrointestinal pathology or dermatopathology, in a recognised centre, which would culminate in the award of the CCST. After this, further training in the sub-specialty may be undertaken. It was recognised that currently trainees were being put off entering such sub-specialties because of lack of information about the future viability of that sub-specialty as a career, i.e. manpower and future funding. This was seen as a significant disincentive to specialise, and without such specialisation the prospects of that individual contributing to academic surgical pathology are limited. Of course, these two programmes are not mutually exclusive and opportunities do exist for individuals to, for example, finish a PhD and then undertake sub-specialty training in preparation for a career in academic surgical pathology.

2.5 It was clear from the several presentations from the grant-giving bodies that there are ample opportunities for young pathologists to apply for competitive fellowships to study for a PhD. However, it was conceded that, at this time, pathology is in such a state that there could be problems about the competitiveness of potential candidates, and the possibility of earmarked fellowships for pathologists was discussed.

It was recognised, therefore, that our problem is not the lack of availability of fellowships at this level but our ability to supply credible candidates.

2.6 The question of clinician scientist appointments is more complex. The Saville Report suggests that 50 such fellowships per year should suffice to underpin a future cadre of clinical academics nationally. It was felt that pathology should bid for five of these.

We heard that funding from the MRC, the Wellcome Trust and the NHS was expected for these and of course pathologists could compete in open competition. Moreover, it was noted that the MRC currently has such a fellowship in conjunction with the Royal College of Physicians, an example we could well emulate with our College. However, because of the special relationship between cancer and pathology, the cancer charities may be interested in funding such fellowships in pathology. Indeed, the CRC has a joint fellowship with the Royal College of Surgeons. However, the CRC has not yet decided whether to support these fellowships more generally, although the ICRF has indeed outlined its support for such a scheme.

2.7 However, all grant-giving bodies present noted that few current grant proposals to their scientific committees originated from pathologists. This is a further contributor to our low hit rate in grant support – the failure to even ask!

2.8 In academic surgical pathology there was some concern about the ability of the system to provide *ad hoc* specialty training post-MRCPath. The example of US fellowships was examined where individuals, usually post-general anatomical pathology Boards, obtain two-year fellowships in gastrointestinal pathology, etc. that consist of a year of training in the subject followed by a research project in the field. This concept was endorsed with the proviso that funding, which in the USA is generally out of private practice, may be difficult.

2.9 It was felt strongly that the RAE had been singularly unhelpful, if not destructive, especially in the sphere of academic surgical pathology. It was also felt that such activities, published perforce in journals with low impact factors and relying on classical morphological techniques, are not rated by our peers/assessors. It was felt, too, that this was one important reason why surgical pathological research is no longer regarded as being important in this country, why the USA is now the centre of such activity and why we have lost a number of our leading surgical pathologists to the USA in recent years. It is possible for academic surgical pathologists to be international leaders in their field and yet be considered to be barely returnable in the RAE.

It was also felt that the RAE has been responsible for the selection policy for chairs of pathology in this country with, in the main, researchers in basic/translational research being selected for such positions. We had signally failed to produce a cadre of pathologists who could pursue such research from a firm basis of surgical pathology.

The majority opinion was that the last RAE had done a severe disservice to pathology: those Higher Education Institutions who did achieve 5^* in UoA 1 were those without significant commitments to clinical work or undergraduate teaching. If similar criteria were applied in the next RAE, given the heavy clinical and teaching loads that many academic departments of pathology carry, then we are likely to see a further reduction in the profile and content of these departments in the next quinquennium.

2.10 It was recognised that, although pathologists are important in supporting the research of Trusts that receive portfolio funding (‘Support for Science’) from the NHS R&D Budget, there are limited opportunities for pathologists to benefit directly from such monies. However, the announcement of the ‘Needs and Priorities’, previously Budget 2, may provide such opportunities.

It was clear that neither paper (‘Support for Science’ nor ‘Needs and Priorities’) provided anything in the way of infrastructure or support of the research culture and ethos in Trusts to promote research as a core activity rather than a marginal pursuit. Pathology services are very much part of this infrastructure and it was again clear that in few, if any, places are NHS R&D Directors correctly identifying the resource implications for projects that require pathological support. In fact, the same criticism can be made of grant proposals to, for example, the research councils. Members were urged to press for such resources to be identified in both Culyer-type and grant-funded research.

2.11 It was recognised that probably the single most important factor impeding successful research by clinical academics in pathology is lack of protected time. It was agreed that senior lecturers or equivalent must have a strictly controlled job plan, preferably within the context of a Departmental Job Plan. Of course, it is one thing to argue this and quite another to ensure that it happens in the face of increased clinical load, staff shortages and burgeoning numbers of medical students. Nevertheless, this was regarded as a *sine qua non.*

2.12 It was established that, although the Wellcome Trust does not support overtly clinical cancer research, there is no reason why applications for basic or translational research related to cancer should not be funded.

Action points

(i) Enter discussions with the CRC and the ICRF about the possibility of supporting Clinician Scientist Fellowships targeted in specific areas such as transgenic mouse pathology, etc.: bring this to the attention of the National Cancer Research Institute chaired by Sir George Radda. The importance to the Wellcome Trust of mouse phenotyping should be noted (*PathSoc*).

(ii) Enter discussions with the major funding bodies for a quota of fellowships at doctoral and Clinician Scientist level to rejuvenate the discipline (*PathSoc*).

(iii) Open discussions with the newly established RCPath Research Committee, the Committee of The Pathological Society and the MRC, Wellcome Trust, CRC and ICRF about the possibility of joint fellowships (*RCPath/PathSoc*).

(iv) Establish a register of specialist positions within the country, together with an indication of expected future needs (*RCPath*).

(v) Explore the possibility of earmarking some of the presently available fully funded SpR positions to provide specialty training positions or fellowships in selected centres throughout the country (*RCPath*).

(vi) Strive to re-establish the Clinical Lecturer grade in pathology: this could be pursued at the local level through the Medical School Deans and also at the national level through the CHMS. The possibility of requesting that such a position should only count 0.5 FTE in the RAE was also raised to take into account the clinical training component of the post (*Profs/Deans/CHMS*).

(vii) Representations should be made to the Chairmen of UoA 1 and 3 that due recognition of the contribution of pathology departments to clinical service and teaching is very important in preserving the discipline as an academic subject (*PathSoc*).

(viii) Every effort should be made to identify the appropriate resource implications for collaborative projects that require pathological input in both NHS R&D and grant-funded research (*Profs/Directors of R&D*).

(ix) There must be a concerted effort to ensure that academics do not do more than three fixed sessions per week and that protected time for research is mandatory (*Profs/Deans*).

(x) There should be a concerted campaign to ensure that academic pathologists be proposed for the Fellowship of the Academy of Medical Sciences (*Fellows of the Academy*).

3. The relationship with the NHS

3.1 As in academic departments, a crisis exists in District General Hospitals (DGHs) with increasing workload, reduction in manpower and a reduction in time available for those individuals in post. A major component of this problem is the lack of agreement about the workload suitable for pathologists working in different environments: for example, the RCPath guidelines suggest that consultant pathologists in DGHs should do 4000 surgicals and in teaching hospitals

2000, although this takes no account of the complexity of the case mix. The latter figure also does not distinguish between clinical academics and NHS consultants. It was agreed that the College guidelines required updating.

3.2 There are other recent developments that impinge on the time pathologists have available for research: with the advent of minimum data sets it is not unusual for a large specimen to take 40 min to dissect. Other constraints include the burgeoning number of endoscopic biopsies, immunohistochemistry, the increase in multi-disciplinary meetings in the wake of the Calman–Hine proposals, the management role of pathologists, Calman training to be equilibrated with the idea of a consultant-led service, Comprehensive Performance Assessment, audit, Environmental Quality Assessment, Continuing Professional Development and undergraduate teaching and service reviews, which all militate against an active research career once a consultant position is attained. Professor Richards pointed out that, with the increase in screening, this workload will rise further. Presently a paper by Professor Lowe is being considered by the RCPath that sets out the problems pathologists face with an increasing workload and suggests ways of regulating it.

3.3 It was agreed that a good deal of academic activity, particularly in surgical pathology, is carried out by NHS consultants, some of whom are in DGHs, and that a problem exists in harnessing and enfranchising NHS pathologists into academia. Academics and NHS pathologists can live in the same cage.

3.4 There is a need to acknowledge the contributions that DGH pathologists make to surgical pathology research and to bring them on board.

3.5. Histopathology in the UK, unlike others such as the USA, does not have a national referral centre to which difficult cases may be sent for an opinion, which is often needed urgently. Currently, pathologists all over the country and abroad have a list of individuals to whom they refer such cases, from whom experience has shown that an early response is usually obtained and a helpful consultation results. A survey carried out of members of the Association revealed that a large number of referred cases are being carried out by academic departments all over the country. The load varies from 150 to 740 cases per annum per individual and was thought to amount to a minimum of one session a week per pathologist. It must be emphasised that this work is carried out, in the main, for the benefit of patients in the NHS and in addition to any other duties that the pathologist has.

3.6 In most instances this activity is not funded by the department referring the case and experience has shown that the introduction of charging for this service results in a sharp reduction in referrals. The singular attempt to fund this service via ‘extra-contractual referrals’ has transparently failed. It is certainly time that this country regularised this ludicrously *ad hoc* system.

Action points

(i) NHS pathologists must be enfranchised into academic pathology and feel that they are very much part of the system (*Everyone/PathSoc*).

(ii) Centres where referrals are currently made should be listed and a database set up showing the experts available, with their sub-specialty (*Prof Elston et al*).

(iii) These centres should form a Virtual Institute of Pathology that should be funded by top-slicing the regional budget. In addition to paying for materials and technical time, consultant sessions should be charged to this budget. The example of Cardiff was noted, where one consultant FTE is available to provide support for the referral service. We should engage with Specialist Commissioning Agencies and also determine whether the National Specialist Commissioniry Advisory Group would be interested in funding at least part of this venture (*Prof Elston et al*).

(iv) It is suggested that the money earmarked for cancer, which Health Authorities have been charged with releasing, is an appropriate source of such funding. In this respect, members were encouraged to approach this source as a means of supporting the infrastructure, such as personal assistants, etc. (*Prof Elston et al.*).

4. Appraisal and revalidation

4.1 Although the GMC's thinking about the revalidation of clinical academics had not fully crystallised, it was expected that pathologists would be revalidated upon what they returned: for example, if they stated that they were a gynaecological pathologist then that is what they would be assessed on to remain on the general register, and so on. It was felt that this was a constructive way forward.

4.2 However, it was appreciated that there was a great gulf between the so-called craft specialties, such as pathology, where endpoints are easily measured, and the non-craft specialties, such as dermatology, where measurement is not so easy.

5. Manpower

5.1 The reasons for the crisis in manpower were rehearsed (again!). Unless something is done, and now, there will be a tremendous shortage of pathologists. Negotiations between the College and the Department of Health has led to the provision of 160 fully funded SpRs over the next three years. A way around the provision of microscopes for these individuals has been found in that once the post has been approved the money is available; any lead-time funding until the position is filled can be used for the purchase of a microscope. Unfortunately, there is no provision of funds for overtime and it was calculated that each SpR on 1B payments would cost a department £8000 a year. Although this is good news, there is evidently a long way to go because we are probably some 460–560 SpR positions short.

5.2 Enquiries among members showed that a major constraint to increasing the number of trainees in histopathology was the 'ability to train'. Leaving aside the problems implicit in declining numbers of staff available to train because of shortages and the increase in the clinical load, it was felt strongly that there was just not enough space and facilities to provide placements for further trainees in many departments. Thus an important concept arose, that the need to train was being hindered not by a lack of willingness to train but, in a number of cases, by the lack of facilities.

5.3 The proposal that SHO Schools should be established was supported strongly, as was the concept that retired pathologists should be recruited to teach in these schools.

5.4 The effect of remuneration on recruitment to academic pathology was discussed and it was agreed that there were obviously problems involved here: not only the financial sacrifice that young academic pathologists make in continuing to work in the university environment when colleagues of the same age in the NHS are often earning a great deal more, but also the problems that academics have in winning discretionary points and distinction awards. It was noted that this would not improve owing to the emphasis on service work. Similarly, there was no guarantee that the New Consultant Contract, with its proposal to financially reward new NHS consultants who do not do private practice, would be extended to the academic sector.

Action points

(i) It was proposed that the MADEL budget be considered for the provision of facilities for training. An enquiry of Charles Easmon has suggested that revenue budgets are perhaps not the right place for this and that approaches should be made centrally on this important issue and also locally at the Chief Executive Officer level (*Profs/RCPath/Quirke*).

(ii) It was suggested that the concept of SHO Schools should be extended to SpRs, and that, because of the sharp drop in the exposure of trainees to autopsy pathology, autopsy schools should be established (*Quirke*).

(iii) Members felt that the lack of ability to pay overtime could be an important disincentive to the recruitment of increased numbers of SpRs, and that further representations should be made on this point (*Quirke/Heard*).

(iv) Where provision of a sub-specialist service is concerned, it becomes very important to define the sub-specialist because of the provision of funding (*Quirke*).

(v) The RCPath recovery plan for histopathology should be strongly supported (*Everyone*).

(vi) Every effort should be made to ensure that academic pathologists be put up for discretionary points and proposed for distinction awards at every opportunity. Reassurance should also be sought that the New Consultant Contract will include newly appointed clinical academics (*Everyone/RCPath*).

6. Public profile of pathologists

6.1 It was agreed that pathologists have a problem with the public perception of what they do, particularly in the wake of Alder Hey. It was even suggested that we should consider a change in the name of our discipline but this was rejected in favour of preserving our name and undertaking a programme of public education.

Action points

(i) It was felt that the profession in general does not have a political strategy and that, with the College and the PathSoc, we should evolve a strategy that would incorporate political aims (*PathSoc/College*).

(ii) A number of useful ideas about improving our image were proposed, from commissioning television programmes (at least two programmes on what pathologists do are known to be in production) and also the possibility of other media approaches, via the newspapers or indeed through literature, which is presently limited to forensic pathology (*PathSoc*).

7. Undergraduate medical education

7.1 In the recruitment of individuals into pathology it was agreed that the undergraduate course is of paramount importance. However, it was conceded that the opportunities for undergraduates to see pathologists in action or to understand what it is that pathologists actually do are declining rapidly.

7.2 Everyone present was an advocate of the Intercalated BSc in Pathology, whilst appreciating the decline in resources that are available.

7.3 Despite the enthusiasm for teaching pathology to students and recognition of the important role that this has had in attracting individuals into the profession, it was a constant theme that teachers do not feel valued in the modern medical school setting, where research is rewarded to a much greater degree than teaching achievements in such competitions as the annual promotion round. Currently money does not follow the score in the Quality Assurance Assessment (QAA) as it does in the RAE and universities are not, therefore, currently minded to support and reward individuals who concentrate on teaching or indeed take a major interest in it.

7.4 The pathologist as role model was a recurrent theme and many members said that this was one of the main reasons why they entered pathology. However, the very inclusion of pathology in the undergraduate curriculum is under threat and the potential for senior pathologists to act as such role models is declining.

7.5 This does not mean that there is a decline in the need for pathologists to teach. With the increase in problem-based learning, pathologists are in increasing demand to chair and coordinate such sessions. At the same time, we are seeing a large increase in medical student numbers with a resultant expectation of an increase in contact time.

7.6 It was appreciated that the initial QAA inspections had been advantageous for the development of undergraduate medical education. However, the follow-up from such inspections was viewed with some concern bearing in mind the time and effort expended in such exercises.

Action points

(i) The Intercalated BSc course must be maintained and expanded if possible and methods of financing such courses must be found. The efforts of the PathSoc in supporting these courses were appreciated and the Society was urged to extend its scheme if possible (*PathSoc*).

(ii) In future QAA rounds it would be useful to establish some sort of benchmarking scheme that emphasises pathology (*Underwood/QAA*).

(iii) It is obviously of paramount importance for medical teachers to be recognised and rewarded in the promotion round by appropriate discretionary points and distinction awards (*Deans/Profs*).

(iv) It is considered vitally important to ensure that pathology maintains its identity in the undergraduate curriculum. There must be opportunities for student participation and for students to observe at close quarters what pathologists do and for pathologists to act as role models for students during their undergraduate years. Clinicians should be encouraged to involve pathologists in teaching and pathology should be taught as a block course and be examined separately. Every effort should be made to ensure that pathology remains a core subject and is included in any National Core Curriculum (*Everyone/QAA*).

(v) Autopsy teaching should be promoted (*Everyone*).

(vi) A nationwide inventory of pathology teaching resources would be a good thing. Workforce Confederations should be approached to fund such projects in their future role as 'Educational Trusts' (*West/PathSoc*).

(vii) There was a need to promote our subject in schools and sixth-form colleges and we should consider producing a brochure for use by sixth formers (*West/PathSoc*).

8. Postgraduate education in pathology

8.1 In general the changes in the regulations for the examination of the Royal College of Pathologists were now considered to be appropriate, although some concern was expressed whether individuals could be appropriately assessed for their suitability as histopathologists during the SHO year. Concerns were also expressed about the continuing lack of uniformity in the examination but it was generally recognised that logistics would prevent centralisation.

8.2 Concern was expressed about enabling trainees to obtain sufficient experience in autopsy pathology in the face of the declining post-mortem rate.

8.3 The role of postgraduate diplomas was discussed, with the Diploma in Dermatopathology as a paradigm. It was recognised that the advent of a diploma could galvanise a sub-specialty. On the other hand, it was recognised that organising such a diploma was not a trivial undertaking and, of course, using the Diploma in Dermatopathology as an example, such diplomas would be open to clinicians who are not career pathologists.

8.4 Workforce Confederations were springing up all over the country and although it was not clear how these would work in detail the concept of them as 'Educational Trusts' was important.

8.5 Where academic pathologists are concerned it was considered very important that 'early differentiation' in terms of specialist interest was necessary.

Action points

(i) The concept of an MRCPath examination without the inclusion of a compulsory autopsy should be examined. Failing this, perhaps candidates should be asked to provide a case-book of autopsies carried out rather than carry out an autopsy at the time of the examination, which can be difficult to arrange (*Stamp*).

(ii) The PathSoc should take a larger role in the provision of training of teachers in pathology, possibly sponsoring courses over a weekend on 'how to do it' (*Berry/PathSoc*).

(iii) It would be important to align both medical schools and postgraduate pathology training with the emerging Workforce Confederations (*Deans/Profs*).

(iv) The expansion of the RCPath's portfolio of diplomas in specialist subjects should be (carefully) examined (*RCPath*).

(v) It is important that a culture be developed where differentiation of academic pathologists into sub-specialists be done at an early date to enable concentration on a single part of the discipline and also to constrain the amount of time spent on service work (*Profs/Deans/PathSoc*).

(vi) It was fairly clear that, although there are problems in recruitment in several sub-specialist areas, paediatric pathology was in a desperate strait with no trainees whatsoever! Urgent action was needed to rectify this appalling situation (*BRIPPA/Specialist Committee RCPath*).

(vii) We should work towards a CCST designed specifically for academics (*PathSoc*).

9. Constraints on academic activity

9.1 It was agreed that the expansion in bureaucracy surrounding the granting of personal and project licences to carry out animal experiments, a central technique in experimental pathology, was hindering the rate at which research in competitive areas could be carried out. This included the Ethical Review Process and the often slow rate at which applications were processed in the Home Office.

9.2 There was general support for Nancy Rothwell's initiative, which led to the covert promise from Lord Sainsbury to attempt to streamline the approval process.

9.3 There was also concern expressed about the growing violent opposition to individuals who undertake such work.

9.4 The problems surrounding organ retention, the Alder Hey and Bristol inquiries and the potential and now actual effects on access to material retained at post-mortem and indeed after surgical operations were again rehearsed, with special emphasis on the effects on research, training and the maintenance of standards via examinations, EQA and, indeed, referral of material for diagnosis.

9.5 The emergent MRC guidelines were noted, which, in particular, state that the principle of abandonment after, say, surgical operation is not appropriate and that all tissue has to be individually gifted. It was also noted that these guidelines have specific recommendations for histopathologists seeking to do research on archival material where, even for simple investigations such as re-examination of routinely stained sections, informed consent is needed.

9.6 Although there have been several suggestions for the design of an appropriate consent form, it was clear that different forms were in use all over the country.

Action points

(i) Initiatives to reduce the amount of bureaucracy involved in the granting of animal licences and to increase the security of researchers involved in experiments on animals (*Martin/Wright*).

(ii) Although there was some feeling that we are stuck with the MRC guidelines, some members felt that the principle of abandonment against gifting should be tested and that the guidelines, where they impinge upon simple archival histopathological research, should be challenged. In any case, it was felt that it would be impossible to implement these guidelines without some sort of a grandfather clause that would become operative at some time after the acceptance of the guidelines (*Stamp/Quirke/PathSoc*).

(iii) It was felt very important that the potentially seriously damaging effects on research or lack of access to archival tissues or to properly ordered and classified tissue and organ banks should be made forcibly and publicised (*PathSoc*).

(iv) There should be a movement towards the design and acceptance of a National Ethics and Consent Form as applied to the use of human tissues for teaching and research (*Stamp/Quirke*).

(v) Because of the extreme spin put on the findings of the Alder Hey Inquiry *et sec*, it was felt essential that the profession should engage with Government (*RCPath*).

(vi) Similarly, it was also felt that professional public relations advice should be sought to put over our view on the use of human tissues for research and education (*PathSoc/RCPath*).

(vii) We should also make contact with Pharma UK to explore matters of joint concern and in any campaign underline the potential effects on UK PLCs if research on human tissues is compromised (*Quirke/Stamp/RCPath*).

(viii) A campaign of public education about the use of human tissues in research should be undertaken (*PathSoc*).

(ix) Centres should consider setting up a Tissue Ethics Subcommittee, which already exists in some places, to consider requests for the use of tissues in research (*Profs*).

(x) The possibility of producing a brochure describing the value of the use of human tissues in research, for use in hospitals before and while seeking informed consent, should be explored (*PathSoc*).

10. The role of specialist societies

10.1 It was agreed that the Association of Professors of Pathology had historically done little or nothing for the profession.

10.2 It was appreciated that pathologists, both academic and service-oriented, were all in this together and that great strength lies in us all working together.

Action points

(i) The Association of Professors of Pathology should be dissolved. Instead, a group will be formed within the PathSoc that will include other academics and not only professors. It was agreed that the current gathering was a 'meeting with a future' and that every attempt should be made to hold such a meeting on an annual basis (*Boylston/Wright*).

(ii) The proposal that we should move together towards a Confederation of British Pathology Societies was applauded: we should attempt to move towards a federal annual meeting, where all member societies have their own meeting and come together for plenary sessions and for meetings such as the one we were currently experiencing. It was noted that holding such a meeting would be relatively inexpensive and logistically easy if such a federal meeting was enfranchised (*PathSoc/IAP, etc.*).

The Joint Meeting of the IAP with the PathSoc at Liverpool in July 2001, to which several specialist societies are also committed, would serve as a model for, and introduction to, this process.

Prepared by N.A. Wright, 15 June 2001

APPENDIX 12: THE PATHOLOGICAL SOCIETY: THE WAY FORWARD – A SUMMARY

Based upon the deliberations of the Officers and Committee at the Away Weekend in November 2004 and Committee Meeting of January 2005, the following proposals are made with regard to the Society's future development.

1. *A new image with a clear profile.* The mission of The Pathological Society is to increase the understanding of disease. The focus of The Pathological Society should be '*Understanding Disease*'. This includes the support and encouragement of activities that promote the understanding of disease and disease processes, as well as the furthering of educational activities that promote the understanding of disease, including education of the general public.
2. *A commitment to provide tangible benefits to the members.* The Society's programmes will be designed to help its members promote the mission of understanding disease. This will be by fostering and facilitating research, by developing and supporting programmes for undergraduate and postgraduate teaching and training, and by engaging with the general public so that they also come to *Understand Disease*.
3. *Enhanced transparency of the Society with increased membership involvement.* The Society will develop a structure that allows Members to engage more effectively with the Society's mission and be empowered by the Society to achieve more effectively an understanding of disease. This will involve a reorganisation of the Society's Governance with the creation of subcommittees with specific remits.

4. *Developing partnerships with other organisations to promote pathology.* The Pathological Society wishes to engage with other organisations and, in partnership, develop programmes that are aimed at our goal of understanding disease.

A New Image?

The justification for redefining the Society's Mission Statement comes from the simple point that our current Mission Statement is long, all encompassing and, as a consequence, somewhat vague. It lacks focus and thus does not allow our Society to be distinguished from many others. What are we about? What are we for? Why be a member? It was these issues that led to the realisation that we could define our remit in a very simple way and have a concise two word 'strap line' – *Understanding Disease*. We have already introduced this onto the cover of the *Journal of Pathology* and this defines our focus. Furthermore, that focus can be shared by those interested in the science of mechanisms in pathology, or in the science and art of diagnosis, or in the pedagological aspects of the subject: i.e. the whole range of our membership.

The financial state of the Society is strong, although there remain some uncertainties, including issues such as Open Access, that may influence the income from our Journal. Nevertheless, it was felt that as an organisation we needed to ensure that we spent a substantial fraction of our income on programmes that allow us to accomplish our mission. This we have always done, but the Away Weekend allowed us to take stock of these programmes and ask to what extent they had been effective and how they might develop in the future. Clearly the programmes will be kept on yearly review, based upon changing financial circumstances. One step will be for a 'Finance and General Purposes Committee' chaired by the Treasurer (see below) to define a budget for the coming year. This allocation is then disbursed by the full Committee through a series of subcommittees (Research, Education and Training, Programme, Trainees; see below).

Tangible Benefits?

What programmes should we have?

1. *Meetings and Workshops*. A core programme of the Society is, and will continue to be, the support and running of meetings. The Pathological Society will support four types of meeting:

   - *Annual Meetings* will be held alone or in partnership with other bodies and are the major Scientific Meeting of the Society. These meetings will be organised by the Meetings Secretary together with a Programme Subcommittee. Suggestions for Symposia or other elements of such meetings are welcomed. The major meeting will be in the summer but a winter meeting will also be held. Although the meetings will be research orientated, the needs of Continuing Professional Development and lifelong learning will be core to any programme, as will aspects of training and undergraduate education.
   - *Focused or Themed Meetings or Workshops will be supported, wholly or in part*, on topics of interest to the Membership in any area of pathological science, research and education. Such meetings can be from one to three days in any part of the United Kingdom or Ireland, or on occasions elsewhere in Europe. In addition the Society welcomes proposals for joint events with other organisations and will offer (by negotiation) secretarial support. Proposals should be made by Members in the form of a preliminary outline and costing. Applications must indicate clearly how the Society's image and contribution will be recognised and advertised.
   - *Independent Meetings* are meetings organised entirely by an outside organisation for which The Pathological Society offers support for specific speakers or sessions up to a maximum

of £5000. Proposals should be made by Members in the form of a preliminary outline and costing. Applications must indicate clearly how the Society's image and contribution will be recognised and advertised.

- *Local Scientific Meetings* will be supported up to a maximum of £1000 in order to subsidise the reasonable costs of speakers (but not Honoraria). Proposals should be made by Members in the form of a preliminary outline and costing. Applications must indicate clearly how the Society's image and contribution will be recognised and advertised.

Support for meetings will be determined by the Finance and General Purposes Subcommittee with input from the other subcommittees (Programme, Education and Training, Research and Trainees). Financial support for the latter three categories will come from the Open Scheme (see below) allocation and applications for these three types of meeting will be considered by the Finance and General Purposes Subcommittee on a quarterly basis.

2. *Intercalated Degree Scheme.* Intercalated degrees (both BSc and MSc) continue to be a fertile ground for developing enquiring minds for entry into many aspects of clinical practice, including (but not restricted to) Academia. The Society wishes to support this and proposes to increase the number of awards to eight, with the caveat that there should be some demonstrable pathological component (in the broadest sense). This will be the remit of the Education Subcommittee but awarded by ballot of applicants.

3. *Elective and Vacation Bursary.* The Society currently awards modest sums of money (up to £150 per week for 8 weeks, based upon Wellcome Trust vacation bursary allowances) to undergraduate students for elective and vacation study in the broad area of pathological science. As with the intercalated programme, the Society regards the support of such undergraduate activity as a cornerstone of its activities, potentially encouraging students to pursue pathologically related careers and certainly providing educational opportunities. (Remit of Education Subcommittee)

4. *Pilot Grant Scheme.* We have previously provided modest support (up to £5000) for the development of research projects for trainees in pathology. This has been reasonably popular and successful in that work funded by such support has been presented at Society meetings. We wish to retain and extend this programme and re-badge it as a Pilot Grant Scheme, opening access, to a wider group and emphasising that applications from trainees or recently appointed (within 3 years) Consultants are particularly welcomed. (Remit of Research Subcommittee)

5. *Travel Awards.* The Society will support applications from members to attend Scientific meetings in order to present their work. Support of up to £1000 will be for those who can provide evidence of matching funds from other sources. Applications for smaller sums would be particularly welcomed and applications relating to work that has been presented at Society meetings will be favoured. In addition, a limited number of bursaries (*Conference Bursaries*) to cover the cost of registration will be made available to assist *PhD students* to attend meetings of the Society where they are presenting their research. (Remit of Programme Subcommittee).

6. *Fellowship Scheme.* The purpose of this programme is to provide financial support for travel to learn new techniques in other laboratories. Support can be for travel, accommodation and living allowance or for laboratory expenses (but not bench fees *per se*). (Remit of Research Subcommittee) Note that a requirement of the Charities Commission is that, some awards can be open to non-members and this Scheme is duly advertised biannually in the Biomedical press.

7. *PhD Programme.* On an annual basis, applications from members (in good standing for at least 1 year) will be considered for the award of a three-year PhD Studentship. The award will be competitive and based upon peer review of the scientific proposal and training environment. This will be calculated as MRC stipend plus fees plus a contribution to consumables and travel up to a maximum of £20000 per annum (for three years). (Remit of Research Subcommittee)

8. *Open Scheme.* The purpose of the Open Scheme is to promote any activity that promotes the Mission of the Society that is not covered by the other specified schemes. This will include, but is not restricted to, the range of meetings discussed above. Proposals that promote public awareness and understanding of pathology (in the broadest sense) will be welcomed, including public lectures and similar public awareness schemes. (Remit of Finance and General Purposes Subcommittee)

The range of schemes and programmes will be kept under continual review and the success and their effectiveness (or otherwise) will be monitored continually by the Committee.

New Governance Arrangements?

With regard to the governance of the Society it was felt that this needs to be more transparent, with the roles and responsibilities of different groups being better defined. The proposed structure is out lined below.

The Society Membership elects the President, who is in post for 3 years and can be elected for a maximum of two terms. We propose the introduction of a post of President-elect, which would mean the proleptic appointment of the President 1 year before he/she takes office. The first such election would occur in 2005 because Nick Wright demits office in July 2006. The Society Membership also elects the General Secretary, the Treasurer and the Meetings Secretary, each for a period of 5 years. The membership also elects the 16 members of the Committee, all of whom serve for a maximum of 3 years. The Officers and Committee can co-opt other members and have brought three such persons on to the Committee (again for 3-year periods): Elaine Kay to represent the Republic of Ireland, Paul van der Valk to represent The Netherlands and Paola Domizio to begin a process where we develop Educational and Training Programmes. The webmaster (Jim Lowe, an increasingly important position) and the Editor-in-Chief (Simon Herrington) of our journal, the *Journal of Pathology*, are also in attendance at meetings of the Committee. Officers and members of the Committee have a legal function in that they are Trustees of the Society and answerable to the Charities Commission. The Society and the Committees are ably supported by an administrator (Mrs Ross Pitts) and her deputy (Ms Julie Johnston). The full Committee is responsible for all Society matters and is accountable to the membership.

Previously many decisions were taken by the Officers who formed the Officers Committee (chaired by the President) and met four times a year. It is proposed that this committee is disbanded and replaced by a *Finance and General Purposes Subcommittee* that is chaired by the Treasurer and is constituted by him and the other elected Officers plus the webmaster and Editor-in-Chief who are both in attendance. The function of this Subcommittee is to undertake the general business of the Society and report all activities to the full Committee. A second function is to manage the Society's finances and determine on an annual basis a budget for the support of all Society programmes. The Finance and General Services Subcommittee would meet four times a year.

A *Programme Subcommittee* will be created. This be chaired by the Meetings Secretary and be made up of the lead person from each of the forthcoming venues for Society meetings (summer and winter) for the next 3 years plus the lead person from the immediate past venue. This allows continuity while facilitating turnover, and maximises information transfer about the detail of running meetings, which is one of our key programmes. The IAP Council Meetings Secretary should attend these meetings in order to foster good relations and coordinate joint meetings. As well as being involved in the practicalities of running meetings, the Programme Subcommittee will be responsible for the allocation of travel funds, making recommendations to the full Committee. A final task will be the consideration of all aspects of meetings programmes and bringing proposals to the full Committee. The Programme Subcommittee would meet twice a year at the time of the Society's main meetings.

A *Research Subcommittee* will be created. This will be chaired by a nominee from the Full Subcommittee for 3 years (extending beyond their tenure on the full Subcommittee) and Stewart Fleming has agreed to take this on in the first instance. This will be serviced by the Treasurer and there will be a further six members derived from current committee members (i.e. people go on to the Research Subcommittee while they are on the main committee and stay on even when they are off the main committee). The Research Subcommittee will have the power to co-opt additional members as deemed necessary. The functions will include the development of a research strategy for the Society, and peer review and assessment of those programmes and award schemes of the Society that are research based. In addition, it will endeavour to develop a peer review mechanism for small research projects that have had no peer review by another body. This would only be open to full members in good standing for more than 1 year. The Research Subcommittee would also aspire to develop training programmes with regard to research governance and research ethics advice, perhaps through the use of web-based tutorials. The Research Subcommittee will meet twice a year at the time of the Societies main meetings.

An *Education and Training Subcommittee* will be created. We have not developed this area sufficiently in the past. Prof. Paola Domizio has been co-opted on to the full Committee for 3 years to begin the development of this important Subcommittee, which will have the goal of advising the committee on the development of a strategy for this key area. In addition it will assess those programmes and award schemes of the Society that are education and training based and will liase with the Programme Subcommittee to ensure that educational and training issues are appropriately represented in all Society Meetings. The Sub-subcommittee will be serviced by the President (or President elect) and (eventually) have six additional members who will join the Education and Training Subcommittee while they are on the full Committee (extending beyond their tenure on the full Committee, and as with the Research Subcommittee this then allows turnover). The Education and Training Subcommittee will have the power to co-opt additional members as deemed necessary. The Education and Training Subcommittee would meet twice a year at the time of the Society's main meetings.

The Society has the aspiration of creating a *Trainees Subcommittee* which will have the remit of acting as a forum for trainees, a mechanism for the views of trainees to be brought to the committee, and of liaising with the Research Subcommittee and Education and Training Subcommittee so that the needs of trainees can be fully considered. Discussions are currently taking place on how best to effectively and fairly fill positions on this important committee.

Fostering Links?

Academic medicine and in particular academic pathology has not thrived in recent years and there are many external pressures that have led to this. The Pathological Society can work to promote (in the broadest sense) academic pathology but success will involve concerted action by us and other groups. We already have excellent and developing relations with organisations such at the Royal College of Pathologists and the British Division of the International Academy of Pathology. Partnership with these and other organisations can only be in the best interests of pathology in the broadest sense. We seek to foster and develop such interactions, while being mindful of the need to preserve the identities and traditions of all partner organisations.

Conclusion

The proposals are intended to help the Society to achieve its Mission, in a transparent, timely and financially prudent manner, and to deliver the maximum benefit for its members and the wider community.

Peter Hall
General Secretary, on behalf of Officers and Committee
February 2005

Index

Mouse Models of Human Blood Cancers

Printed in the United States of America
Printed in the United States of America

Shaoguang Li
Editor

Mouse Models of Human Blood Cancers

Basic Research and Pre-Clinical Applications

Springer

Editor
Shaoguang Li
Division of Hematology/Oncology
Department of Medicine
University of Massachusetts
Medical School
Worcester, MA 01605, USA
Shaoguang.Li@umassmed.edu

ISBN: 978-0-387-69130-5 e-ISBN: 978-0-387-69132-9
DOI: 10.1007/978-0-387-69132-9

Library of Congress Control Number: 2008931589

© 2008 Springer Science+Business Media, LLC
All rights reserved. This work may not be translated or copied in whole or in part without the written permission of the publisher (Springer Science + Business Media, LLC, 233 Spring Street, New York, NY 10013, USA), except for brief excerpts in connection with reviews or scholarly analysis. Use in connection with any form of information storage and retrieval, electronic adaptation, computer software, or by similar or dissimilar methodology now known or hereafter developed is forbidden. The use in this publication of trade names, trademarks, service marks, and similar terms, even if they are not identified as such, is not to be taken as an expression of opinion as to whether or not they are subject to proprietary rights.

Printed on acid-free paper

9 8 7 6 5 4 3 2 1

springer.com

Preface

Although it remains an open question among some people whether mice and humans are similar in disease development, the laboratory mouse has emerged as the pre-eminent animal model for human diseases. This is underscored by the recently completed mouse and human genome projects, which have revealed that mice and humans share the vast majority of their genes and thus get many of the same diseases and for the same reasons. For example, many mouse tumor models reflect at least some major characteristics of the corresponding human cancers. It is believed that continuously improved mouse models will play a critical role in understanding disease mechanisms and developing effective therapies for human cancers.

The use of mouse models for cancer research has a long history. In 1929, Dr. Clarence C. Little, a Harvard-trained geneticist, founded The Jackson Laboratory with the vision of generating and using inbred strains of mice to study the genetic basis of cancer. Since then, The Jackson Laboratory has become the world's leading and largest mouse genetics institution for the study and distribution of genetically defined mice, including those that develop cancers. In 1983, the National Institute of Health's National Cancer Institute designated the Laboratory as a National Cancer Center, a status that has been maintained since then. As a cancer researcher at The Jackson Laboratory, I took advantage of the broad range of expertise available here by inviting several Jackson Laboratory cancer researchers to participate in the writing of the book. In addition, to integrate expert opinions from other leading cancer researchers into the book, I invited several outstanding scientists in the blood cancer field outside of The Jackson Laboratory to contribute to the book. I am grateful to have had the opportunity to work with the book contributors, and I have learned a great deal by reading their chapters.

In this book, we emphasize why mouse models are valuable in vivo systems for understanding disease mechanisms and developing therapeutic strategies for human blood cancers. We focus on mouse models of blood cancers with the aim of presenting thorough analyses of the pathological features and the molecular bases of the diseases. However, our intent is not to cover all types of blood cancers; instead, we focus on several major types of blood cancer.

Besides the emphases on the description of variable mouse models of human blood cancers and on the study of disease mechanisms using the models, another focus area of the book is to describe translational research using mouse cancer models, including the models that would be valuable but are not yet available. Such translational research includes identification of critical signaling pathways in cancer cells and the development of novel therapeutic strategies against identified molecular targets. Other important topics are also addressed, including the influence of genome instability and dietary restriction on cancer development, and genetic and virological predisposition to lymphoid cell transformation. Furthermore, a novel method for DNA microarray data analysis is introduced as a potentially valuable method for future research using mouse cancer models. I believe that our areas of research focus will distinguish this book from others currently available that cover topics related to the study of human blood cancers in mouse models.

We acknowledge Stephen Sampson for helpful comments and Patricia Cherry for the secretarial assistance.

Bar Harbor, ME Shaoguang Li

Contents

Contributors

Lura Brianna Caddle
The Jackson Laboratory, Bar Harbor, ME 04609, USA,
brianna.caddle@jax.org

Robin P. Ertl
The Jackson Laboratory, Bar Harbor, ME 04609, USA,
robin.ertl@jax.org

David E. Harrison
The Jackson Laboratory, Bar Harbor, ME 04609, USA,
david.harrison@jax.org

Hiroshi Hiai
Shiga Medical Center Research Institute, 5-4-30 Moriyama, City of Moriyama,
Shiga 524-8524, Japan, hiai@shigamed.jp

Yiguo Hu
The Jackson Laboratory, Bar Harbor, ME, USA,
yiguo.hu@jax.org

Fumihiko Ishikawa
Research Unit for Human Disease Models, RIKEN Research Center for
Allergy and Immunology, Yokohama 230-0045, Japan, f_ishika@rcai.riken.jp

Siegfried Janz
Department of Pathology, Carver College of Medicine, University of Iowa,
500 Newton Road, 1046C ML, Iowa City, IA 52242, USA,
Siegfried-janz@uiowa.edu

Jeffery L. Kutok
Brigham and Women's Hospital, Harvard Medical School, Department of
Pathology, Boston, MA 02115, USA, jkutok@partners.org

Benjamin H. Lee
Brigham and Women's Hospital, Harvard Medical School, Department of
Pathology, Boston, MA 02115, USA, bhlee@partners.org

Francis Lee
Bristol-Myers Squibb Research and Development, Oncology Discovery, Princeton, NJ 08543, USA, francis.lee@bms.com

Dongguang Li
School of Computer and Information Science, Faculty of Computing, Health and Science, Edith Cowan University, Mount Lawley, WA 6050, Australia, d.li@ecu.edu.au

Shaoguang Li
The Jackson Laboratory, Bar Harbor, ME 04609, USA, shaoguang.li@jax.org
Current Address: Division of Hematology/Oncology, Department of Medicine, University of Massachusetts Medical School, Worcester, MA 01605, USA, Shaoguang.Li@umassmed.edu

Sarah A. Maas
The Jackson Laboratory, Bar Harbor, ME 04609, USA, sarah.maas@jax.org

Kevin D. Mills
The Jackson Laboratory, Bar Harbor, ME 04609, USA, kevin.mills@jax.org

Herbert C. Morse
Laboratory of Immunopathology, National Institute of Allergy and Infectious Diseases, National Institutes of Health, Rockville, MD 20852, USA, hmorse@niaid.nih.gov

Yoriko Saito
Research Unit for Human Disease Models, RIKEN Research Center for Allergy and Immunology, Yokohama 230-0045, Japan, ysaito@rcai.riken.jp

Leonard D. Shultz
The Jackson Laboratory, Bar Harbor, ME 04609, USA, lenny.shulta@jax.org

Michael A. Teitell
Department of Pathology and Laboratory Medicine, and Molecular Biology Institute and Jonsson Comprehensive Cancer Center, David Geffen School of Medicine, University of California, Los Angeles, CA 90095, USA, mteitell@ucla.edu

Richard A. Van Etten
Molecular Oncology Research Institute and Division of Hematology/Oncology, Tufts Medical Center, 800 Washington Street, 5609, Boston, MA 02111, USA, rvanetten@tuftsmedicalcenter.org

Roberto Weinmann
Bristol-Myers Squibb Oncology, Princeton, NJ 08543, USA, roberto.weinmann@bms.com

Chapter 1
Mouse Models of Myeloproliferative Disease Associated with Mutant JAK2 Tyrosine Kinase: Insights into Pathophysiology and Therapy

Richard A. Van Etten

Contents

1.1 Dysregulated Tyrosine Kinases are the Hallmark of Chronic Myeloproliferative-Like Syndromes

The classical myeloproliferative diseases (MPDs) include chronic myeloid leukemia (CML), polycythemia vera (PV), essential thrombocythemia (ET), and primary myelofibrosis (PMF, also known as myelofibrosis with myeloid metaplasia or agnogenic myeloid metaplasia). These diseases were first grouped together by Dr. William Dameshek of Tufts-New England Medical Center in

R.A. Van Etten
Molecular Oncology Research Institute and Division of Hematology/Oncology, Tufts Medical Center, 800 Washington Street, 5609, Boston, MA 02111, USA
rvanetten@tuftsmedicalcenter.org

S. Li (ed.), *Mouse Models of Human Blood Cancers*,
DOI: 10.1007/978-0-387-69132-9_1, © Springer Science+Business Media, LLC 2008

a seminal paper in *Blood* in 1951 (Dameshek 1951). The MPDs are clonal disorders of hematopoiesis characterized by overproduction of mature myeloerythroid cells, abnormalities of hemostasis and thrombosis, and tendency to progress to acute leukemia (Van Etten and Shannon 2004). In the 2001 WHO classification, chronic eosinophilic leukemia (CEL) was included among the MPDs while a closely related group of diseases with mixed myelodysplastic/myeloproliferative features was also recognized (Vardiman et al. 2002). Over the last several years, there has been a revolution in our understanding of the pathogenesis of these disorders, with the recognition that somatic activating mutations in tyrosine kinases (TKs) are found in a subset of patients from each disease category (Fig. 1.1) (Krause and Van Etten 2005). Some cases of chronic myelomonocytic leukemia (CMML) are associated with activation of platelet-derived growth factor receptor beta (PDGFRβ) through chromosome 5q translocations that fuse PDGFRβ with TEL (Golub et al. 1994) or many other partners (Jones and Cross 2004). Fusion of PDGFRα to FIP1L1 through interstitial deletions on chromosome 4q is found in a subset of patients with CEL/hypereosinophilic syndrome (Cools et al. 2003; Griffin et al. 2003), whereas activating point mutations in c-KIT are found in some patients with systemic mast cell disease (Furitsu et al. 1993). Patients with 8p11 myeloproliferative syndrome (EMS) (Macdonald et al. 2002) have myeloproliferation frequently accompanied by non-Hodgkin's lymphoma. Both myeloid and lymphoma cells share translocations involving chromosome 8p, which lead to fusion of the receptor TK fibroblast growth factor receptor-1 (FGFR-1) to multiple partners, including ZNF198 (Xiao et al. 1998). Together, these

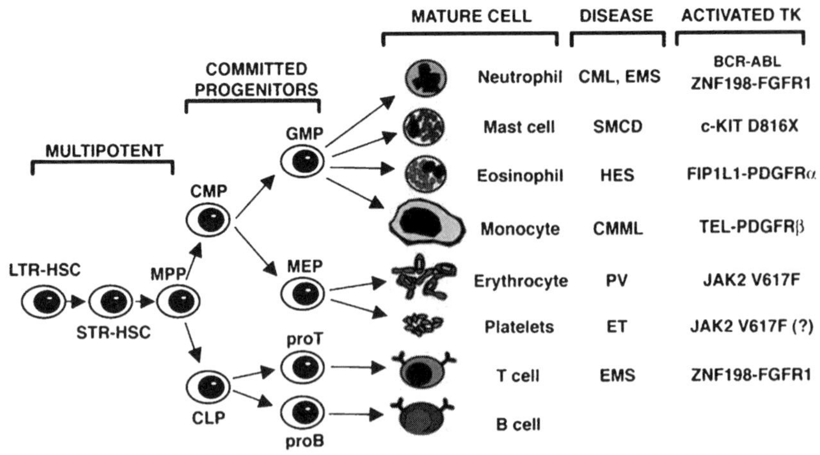

Fig. 1.1 Dysregulated tyrosine kinases (TKs) in the myeloproliferative syndromes. Multi-potent stem cells are depicted at *left*, committed progenitors in the *middle*, and mature blood cells at *right*. Each mature myeloid element is overproduced in a distinct myeloproliferative-like syndrome that is associated with a specific activated tyrosine kinase (far *right*)

observations indicate that dysregulated TKs are found in the majority of the chronic myeloproliferative-like syndromes. This new understanding is reflected in the new 2008 WHO classification of the chronic myeloid neoplasms, which recognizes a novel category of chronic myeloid disease with eosinophila and mutations in PDGFRα/β or FGFR-1 (Tefferi and Vardiman 2008).

Until recently, the pathogenesis of PV, ET, and PMF was less clear. PV is characterized by overproduction of mature erythrocytes, increased hematocrit and red cell mass, splenomegaly due to extramedullary hematopoiesis (Spivak 2002), and often increased circulating granulocytes and platelets. The clinical course of PV is complicated by abnormalities of hemostasis, including platelet dysfunction and bleeding, as well as arterial and venous thrombosis. The disease evolves to acute myeloid leukemia in about 20% of patients while progression to a "spent" phase, characterized by myelofibrosis and normal or low hematocrit, is more common. A hallmark of PV is the presence of endogenous erythroid colonies (EECs), erythroid progenitors that form colonies in vitro in the absence of exogenous erythropoietin (Epo) (Prchal and Axelrad 1974). Molecular studies in PV revealed no mutations in the Epo receptor, but PV granulocytes have increased transcripts for the urokinase plasminogen activator receptor PRV-1 (Temerinac et al. 2000), whereas PV platelets show decreased expression of c-Mpl, the receptor for thrombopoietin (Moliterno et al. 1998). However, whether these abnormalities are fundamental to the pathogenesis of PV was unclear.

JAK2 is a member of the Janus family of nonreceptor TKs and is required for signaling from the Epo receptor and other type I cytokine receptors (Parganas et al. 1998). In 2005, studies of erythroid progenitors from PV patients demonstrated that Epo-independent erythroid maturation was impaired by a JAK2 inhibitor (Ugo et al. 2004) and by siRNA knockdown of JAK2 (James et al. 2005). This prompted sequencing of the *JAK2* gene, which identified a G to A point mutation, resulting in substitution of phenylalanine for valine at amino acid 617 (V617F), in the JAK2 pseudokinase domain in the majority of PV patients (James et al. 2005). The JAK2-V617F mutant had constitutive kinase activity in vivo in the absence of Epo stimulation, and retroviral expression in murine bone marrow (BM) caused erythrocytosis (James et al. 2005). The JAK2-V617F mutation was independently identified through genomic sequencing of TKs in MPD patients (Baxter et al. 2005; Levine et al. 2005), and by investigation of loss of heterozygosity involving the *JAK2* gene on chromosome 9p (Kralovics et al. 2005). The JAK2-V617F mutation is found in nearly every patient with PV and is present in homozygous form through mitotic recombination in up to 30% of patients. The mutation is also found in 30–60% of ET and CIMF patients but is rarely found outside the MPDs (Jones et al. 2005a; Scott et al. 2005; Steensma et al. 2005). The widespread finding of JAK2-V617F in the non-CML MPDs suggested that it may contribute to the pathogenesis of these diseases. However, it was not clear from these human studies whether JAK2-V617F could be implicated as the direct and primary cause of PV, ET, or

CIMF nor was the relationship between the different MPDs that share the JAK2 mutation understood.

1.2 Mouse Models of Hematologic Malignancies Induced by Dysregulated TKs

How do we know that the dysregulated TKs depicted in Fig. 1.1 play a role in the pathogenesis of these distinctly different diseases? Biochemical studies in vitro, in cell lines, and in primary patient cells can confirm that these TKs are dysregulated and can give insight into the signaling pathways that they activate. However, a role of a TK in disease pathogenesis can only be established by the expression of that TK in the hematopoietic system in vivo. Over the past decade, several laboratories have pioneered the use of laboratory mice as model systems for studying the genetics and pathophysiology of human leukemia. The strategy is conceptually straightforward and involves expression, in BM of mice, of genes that are mutated or dysregulated in human leukemia cells. A primary motivation for this effort is to determine whether and how a particular genetic abnormality that is identified in a leukemic cell contributes to the malignant phenotype. If one is successful in recapitulating some or all of the leukemia phenotype in mice, then the system can then be used for studying the molecular pathophysiology of that disease, where the goal is a description, in biochemical terms, of the specific cellular abnormalities that explain the development and clinical course of the malignancy and its response to treatment. Finally, an accurate mouse model of leukemia can serve as a platform for testing potential new therapies, particularly those directed at specific molecular targets. The power of mouse models derives from their ability to accurately recapitulate the malignant phenotype in primary cells in vivo. However, this accuracy comes at the price of significant complexity, and careful pathological and molecular analysis is required in order to reach correct conclusions [for review, see Van Etten (2002); see also the section on "Pathological Analysis and Characterization of Mouse Models of Hematopoietic Disease"]. If these precautions are heeded, then mouse models can be used to answer important questions about the pathophysiology of human leukemia that are difficult if not impossible to approach through studies of human primary cells and cell lines.

There are two different strategies to express dysregulated TKs in the mouse hematopoietic system: transgenic mice and retroviral gene transfer into the BM followed by transplantation. Both methods have their own advantages and limitations [reviewed in Van Etten (2001)]. Transgenic mice allow production of a uniform cohort of diseased mice by breeding, but multiple new transgenic lines must be generated for each new TK mutant to be studied, and the transgene is present in all tissues in the embryo and adult. As activated TKs can have deleterious effects during development, attempts to express BCR–ABL via a traditional transgene or knock-in have encountered problems with toxicity and silencing (Heisterkamp et al. 1991; Jaiswal et al. 2003). With JAK2-V617F, similar difficulties have been observed. Attempts to express JAK2-V617F via a 190-kb human BAC transgene led to early lethality in three transgenic pups while a fourth viable transgenic mouse that expressed mutant JAK2 at very low levels had no erythroid phenotype (R. Skoda, personal communication). These observations suggest that more sophisticated conditional transgenic approaches [for example, see Huettner et al. (2000)] may be necessary to express dysregulated TKs in mice. By contrast, in the retroviral BM transduction/transplantation system, it is easy to test the leukemogenicity of new TKs and TK mutants by simply making new retroviral stocks. Furthermore, the effect of expression of a TK in distinct subsets of BM progenitors can be assessed. The major drawback is the labor-intensive and technically demanding nature of the experiments. This retroviral model system is now widely used by scientists across the molecular oncology field to investigate the pathogenetic role of genetic abnormalities identified in cancer cells.

1.3 The Retroviral BM Transduction/Transplantation Model of CML

The causative role of BCR–ABL in CML was demonstrated 17 years ago when expression of this TK by retroviral transduction in mouse BM induced MPD in recipients that closely resembled human CML (Daley et al. 1990; Kelliher et al. 1990). Subsequently, several laboratories exploited transient retroviral packaging systems to achieve efficient induction of CML-like leukemia in mice (Li et al. 1999; Pear et al. 1998; Zhang and Ren 1998), allowing the model to be used as an assay for the first time (for a detailed experimental protocol, see Gavrilescu and Van Etten (2008). It is now possible to routinely induce CML-like leukemia in 100% of recipient mice within 4–5 weeks after transplantation when the donors are pretreated with 5-fluorouracil (5-FU) and transduced in the presence of myeloid cytokines (Fig. 1.2). Myeloid cells from these mice carry the retroviral provirus, express BCR–ABL, and exhibit increased levels of tyrosyl-phosphorylated proteins and activation of multiple cell signaling pathways (Li et al. 1999; Roumiantsev et al. 2001). Analysis of the proviral integration pattern by Southern blotting reveals that the CML-like disease is polyclonal, with the same spectrum of proviral clones present in neutrophils, macrophages, erythroid progenitors, B lymphocytes, and in some cases T lymphocytes (Li et al. 1999; Million et al. 2002). This demonstrates that the *BCR–ABL*-transduced BM cells that initiate the CML-like disease in primary recipients have multi-lineage repopulating ability, a feature of hematopoietic stem cells. The polyclonal nature and short latency of murine CML-like leukemia differ from human CML, which is monoclonal and more chronic. However, these are not important pathophysiological differences but merely reflect transplantation of multiple *BCR–ABL*-transduced progenitors into each

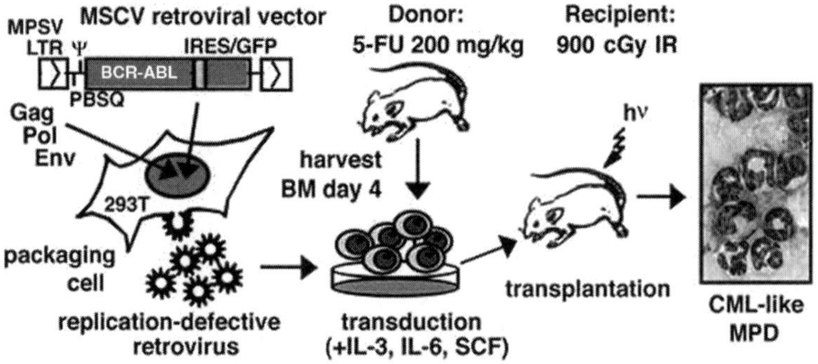

Fig. 1.2 Retroviral BM transduction-transplantation model of BCR–ABL-induced chronic myeloid leukemia (CML)-like myeloproliferative disease (MPD). The *BCR-ABL* oncogene is cloned in the MSCV retroviral vector, which co-expresses green fluorescent protein (GFP) from an internal ribosome entry site (IRES). For induction of CML-like disease, donors are pretreated with 5-FU, bone marrow (BM) is harvested and transduced ex vivo in the presence of myeloid cytokines, followed by transplantation into irradiated syngeneic recipient mice. All recipients develop fatal MPD within 5 weeks, characterized by leukocytosis with maturing neutrophils, as illustrated by the peripheral blood smear

recipient. When lower titer virus is used or limiting numbers of transduced cells are transplanted, oligo- to monoclonal disease with a longer latency is observed (Daley et al. 1990; Jiang et al. 2003).

The CML-like disease induced by BCR–ABL is efficiently transplanted to irradiated secondary recipient mice with BM or spleen cells from primary diseased mice and secondary leukemic recipients also demonstrate multi-lineage involvement (Li et al. 1999). Unless treated by allogeneic hematopoietic stem cell transplantation or ABL kinase inhibitor drugs, CML patients inevitably progress to acute myeloid or lymphoid leukemia, known as blast crisis. Mice with CML-like leukemia die soon after reconstituting hematopoiesis from overwhelming granulocytosis and organ infiltration and dysfunction, and we generally do not observe evidence of progression to blast crisis in these primary recipients. However, acute leukemias of myeloid, and, more commonly, lymphoid origin are observed upon serial transplantation of CML-like disease to secondary and tertiary recipients (Daley et al. 1991; Gishizky et al. 1993; Pear et al. 1998). Analysis of proviral integration patterns demonstrates that these acute leukemias are oligo- to monoclonal and arise from clone(s) found in the primary animal with CML-like leukemia. This is evidence of clonal disease progression and demonstrates that the model recapitulates this important feature of human CML. Finally, the murine CML-like disease responds to treatment with the ABL kinase inhibitor imatinib (Hu et al. 2004; Wolff and Ilaria 2001) and to immunotherapy with allogeneic donor leukocyte infusions (Krause and Van Etten 2004).

To summarize, the murine CML-like disease induced by BCR–ABL upon retroviral transduction of BM is a very close pathophysiological match to the human illness in terms of the cell of origin, transplantability, disease progression, and response to both kinase inhibitor and immunological therapies. However, the retroviral model system does have some drawbacks and limitations [reviewed in Van Etten (2001)]. The issues of disease latency and clonality were mentioned earlier. In addition, BCR–ABL is expressed from the proviral LTR at several-fold higher levels than are typically found in chronic phase CML cells (Barnes et al. 2005; Li et al. 1999), which may also affect disease latency. In addition, human CML cells are typically haploid for the *BCR* and c-*ABL* genes and can express the reciprocal ABL–-BCR fusion product. However, the fact that BCR–ABL expression alone recapitulates the disease in mice argues that these differences are not critical for leukemogenesis.

1.4 Strategies to Study Mechanisms of Leukemogenesis in Mice

Once an accurate retroviral transplant model of human leukemia or MPD is established, there are several complementary strategies that can be used to analyze the molecular pathogenesis of the disease (Fig. 1.3). First, one can introduce mutants of the TK into BM to assess their affect on leukemogenesis. The most informative mutants are point mutations or small deletions that selectively affect the phosphorylation, protein–protein interactions, subcellular localization, or regulatory properties of the TK. Second, the investigator can utilize mice with naturally occurring or targeted mutations in signaling molecules as BM donors in the retroviral transduction/transplantation model to determine whether a given molecule plays a role in leukemogenesis. This strategy works best when the mutant mice have relatively normal baseline hematopoiesis, because it can be difficult to interpret defects in leukemogenesis when a mutation profoundly affects the production of blood cells. In a third scenario, if signaling within the BM microenvironment plays a role in leukemia development, mutant mice can be utilized as the recipients for transduced BM from either normal or mutant donors. Fourth, one can co-express other genes along with the dysregulated TK in the BM. This can be done either using a separate retroviral vector to co-transduce the BM or by co-expressing the second gene downstream of the IRES in place of GFP, in the same vector used to express the TK. The first

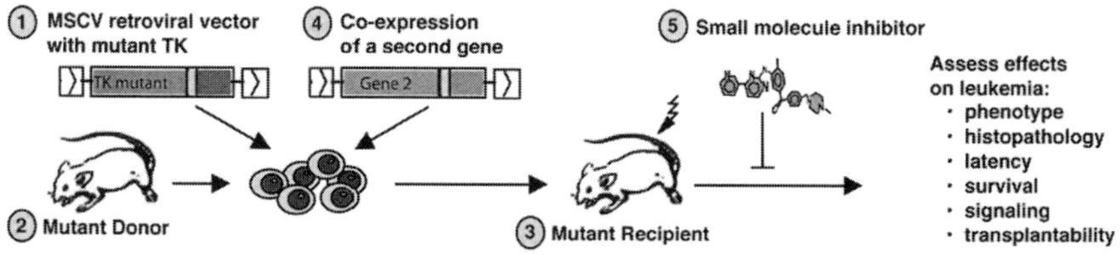

Fig. 1.3 Strategies to study mechanisms of leukemogenesis by dysregulated tyrosine kinases (TKs) in the retroviral transduction model. Five complementary approaches can be employed to study the pathogenesis of leukemias induced by dysregulated TKs. See text

approach can be useful for assessing the effect of dominantly acting genes that potentiate leukemogenesis [for example, see Dash et al. (2002)], but it is difficult to detect negative effects (such as expression of a dominant-negative mutant) because of the low probability of transducing individual HSC with more than one virus. The alternative approach, using the IRES to co-express the second gene, forces each transduced cell to express both genes and does allow negative effects to be demonstrated (Hao and Ren 2000). The latter approach can also be used in a "rescue" experiment to complement a leukemogenic defect in mutant BM cells (Ayton and Cleary 2003). Finally, the investigator can treat recipient mice with small molecule inhibitors of various signaling pathways to determine whether that pathway contributes to leukemogenesis. In order to dose the drug properly, one must know the pharmacokinetic profile of the compound in rodents, but this information is usually available for drugs that are candidates for clinical development. Using drugs to study leukemia signaling in mice is subject to the same concerns about specificity and off-target effects that are encountered in cell-culture experiments. With molecularly targeted drugs, one has the advantage of being able to assess the target directly and of using genetic approaches for target validation [for example, see Hu et al. (2004)]. With all these strategies, the endpoints that can be assessed are quantitative effects on the disease phenotype, including histopathology, latency, survival, signaling abnormalities, and transplantability.

1.5 Studies of MPD Induced by JAK2-V617F in the Mouse Retroviral Transduction/Transplantation Model

To investigate the molecular pathogenesis of MPD induced by JAK2-V617F, several research groups have expressed murine JAK2 WT or JAK2-V617F in the hematopoietic system of mice using the retroviral transduction/transplantation approach (Bumm et al. 2006; Lacout et al. 2006; Wernig et al. 2006; Zaleskas et al. 2006). Two of the studies further compared the phenotype of the disease in two different inbred strains of mice, Balb/c and C57Bl/6 (B6) (Wernig et al. 2006; Zaleskas et al. 2006).

1.5.1 JAK2-V617F Induces Polycythemia in Mice by Overproduction of Erythrocytes that is Independent of Epo

In both strains of mice, recipients of JAK2-V617F-transduced BM exhibited markedly increased blood hematocrit and hemoglobin levels that were evident by three weeks after transplantation and sustained for months, whereas recipients of JAK2 WT- or vector-transduced BM were normal. Polycythemia was accompanied by a striking increase in circulating reticulocytes, representing the newest population of circulating red cells. Plasma Epo levels were suppressed in the polycythemic mice, demonstrating that the erythropoiesis in these mice was autonomous and not driven by overproduction of Epo. CFU-E from BM or spleen of these recipients showed increased sensitivity to Epo, with around 25% of CFU-E growing in the absence of exogenous Epo. This demonstrates that EECs are found in these polycythemic mice, similar to human PV patients. Taken together, these results indicate that JAK2-V617F expression directly induces polycythemia in mice through Epo-independent overproduction of erythrocytes (Fig. 1.4). The fact that the principal erythroid features of PV are recapitulated by expression of JAK2-V617F argues that it is the primary and direct cause of human PV.

1.5.2 JAK2-V617F Induces Strain-Dependent Leukocytosis In Mice, but not Thrombocytosis

In contrast to the polycythemia, the effects of JAK2-V617F expression on leukocyte and platelet counts in the retroviral model were more variable.

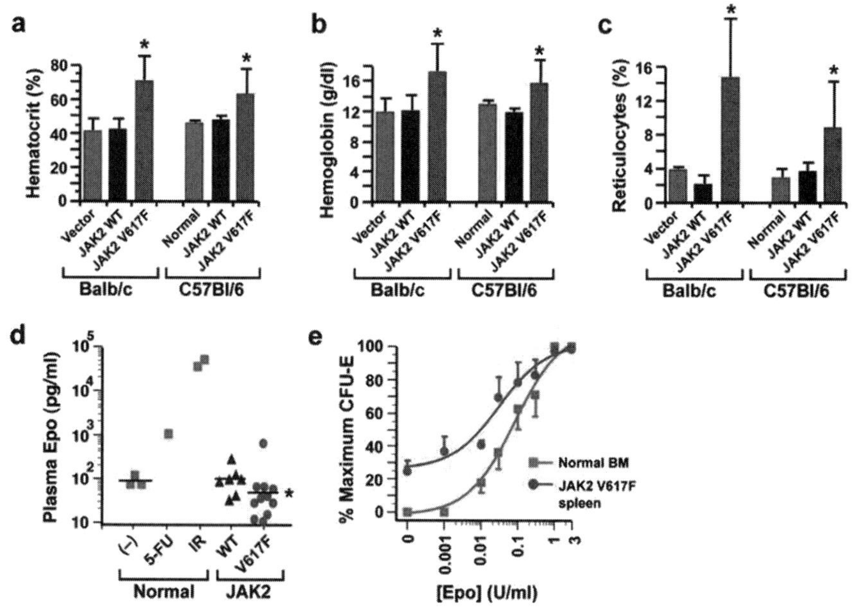

Fig. 1.4 JAK2-V617F induces polycythemia through autonomous overproduction of erythrocytes. (**a**) Hematocrit, (**b**) blood hemoglobin, and (**c**) reticulocyte counts from cohorts of Balb/c or B6 mice transplanted with syngeneic BM cells transduced with empty vector (*green*), or retrovirus expressing murine JAK2 WT (*blue*) or JAK2-V617F (*red*). In the case of the B6 cohorts, untransplanted mice ("normal") were used as controls. (**d**) Plasma Epo levels for the three groups (B6 background). (**e**) Percent maximal CFU-E from normal BM (*green*) or spleen of JAK2-V617F recipients (*red*). The asterisks in the figure indicate that the differences between JAK2-V617F and JAK2 WT in each panel were statistically ($P^2$0.05, t-test) Adapted from Zaleskas et al. (2006). (See color insert)

JAK2-V617F induced significant leukocytosis in Balb/c mice, but only a modest increase in B6 mice. These results suggest that genetic differences between the two mouse strains affect the leukocytosis induced by JAK2-V617F. JAK2-V617F expression did not affect the platelet count in either strain despite evidence of proviral expression of GFP in megakaryocytes, which was associated with a significant decrease in the DNA ploidy of the megakaryocytes (Wernig et al. 2006). However, JAK2-V617F recipients had a marked defect in platelet function, with significantly prolonged tail bleeding time (Zaleskas et al. 2006). The lack of thrombocytosis suggests that additional events may be required for JAK2-V617F to cause ET, which is consistent with human studies that suggest that there may be a predisposing mutation(s) distinct from JAK2-V617F that influence the development and phenotype of the MPD (Kralovics et al. 2006). These mouse studies further suggest that qualitative platelet abnormalities induced by JAK2-V617F may contribute to the hemostatic complications of PV patients.

1.5.3 Histopathology of MPD Induced in Mice by JAK2-V617F

Despite the marked polycythemia, the MPD induced by JAK2-V617F was not fatal in either strain, with most recipients surviving for many months. This is in sharp contrast to BCR–ABL-induced CML-like MPD, which is rapidly fatal in mice because of massive infiltration of the lungs, liver, and spleen with maturing neutrophils (Roumiantsev et al. 2004). At necropsy, JAK2-V617F recipients had significant splenomegaly, particularly in Balb/c mice, but no involvement of lymph nodes or thymus and no pulmonary hemorrhages. The marrow of JAK2-V617F recipients was hypercellular, with a predominance of myeloid over erythroid cells and less than 5% blasts. Spleens exhibited massively increased erythroid precursors with partial disruption of follicular architecture and infiltration with mature myeloid cells. Livers showed moderate periportal extramedullary myeloerythropoiesis, whereas lungs had only minimal myeloid infiltration. There were increased numbers of abnormal megakaryocytes present in BM and spleen, with clustering.

The polycythemia induced by JAK2-V617F was maximal at about 4 months following transplantation but tended to decrease with time in both strains, with hematocrit and reticulocyte counts returning to nearly normal ranges by 7–8 months after transplantation and some mice developing frank anemia. This coincided with a gradual but marked increase in fibrosis in the BM and spleen of JAK2-V617F recipients that was not observed in JAK2 WT recipients (Lacout et al. 2006; Wernig et al. 2006; Zaleskas et al. 2006) (Fig. 1.5). This is reminiscent of evolution of human PV to a "spent phase" resembling PMF. In one study, polycythemia and reticulocytosis could be resurrected in secondary mice through transplantation of BM or spleen cells from primary JAK2-V617F recipients harvested either in the early

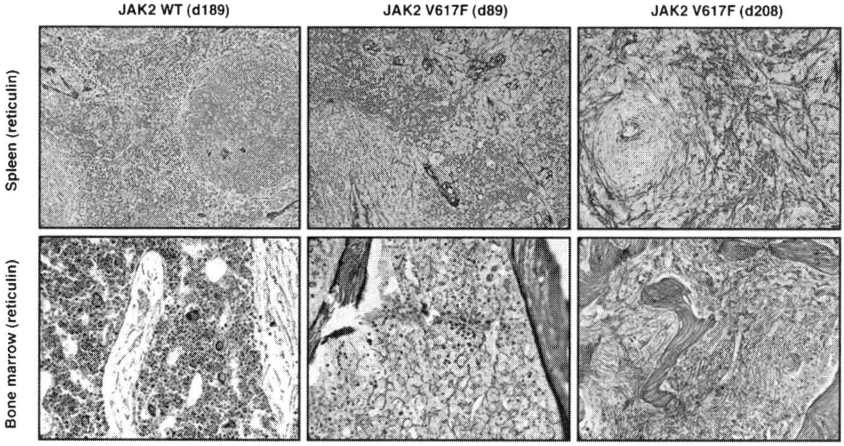

Fig. 1.5 Development of myelofibrosis in JAK2-V617F recipient mice. Increasing fibrosis (demonstrated by reticulin staining) in spleen (*top panels*) and bone marrow (BM) (*bottom panels*) of representative JAK2-V617F recipients at about 3 (middle panels) and 7 months (*right panels*) after transplantation. Note the marked increase in reticulin staining at 7 months in the JAK2-V617F recipients, but not in recipients of JAK2 wild-type (WT)-transduced BM (*left panels*). Adapted from Zaleskas et al. (2006). (See color insert)

polycythemic phase of the disease or in the later myelofibrotic stage (Zaleskas et al. 2006). These findings suggest that JAK2-V617F expression induces myelofibrosis, but the resulting impairment of erythropoiesis is due to a defect of the hematopoietic microenvironment rather than a deficiency of malignant hematopoietic stem cells.

1.6 Studying Signaling Mechanisms of JAK2-V617F-Induced Polycythemia in Mice

The retroviral model of JAK2-V617F-induced polycythemia provides an excellent tool to investigate the signaling pathways critical for disease pathogenesis and to identify new potential targets for therapy. Stimulation of erythroid cells with Epo leads to activation of several Src family kinases, including Lyn (Richmond et al. 2005). Interestingly, previous studies demonstrated that a relatively nonselective Src kinase inhibitor, PP2, impaired the Epo-independent differentiation of erythroid progenitors from PV patients (Ugo et al. 2004), suggesting a role for Src kinases in the pathogenesis of PV. This has clinical relevance, because dasatinib, a dual ABL/SRC kinase inhibitor, has been approved by the FDA for the treatment of CML but could be redirected for therapy of PV. One approach to investigate the role of Src kinases in the polycythemia induced by JAK2-V617F (strategy #2 in Fig. 1.3) is to employ donor mice lacking Lyn, Hck, and Fgr, the three principal Src kinases in myeloerythroid progenitor cells (Hu et al. 2004; Meng and Lowell 1997), as the donors for BM for transduction with JAK2-V617F. These triple Src-deficient mice have normal steady-state hematopoiesis but exhibit impaired erythropoietic responses to hemolysis as a consequence of Lyn deficiency (Ingley et al. 2005). Interestingly, recipients of *Lyn*$^{-/-}$*Hck*$^{-/-}$*Fgr*$^{-/-}$ BM transduced with JAK2-V617F developed polycythemia and reticulocytosis that tended to be greater than recipients of JAK2-V617F-transduced WT donor BM (Fig. 1.6) although this did not reach statistical significance. The results demonstrate that these particular Src kinases are not required for polycythemia induced by JAK2-V617F and might even play a negative role in JAK2-V617F signaling.

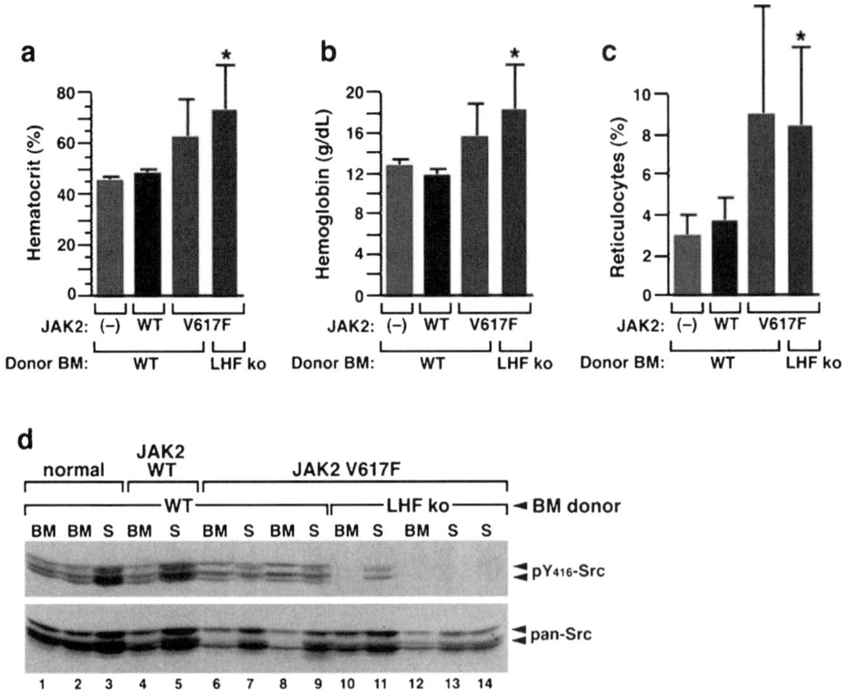

Fig. 1.6 Polycythemia induced by JAK2-V617F is independent of Src family kinases. (**a**) Hematocrit, (**b**) blood hemoglobin, and (**c**) reticulocyte counts from normal (–) B6 mice (*green*), B6 recipients of B6 wild-type (WT) bone marrow (BM) transduced with retrovirus expressing murine JAK2 WT (*blue*) or JAK2-V617F (*red*), and B6 *Lyn*$^{-/-}$*Hck*$^{-/-}$*Fgr*$^{-/-}$ BM transduced with retrovirus expressing JAK2-V617F (*orange*). (**d**) Western blot analysis of extracts of primary myeloerythroid cells from individual normal (lanes 1–3) B6 mice, recipients of WT BM transduced with JAK2 WT retrovirus (lanes 4–5), recipients of WT BM transduced with JAK2-V617F retrovirus (lanes 6–9), and recipients of *Lyn*$^{-/-}$*Hck*$^{-/-}$*Fgr*$^{-/-}$ BM transduced with JAK2-V617F retrovirus (lanes 10–14). The membrane was blotted with antibody recognizing the phosphorylated activation loop tyrosine (Y146 homolog) of c-Src, Lyn, Hck, Fyn, Lck, and Yes (*top panel*) and subsequently with antibody against total c-Src, Fyn, Yes, and Fgr (*bottom panel*). The asterisks in the figure indicate that the differences between JAK2-V617F and JAK2 WT in each panel were statistically ($P^2$0.05, t-test) Adapted from Zaleskas et al. (2006). (See color insert)

There is a formal possibility that one or more of the other six vertebrate Src family kinases might compensate for the lack of Lyn/Hck/Fgr, particularly Fyn, Yes, and c-Src, which are expressed in myeloid cells. However, there was no overexpression of Fyn, Yes, or c-Src in myeloerythroid cells from polycythemic recipients of JAK2-V617F-transduced $Lyn^{-/-}Hck^{-/-}Fgr^{-/-}$ BM and little or no detectable activation of these Src kinases, as assessed by an antibody against the phosphorylated activation loop tyrosine in Src (Fig. 1.6). These results suggest that compensation by other Src family members is unlikely to play a role in polycythemia induced by JAK2-V617F in the mutant cells.

1.7 Testing the Response of JAK2-V617F-Induced Polycythemia to Kinase Inhibitor Therapy

The retroviral model of JAK2-V617F-induced MPD is also an excellent platform for preclinical testing of new therapies, particularly molecularly targeted drugs. By analogy to BCR–ABL in CML, JAK2 is a rational therapeutic target in PV. Several published studies have already begun to address this topic (Pardanani 2008). In one study, cohorts of polycythemic JAK2-V617F recipient mice were treated for a 2-week period with small molecule TK inhibitors, including imatinib and the dual ABL/Src inhibitor dasatinib (Zaleskas et al. 2006). Imatinib therapy can reduce the hematocrit in some human PV patients but has minimal effects on the level of JAK2-V617F (Jones et al. 2005b). Relative to vehicle-treated controls, imatinib-treated mice demonstrated significant decreases in hematocrit and reticulocyte counts, while the corresponding responses to dasatinib were less robust and did not reach statistical significance (Fig. 1.7a, b). These results suggest that imatinib impairs JAK2-V617F-induced erythropoiesis through inhibition of a target other than ABL or c-Kit and confirm the genetic data that Src kinases may not be good targets for therapy in PV. AG-490 is a parenteral kinase inhibitor of the tyrphostin family that inhibits JAK2 but is relatively nonspecific. The compound is not orally bioavailable, and parenteral administration is complicated by its short half-life and low solubility, but it has been previously shown to be efficacious against acute lymphoid leukemia cells in a mouse xenotransplant model (Meydan et al. 1996). Continuous parenteral administration of AG-490 to mice with JAK2-V617F-induced polycythemia over a 2-week period caused a modest but significant decrease in hematocrit with a more pronounced drop in reticulocytes (Fig. 1.7b), suggesting that chronic treatment with a JAK2 inhibitor would have therapeutic benefit in PV (Zaleskas et al. 2006).

A second study employed an orally bioavailable small molecule JAK2 inhibitor, TG101209, in mice transplanted with cell lines expressing JAK2-V617F (Pardanani et al. 2007). Pharmacodynamic studies documented a marked inhibition of Stat5 phosphorylation in the leukemic cells following a single oral 100 mg/kg dose, and sustained daily therapy was associated with

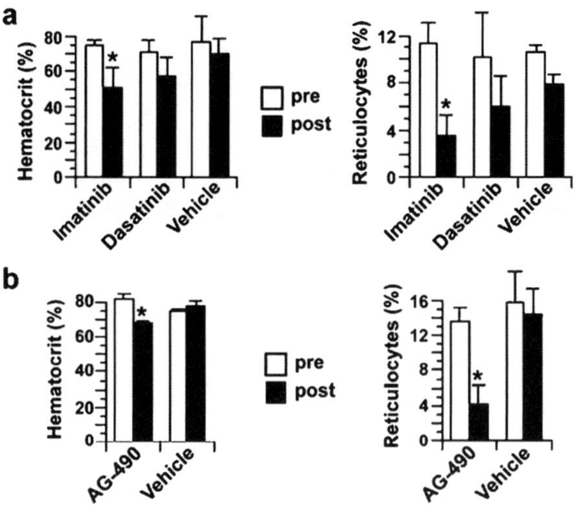

Fig. 1.7 Polycythemia and reticulocytosis induced by JAK2-V617F responds to kinase inhibitor therapy. (**a**) Hematocrit (*left panel*) and reticulocyte counts (right panel) of cohorts of mice treated with twice daily oral gavage with 100 mg/kg imatinib, 10 mg/kg dasatinib, or vehicle, determined before initiation of therapy (*white bars*, "pre") or after 2 weeks of treatment (*black bars*, "post"). The hematocrit and reticulocyte count were significantly decreased in response to imatinib therapy, whereas imatinib had no effect on these parameters in normal mice (data not shown). (**b**) Hematocrit (*left panel*) and reticulocyte counts (*right panel*) of mice treated with continuous parenteral ad ministration of 300 μg/day AG-490 or vehicle, determined before initiation of therapy (*white bars*) or after 2 weeks of treatment (*black bars*). The hematocrit and reticulocyte count were significantly decreased in response to AG-490 therapy. The asterisks in the figure indicate that the difference between pre- and post-treatment values in each panel were statistically significant ($P^{2}0.05$, t-test) Adapted from Zaleskas et al. (2006)

a significant decrease in leukemic cell burden and with prolonged survival. Together, these studies demonstrate that JAK2-V617F is a very promising target for rational therapy of PV. However, several critical questions have not yet been addressed in the model. Initially, there is great interest in determining whether erythropoiesis driven by JAK2-V617F may be particularly sensitive to pharmacological inhibition of JAK2, relative to normal Epo-dependent erythropoiesis. In CML, depending on the cytokine conditions used, Ph^{+} myeloid progenitors are selectively killed in vitro by ABL kinase inhibitors such as imatinib (Deininger et al. 1997; Druker et al. 1996), a phenomenon referred to as "oncogene addiction" (Weinstein 2002). If JAK2-V617F^{+} erythroid progenitors also exhibit heightened sensitivity to a JAK2 inhibitor, this may create a therapeutic "window" that allows elimination of the malignant clone in PV without causing generalized myelosuppression. Another important question is whether inhibition of JAK2-V617F will reverse the nonerythroid phenotypic abnormalities found in PV, such as myelofibrosis, platelet dysfunction, and predisposition to thrombosis. This is a critical question for clinical trial design, because it is very likely that JAK2 inhibitors will enter human trials in patients with PMF, not classical PV, because of the dismal prognosis of the former patients. We may expect these important preclinical questions to be addressed in the retroviral model system in the near future.

1.8 Modeling MPDs Associated with Other Mutant TKs

Although the great majority of patients with the clinical diagnosis of PV have the JAK2-V617F mutation if the analysis is done with sensitive allele-specific PCR, a small subset of patients are negative for this mutation, which prompted a search for mutations elsewhere in the JAK2 molecule. This led to the identification of a cluster of somatic mutations in exon 12 of the JAK2 gene, including a point mutation (K539L) and several small amino acid deletions and insertions (Scott et al. 2007). These exon 12 mutant JAK2 kinases, when co-expressed in cytokine-dependent hematopoietic cell lines with Epo-R, transformed the cells to cytokine-independent growth. When expressed in murine BM via the retroviral transduction/transplantation model, the JAK2 exon 12 mutants induced MPD that was indistinguishable from that induced by JAK2-V617F, with erythrocytosis and polycythemia, leukocytosis, and splenomegaly. Interestingly, although a subset of patients with JAK2 exon 12 mutations had a clinical phenotype of isolated erythrocytosis (i.e., without leukocytosis or thrombocytosis), this was not completely reproduced in mice, as the leukocyte counts were increased in mice that received either JAK2-V167F or K539L although the latter cohort did have significantly lower leukocyte levels (Scott et al. 2007). These studies suggest that mutant JAK2 kinases are the fundamental cause of virtually all cases of clinical PV that present with an increased red cell mass.

By contrast, about half of patients with ET or PMF lack JAK2 mutations, and genomic sequencing of the other JAK family kinases or of the Stat5 genes has failed to reveal any mutations in these signaling molecules. Inherited mutations in EpoR and MPL, the receptor for thrombopoietin, are found in patients with familial erythrocytosis and thrombocytosis, respectively (Kralovics et al. 1997), suggesting that these cytokine receptors might also be targets for somatic mutation in the MPDs. Indeed, systematic exonic sequencing of the MPL gene revealed a somatic juxtamembrane mutation (W515K or L) in about 6–8% of patients with JAK2-V617F-negative PMF and a smaller proportion of JAK2-negative ET patients (Pardanani et al. 2006; Pikman et al. 2006). Once again, the mutant MPL receptor transformed cytokine-dependent hematopoietic cells to cytokine independence. In the retroviral BM transduction/transplantation model, MPL W515K/L induced marked megakaryocytic hyperplasia with thrombocytosis and myelofibrosis. The recipients also developed leukocytosis with very high white blood cell counts reminiscent of BCR–ABL-induced CML-like disease but no polycythemia (Pikman et al. 2006). Interestingly, the mice were found to have frequent infarcts in the spleen at necropsy, but because similar infarcts are observed in mice with BCR–ABL-induced disease (where the platelet count is normal), it is not clear whether this can be attributed to the increased leukocytes or platelets.

1.9 Emerging Transgenic Mouse Models of JAK2-V617F-Induced MPD

Although the retroviral models of JAK2-induced MPD have already proven very valuable, transgenic mice offer an alternative that is attractive because of the ease of generation of diseased mice, and the more uniform phenotype of disease within a cohort. As mentioned in Section 1.2, successful generation of transgenic mice expressing JAK2-V617F within the hematopoietic system may require a system to conditionally express the transgene in order to avoid deleterious effects of the dysregulated TK on embryonic development. One method to accomplish this is to use tissue-specific or conditional expression of a transgene expressing Cre recombinase to modify the genomic structure of the TK transgene allowing expression. Most commonly, this is done by inserting a transcriptional "stop" cassette flanked by loxP sites upstream of the TK gene. In a recently published study, the authors took a slightly different approach. They generated *JAK2*-V617F transgenic mice where the sequences encoding the JAK2 kinase domain were in the inverse orientation, flanked by antiparallel loxP sites. These JAK2 transgenic mice were then crossed with a second transgenic strain expressing Cre recombinase under the control of the hematopoiesis-specific *Vav* promoter. In these double transgenic offspring, the level of expression of *JAK2*-V617F was lower than the endogenous wild-type (WT) JAK2, and the mice developed a phenotype resembling ET with strongly elevated platelet counts and moderate neutrophilia (Tiedt et al. 2008). By contrast, when the same JAK2-V617F transgenic mice were crossed to Mx–Cre transgenic mice and Cre expression induced by poly-I : C injection, this resulted in expression of *JAK2*-V617F that was approximately equal to WT JAK2 and resulted in a PV-like phenotype, with increased hemoglobin, thrombocytosis, and neutrophilia (Tiedt et al. 2008). These studies suggest that the ratio of mutant to WT JAK2 influences the MPD phenotype that results in vivo.

1.10 Summary and Future Directions

Mouse models of the MPDs have already proven their worth by allowing novel insights into the molecular pathogenesis of these diseases, an understanding of disease pathophysiology and identification of new potential targets for therapy. This knowledge would be difficult if not impossible to obtain if one was limited to studying primary human cells or cell lines. Going forward, we should expect to see continued use of these model systems for validation of new molecular targets and for the preclinical testing of targeted therapeutic agents, particularly combinations of agents. The diversity of inbred mouse strains and the ongoing Mouse Phenome Project at The Jackson Laboratory also offer a unique opportunity to identify genetic modifiers of the MPD phenotype in mice, which may have clinical relevance in human MPD patients.

References

Ayton PM, Cleary ML (2003) Transformation of myeloid progenitors by MLL oncoproteins is dependent on Hoxa7 and Hoxa9. Genes Dev 17:2298–2307

Barnes DJ, Schultheis B, Adedeji S, Melo JV (2005) Dose-dependent effects of Bcr-Abl in cell line models of different stages of chronic myeloid leukemia. Oncogene 24:6432–6440

Baxter EJ, Scott LM, Campbell PJ, East C, Fourouclas N, Swanton S, Vassiliou GS, Bench AJ, Boyd EM, Curtin N et al. (2005) Acquired mutation of the tyrosine kinase JAK2 in human myeloproliferative disorders. Lancet 365:1054–1061

Bumm TG, Elsea C, Corbin AS, Loriaux M, Sherbenou D, Wood L, Deininger J, Silver RT, Druker BJ, Deininger MW (2006) Characterization of murine JAK2V617F-positive myeloproliferative disease. Cancer Res 66:11156–11165

Cools J, DeAngelo DJ, Gotlib J, Stover EH, Lagare RD, Cottes J, Kutok J, Clark J, Galinsky I, Griffin JD et al. (2003) A tyrosine kinase created by fusion of the PDGFA and FIP1L1 genes as a therapeutic target of imatinib in idiopathic hypereosinophilic syndrome. N Engl J Med 348:1201–1214

Daley GQ, Van Etten RA, Baltimore D (1990) Induction of chronic myelogenous leukemia in mice by the P210$^{bcr/abl}$ gene of the Philadelphia chromosome. Science 247:824–830

Daley GQ, Van Etten RA, Baltimore D (1991) Blast crisis in a murine model of chronic myelogenous leukemia. Proc Natl Acad Sci USA 88:11335–11338

Dameshek W (1951) Some speculations on the myeloproliferative disorders. Blood 6:372–375

Dash AB, Williams IR, Kutok JL, Tomasson MH, Anastasiadou E, Lindahl K, Li S, Van Etten RA, Borrow J, Housman D et al. (2002) A murine model of CML blast crisis induced by cooperation between *BCR/ABL* and *NUP98/HOX49*. Proc Natl Acad Sci USA 99:7622–7627

Deininger MW, Goldman JM, Lydon N, Melo JV (1997) The tyrosine kinase inhibitor CGP57148B selectively inhibits the growth of BCR-ABL-positive cells. Blood 90:3691–3698

Druker BJ, Tamura S, Buchdunger E, Ohno S, Segal GM, Fanning S, Zimmermann J, Lydon NB (1996) Effects of a selective inhibitor of the Abl tyrosine kinase on the growth of Bcr-Abl positive cells. Nat Med 2:561–566

Furitsu T, Tsujimura T, Tono T, Ikeda H, Kitayama H, Koshimizu U, Sugahara H, Butterfield JH, Ashman LK, Kanayama Y (1993) Identification of mutations in the coding sequence of the proto-oncogene c-kit in a human mast cell leukemia cell line causing ligand-independent activation of c-kit product. J Clin Invest 92:1736–1744

Gavrilescu LC, Van Etten RA (2008). Applications of murine retroviral bone marrow transplantation models for the study of human myeloproliferative disorders. In: Enna SJ, Williams M, Ferkany JW, Kenakin T, Moser P, Ruggeri B (eds) Current protocols in pharmacology, John Wiley & Sons, Inc., Pagosa Springs, CO

Gishizky MI, Johnson-White J, Witte ON (1993) Efficient transplantation of *BCR-ABL*-induced chronic myelogenous leukemia-like syndrome in mice. Proc Natl Acad Sci USA 90:3755–3759

Golub TR, Barker GF, Lovett M, Gilliland DG (1994) Fusion of the PDGF receptor β to a novel ets-like gene, tel, in chronic myelomonocytic leukemia with t(5;12) chromosomal translocation. Cell 77:307–316

Griffin JH, Leung J, Bruner RJ, Caligiuri MA, Briesewitz R (2003) Discovery of a fusion kinase in EOL-1 cells and idiopathic hypereosinophilic syndrome. Proc Natl Acad Sci USA 100:7830–7835

Hao SX, Ren R (2000) Expression of interferon consensus sequence binding protein (ICSBP) is downregulated in Bcr-Abl-induced murine chronic myelogenous leukemia-like disease, and enforced coexpression of ICSBP inhibits Bcr-Abl induced myeloproliferative disorder. Mol Cell Biol 20:1149–1161

Heisterkamp N, Jenster G, Kioussis D, Pattengale PK, Groffen J (1991) Human *bcr-abl* gene has a lethal effect on embryogenesis. Transgenic Res 1:45–53

Hu Y, Liu Y, Pelletier S, Buchdunger E, Warmuth M, Fabbro D, Hallek M, Van Etten RA, Li S (2004) Requirement of Src kinases Lyn, Hck and Fgr for *BCR-ABL1*-induced B-lymphoblastic leukemia but not chronic myeloid leukemia. Nat Genet 36:453–461

Huettner CS, Zhang P, Van Etten RA, Tenen DG (2000) Reversibility of acute B-cell leukaemia induced by *BCR-ABL1*. Nat Genet 24:57–60

Ingley E, McCarthy DJ, Pore JR, Sarna MK, Adenan AS, Wright MJ, Erber W, Tilbrook PA, Klinken SP (2005) Lyn deficiency reduces GATA-1, EKLF and STAT5, and induces extramedullary stress erythropoiesis. Oncogene 24:336–343

Jaiswal S, Traver D, Miyamoto T, Akashi K, Lagasse E, Weissman IL (2003) Expression of BCR/ABL and BCL2 in myeloid progenitors leads to myeloid leukemias. Proc Natl Acad Sci USA 100:10002–10007

James C, Ugo V, Le Couedic JP, Staerk J, Delhommeau F, Lacout C, Garcon L, Raslova H, Berger R, Bennaceur-Griscelli A et al. (2005) A unique clonal JAK2 mutation leading to constitutive signalling causes polycythaemia vera. Nature 434:1144–1148

Jiang X, Stuible M, Chalandon Y, Li A, Chan WY, Eisterer W, Krystal G, Eaves A, Eaves C (2003) Evidence for a positive role of SHIP in BCR-ABL-mediated transformation of primitive murine hematopoietic cells and in human chronic myeloid leukemia. Blood 102:2976–2984

Jones AV, Cross NC (2004) Oncogenic derivatives of platelet-derived growth factor receptors. Cell Mol Life Sci 61:2912–2923

Jones AV, Kreil S, Zoi K, Waghorn K, Curtis C, Zhang L, Score J, Seear R, Chase AJ, Grand FH et al. (2005a) Widespread occurrence of the JAK2 V617F mutation in chronic myeloproliferative disorders. Blood 106:2162–2168

Jones AV, Silver RT, Waghorn K, Curtis C, Kreil S, Zoi K, Hochhaus A, Oscier D, Metzgeroth G, Lengfelder E et al. (2005b) Minimal molecular response in polycythemia vera patients treated with imatinib or interferon alpha. Blood 107:3339–3341

Kelliher MA, McLaughlin J, Witte ON, Rosenberg N (1990) Induction of a chronic myelogenous leukemia-like syndrome in mice with v-abl and bcr/abl. Proc Natl Acad Sci USA 87:6649–6653

Kralovics R, Indrak K, Stopka T, Berman BW, Prchal JF, Prchal JT (1997) Two new EPO receptor mutations: truncated EPO receptors are most frequently associated with primary familial and congenital polycythemias. Blood 90:2057–2061

Kralovics R, Passamonti F, Buser AS, Teo SS, Tiedt R, Passweg JR, Tichelli A, Cazzola M, Skoda RC (2005) A gain-of-function mutation of JAK2 in myeloproliferative disorders. N Engl J Med 352:1779–1790

Kralovics R, Teo SS, Li S, Theocharides A, Buser AS, Tichelli A, Skoda RC (2006) Acquisition of the V617F mutation of JAK2 is a late genetic event in a subset of patients with myeloproliferative disorders. Blood 108:1377–1380

Krause DS, Van Etten RA (2004) Adoptive immunotherapy of *BCR-ABL*-induced chronic myeloid leukemia-like myeloproliferative disease in a murine model. Blood 104:4236–4244

Krause DS, Van Etten RA (2005) Tyrosine kinases as targets for cancer therapy. N Engl J Med 353:172–187

Lacout C, Pisani DF, Tulliez M, Gachelin FM, Vainchenker W, Villeval JL (2006) JAK2V617F expression in murine hematopoietic cells leads to MPD mimicking human PV with secondary myelofibrosis. Blood 108:1652–1660

Levine RL, Wadleigh M, Cools J, Ebert BL, Wernig G, Huntly BJ, Boggon TJ, Wlodarska I, Clark JJ, Moore S et al. (2005) Activating mutation in the tyrosine kinase JAK2 in polycythemia vera, essential thrombocythemia, and myeloid metaplasia with myelofibrosis. Cancer Cell 7:387–397

Li S, Ilaria RL, Million RP, Daley GQ, Van Etten RA (1999) The P190, P210, and P230 forms of the *BCR/ABL* oncogene induce a similar chronic myeloid leukemia-like syndrome in mice but have different lymphoid leukemogenic activity. J Exp Med 189:1399–1412

Macdonald D, Reiter A, Cross NCP (2002) The 8p11 myeloproliferative syndrome: a distinct clinical entity caused by constitutive activation of FGFR1. Acta Haematol 107:101–107

Meng F, Lowell CA (1997) Lipopolysaccharide (LPS)-induced macrophage activation and signal transduction in the absence of Src-family kinases Hck, Fgr, and Lyn. J Exp Med 185:1661–1670

Meydan N, Grunberger T, Dadi H, Shahar M, Arpaia E, Lapidot Z, Leeder JS, Freedman M, Cohen A, Gazit A et al. (1996) Inhibition of acute lymphoblastic leukaemia by a Jak-2 inhibitor. Nature 379:645–648

Million RP, Aster J, Gilliland DG, Van Etten RA (2002) The Tel-Abl (ETV6-Abl) tyrosine kinase, product of complex (9;12) translocations in human leukemia, induces distinct myeloproliferative disease in mice. Blood 99:4568–4577

Moliterno AR, Hankins WD, Spivak JL (1998) Impaired expression of the thrombopoietin receptor by platelets from patients with polycythemia vera. N Engl J Med 338:572–580

Pardanani A (2008) JAK2 inhibitor therapy in myeloproliferative disorders: rationale, preclinical studies and ongoing clinical trials. Leukemia 22:23–30

Pardanani A, Hood J, Lasho T, Levine RL, Martin MB, Noronha G, Finke C, Mak CC, Mesa R, Zhu H et al. (2007) TG101209, a small molecule JAK2-selective kinase inhibitor potently inhibits myeloproliferative disorder-associated JAK2V617F and MPLW515L/K mutations. Leukemia 21:1658–1668

Pardanani AD, Levine RL, Lasho T, Pikman Y, Mesa RA, Wadleigh M, Steensma DP, Elliott MA, Wolanskyj AP, Hogan WJ et al. (2006) MPL515 mutations in myeloproliferative and other myeloid disorders: a study of 1182 patients. Blood 108:3472–3476

Parganas E, Wang D, Stravopodis D, Topham DJ, Marine JC, Teglund S, Vanin EF, Bodner S, Colamonici OR, van Deursen JM et al. (1998) Jak2 is essential for signaling through a variety of cytokine receptors. Cell 93:385–395

Pear WS, Miller JP, Xu L, Pui JC, Soffer B, Quackenbush RC, Pendergast AM, Bronson R, Aster JC, Scott ML, Baltimore D (1998) Efficient and rapid induction of a chronic myelogenous leukemia-like myeloproliferative disease in mice receiving P210 bcr/abl-transduced bone marrow. Blood 92:3780–3792

Pikman Y, Lee BH, Mercher T, McDowell E, Ebert BL, Gozo M, Cuker A, Wernig G, Moore S, Galinsky I et al. (2006) MPLW515L Is a novel somatic activating mutation in myelofibrosis with myeloid metaplasia. PLoS Med 3:e270

Prchal JF, Axelrad AA (1974) Letter: bone-marrow responses in polycythemia vera. N Engl J Med 290:1382

Richmond TD, Chohan M, Barber DL (2005) Turning cells red: signal transduction mediated by erythropoietin. Trends Biochem Sci 15:146–155

Roumiantsev S, de Aos I, Varticovski L, Ilaria RL, Van Etten RA (2001) The Src homology 2 domain of Bcr/Abl is required for efficient induction of chronic myeloid leukemia-like disease in mice but not for lymphoid leukemogenesis or activation of phosphatidylinositol 3-kinase. Blood 97:4–13

Roumiantsev S, Krause DS, Neumann CA, Dimitri CA, Asiedu F, Cross NC, Van Etten RA (2004) Distinct stem cell myeloproliferative/T lymphoma syndromes induced by ZNF198-FGFR1 and BCR-FGFR1 fusion genes from 8p11 translocations. Cancer Cell 5:287–298

Scott LM, Campbell PJ, Baxter EJ, Todd T, Stephens P, Edkins S, Wooster R, Stratton MR, Futreal PA, Green AR (2005) The V617F JAK2 mutation is uncommon in cancers and in myeloid malignancies other than the classic myeloproliferative disorders. Blood 106:2920–2921

Scott LM, Tong W, Levine RL, Scott MA, Beer PA, Stratton MR, Futreal PA, Erber WN, McMullin MF, Harrison CN et al. (2007) JAK2 exon 12 mutations in polycythemia vera and idiopathic erythrocytosis. N Engl J Med 356:459–468

Spivak JL (2002) Polycythemia vera: myths, mechanisms, and management. Blood 100:4272–4290

Steensma DP, Dewald GW, Lasho TL, Powell HL, McClure RF, Levine RL, Gilliland DG, Tefferi A (2005) The JAK2 V617F activating tyrosine kinase mutation is an infrequent event in both "atypical" myeloproliferative disorders and myelodysplastic syndromes. Blood 106:1207–1209

Tefferi A, Vardiman JW (2008) Classification and diagnosis of myeloproliferative neoplasms: the 2008 World Health Organization criteria and point-of-care diagnostic algorithms. Leukemia 22:14–22

Temerinac S, Klippel S, Strunck E, Roder S, Lubbert M, Lange W, Azemar M, Meinhardt G, Schaefer HE, Pahl HL (2000) Cloning of PRV-1, a novel member of the uPAR receptor superfamily, which is overexpressed in polycythemia rubra vera. Blood 95:2569–2576

Tiedt R, Hao-Shen H, Looser R, Dirnhofer S, Schwaller J, Skoda RC (2008) Ratio of mutant JAK2-V617F to wild type Jak2 determines the MPD phenotypes in transgenic mice. Blood 111:3931–3940

Ugo V, Marzac C, Teyssandier I, Larbret F, Lecluse Y, Debili N, Vainchenker W, Casadevall N (2004) Multiple signaling pathways are involved in erythropoietin-independent differentiation of erythroid progenitors in polycythemia vera. Exp Hematol 32:179–187

Van Etten RA (2001) Models of chronic myeloid leukemia. Curr Oncol Rep 3:228–237

Van Etten RA (2002) Studying the pathogenesis of *BCR-ABL*$^{+}$ leukemia in mice. Oncogene 21:8643–8651

Van Etten RA, Shannon KM (2004) Focus on myeloproliferative diseases and myelodysplastic syndromes. Cancer Cell 6:547–552

Vardiman JW, Harris NL, Brunning RD (2002) The World Health Organization (WHO) classification of the myeloid neoplasms. Blood 100:2292–2302

Weinstein IB (2002) Addiction to oncogenes-the Achilles heal of cancer. Science 297:63–64

Wernig G, Mercher T, Okabe R, Levine RL, Lee BH, Gilliland DG (2006) Expression of Jak2V617F causes a polycythemia vera-like disease with associated myelofibrosis in a murine bone marrow transplant model. Blood 107:4274–4281

Wolff NC, Ilaria RL Jr (2001) Establishment of a murine model for therapy-treated chronic myelogenous leukemia using the tyrosine kinase inhibitor STI571. Blood 98:2808–2816

Xiao S, Nalabolu SR, Aster JC, Ma J, Abruzzo L, Jaffe ES, Stone R, Weissman SM, Hudson TJ, Fletcher JA (1998) *FGFR1* is fused with a novel zinc-finger gene, *ZNF198*, in the t(8;13) leukaemia/lymphoma syndrome. Nature Genet 18:84–87

Zaleskas VM, Krause DS, Lazarides K, Patel N, Hu Y, Li S, Van Etten RA (2006) Molecular Pathogenesis and Therapy of Polycythemia Induced in Mice by JAK2 V617F. PLoS ONE 1:e18

Zhang X, Ren R (1998) Bcr-Abl efficiently induces a myeloproliferative disease and production of excess interleukin-3 and granulocyte-macrophage colony-stimulating factor in mice: a novel model for chronic myelogenous leukemia. Blood 92:3829–3840

Chapter 2
Genetic Modeling of Human Blood Cancers in Mice

Yiguo Hu and Shaoguang Li

Contents

2.1 Introduction

Leukemia is a broad term describing a spectrum of diseases involving white blood cells and is divided into four categories: acute or chronic myelogenous and acute or chronic lymphocytic leukemia (CLL). Acute leukemia is characterized by the rapid proliferation of immature blood cells that cannot carry out their normal functions. Acute leukemia generally occurs in children and young adults and needs immediate treatment because of the rapid progression and accumulation of the malignant cells in the body. Chronic leukemia is distinguished by the excessive and slow build-up of relatively mature white blood cells, which can still carry out some of their normal functions. Chronic leukemia mostly occurs in older people but can theoretically occur in any age group. Whereas acute leukemia must be treated immediately, chronic forms are sometimes monitored for some time before treatment to ensure maximum effectiveness of therapy. Classification of leukemia into myeloid or lymphoid form is based on the type of abnormal white blood cells found most in the blood or bone marrow. Acute lymphocytic leukemia (also known as acute lymphoblastic leukemia, or ALL) is the most common type of leukemia in young children and

---

S. Li
Division of Hematology/Oncology, Department of Medicine, University of Massachusetts Medical School, Worcester, MA 010605, USA
Shaoguang.Li@umassmed.edu

S. Li (ed.), *Mouse Models of Human Blood Cancers*,
DOI: 10.1007/978-0-387-69132-9_2, © Springer Science+Business Media, LLC 2008

also affects adults, especially those age 65 and older. CLL most often affects adults over the age of 55. CLL sometimes occurs in younger adults, but it almost never affects children.

There is no single known cause for all different types of leukemia. Four possible causes are (1) natural or artificial ionizing radiation, (2) certain kinds of chemicals, (3) some viruses, and (4) genetic predispositions. Leukemia, like other cancers, can result from somatic mutations in the DNA, which leads to disruption of the regulation of cell death, proliferation, and differentiation. These mutations may occur spontaneously or as a result of exposure to radiation or carcinogenic substances (such as benzene, hair dyes, etc.), and sensitivity of humans to these cancer-causing agents are likely to be influenced by genetic factors. Viruses have also been linked to some forms of leukemia. For example, certain cases of ALL are associated with viral infections by either the human immunodeficiency virus (HIV, responsible for AIDS) (Murray et al., 1999) or human T-lymphotropic virus [HTLV-1 and HTLV-2, causing adult T-cell leukemia/lymphoma (TCL)] (Poiesz et al., 2001). Fanconi anemia is also a risk factor for developing acute myelogenous leukemia (Bhatia et al., 2007). All these risk factors end up causing aberrant activation or inactivation of cellular genes that control normal cell proliferation and differentiation. In human blood cancers, formation of a fusion gene from two normal cellular genes, which is caused by chromosomal translocation, is a frequent way to abnormally activate a cellular gene that becomes oncogenic after forming a chimeric gene with another cellular gene. Large numbers of mouse models of human blood cancers are generated by expressing these chimeric or active oncogenes in mice. Mouse leukemia models provide powerful tools to investigate the disease mechanisms and help to develop new therapies.

2.2 Mouse Leukemia Models

In principle, leukemia mouse models are generated based on three major mechanisms: (1) expressing human oncogene(s) in hematopoietic progenitor cells, (2) inactivating tumor suppressor gene(s) (including DNA repair genes) in hematopoietic cells, and (3) combining these two methods. Described below are examples of established mouse models for different forms of human blood cancers.

2.2.1 Modeling Acute Myeloid Leukemia

Expression of a human acute myeloid leukemia-inducing gene in mouse bone marrow cells using retrovirus. Fusion genes involving transcriptional coactivators and generated through chromosomal translocations are frequently found in human acute myeloid leukemia (AML). Examples of these fusion genes are MLL/CBP (Satake et al., 1997; Sobulo et al., 1997; Taki et al., 1997), MLL/

p300 (Ida et al., 1997), MOZ (monocytic leukemia zinc finger)/CBP (Borrow et al., 1996), MOZ/p300 (Chaffanet et al., 2000; Kitabayashi et al., 2001b), MORF/CBP (Panagopoulos et al., 2001), and MOZ–TIF2 (Carapeti et al., 1998; Liang et al., 1998). Each of these fusion proteins contains one or more histone acetyltransferase (HAT) domain(s) that function to modify chromatin by acetylation of the N-terminal histone tail. Because MOZ–TIF2 is a common and well-understood fusion oncogene causing human AML, here we use this fusion gene as an example to describe the retroviral bone marrow transduction/transplantation mouse model of AML induced by MOZ–TIF2.

MOZ belongs to the MYST family of HATs and was first cloned as a fusion partner of CBP as a consequence of t(8;16)(p11;p13) chromosomal translocation associated with the French–American–British M4/M5 subtype of AML (Borrow et al., 1996). MOZ regulates transcriptional activation mediated by the hematopoietic transcription factor, Runx1 (AML1) (Kitabayashi et al., 2001a), and a related osteogenic transcriptional factor, Runx2 (Kitabayashi et al., 2001a). TIF2 belongs to p160 nuclear receptor transcriptional coactivator family (NRCoAs) (Glass et al., 1997; Horwitz et al., 1996), which includes SRC-1, TIF2/GRIP1, and ACTR/RAC3/pCIP/AIB-1. p160 family coactivators have a conserved N-terminal bHLH–PAS domain, a centrally located receptor interaction domain (RID), and a C-terminal transcriptional activation domain (AD). The RID contains three conserved motifs, LXXLL (where L is leucine and X is any amino acid), that are required to mediate interactions between coactivators and liganded nuclear receptors (Ding et al., 1998; Heery et al., 1997; Torchia et al., 1997). TIF2 can directly interact with CBP via its three conserved LXXLL motifs (Demarest et al., 2002; Torchia et al., 1997). P160 family members interact with nuclear receptors and enhance transcriptional activation by the receptor via histone acetylation/methylation (Leo and Chen, 2000).

In the MOZ–TIF2 fusion protein, MOZ retains the C4HC3-type PHD zinc finger domain and the HAT (MYST) domain and TIF2 retains the CBP interaction domain (CID) and CBP-independent activation domain (called AD2) of TIF2. MOZ–TIF2 lacks the C-terminus of MOZ and the PAS–bHLH DNA-binding/protein heterodimerization domain, and nuclear RID of TIF2 (Deguchi et al., 2003). To assess the transforming properties of MOZ–TIF2 in vivo, the *MOZ–TIF2* gene was cloned into the MSCV retroviral vector (see Fig. 1.2 in Chapter 1 for the viral vector structure); mouse bone marrow cells transduced with the MOZ–TIF2 containing retrovirus were transplanted into irradiated syngeneic mice (Deguchi et al., 2003). Recipients receiving bone marrow transduced with either the *MOZ–TIF2(I)* or the *MOZ–TIF2(II)* variant fusion genes developed fatal hematopoietic malignant disease, with high white blood cell (WBC) counts and splenomegaly. In addition, the mice demonstrated the presence of peripheral blood and bone marrow blasts and extensive tissue infiltration of organs including the liver, spleen, and lungs by leukemic blasts (Deguchi et al., 2003). This study provides sufficient evidence showing that MOZ–TIF2, which is associated with human AML, induces similar disease in mice.

Transgenic AML mouse model. A good example of transgenic AML model is to express the *CBFβ–SMMHC* gene in mice. *CBFβ–SMMHC* resulted from the inversion of chromosome 16 inv(16)(p13.1;1q22), which breaks and joins the *CBFβ* gene with the myosin gene *MYH11* (Liu et al., 1993, 1996) and causes about 12% of human AML. To avoid embryonic lethality caused by expression of the *CBFβ–SMMHC* gene[6–10], a conditional *CBFβ–SMMHC* knock-in mouse was generated to analyze the preleukemic effects of CBFβ–SMMHC in hematopoiesis and AML development in adult mice. The *CBFβ–SMMHC* gene caused appearance of abnormal progenitor cells that are leukemic precursors. Mice expressing CBFβ–SMMHC developed AML with a median latency of approximately 5 months. Interestingly, the number of CBFβ–SMMHC-expressing hematopoietic stem cells (HSCs) was maintained at a normal level, but their ability to differentiate into multiple lineages of blood cells was severely impaired. This AML model is key for the study of early target genes in progenitor cells and provides an in vivo validation system for studying cooperative oncogenes and for testing candidate drugs for improved treatment of AML.

Collaborative induction of AML with multiple oncogenes. It is generally believed that multiple genetic alterations are required for the initiation and progression of malignant diseases. There are many examples that show the failure of a single AML-inducing oncogene to efficiently induce AML, as evident by no induction of leukemia or induction of leukemia with low penetrance and long latency. Additional genetic events (secondary "hits") are needed to promote the pathogenesis of leukemia. In this case, coexpression of more than one oncogene in the same hematopoietic progenitor cells helps to successfully induce human AML in mice.

The PML–RAPα fusion oncogene is found in acute promyelocytic leukemia (APL). APL comprises about 5–10% of cases of AML, and approximately 90% of APL patients are associated with a balanced t(15;17)(q22;q21) reciprocal chromosomal translocation. This translocation results in the fusion of the *PML* gene on chromosome 15 to the retinoic acid receptor alpha (*RARα*) gene on chromosome 17, forming two new oncogenes, PML–RARα and RARα–PML. The *RARα* gene encodes a hormone-inducible nuclear receptor that has been shown to be involved in myeloid development (Collins et al., 1990; Dawson et al., 1994; Onodera et al., 1995; Tsai and Collins, 1993). Both PML–RARα and RARα–PML play roles in APL phathogenesis.

To induce APL in mice, a transgene containing a human PML–RARα cDNA under the control of sequence that regulates the promyelocyte-specific expression of the human CG gene allows expression of PML–RARα in the early myeloid cells of the transgenic mice (Grisolano et al., 1997). At the early stage, these transgenic mice were found to have altered myeloid development with an expansion of myeloid cells in their bone marrows and spleens. After a long latent period, approximately 30% of the transgenic mice developed leukemia, with massive splenomegaly, high percentage of immature myeloid cells in peripheral blood and bone marrow of the mice (Grisolano et al., 1997). In addition, approximately 40% of human APL patients are found to contain an activating mutation in the *FLT3* gene, containing internal tandem duplication (ITD) in the juxtamembrane domain. ITDs in FLT3 (FLT3–ITD) are found in 27% of all AML cases (Stirewalt et al., 2001; Yamamoto et al., 2001; Yokota et al., 1997) and 37% of APL patients (Kottaridis et al., 2001). FLT3–ITDs induce a myeloproliferative disease in a murine bone marrow transplantation model but are insufficient to induce AML (Kelly et al., 2002b). This low frequency and long latency of APL pathogenesis induced by PML–RARα or FLT3–ITDs can be overcome by coexpression of both genes in the same animal. In this model, bone marrow cells derived from hCG-PML–RARα transgenic mice (Grisolano et al., 1997) were transducted with the FLT3–ITD retrovirus, followed by transplantation of transduced cells into lethally irradiated syngeneic recipient mice. These recipients developed APL-like disease with complete penetrance and a short latency. The pathogenesis of this disease resembles the APL-like disease that occurs with a long latency in the PML/RARα transgenic mice, suggesting that activating mutations in FLT3–ITD services as the additional mutations in APL progression in the hCG-PML–RARα transgenic mice.

Another example is the Ras oncogene. Ras mutations are commonly found in AML. N-ras and K-ras mutations are found in 4 (Callens et al., 2005) and 10% of APL patients (Bowen et al., 2005), respectively. Overexpressing oncogenic K-ras under the control of its endogenous promoter in the mouse hematopoietic system, K-ras induces a myeloproliferative disease, but it is not sufficient to induce AML (Braun et al., 2004; Chan et al., 2004). To test whether K-ras serves as a cooperative secondary genetic event in induction of AML, LSL-K-ras G12D mice (Jackson et al., 2001), in which K-ras expression is controlled by the conditional knock-in Lox-stop-Lox, were crossed with cathepsin G-PML–RARα mice (Grisolano et al., 1997) to generate LSL-K-ras G12D$^{+/-}$/cathepsin G-PML–RARα$^{+/-}$ mice (KP mice). Subsequently, these mice were crossed with Mx-1–Cre mice (Kuhn et al., 1995) to generate triple-transgenic LSL-K-ras G12D$^{+/-}$/cathepsin G-PML–RARα$^{+/-}$/Mx-1–Cre$^{+/-}$ mice (KPM mice). K-ras expression was induced by deletion of the Lox-stop-Lox with Cre, whose expression was induced with polyinosinic–polycytidylic acid (pI–pC) (Chan et al., 2006). Mice expressing oncogenic K-ras and PML–RARα developed an APL-like disease with a high penetrance and short latency compared to cathepsin G-PML–RARα transgene mice (Chan et al., 2006).

Acceleration of AML development with a chemical mutagen. As pointed out above, some oncogenes are, by themselves, insufficient to transform cells and induce leukemia. However, genetic modifications or changes of the model-making procedures, or the oncogene itself, or even mouse background would dramatically increase the penetrance of leukemogenesis. Mouse model of *AML1–ETO*-induced AML is such an example.

AML1–ETO (also known as RUNX1-ETO) is a fusion gene resulted from translocation between chromosomes 8 and 21. The translocation is highly associated with human AML and is present in up to 40% of leukemias of the French–American–British M2 subtype (Hess and Hug, 2004). AML1 is a key regulator of normal blood formation and is frequently altered in leukemias. However, it has been difficult to clarify the role of AML1–ETO in leukemogenesis, because AML1–ETO alone is not sufficient to cause AML, and AML1–ETO transgene causes embryonic lethality (Okuda et al., 1998, 2000). To bypass the embryonic lethality caused by AML1–ETO, conditional and inducible transgenic models, and bone marrow transplantation system were used to express AML1–ETO in mice; all these strategies were unable to reliably induce AML even after 24 months (de Guzman et al., 2002; Fenske et al., 2004; Higuchi et al., 2002; Rhoades et al., 2000), suggesting that induction of AML by AML1–ETO requires additional genetic events. However, when stem cells were transduced with AML1–ETO and transplanted into lethally irradiated recipient animals, the stem cell compartment expanded dramatically (de Guzman et al., 2002). Similarly, direct targeting of AML1–ETO expression to stem cells by using the SCA-1 promoter enhanced myeloid progenitor expansion (Fenske et al., 2004). These results imply that retroviral insertion sites or large numbers of leukemia-initiating progenitors provide the additional "hits" for AML1–ETO-induced leukemia. To assess the ability of AML1–ETO to induce leukemia in the context of cooperating mutations, animals expressing AML1–ETO were mutagenized with the alkylating agent *N*-ethyl-*N*-nitrosourea (ENU). In two independent systems, mutagenized AML1–ETO-expressing mice developed myeloid leukemia or granulocytic sarcoma at frequencies greater than ENU-treated wild-type animals (Higuchi et al., 2002; Yuan et al., 2001). These results confirm that AML1–ETO predisposes a myeloid precursor population to cellular transformation (Hess et al., 2004).

The AML1–ETO mouse model provides an excellent assay system to investigate AML1–ETO downstream signaling pathways. AML1–ETO was found to suppress cell proliferation by inhibiting its targeting genes, including cyclin D3 and CDK4 (Bernardin-Fried et al., 2004; Burel et al., 2001; Lou et al., 2000), and impair cell cycle in the transition of G1 to S phase (Burel et al., 2001). In addition, an AML1–ETO truncated protein (loss of C-terminal Nervy homology regions 3 and 4 domain), which binds the corepressor complexes associated with N-CoR (nuclear receptor corepressor) and SMRT (silencing mediator for retinoid and thyroid hormone receptor) (Lutterbach et al., 1998), can induce high penetrance of leukemia with a short disease latency (mean survival of 20 weeks) in the retroviral transduction/transplantation model (Yan et al., 2004). In this study, the results also showed that expression of cyclin A and D3 was increased in truncated AML1–ETO-transformed cells compared with full-length AML1–ETO-transformed cells. Taken together, these studies demonstrate that AML1–ETO alone is not sufficient to cause leukemia, and additional genetic changes that cooperate with AML1–ETO are required for the development of AML. Obviously, AML1–ETO mouse models of AML will be helpful in study of genetic pathways involved in AML development.

Deletion of a tumor suppressor gene causes AML. Tumor suppressor genes play critical roles in regulating biological properties of cells, including cell cycle control, apoptosis, proliferation and differentiation, detecting and repairing DNA damage, and protein ubiquitination and degradation (Sherr, 2004). Deletions of tumor suppressor genes are associated with many types of tumors, and examples of tumor suppressor genes are *P53*, *RB*, *INK4a*, *ARF*, *APC*, *PTCH*, *SAMAD4/DPC4*, *PTEN*, *TSC1/2*, *NF1*, *WT1*, *MSH2*, *MLH1*, *ATM*, *NBS1*, *CHK2*, *BRCA1/2*, *FA*, and *VHL* (Sherr, 2004). The best AML model established by the deletion of a tumor suppressor gene is the removal of the *PTEN* gene in mice.

The *PTEN* gene was initially identified based on the observation that a loss of heterozygosity (LOH) at 10q23 was frequently detected in a variety of human tumors, and PTEN was later identified as the corresponding gene (Li et al., 1997). Further studies indicate that PTEN suppresses tumor cell growth by modulating G1 cell cycle progression through negatively regulating the PI3 K/Akt signaling pathway, and a critical target gene of this pathway is the cyclin-dependent kinase inhibitor p27 (KIP1) (Li and Sun, 1998). PTEN has been found to be associated with a series of primary acute leukemias and non-Hodgkin lymphomas (NHLs) as well as many tumor cell lines, and 40% of these cell lines carried PTEN mutations or hemizygous PTEN deletions. On the other hand, one-third of these cell lines had low PTEN transcript levels, and 60% of them had low or absent PTEN protein. Furthermore, a smaller number of primary hematologic malignancies, in particular NHLs, carried PTEN mutations (Dahia et al., 1999). To model AML induced by the deletion of the *PTEN* gene,

Ptenfl/fl mice (Lessard and Sauvageau, 2003) were crossed with Ptenfl/+ mice carrying an Mx-1–Cre (Park et al., 2003) transgene to generate litters containing Mx-1–Cre^+ and Ptenfl/fl. PTEN deletion was induced by injection of pI–pC to mice at weaning. After the induction of PTEN deletion, mice had an increased representation of myeloid and T-lymphoid lineages in bone marrow and developed myeloproliferative disorder. Notably, the cell populations that expanded in PTEN-deficient mice matched those that became dominant in the acute myeloid/lymphoid leukemia that developed in later stages of myeloproliferative disorder. This study demonstrates that PTEN has essential roles in restricting the activation of HSCs, in lineage fate determination, and in the prevention of leukemogenesis (Zhang et al., 2006).

2.2.2 *Modeling Chronic Myeloid Leukemia-Like Diseases*

Chronic myeloid leukemia (CML) is represented by myeloproliferative disease induced by the BCR–ABL oncogene that results from the t(9;22)(q34;q22)

chromosomal translocation. Other CML-like diseases are induced by the fusion genes *TEL/PDGFβR* (Golub et al., 1994), *TEL/ABL* (Golub et al., 1995), *TEL/JAK2* (Lacronique et al., 1997), and *H4/PDGFβR* (Kulkarni et al., 2000; Schwaller et al., 2001), which are associated with t(5;12)(q33;p13), t(9;12)(q34;p13), t(9;12)(p24;p13), and t(5;10)(q33;q11.2) translocations, respectively. These fusion genes encode constitutively activated tyrosine kinases and are sufficient to induce myeloproliferative diseases in mice (Daley et al., 1990; Schwaller et al., 1998; Tomasson et al., 2000). Because BCR–ABL oncogene is associated with over 95% of human CML, we describe BCR–ABL-induced mouse CML models in detail in Chapter 7.

2.2.3 Modeling Acute Lymphoblastic Leukemia

ETV6/RUNX1 (TEL/AML1) results from a t(12;21)(p13;q22) chromosomal translocation and is the most common known gene rearrangement in childhood cancer. Twenty-seven percent of childhood ALL samples contain an ETV6/RUNX1 fusion transcript detected by the PCR screening. RUNX1 is a member of the heterodimeric core-binding factor (CBF) family of transcription factors and has been shown to regulate a number of genes relevant to myeloid and lymphoid development (Tenen et al., 1997). RUNX1 contains conserved Runt homology domain (RHD) in the N-terminal half, which can bind to DNA, and this DNA-binding activity is enhanced by interaction with the C-terminal portion of the CBF beta subunit (Fenrick et al., 1999; Kitabayashi et al., 1998; Levanon et al., 1998; Meyers et al., 1993). Recruitment of the AML1 complex to the enhancers of its target genes can be direct or cooperatively with other proteins (Pabst et al., 2001). ETV6 protein contains a helix-loop-helix (HLH) motif and an ETS DNA-binding domain. 12p13 translocations and deletions are highly associated with childhood ALL, suggesting that there is a tumor suppressor gene that is disturbed by these chromosomal changes. Detailed examination shows that the critically deleted region includes two candidate suppressor genes: *ETV6* and *KIP* (Stegmaier et al., 1995). ETV6/RUNX1 forms homodimers and forms heterodimers with the normal ETV6 protein when the two proteins were expressed together (Hess and Hug, 2004). Besides ETV6/RUNX1, ETV6 variably forms fusion genes with other genes, including *ETV6/MN1* (Raynaud et al., 1996), *ETV6/AML1* (Ford et al., 1998), *ETV6/JAK2* (Schwaller et al., 2000), *ETV6/ARNT* (Salomon-Nguyen et al., 2000b), *ETV6/MDS2* (Odero et al., 2002), *ETV6/PER1*, and *ETV6/ABL* (Papadopoulos et al., 1995).

To elucidate the mechanism of lymphoid transformation by ETV6/RUNX1, the ETV6/AML1 coding region was inserted into retroviral vector to allow expression of ETV6/AML1 in lineage-negative donor bone marrow cells in mice (Fischer et al., 2005). Although mice receiving ETV6/RUNX1-transduced bone morrow cells did not develop B cell ALL, ETV6/RUNX1 perturbed B-cell differentiation by increasing the proportion of pro-B cells with low level of mature lymphoid cells in the blood and spleen, which is consistent with human precursor B cell ALL at an early stage. This mouse ALL model can be used for studying the mechanism of early stage of ETV6/RUNX1-induced ALL. Apparently, better disease models need to be developed with *ETV6/RUNX1* or other *ETV6*-related fusion genes to study the molecular basis of ALL.

2.2.4 Modeling Chronic Lymphocytic Leukemia

CLL is a common type of leukemia. There are about 10,000 new CLL cases in United States every year (Bichi et al., 2002; Landis et al., 1998), and CLL accounts for almost 30% of all adult leukemia cases. Most cases of CLL are of B-cell origin, and a few are of T-cell origin. B-CLL is believed to be derived from $CD5^+$ B lymphocyte through clonal expansion. Several common genomic abnormalities in CLL have been identified, and TCL1 is involved in the pathogenesis of CLL. The *TCL1* gene locates at chromosome 14q32.1 (Virgilio et al., 1994) and is commonly activated by inversions or translocations that juxtapose it to a T-cell receptor locus at 14q11 or 7q35. TCL1 has been found to be overexpressed in sporadic and ataxia telangiectasia-associated T-prolymphocytic leukemia (T-PLL) (Narducci et al., 1997; Thick et al., 1996). TCL1 is also highly expressed in a broad variety of human tumor-derived B-cell lines and in many cases of B-cell neoplasias (Narducci et al., 2000; Takizawa et al., 1998). To elucidate the role of *TCL1* in B-cell development and in B-cell leukemia pathogenesis, TCL1 transgenic mouse has been generated by cloning human *TCL1* coding region into the pBSVE6BK (pEμ) plasmid containing a mouse VH promoter (V186.2) and the IgH-μ enhancer along with the 3′-untranslated region and the poly(A) site of the human beta-globin gene, followed by injecting the *TCL1*-containing construct free from vector sequences into fertilized oocytes from B6C3 mice. In this model, *TCL1* was under the control of a promoter and enhancer whose activity specifically targets expression of the *TCL1* transgene to the B-cell compartment. Eμ-TCL1 transgenic mice developed a disease similar to human CLL. The mice first developed a preleukemic phenotype and later developed a frank leukemia with all characteristics of CLL (Bichi et al., 2002).

TNF receptor-associated factors (TRAFs) are a family of adapter proteins that link TNF-family receptors (TNFRs) to intracellular signaling pathways. It has been demonstrated that TRAF-family members participate in signaling cascades involved in gene expression, cell proliferation, and control of apoptosis. Elevated expression of some TRAF-family proteins, in particular TRAF1, is found in hematopoietic malignancies such as CLL and NHL (Munzert et al., 2002; Zapata et al., 2000). A study shows that TRAF1 and TRAF2 mediated apoptosis protection (Arron et al., 2002; Lin et al., 2003; Wang et al., 1998), suggesting that these TRAF family members could participate in the

Table 2.1 Examples of mouse models of human blood cancers

Chromosomal translocation	Fusion gene	Leukemia type	Disease frequency	Mouse models (approaches)	Citations
t(15;17)(q22-q11.2-12)	*PML–RARα*	AML	10% (98%)	Transgene, retroviral transduction of bone marrow cells	(Chan et al., 2006; Grisolano et al., 1997; Kelly et al., 2000a; Westervelt et al., 2003)
t(8;21)(q22;q22)	*AML1–ETO*	AML	18% (30%)	Transgene, retroviral transduction of bone marrow cells	(de Guzman et al., 2002; Fenske et al., 2004; Yan et al., 2004)
t(11;17)(q23;q21)	*PLZF–RARα*	AML	Rare	Transgene	(Rego et al., 2006)
inv(16) or t(16;16)	*CBFβ–MYH11*	AML	8% (~100%)	Conditional transgene	(Kuo et al., 2006)
t(9;11)(p22;q23)	*MLL–AF9*	AML	11% (30%)	Knock-in	(Dobson et al., 1999)
t(6;11)(q27;q23)	*MLL–AF6*	AML	11q23 abnormalities are detected in ~35% of all AML		(Joh et al., 1997; Poirel et al., 1996)
t(10;11)	*MLL–AF10, CALM–AF10*				(Borkhardt et al., 1995a)
t(11;17)(q23;q21)	*MLL–AF17*				(Suzukawa et al., 2005)
t(11;19)(q23;p13.3)	*MLL–ENL/ENL/EEN*			Retroviral transduction of bone marrow cell	(DiMartino et al., 2000; Rubnitz et al., 1999)
t(4;11)(q21;q23)	*MLL–AF4*			Knock-in	(Chen et al., 2006; Domer et al., 1993)
t(6;9)(p23;q34)	*DEK–CAN*	AML	1%		(Soekarman et al., 1992; von Lindern et al., 1992)

Table 2.1 (continued)

Chromosomal translocation	Fusion gene	Leukemia type	Disease frequency	Mouse models (approaches)	Citations
t(16;21)(p11;q22)	*TLS (FUS)–ERG*	AML	<1%		(Ichikawa et al., 1994; Kong et al., 1997; Panagopoulos et al., 1994)
t(16;21)(q24;q22)	*AML1–MTG16*	t-AML, MDS	<1%		(La Starza et al., 2001; Salomon-Nguyen et al., 2000a)
t(3;21)	*AML1–EVI1* *AML1–EAP* *AML1–MDS1*	AML	<1%	Knock-in	(Maki et al., 2005)
t(7;11)(p15;p15)	*NUP98–HOXA9*	AML	<1%	Retroviral transduction of bone marrow cells	(Kroon et al., 2001; Nakamura et al., 1996)
t(1;11)(q23;p15)	*NUP98–PMX1*	AML			
t(8;16)(p11;p13.3)	*MOZ–CBP*	AML	<1%		(Borrow et al., 1996)
inv(8)(p11q13)	*MOZ–TIF2*	AML	<1%	Retroviral transduction of bone marrow cells	(Deguchi et al., 2003)
t(8;22)(p11;p13)	*MOZ–p300*	AML	<1%		(Imamura et al., 2003; Kitabayashi et al., 2001b)
t(12;22)(p12;q23)	*TEL–MN1*	AML, CML	<1%		(Buijs et al., 1995; Nakazato et al., 2001)

Table 2.1 (continued)

Chromosomal translocation	Fusion gene	Leukemia type	Disease frequency	Mouse models (approaches)	Citations
t(1;229)(p13;q13)	*OTT–MAL*	AML	<1%		(Ma et al., 2001; Mercher et al., 2001)
t(5;12)(q33;p12)	*TEL–PDGFRβ*	CMMoL	2–5%	Transgene; retroviral transduction of bone marrow cells	(Ritchie et al., 1999; Sawyers and Denny, 1994; Tomasson et al., 2000; Wlodarska et al., 1995)
t(9;22)(q34;q11.2)	*BCR–ABL*	CML	~ 98%	Retroviral transduction of bone marrow cells; tetracycline inducible system	(Koschmieder et al., 2005; Li et al., 1999)
t(1;19)(q23;p13.3)	*E2A–PBX1*	Pre-B ALL	6% (30%)		(Kamps et al., 1991)
t(17;19)(q22;p13.3)	*E2A–HLF*	Pro-B ALL	1%	Transgene	(Honda et al., 1999; Hunger et al., 1992)
t(12;21)(p12;q22)	*TEL–AML1*	Pre-B ALL	25%	Retroviral transduction of bone marrow cells	(Bernardin et al., 2002; Tsuzuki et al., 2004)
t(9;22)(q34;q11.2)	*BCR–ABL*	ALL	~5% of childhood ALL; 30% of adult B-ALL	retroviral transduction of bone marrow cells; knock-in	(Castellanos et al., 1997; Li et al., 1999)
t(4;11)(q21;q23)	*MLL–AF4*	Pre-B ALL	5%	Knock-in	(Chen et al., 2006; Domer et al., 1993)

Table 2.1 (continued)

Chromosomal translocation	Fusion gene	Leukemia type	Disease frequency	Mouse models (approaches)	Citations
t(9;11)(p22;q23)	*MLL–AF9*	Pre-B ALL	<1%	Knock-in	(Dobson et al., 1999)
t(11;19)(q23;p13.3)	*MLL–ENL*	Pre-B ALL, T-ALL	1%	Retroviral transduction of bone marrow cell	(DiMartino et al., 2000; Rubnitz et al., 1999)
t(X;11)(q13;q23)	*MLL–AFX1*	T-ALL	<1%		(Corral et al., 1993)
t(1;11)(p32;q23)	*MLL–AFP1*	ALL	<1%		(Borkhardt et al., 1995b)
t(6;11)(q27;q23)	*MLL–AF6*	ALL	<1%		(Joh et al., 1997; Poirel et al., 1996)
t(2;5(2p23;q35)	*NPM–ALK*	Lymphoma ALCL, NHL	75%	Retroviral transduction of bone marrow cell; transgene	(Chiarle et al., 2003; Jager et al., 2005; Kuefer et al., 1997; Miething et al., 2003)

The percentage refers to the frequency of the translocations within the disease overall. The values within parentheses refer to the frequency within the morphologic or immunologic subtype of the disease. ALCL, anaplastic large cell lymphoma; ALL, acute lymphoblastic leukemia; AML, acute myelogenous leukemia; CML, chronic myelogenous leukemia; CMMoL, chronic myelomonocytic leukemia; MDS, myelodysplastic syndrome; NHL, non-HodgkinÂ's lymphoma. (Referred and modified from http://emice.nci.nih.gov/emice/mouse_models/organ_models/hema_models/hema_appendix_two.)

apoptosis-resistant phenotype of CLL and NHL. To model TRAF-mediated CLL, transgenic mice, which expressed in lymphocytes a TRAF2 mutant lacking the RING and zinc finger domains located at the N-terminus of TRAF2 (TRAF2DN), developed splenomegaly and lymphadenopathy, as a result of a polyclonal expansion of B lymphocytes (Lee et al., 1997). In addition, transgenic mouse expressing Bcl-2 in B lymphocytes developed age-dependent lymphadenopathy and splenomegaly (Katsumata et al., 1992), associated with lymphoid cell expansions resembling certain human low-grade B-cell malignancies (Katsumata et al., 1992; Strasser et al., 1993). When both TRAF2DN and Bcl-2 transgenic mice were crossed to generate double transgenic mice, the double homozygous mice develop an age-dependent B-cell leukemia and lymphoma, with striking similarities to human CLL. These findings also provide direct evidence that TRAFs contribute to CLL development and that the high coexpression levels of TRAF1 and Bcl-2 commonly found in human CLL contribute to the pathogenesis of this leukemia (Zapata et al., 2000).

2.3 Conclusion

Although many mouse models of human blood cancers (Table 2.1) are available for the study of disease mechanisms and the development of new therapeutic strategies, improvements are needed to more accurately mimic human blood cancers. On the other hand, mouse models of many types of human leukemia induced or accelerated by fusion genes and other mutated genes are not yet available (Table 2.1), and generation of these disease models will be of important value.

References

Arron, J.R., Pewzner-Jung, Y., Walsh, M.C., Kobayashi, T., and Choi, Y. (2002). Regulation of the subcellular localization of tumor necrosis factor receptor-associated factor (TRAF)2 by TRAF1 reveals mechanisms of TRAF2 signaling. J Exp Med *196*, 923–934.

Bernardin, F., Yang, Y., Cleaves, R., Zahurak, M., Cheng, L., Civin, C.I., and Friedman, A.D. (2002). TEL-AML1, expressed from t(12;21) in human acute lymphocytic leukemia, induces acute leukemia in mice. Cancer Res *62*, 3904–3908.

Bernardin-Fried, F., Kummalue, T., Leijen, S., Collector, M.I., Ravid, K., and Friedman, A.D. (2004). AML1/RUNX1 increases during G1 to S cell cycle progression independent of cytokine-dependent phosphorylation and induces cyclin D3 gene expression. J Biol Chem *279*, 15678–15687.

Bhatia, A., Dash, S., Varma, N., and Marwaha, R.K. (2007). Fanconi anemia presenting as acute myeloid leukemia: a case report. Indian J Pathol Microbiol *50*, 441–443.

Bichi, R., Shinton, S.A., Martin, E.S., Koval, A., Calin, G.A., Cesari, R., Russo, G., Hardy, R.R., and Croce, C.M. (2002). Human chronic lymphocytic leukemia modeled in mouse by targeted TCL1 expression. Proc Natl Acad Sci USA *99*, 6955–6960.

Borkhardt, A., Haas, O.A., Strobl, W., Repp, R., Mann, G., Gadner, H., and Lampert, F. (1995a). A novel type of MLL/AF10 fusion transcript in a child with acute megakaryocytic leukemia (AML-M7). Leukemia *9*, 1796–1797.
Borkhardt, A., Mitteis, M., Brettreich, S., Schlieben, S., Hammermann, J., Repp, R., Kreuder, J., Buchen, U., and Lampert, F. (1995b). Rapid synthesis of hybrid RNA molecules associated with leukemia-specific chromosomal translocations. Leukemia *9*, 719–722.
Borrow, J., Stanton, V.P., Jr., Andresen, J.M., Becher, R., Behm, F.G., Chaganti, R.S., Civin, C.I., Disteche, C., Dube, I., Frischauf, A.M., et al. (1996). The translocation t(8;16)(p11;p13) of acute myeloid leukaemia fuses a putative acetyltransferase to the CREB-binding protein. Nat Genet *14*, 33–41.
Bowen, D.T., Frew, M.E., Hills, R., Gale, R.E., Wheatley, K., Groves, M.J., Langabeer, S.E., Kottaridis, P.D., Moorman, A.V., Burnett, A.K., et al. (2005). RAS mutation in acute myeloid leukemia is associated with distinct cytogenetic subgroups but does not influence outcome in patients younger than 60 years. Blood *106*, 2113–2119.
Braun, B.S., Tuveson, D.A., Kong, N., Le, D.T., Kogan, S.C., Rozmus, J., Le Beau, M.M., Jacks, T.E., and Shannon, K.M. (2004). Somatic activation of oncogenic Kras in hematopoietic cells initiates a rapidly fatal myeloproliferative disorder. Proc Natl Acad Sci USA *101*, 597–602.
Buijs, A., Sherr, S., van Baal, S., van Bezouw, S., van der Plas, D., Geurts van Kessel, A., Riegman, P., Lekanne Deprez, R., Zwarthoff, E., Hagemeijer, A., et al. (1995). Translocation (12;22)(p13;q11) in myeloproliferative disorders results in fusion of the ETS-like TEL gene on 12p13 to the MN1 gene on 22q11. Oncogene *10*, 1511–1519.
Burel, S.A., Harakawa, N., Zhou, L., Pabst, T., Tenen, D.G., and Zhang, D.E. (2001). Dichotomy of AML1-ETO functions: growth arrest versus block of differentiation. Mol Cell Biol *21*, 5577–5590.
Callens, C., Chevret, S., Cayuela, J.M., Cassinat, B., Raffoux, E., de Botton, S., Thomas, X., Guerci, A., Fegueux, N., Pigneux, A., et al. (2005). Prognostic implication of FLT3 and Ras gene mutations in patients with acute promyelocytic leukemia (APL): a retrospective study from the European APL Group. Leukemia *19*, 1153–1160.
Carapeti, M., Aguiar, R.C., Goldman, J.M., and Cross, N.C. (1998). A novel fusion between MOZ and the nuclear receptor coactivator TIF2 in acute myeloid leukemia. Blood *91*, 3127–3133.
Castellanos, A., Pintado, B., Weruaga, E., Arevalo, R., Lopez, A., Orfao, A., and Sanchez-Garcia, I. (1997). A BCR-ABL(p190) fusion gene made by homologous recombination causes B-cell acute lymphoblastic leukemias in chimeric mice with independence of the endogenous bcr product. Blood *90*, 2168–2174.
Chaffanet, M., Gressin, L., Preudhomme, C., Soenen-Cornu, V., Birnbaum, D., and Pebusque, M.J. (2000). MOZ is fused to p300 in an acute monocytic leukemia with t(8;22). Genes Chromosomes Cancer *28*, 138–144.
Chan, I.T., Kutok, J.L., Williams, I.R., Cohen, S., Kelly, L., Shigematsu, H., Johnson, L., Akashi, K., Tuveson, D.A., Jacks, T., et al. (2004). Conditional expression of oncogenic K-ras from its endogenous promoter induces a myeloproliferative disease. J Clin Invest *113*, 528–538.
Chan, I.T., Kutok, J.L., Williams, I.R., Cohen, S., Moore, S., Shigematsu, H., Ley, T.J., Akashi, K., Le Beau, M.M., and Gilliland, D.G. (2006). Oncogenic K-ras cooperates with PML-RAR alpha to induce an acute promyelocytic leukemia-like disease. Blood *108*, 1708–1715.
Chen, W., Li, Q., Hudson, W.A., Kumar, A., Kirchhof, N., and Kersey, J.H. (2006). A murine Mll-AF4 knock-in model results in lymphoid and myeloid deregulation and hematologic malignancy. Blood *108*, 669–677.
Chiarle, R., Gong, J.Z., Guasparri, I., Pesci, A., Cai, J., Liu, J., Simmons, W.J., Dhall, G., Howes, J., Piva, R., et al. (2003). NPM-ALK transgenic mice spontaneously develop T-cell lymphomas and plasma cell tumors. Blood *101*, 1919–1927.

Collins, S.J., Robertson, K.A., and Mueller, L. (1990). Retinoic acid-induced granulocytic differentiation of HL-60 myeloid leukemia cells is mediated directly through the retinoic acid receptor (RAR-alpha). Mol Cell Biol *10*, 2154–2163.

Corral, J., Forster, A., Thompson, S., Lampert, F., Kaneko, Y., Slater, R., Kroes, W.G., van der Schoot, C.E., Ludwig, W.D., Karpas, A., et al. (1993). Acute leukemias of different lineages have similar MLL gene fusions encoding related chimeric proteins resulting from chromosomal translocation. Proc Natl Acad Sci USA *90*, 8538–8542.

Dahia, P.L., Aguiar, R.C., Alberta, J., Kum, J.B., Caron, S., Sill, H., Marsh, D.J., Ritz, J., Freedman, A., Stiles, C., et al. (1999). PTEN is inversely correlated with the cell survival factor Akt/PKB and is inactivated via multiple mechanisms in haematological malignancies. Hum Mol Genet *8*, 185–193.

Daley, G.Q., Van Etten, R.A., and Baltimore, D. (1990). Induction of chronic myelogenous leukemia in mice by the P210bcr/abl gene of the Philadelphia chromosome. Science *247*, 824–830.

Dawson, M.I., Elstner, E., Kizaki, M., Chen, D.L., Pakkala, S., Kerner, B., and Koeffler, H.P. (1994). Myeloid differentiation mediated through retinoic acid receptor/retinoic X receptor (RXR) not RXR/RXR pathway. Blood *84*, 446–452.

de Guzman, C.G., Warren, A.J., Zhang, Z., Gartland, L., Erickson, P., Drabkin, H., Hiebert, S.W., and Klug, C.A. (2002). Hematopoietic stem cell expansion and distinct myeloid developmental abnormalities in a murine model of the AML1-ETO translocation. Mol Cell Biol *22*, 5506–5517.

Deguchi, K., Ayton, P.M., Carapeti, M., Kutok, J.L., Snyder, C.S., Williams, I.R., Cross, N.C., Glass, C.K., Cleary, M.L., and Gilliland, D.G. (2003). MOZ-TIF2-induced acute myeloid leukemia requires the MOZ nucleosome binding motif and TIF2-mediated recruitment of CBP. Cancer Cell *3*, 259–271.

Demarest, S.J., Martinez-Yamout, M., Chung, J., Chen, H., Xu, W., Dyson, H.J., Evans, R.M., and Wright, P.E. (2002). Mutual synergistic folding in recruitment of CBP/p300 by p160 nuclear receptor coactivators. Nature *415*, 549–553.

DiMartino, J.F., Miller, T., Ayton, P.M., Landewe, T., Hess, J.L., Cleary, M.L., and Shilatifard, A. (2000). A carboxy-terminal domain of ELL is required and sufficient for immortalization of myeloid progenitors by MLL-ELL. Blood *96*, 3887–3893.

Ding, X.F., Anderson, C.M., Ma, H., Hong, H., Uht, R.M., Kushner, P.J., and Stallcup, M.R. (1998). Nuclear receptor-binding sites of coactivators glucocorticoid receptor interacting protein 1 (GRIP1) and steroid receptor coactivator 1 (SRC-1): multiple motifs with different binding specificities. Mol Endocrinol *12*, 302–313.

Dobson, C.L., Warren, A.J., Pannell, R., Forster, A., Lavenir, I., Corral, J., Smith, A.J., and Rabbitts, T.H. (1999). The mll-AF9 gene fusion in mice controls myeloproliferation and specifies acute myeloid leukaemogenesis. Embo J *18*, 3564–3574.

Domer, P.H., Fakharzadeh, S.S., Chen, C.S., Jockel, J., Johansen, L., Silverman, G.A., Kersey, J.H., and Korsmeyer, S.J. (1993). Acute mixed-lineage leukemia t(4;11)(q21;q23) generates an MLL-AF4 fusion product. Proc Natl Acad Sci USA *90*, 7884–7888.

Fenrick, R., Amann, J.M., Lutterbach, B., Wang, L., Westendorf, J.J., Downing, J.R., and Hiebert, S.W. (1999). Both TEL and AML-1 contribute repression domains to the t(12;21) fusion protein. Mol Cell Biol *19*, 6566–6574.

Fenske, T.S., Pengue, G., Mathews, V., Hanson, P.T., Hamm, S.E., Riaz, N., and Graubert, T.A. (2004). Stem cell expression of the AML1/ETO fusion protein induces a myeloproliferative disorder in mice. Proc Natl Acad Sci USA *101*, 15184–15189.

Fischer, M., Schwieger, M., Horn, S., Niebuhr, B., Ford, A., Roscher, S., Bergholz, U., Greaves, M., Lohler, J., and Stocking, C. (2005). Defining the oncogenic function of the TEL/AML1 (ETV6/RUNX1) fusion protein in a mouse model. Oncogene *24*, 7579–7591.

Ford, A.M., Bennett, C.A., Price, C.M., Bruin, M.C., Van Wering, E.R., and Greaves, M. (1998). Fetal origins of the TEL-AML1 fusion gene in identical twins with leukemia. Proc Natl Acad Sci USA *95*, 4584–4588.

Glass, C.K., Rose, D.W., and Rosenfeld, M.G. (1997). Nuclear receptor coactivators. Curr Opin Cell Biol *9*, 222–232.

Golub, T.R., Barker, G.F., Bohlander, S.K., Hiebert, S.W., Ward, D.C., Bray-Ward, P., Morgan, E., Raimondi, S.C., Rowley, J.D., and Gilliland, D.G. (1995). Fusion of the TEL gene on 12p13 to the AML1 gene on 21q22 in acute lymphoblastic leukemia. Proc Natl Acad Sci USA *92*, 4917–4921.

Golub, T.R., Barker, G.F., Lovett, M., and Gilliland, D.G. (1994). Fusion of PDGF receptor beta to a novel ets-like gene, tel, in chronic myelomonocytic leukemia with t(5;12) chromosomal translocation. Cell *77*, 307–316.

Grisolano, J.L., Wesselschmidt, R.L., Pelicci, P.G., and Ley, T.J. (1997). Altered myeloid development and acute leukemia in transgenic mice expressing PML-RAR alpha under control of cathepsin G regulatory sequences. Blood *89*, 376–387.

Heery, D.M., Kalkhoven, E., Hoare, S., and Parker, M.G. (1997). A signature motif in transcriptional co-activators mediates binding to nuclear receptors. Nature *387*, 733–736.

Hess, J.L., and Hug, B.A. (2004). Fusion-protein truncation provides new insights into leukemogenesis. Proc Natl Acad Sci USA *101*, 16985–16986.

Hess, M., Huggins, M.B., Mudzamiri, R., and Heincz, U. (2004). Avian metapneumovirus excretion in vaccinated and non-vaccinated specified pathogen free laying chickens. Avian Pathol *33*, 35–40.

Higuchi, M., O'Brien, D., Kumaravelu, P., Lenny, N., Yeoh, E.J., and Downing, J.R. (2002). Expression of a conditional AML1-ETO oncogene bypasses embryonic lethality and establishes a murine model of human t(8;21) acute myeloid leukemia. Cancer Cell *1*, 63–74.

Honda, H., Inaba, T., Suzuki, T., Oda, H., Ebihara, Y., Tsuiji, K., Nakahata, T., Ishikawa, T., Yazaki, Y., and Hirai, H. (1999). Expression of E2A-HLF chimeric protein induced T-cell apoptosis, B-cell maturation arrest, and development of acute lymphoblastic leukemia. Blood *93*, 2780–2790.

Horwitz, K.B., Jackson, T.A., Bain, D.L., Richer, J.K., Takimoto, G.S., and Tung, L. (1996). Nuclear receptor coactivators and corepressors. Mol Endocrinol *10*, 1167–1177.

Hunger, S.P., Ohyashiki, K., Toyama, K., and Cleary, M.L. (1992). Hlf, a novel hepatic bZIP protein, shows altered DNA-binding properties following fusion to E2A in t(17;19) acute lymphoblastic leukemia. Genes Dev *6*, 1608–1620.

Ichikawa, H., Shimizu, K., Hayashi, Y., and Ohki, M. (1994). An RNA-binding protein gene, TLS/FUS, is fused to ERG in human myeloid leukemia with t(16;21) chromosomal translocation. Cancer Res *54*, 2865–2868.

Ida, K., Kitabayashi, I., Taki, T., Taniwaki, M., Noro, K., Yamamoto, M., Ohki, M., and Hayashi, Y. (1997). Adenoviral E1A-associated protein p300 is involved in acute myeloid leukemia with t(11;22)(q23;q13). Blood *90*, 4699–4704.

Imamura, T., Kakazu, N., Hibi, S., Morimoto, A., Fukushima, Y., Ijuin, I., Hada, S., Kitabayashi, I., Abe, T., and Imashuku, S. (2003). Rearrangement of the MOZ gene in pediatric therapy-related myelodysplastic syndrome with a novel chromosomal translocation t(2;8)(p23;p11). Genes Chromosomes Cancer *36*, 413–419.

Jackson, E.L., Willis, N., Mercer, K., Bronson, R.T., Crowley, D., Montoya, R., Jacks, T., and Tuveson, D.A. (2001). Analysis of lung tumor initiation and progression using conditional expression of oncogenic K-ras. Genes Dev *15*, 3243–3248.

Jager, R., Hahne, J., Jacob, A., Egert, A., Schenkel, J., Wernert, N., Schorle, H., and Wellmann, A. (2005). Mice transgenic for NPM-ALK develop non-Hodgkin lymphomas. Anticancer Res *25*, 3191–3196.

Joh, T., Yamamoto, K., Kagami, Y., Kakuda, H., Sato, T., Yamamoto, T., Takahashi, T., Ueda, R., Kaibuchi, K., and Seto, M. (1997). Chimeric MLL products with a Ras binding cytoplasmic protein AF6 involved in t(6;11)(q27;q23) leukemia localize in the nucleus. Oncogene *15*, 1681–1687.

Kamps, M.P., Look, A.T., and Baltimore, D. (1991). The human t(1;19) translocation in pre-B ALL produces multiple nuclear E2A-Pbx1 fusion proteins with differing transforming potentials. Genes Dev *5*, 358–368.

Katsumata, M., Siegel, R.M., Louie, D.C., Miyashita, T., Tsujimoto, Y., Nowell, P.C., Greene, M.I., and Reed, J.C. (1992). Differential effects of Bcl-2 on T and B cells in transgenic mice. Proc Natl Acad Sci USA *89*, 11376–11380.

Kelly, L.M., Kutok, J.L., Williams, I.R., Boulton, C.L., Amaral, S.M., Curley, D.P., Ley, T.J., and Gilliland, D.G. (2000a). PML/RARalpha and FLT3-ITD induce an APL-like disease in a mouse model. Proc Natl Acad Sci USA *99*, 8283–8288.

Kelly, L.M., Liu, Q., Kutok, J.L., Williams, I.R., Boulton, C.L., and Gilliland, D.G. (2002b). FLT3 internal tandem duplication mutations associated with human acute myeloid leukemias induce myeloproliferative disease in a murine bone marrow transplant model. Blood *99*, 310–318.

Kitabayashi, I., Aikawa, Y., Nguyen, L.A., Yokoyama, A., and Ohki, M. (2001a). Activation of AML1-mediated transcription by MOZ and inhibition by the MOZ-CBP fusion protein. Embo J *20*, 7184–7196.

Kitabayashi, I., Aikawa, Y., Yokoyama, A., Hosoda, F., Nagai, M., Kakazu, N., Abe, T., and Ohki, M. (2001b). Fusion of MOZ and p300 histone acetyltransferases in acute monocytic leukemia with a t(8;22)(p11;q13) chromosome translocation. Leukemia *15*, 89–94.

Kitabayashi, I., Yokoyama, A., Shimizu, K., and Ohki, M. (1998). Interaction and functional cooperation of the leukemia-associated factors AML1 and p300 in myeloid cell differentiation. Embo J *17*, 2994–3004.

Kong, X.T., Ida, K., Ichikawa, H., Shimizu, K., Ohki, M., Maseki, N., Kaneko, Y., Sako, M., Kobayashi, Y., Tojou, A., et al. (1997). Consistent detection of TLS/FUS-ERG chimeric transcripts in acute myeloid leukemia with t(16;21)(p11;q22) and identification of a novel transcript. Blood *90*, 1192–1199.

Koschmieder, S., Gottgens, B., Zhang, P., Iwasaki-Arai, J., Akashi, K., Kutok, J.L., Dayaram, T., Geary, K., Green, A.R., Tenen, D.G., et al. (2005). Inducible chronic phase of myeloid leukemia with expansion of hematopoietic stem cells in a transgenic model of BCR-ABL leukemogenesis. Blood *105*, 324–334.

Kottaridis, P.D., Gale, R.E., Frew, M.E., Harrison, G., Langabeer, S.E., Belton, A.A., Walker, H., Wheatley, K., Bowen, D.T., Burnett, A.K., et al. (2001). The presence of a FLT3 internal tandem duplication in patients with acute myeloid leukemia (AML) adds important prognostic information to cytogenetic risk group and response to the first cycle of chemotherapy: analysis of 854 patients from the United Kingdom Medical Research Council AML 10 and 12 trials. Blood *98*, 1752–1759.

Kroon, E., Thorsteinsdottir, U., Mayotte, N., Nakamura, T., and Sauvageau, G. (2001). NUP98-HOXA9 expression in hemopoietic stem cells induces chronic and acute myeloid leukemias in mice. Embo J *20*, 350–361.

Kuefer, M.U., Look, A.T., Pulford, K., Behm, F.G., Pattengale, P.K., Mason, D.Y., and Morris, S.W. (1997). Retrovirus-mediated gene transfer of NPM-ALK causes lymphoid malignancy in mice. Blood *90*, 2901–2910.

Kuhn, R., Schwenk, F., Aguet, M., and Rajewsky, K. (1995). Inducible gene targeting in mice. Science *269*, 1427–1429.

Kulkarni, S., Heath, C., Parker, S., Chase, A., Iqbal, S., Pocock, C.F., Kaeda, J., Cwynarski, K., Goldman, J.M., and Cross, N.C. (2000). Fusion of H4/D10S170 to the platelet-derived growth factor receptor beta in BCR-ABL-negative myeloproliferative disorders with a t(5;10)(q33;q21). Cancer Res *60*, 3592–3598.

Kuo, Y.H., Landrette, S.F., Heilman, S.A., Perrat, P.N., Garrett, L., Liu, P.P., Le Beau, M.M., Kogan, S.C., and Castilla, L.H. (2006). Cbf beta-SMMHC induces distinct abnormal myeloid progenitors able to develop acute myeloid leukemia. Cancer Cell *9*, 57–68.

La Starza, R., Sambani, C., Crescenzi, B., Matteucci, C., Martelli, M.F., and Mecucci, C. (2001). AML1/MTG16 fusion gene from a t(16;21)(q24;q22) translocation in treatment-induced leukemia after breast cancer. Haematologica *86*, 212–213.

Lacronique, V., Boureux, A., Valle, V.D., Poirel, H., Quang, C.T., Mauchauffe, M., Berthou, C., Lessard, M., Berger, R., Ghysdael, J., et al. (1997). A TEL-JAK2 fusion protein with constitutive kinase activity in human leukemia. Science *278*, 1309–1312.

Landis, S.H., Murray, T., Bolden, S., and Wingo, P.A. (1998). Cancer statistics, 1998. CA Cancer J Clin *48*, 6–29.

Lee, S.Y., Reichlin, A., Santana, A., Sokol, K.A., Nussenzweig, M.C., and Choi, Y. (1997). TRAF2 is essential for JNK but not NF-kappaB activation and regulates lymphocyte proliferation and survival. Immunity *7*, 703–713.

Leo, C., and Chen, J.D. (2000). The SRC family of nuclear receptor coactivators. Gene *245*, 1–11.

Lessard, J., and Sauvageau, G. (2003). Bmi-1 determines the proliferative capacity of normal and leukaemic stem cells. Nature *423*, 255–260.

Levanon, D., Goldstein, R.E., Bernstein, Y., Tang, H., Goldenberg, D., Stifani, S., Paroush, Z., and Groner, Y. (1998). Transcriptional repression by AML1 and LEF-1 is mediated by the TLE/Groucho corepressors. Proc Natl Acad Sci USA *95*, 11590–11595.

Li, D.M., and Sun, H. (1998). PTEN/MMAC1/TEP1 suppresses the tumorigenicity and induces G1 cell cycle arrest in human glioblastoma cells. Proc Natl Acad Sci USA *95*, 15406–15411.

Li, S., Ilaria, R.L., Jr., Million, R.P., Daley, G.Q., and Van Etten, R.A. (1999). The P190, P210, and p230 forms of the *BCR/ABL* oncogene induce a similar chronic myeloid leukemia-like syndrome in mice but have different lymphoid leukemogenic activity. J Exp Med *189*, 1399–1412.

Li, J., Yen, C., Liaw, D., Podsypanina, K., Bose, S., Wang, S.I., Puc, J., Miliaresis, C., Rodgers, L., McCombie, R., et al. (1997). PTEN, a putative protein tyrosine phosphatase gene mutated in human brain, breast, and prostate cancer. Science *275*, 1943–1947.

Liang, J., Prouty, L., Williams, B.J., Dayton, M.A., and Blanchard, K.L. (1998). Acute mixed lineage leukemia with an inv(8)(p11q13) resulting in fusion of the genes for MOZ and TIF2. Blood *92*, 2118–2122.

Lin, Y., Ryan, J., Lewis, J., Wani, M.A., Lingrel, J.B., and Liu, Z.G. (2003). TRAF2 exerts its antiapoptotic effect by regulating the expression of Kruppel-like factor LKLF. Mol Cell Biol *23*, 5849–5856.

Liu, P., Tarle, S.A., Hajra, A., Claxton, D.F., Marlton, P., Freedman, M., Siciliano, M.J., and Collins, F.S. (1993). Fusion between transcription factor CBF beta/PEBP2 beta and a myosin heavy chain in acute myeloid leukemia. Science *261*, 1041–1044.

Liu, P.P., Wijmenga, C., Hajra, A., Blake, T.B., Kelley, C.A., Adelstein, R.S., Bagg, A., Rector, J., Cotelingam, J., Willman, C.L., et al. (1996). Identification of the chimeric protein product of the CBFβ-MYH11 fusion gene in inv(16) leukemia cells. Genes Chromosomes Cancer *16*, 77–87.

Lou, J., Cao, W., Bernardin, F., Ayyanathan, K., Rauscher, I.F., and Friedman, A.D. (2000). Exogenous cdk4 overcomes reduced cdk4 RNA and inhibition of G1 progression in hematopoietic cells expressing a dominant-negative CBF – a model for overcoming inhibition of proliferation by CBF oncoproteins. Oncogene *19*, 2695–2703.

Lutterbach, B., Westendorf, J.J., Linggi, B., Patten, A., Moniwa, M., Davie, J.R., Huynh, K.D., Bardwell, V.J., Lavinsky, R.M., Rosenfeld, M.G., et al. (1998). ETO, a target of t(8;21) in acute leukemia, interacts with the N-CoR and mSin3 corepressors. Mol Cell Biol *18*, 7176–7184.

Ma, Z., Morris, S.W., Valentine, V., Li, M., Herbrick, J.A., Cui, X., Bouman, D., Li, Y., Mehta, P.K., Nizetic, D., et al. (2001). Fusion of two novel genes, RBM15 and MKL1, in the t(1;22)(p13;q13) of acute megakaryoblastic leukemia. Nat Genet *28*, 220–221.

Maki, K., Yamagata, T., Asai, T., Yamazaki, I., Oda, H., Hirai, H., and Mitani, K. (2005). Dysplastic definitive hematopoiesis in AML1/EVI1 knock-in embryos. Blood *106*, 2147–2155.

Mercher, T., Coniat, M.B., Monni, R., Mauchauffe, M., Nguyen Khac, F., Gressin, L., Mugneret, F., Leblanc, T., Dastugue, N., Berger, R., et al. (2001). Involvement of a human gene related to the Drosophila spen gene in the recurrent t(1;22) translocation of acute megakaryocytic leukemia. Proc Natl Acad Sci USA *98*, 5776–5779.

Meyers, S., Downing, J.R., and Hiebert, S.W. (1993). Identification of AML-1 and the (8;21) translocation protein (AML-1/ETO) as sequence-specific DNA-binding proteins: the Runt homology domain is required for DNA binding and protein-protein interactions. Mol Cell Biol *13*, 6336–6345.

Miething, C., Grundler, R., Fend, F., Hoepfl, J., Mugler, C., von Schilling, C., Morris, S.W., Peschel, C., and Duyster, J. (2003). The oncogenic fusion protein nucleophosmin-anaplastic lymphoma kinase (NPM-ALK) induces two distinct malignant phenotypes in a murine retroviral transplantation model. Oncogene *22*, 4642–4647.

Munzert, G., Kirchner, D., Stobbe, H., Bergmann, L., Schmid, R.M., Dohner, H., and Heimpel, H. (2002). Tumor necrosis factor receptor-associated factor 1 gene overexpression in B-cell chronic lymphocytic leukemia: analysis of NF-kappa B/Rel-regulated inhibitors of apoptosis. Blood *100*, 3749–3756.

Murray, R.J., O'ReillyR.J., Cannell, P, French, M.A. (1999). B-cell acute lymphoblastic leukaemia in HIV infection. Annu Conf Australas Soc HIV Med, 11.

Nakamura, T., Largaespada, D.A., Lee, M.P., Johnson, L.A., Ohyashiki, K., Toyama, K., Chen, S.J., Willman, C.L., Chen, I.M., Feinberg, A.P., et al. (1996). Fusion of the nucleoporin gene NUP98 to HOXA9 by the chromosome translocation t(7;11)(p15;p15) in human myeloid leukaemia. Nat Genet *12*, 154–158.

Nakazato, H., Shiozaki, H., Zhou, M., Nakatsu, M., Motoji, T., Mizoguchi, H., Miyawaki, S., and Sato, Y. (2001). TEL/MN1 fusion in a de novo acute myeloid leukaemia-M2 patient who showed strong resistance to treatment. Br J Haematol *113*, 1079–1081.

Narducci, M.G., Pescarmona, E., Lazzeri, C., Signoretti, S., Lavinia, A.M., Remotti, D., Scala, E., Baroni, C.D., Stoppacciaro, A., Croce, C.M., et al. (2000). Regulation of TCL1 expression in B- and T-cell lymphomas and reactive lymphoid tissues. Cancer Res *60*, 2095–2100.

Narducci, M.G., Stoppacciaro, A., Imada, K., Uchiyama, T., Virgilio, L., Lazzeri, C., Croce, C.M., and Russo, G. (1997). TCL1 is overexpressed in patients affected by adult T-cell leukemias. Cancer Res *57*, 5452–5456.

Odero, M.D., Vizmanos, J.L., Roman, J.P., Lahortiga, I., Panizo, C., Calasanz, M.J., Zeleznik-Le, N.J., Rowley, J.D., and Novo, F.J. (2002). A novel gene, MDS2, is fused to ETV6/TEL in a t(1;12)(p36.1;p13) in a patient with myelodysplastic syndrome. Genes Chromosomes Cancer *35*, 11–19.

Okuda, T., Cai, Z., Yang, S., Lenny, N., Lyu, C.J., van Deursen, J.M., Harada, H., and Downing, J.R. (1998). Expression of a knocked-in AML1-ETO leukemia gene inhibits the establishment of normal definitive hematopoiesis and directly generates dysplastic hematopoietic progenitors. Blood *91*, 3134–3143.

Okuda, T., Takeda, K., Fujita, Y., Nishimura, M., Yagyu, S., Yoshida, M., Akira, S., Downing, J.R., and Abe, T. (2000). Biological characteristics of the leukemia-associated transcriptional factor AML1 disclosed by hematopoietic rescue of *AML1*-deficient embryonic stem cells by using a knock-in strateby. Mol Cell Biol *20*, 319–328.

Onodera, M., Kunisada, T., Nishikawa, S., Sakiyama, Y., Matsumoto, S., and Nishikawa, S. (1995). Overexpression of retinoic acid receptor alpha suppresses myeloid cell differentiation at the promyelocyte stage. Oncogene *11*, 1291–1298.

Pabst, T., Mueller, B.U., Harakawa, N., Schoch, C., Haferlach, T., Behre, G., Hiddemann, W., Zhang, D.E., and Tenen, D.G. (2001). AML1-ETO downregulates the granulocytic differentiation factor C/EBPalpha in t(8;21) myeloid leukemia. Nat Med *7*, 444–451.

Panagopoulos, I., Aman, P., Fioretos, T., Hoglund, M., Johansson, B., Mandahl, N., Heim, S., Behrendtz, M., and Mitelman, F. (1994). Fusion of the FUS gene with ERG in acute myeloid leukemia with t(16;21)(p11;q22). Genes Chromosomes Cancer *11*, 256–262.

Panagopoulos, I., Fioretos, T., Isaksson, M., Samuelsson, U., Billstrom, R., Strombeck, B., Mitelman, F., and Johansson, B. (2001). Fusion of the MORF and CBP genes in acute myeloid leukemia with the t(10;16)(q22;p13). Hum Mol Genet *10*, 395–404.

Papadopoulos, P., Ridge, S.A., Boucher, C.A., Stocking, C., and Wiedemann, L.M. (1995). The novel activation of ABL by fusion to an ets-related gene, TEL. Cancer Res *55*, 34–38.

Park, I.K., Qian, D., Kiel, M., Becker, M.W., Pihalja, M., Weissman, I.L., Morrison, S.J., and Clarke, M.F. (2003). Bmi-1 is required for maintenance of adult self-renewing haematopoietic stem cells. Nature *423*, 302–305.

Poiesz, B.J., Papsidero, L.D., Ehrlich, G., Sherman, M., Dube, S., Poiesz, M., Dillon, K., Ruscetti, F.W., Slamon, D., Fang, C., et al. (2001). Prevalence of HTLV-I-associated T-cell lymphoma. Am J Hematol *66*, 32–38.

Poirel, H., Rack, K., Delabesse, E., Radford-Weiss, I., Troussard, X., Debert, C., Leboeuf, D., Bastard, C., Picard, F., Veil-Buzyn, A., et al. (1996). Incidence and characterization of MLL gene (11q23) rearrangements in acute myeloid leukemia M1 and M5. Blood *87*, 2496–2505.

Raynaud, S.D., Baens, M., Grosgeorge, J., Rodgers, K., Reid, C.D., Dainton, M., Dyer, M., Fuzibet, J.G., Gratecos, N., Taillan, B., et al. (1996). Fluorescence in situ hybridization analysis of t(3; 12)(q26; p13): a recurring chromosomal abnormality involving the TEL gene (ETV6) in myelodysplastic syndromes. Blood *88*, 682–689.

Rego, E.M., Ruggero, D., Tribioli, C., Cattoretti, G., Kogan, S., Redner, R.L., and Pandolfi, P.P. (2006). Leukemia with distinct phenotypes in transgenic mice expressing PML/RAR alpha, PLZF/RAR alpha or NPM/RAR alpha. Oncogene *25*, 1974–1979.

Rhoades, K.L., Hetherington, C.J., Harakawa, N., Yergeau, D.A., Zhou, L., Liu, L.Q., Little, M.T., Tenen, D.G., and Zhang, D.E. (2000). Analysis of the role of AML1-ETO in leukemogenesis, using an inducible transgenic mouse model. Blood *96*, 2108–2115.

Ritchie, K.A., Aprikyan, A.A., Bowen-Pope, D.F., Norby-Slycord, C.J., Conyers, S., Bartelmez, S., Sitnicka, E.H., and Hickstein, D.D. (1999). The Tel-PDGFRbeta fusion gene produces a chronic myeloproliferative syndrome in transgenic mice. Leukemia *13*, 1790–1803.

Rubnitz, J.E., Camitta, B.M., Mahmoud, H., Raimondi, S.C., Carroll, A.J., Borowitz, M.J., Shuster, J.J., Link, M.P., Pullen, D.J., Downing, J.R., et al. (1999). Childhood acute lymphoblastic leukemia with the MLL-ENL fusion and t(11;19)(q23;p13.3) translocation. J Clin Oncol *17*, 191–196.

Salomon-Nguyen, F., Busson-Le Coniat, M., Lafage Pochitaloff, M., Mozziconacci, J., Berger, R., and Bernard, O.A. (2000a). AML1-MTG16 fusion gene in therapy-related acute leukemia with t(16;21)(q24;q22): two new cases. Leukemia *14*, 1704–1705.

Salomon-Nguyen, F., Della-Valle, V., Mauchauffe, M., Busson-Le Coniat, M., Ghysdael, J., Berger, R., and Bernard, O.A. (2000b). The t(1;12)(q21;p13) translocation of human acute myeloblastic leukemia results in a TEL-ARNT fusion. Proc Natl Acad Sci USA *97*, 6757–6762.

Satake, N., Ishida, Y., Otoh, Y., Hinohara, S., Kobayashi, H., Sakashita, A., Maseki, N., and Kaneko, Y. (1997). Novel MLL-CBP fusion transcript in therapy-related chronic myelomonocytic leukemia with a t(11;16)(q23;p13) chromosome translocation. Genes Chromosomes Cancer *20*, 60–63.

Sawyers, C.L., and Denny, C.T. (1994). Chronic myelomonocytic leukemia: Tel-a-kinase what Ets all about. Cell *77*, 171–173.

Schwaller, J., Anastasiadou, E., Cain, D., Kutok, J., Wojiski, S., Williams, I.R., LaStarza, R., Crescenzi, B., Sternberg, D.W., Andreasson, P., et al. (2001). H4(D10S170), a gene frequently rearranged in papillary thyroid carcinoma, is fused to the platelet-derived growth factor receptor beta gene in atypical chronic myeloid leukemia with t(5;10)(q33;q22). Blood *97*, 3910–3918.

Schwaller, J., Frantsve, J., Aster, J., Williams, I.R., Tomasson, M.H., Ross, T.S., Peeters, P., Van Rompaey, L., Van Etten, R.A., Ilaria, R., Jr., et al. (1998). Transformation of hematopoietic cell lines to growth-factor independence and induction of a fatal myelo- and lymphoproliferative disease in mice by retrovirally transduced TEL/JAK2 fusion genes. Embo J *17*, 5321–5333.

Schwaller, J., Parganas, E., Wang, D., Cain, D., Aster, J.C., Williams, I.R., Lee, C.K., Gerthner, R., Kitamura, T., Frantsve, J., et al. (2000). Stat5 is essential for the myelo- and lymphoproliferative disease induced by TEL/JAK2. Mol Cell *6*, 693–704.

Sherr, C.J. (2004). Principles of tumor suppression. Cell *116*, 235–246.

Sobulo, O.M., Borrow, J., Tomek, R., Reshmi, S., Harden, A., Schlegelberger, B., Housman, D., Doggett, N.A., Rowley, J.D., and Zeleznik-Le, N.J. (1997). MLL is fused to CBP, a histone acetyltransferase, in therapy-related acute myeloid leukemia with a t(11;16)(q23;p13.3). Proc Natl Acad Sci USA *94*, 8732–8737.

Soekarman, D., von Lindern, M., Daenen, S., de Jong, B., Fonatsch, C., Heinze, B., Bartram, C., Hagemeijer, A., and Grosveld, G. (1992). The translocation (6;9)(p23;q34) shows consistent rearrangement of two genes and defines a myeloproliferative disorder with specific clinical features. Blood *79*, 2990–2997.

Stegmaier, K., Pendse, S., Barker, G.F., Bray-Ward, P., Ward, D.C., Montgomery, K.T., Krauter, K.S., Reynolds, C., Sklar, J., Donnelly, M., et al. (1995). Frequent loss of heterozygosity at the TEL gene locus in acute lymphoblastic leukemia of childhood. Blood *86*, 38–44.

Stirewalt, D.L., Kopecky, K.J., Meshinchi, S., Appelbaum, F.R., Slovak, M.L., Willman, C.L., and Radich, J.P. (2001). FLT3, RAS, and TP53 mutations in elderly patients with acute myeloid leukemia. Blood *97*, 3589–3595.

Strasser, A., Harris, A.W., and Cory, S. (1993). E mu-bcl-2 transgene facilitates spontaneous transformation of early pre-B and immunoglobulin-secreting cells but not T cells. Oncogene *8*, 1–9.

Suzukawa, K., Shimizu, S., Nemoto, N., Takei, N., Taki, T., and Nagasawa, T. (2005). Identification of a chromosomal breakpoint and detection of a novel form of an MLL-AF17 fusion transcript in acute monocytic leukemia with t(11;17)(q23;q21). Int J Hematol *82*, 38–41.

Taki, T., Sako, M., Tsuchida, M., and Hayashi, Y. (1997). The t(11;16)(q23;p13) translocation in myelodysplastic syndrome fuses the MLL gene to the CBP gene. Blood *89*, 3945–3950.

Takizawa, J., Suzuki, R., Kuroda, H., Utsunomiya, A., Kagami, Y., Joh, T., Aizawa, Y., Ueda, R., and Seto, M. (1998). Expression of the TCL1 gene at 14q32 in B-cell malignancies but not in adult T-cell leukemia. Jpn J Cancer Res *89*, 712–718.

Tenen, D.G., Hromas, R., Licht, J.D., and Zhang, D.E. (1997). Transcription factors, normal myeloid development, and leukemia. Blood *90*, 489–519.

Thick, J., Metcalfe, J.A., Mak, Y.F., Beatty, D., Minegishi, M., Dyer, M.J., Lucas, G., and Taylor, A.M. (1996). Expression of either the TCL1 oncogene, or transcripts from its homologue MTCP1/c6.1B, in leukaemic and non-leukaemic T cells from ataxia telangiectasia patients. Oncogene *12*, 379–386.

Tomasson, M.H., Sternberg, D.W., Williams, I.R., Carroll, M., Cain, D., Aster, J.C., Ilaria, R.L., Jr., Van Etten, R.A., and Gilliland, D.G. (2000). Fatal myeloproliferation, induced in mice by TEL/PDGFbetaR expression, depends on PDGFbetaR tyrosines 579/581. J Clin Invest *105*, 423–432.

Torchia, J., Rose, D.W., Inostroza, J., Kamei, Y., Westin, S., Glass, C.K., and Rosenfeld, M.G. (1997). The transcriptional co-activator p/CIP binds CBP and mediates nuclear-receptor function. Nature *387*, 677–684.

Tsai, S., and Collins, S.J. (1993). A dominant negative retinoic acid receptor blocks neutrophil differentiation at the promyelocyte stage. Proc Natl Acad Sci USA *90*, 7153–7157.

Tsuzuki, S., Seto, M., Greaves, M., and Enver, T. (2004). Modeling first-hit functions of the t(12;21) TEL-AML1 translocation in mice. Proc Natl Acad Sci USA *101*, 8443–8448.

Virgilio, L., Narducci, M.G., Isobe, M., Billips, L.G., Cooper, M.D., Croce, C.M., and Russo, G. (1994). Identification of the TCL1 gene involved in T-cell malignancies. Proc Natl Acad Sci USA *91*, 12530–12534.

von Lindern, M., Fornerod, M., van Baal, S., Jaegle, M., de Wit, T., Buijs, A., and Grosveld, G. (1992). The translocation (6;9), associated with a specific subtype of acute myeloid leukemia, results in the fusion of two genes, dek and can, and the expression of a chimeric, leukemia-specific dek-can mRNA. Mol Cell Biol *12*, 1687–1697.

Wang, C.Y., Mayo, M.W., Korneluk, R.G., Goeddel, D.V., and Baldwin, A.S., Jr. (1998). NF-kappaB antiapoptosis: induction of TRAF1 and TRAF2 and c-IAP1 and c-IAP2 to suppress caspase-8 activation. Science *281*, 1680–1683.

Westervelt, P., Lane, A.A., Pollock, J.L., Oldfather, K., Holt, M.S., Zimonjic, D.B., Popescu, N.C., DiPersio, J.F., and Ley, T.J. (2003). High-penetrance mouse model of acute promyelocytic leukemia with very low levels of PML-RARalpha expression. Blood *102*, 1857–1865.

Wlodarska, I., Mecucci, C., Marynen, P., Guo, C., Franckx, D., La Starza, R., Aventin, A., Bosly, A., Martelli, M.F., Cassiman, J.J., et al. (1995). TEL gene is involved in myelodysplastic syndromes with either the typical t(5;12)(q33;p13) translocation or its variant t(10;12)(q24;p13). Blood *85*, 2848–2852.

Yamamoto, Y., Kiyoi, H., Nakano, Y., Suzuki, R., Kodera, Y., Miyawaki, S., Asou, N., Kuriyama, K., Yagasaki, F., Shimazaki, C., et al. (2001). Activating mutation of D835 within the activation loop of FLT3 in human hematologic malignancies. Blood *97*, 2434–2439.

Yan, M., Burel, S.A., Peterson, L.F., Kanbe, E., Iwasaki, H., Boyapati, A., Hines, R., Akashi, K., and Zhang, D.E. (2004). Deletion of an AML1-ETO C-terminal NcoR/SMRT-interacting region strongly induces leukemia development. Proc Natl Acad Sci USA *101*, 17186–17191.

Yokota, S., Kiyoi, H., Nakao, M., Iwai, T., Misawa, S., Okuda, T., Sonoda, Y., Abe, T., Kahsima, K., Matsuo, Y., et al. (1997). Internal tandem duplication of the FLT3 gene is preferentially seen in acute myeloid leukemia and myelodysplastic syndrome among various hematological malignancies. A study on a large series of patients and cell lines. Leukemia *11*, 1605–1609.

Yuan, Y., Zhou, L., Miyamoto, T., Iwasaki, H., Harakawa, N., Hetherington, C.J., Burel, S.A., Lagasse, E., Weissman, I.L., Akashi, K., et al. (2001). AML1-ETO expression is directly involved in the development of acute myeloid leukemia in the presence of additional mutations. Proc Natl Acad Sci USA *98*, 10398–10403.

Zapata, J.M., Krajewska, M., Krajewski, S., Kitada, S., Welsh, K., Monks, A., McCloskey, N., Gordon, J., Kipps, T.J., Gascoyne, R.D., et al. (2000). TNFR-associated factor family protein expression in normal tissues and lymphoid malignancies. J Immunol *165*, 5084–5096.

Zhang, J., Grindley, J.C., Yin, T., Jayasinghe, S., He, X.C., Ross, J.T., Haug, J.S., Rupp, D., Porter-Westpfahl, K.S., Wiedemann, L.M., et al. (2006). PTEN maintains haematopoietic stem cells and acts in lineage choice and leukaemia prevention. Nature *441*, 518–522.

Chapter 3
Murine Models of Hematopoietic Disease: Pathologic Analysis and Characterization

Benjamin H. Lee and Jeffery L. Kutok

Contents

3.1 Introduction

The pathologic evaluation of murine hematologic disease can be considerably more challenging than the assessment of human hematopoietic malignancies. Diagnoses in humans that may be difficult based solely on histology are often straightforward with careful review of the patient's laboratory data or after specialized ancillary testing. Unfortunately, such luxuries do not always exist in the workup of a mouse. Obtaining important clinical and laboratory data for each mouse in a cohort is often difficult and costly. Peripheral blood counts and cytologic findings in the blood and marrow play a critical role in the diagnosis of disease in both mice and humans; however, quite often, a mouse is simply

---

J.L. Kutok
Brigham and Women's Hospital, Harvard Medical School, Department of Pathology, Boston, MA 02115, USA
jkutok@partners.org

S. Li (ed.), *Mouse Models of Human Blood Cancers*,
DOI: 10.1007/978-0-387-69132-9_3,

© Springer Science+Business Media, LLC 2008

fixed in formalin enabling only histopathologic review. Immunophenotyping by flow cytometry or cytochemical studies require fresh cells and are necessary to confirm morphologic impressions. This testing should be a part of all murine hematopoietic workups but needs to be planned and performed soon after the time of euthanasia. Genetic testing, such as karyotyping and Southern blotting for clonality, also require unfixed cells obtained at the time of euthanasia. These studies are difficult and infrequently performed and, additionally, may be of limited value in some murine genetic models where monoclonality may not necessarily be synonymous with aggressive disease. Finally, while the objective of the analysis is often to compare the murine findings to the corresponding human diseases, this is not always possible. The genetic backgrounds created in some experimental mice may be sufficient to induce hematologic abnormalities but may not result in phenocopies of the human diseases. In addition, variations in murine strains can contribute greatly to the observed hematologic abnormalities. With all of these inherent difficulties in mind, a recent attempt to standardize the classification of nonlymphoid and lymphoid murine hematopoietic malignancies has been undertaken (Kogan et al. 2002; Morse et al. 2002). The goals of these classification systems are to allow investigators to diagnose murine hematopoietic neoplasms as well-defined entities according to accepted criteria. They emphasize the need to incorporate peripheral blood findings, cytologic features of hematopoietic cells, histopathology of hematopoietic tissues, immunophenotypic and genetic features, and the clinical course into each diagnosis. In addition, the differences between the murine and the human diseases are reflected in the nomenclature and methods used in these classifications.

This chapter will provide an overview of the general approach to the pathologic characterization of murine hematopoietic diseases. A review of the normal histology of the murine system will be provided and attention will be paid to the pathologic differences and similarities between the murine and the human hematopoietic systems. Specific emphasis will be placed on nonlymphoid leukemias, myeloproliferative-like leukemias, and myeloid proliferations, and the application of existing classification guidelines in their diagnosis will be highlighted.

3.2 General Approach to the Analysis of a Mouse

3.2.1 Physical Findings

The hallmark of neoplastic hematopoietic disease is the infiltration or proliferation of myeloid or lymphoid cells into the hematolymphoid organs. The hematolymphoid organs include the bone marrow, spleen, lymph nodes, Peyer's patches, and thymus. The neoplastic infiltration typically leads to hematopoietic failure secondary to the replacement of normal hematopoietic cells within the marrow, that is, lack of normal red blood cells (RBCs), white blood cells (WBCs), and platelets. In humans, the clinical presentations that result from the loss of normal hematopoietic cells include anemia (due to RBC loss), infection (due to lymphocyte and granulocyte loss), and bleeding (due to platelet loss). In mice, however, the spectrum of clinical signs may be much more limited. The sterile environment in which laboratory mice are kept reduces the infectious complications resulting from leukopenia, and spontaneous bleeding due to platelet deficiencies is uncommon. Anemia is often the most consistent indicator of hematopoietic failure, but the clinical appearance of anemia in mice can be subtle. Enlarged organs and tissues are frequent signs of disease, as mice can survive with a marked degree of tumor burden, but organomegaly often occurs later in the disease process. Sites of neoplastic cell dissemination into nonhematolymphoid organs include the liver, kidneys, lungs, and bowel. Given these issues, routine observation to identify the onset of a disease phenotype should be undertaken. Once a mouse dies, the clotting of blood and autolysis of the marrow and lymphoid organs precludes meaningful evaluation. Daily observation and weekly physical examination is, therefore, a useful practice. Observable signs of systemic disease include lethargy or inactivity, poor grooming with unkempt fur, weight loss, respiratory difficulties (often associated with a mediastinal mass), hind-limb paralysis (associated with spinal cord infiltrates), or a visible mass. Anemic mice often have pale ears and feet. On physical examination, careful palpation can reveal enlargement of the spleen, liver, or lymph nodes, particularly the nodes of the axilla or neck. It is critical to realize that the spleen is a functioning hematopoietic organ throughout the life of a mouse and is often a primary site of hematopoietic disease (much like the bone marrow). If available, small animal noninvasive imaging modalities, including high-frequency ultrasound and FDG PET/CT, may also assist in following tumor development (Tatsumi et al. 2003; Liao et al. 2005).

3.2.2 Laboratory Findings

Very commonly, the composition of the peripheral blood will mirror systemic infiltrates, and monthly blood draws are suggested to monitor for abnormalities. Blood collection from the saphenous or dorsal pedal vein do not require anesthesia, whereas anesthesia is necessary for tail vein, orbital sinus, or jugular vein blood draws (Hoff 2000). Blood should not be collected from the orbital sinus more frequently than once every 2 weeks; other venous sites can be used as often as needed (Hoff 2000). Of note, packed cell volume and hemoglobin measurements have been reported to be higher from tail vein draws compared to other sites (Sakaki 1961). Automated cell differential counts can be performed in a veterinary blood analyzer with software capable of evaluating murine blood (e.g., HemaVet Vet950FS, Drew Scientific). Such analyzers are capable of recording hemoglobin, hematocrit, platelet counts, and white cell counts and automated differentials. EDTA spray-coated tubes are recommended to avoid dilutional effects of the anticoagulant in the small blood volumes obtained. Considerable strain variation exists in normal hematologic parameters, so it is important to consult reference databases to determine whether the blood in question is outside of the normal range. The Mouse Phenome Database is one such database that provides a continually growing repository of phenotypic and genotypic data, including blood hematology values, for many commonly studied inbred strains that are easily accessed through the Mouse Phenome Database website (http://www.jax.org/phenome) maintained by the Jackson Laboratory (Bogue et al. 2007). Once peripheral blood is obtained, air-dried smears on glass slides should be made. Wright–Giemsa staining is preferred for confirming nucleated cell differential counts and observing morphologic abnormalities. Just prior to euthanasia, additional blood can be obtained from the anesthetized animal's heart, the posterior vena cava, the axillary vessels, or the orbital sinus (Hoff 2000). If the blood is thick or clotting occurs, a small amount of normal saline can be added for the purposes of preparing blood smears.

3.2.3 Necropsy Findings

Once the animal is euthanized, macroscopic or gross examination of the internal organs can be valuable in identifying pathology. An excellent resource for the necroscopic evaluation of a mouse for hematopoietic disease is found at the National Cancer Institute (NCI)-sponsored website (http://emice.nci.nih.gov/) that contains the supplemental materials to Bethesda classification articles (Kogan et al. 2002; Morse et al. 2002), as well as the on-line Virtual Mouse Necropsy site (http://geocities.com/virtualbiology/necropsy.html). Attention should be paid to the size of the spleen, thymus, lymph nodes, and liver, and recording the weights of enlarged organs can be helpful in documenting abnormalities. The organs should be sectioned before fixation and examined for color and the presence of macroscopic lesions. A greenish or brownish hue to lymph nodes or spleen can occasionally be seen in myeloid leukemia, and white nodules or a lacy pattern observed in lymphomatous involvement of organs. The presence of abnormalities in the cut surface of the liver can be a sensitive indicator of neoplastic disease, since reactive conditions do not normally cause visible abnormalities. The sternum and hind limbs can be pale in color, as opposed to red, when the marrow is infiltrated by WBCs. An enlarged thymus is usually associated with T-lymphoblastic leukemia/lymphoma.

Sections of spleen, lymph nodes, thymus, liver, bone marrow (sternum or femur), lungs, and any tumor masses should be placed in 10% buffered formalin for 24–48 h and then processed for paraffin sections as soon as possible. Formalin is the best fixative to maintain antigenicity for subsequent immunohistochemical analysis. In addition, single-cell suspensions should be prepared from disaggregated tissues and flushed bone marrow to be used for flow cytometric analysis, cytospin slides (for morphology or cytochemical stains), or as a source of DNA, RNA, and protein. Unused cells can be stored in an RPMI, 20% fetal calf serum, and 10% DMSO solution at –80°C for long periods.

3.3 Histology of Normal Murine Hematopoietic Tissue

In order to determine whether the presence of a hematological disorder exists, careful cytologic and histologic examination must be undertaken. This requires knowledge of the normal cytology and histology of the murine system one is working with. Importantly, several distinct differences exist in the normal anatomy of the murine hematopoietic system compared to humans. It is necessary to keep these dissimilarities in mind when evaluating for hematologic disease. A detailed description of normal histology and cytology can be found in several fine atlases including the *Atlas of Mouse Hematopathology* by Fredrickson and Harris (Fredrickson and Harris 2000).

Bone marrow. In contrast to other mammalian species, the bone marrow of mice contains very little medullary fat and, therefore, appears quite cellular throughout life (Fig. 3.1A,B). Careful inspection of the medullary cavity does reveal a prominent network of endothelial-lined sinusoidal channels. In the normal state, these channels are open and filled with mature RBCs. When marrow hypercellularity occurs, it can be difficult to identify. One typical finding in these cases is that the sinuses become compressed and inconspicuous. In contrast, hypercellularity in humans manifests itself by the replacement of medullary fat with hematopoietic cells. Interestingly, when compared to human marrow, monocytes and lymphocytes comprise a significant proportion of murine marrow cellularity. In the mouse, granulocytes typically comprise 30–40% of the marrow nucleated cells (Fig. 3.1C), with the remaining cellularity comprised of erythroid precursors (20%) (Fig. 3.1D), monocytes (10–20%), and lymphoid cells (25–30%). In contrast, the relative proportion of cell types in human marrow is 67% granulocytes, 19% erythroid, 1% monocytes, 3% myeloblasts, and 10% lymphocytes (Brunning and McKenna 1994). Megakaryocytes are readily identifiable throughout the marrow cavity and are in similar proportions to that seen in the human (Fig. 3.1B,D).

Spleen.As mentioned above, the splenic red pulp is a site of primary hematopoiesis throughout the life of a mouse (Fig. 3.2). This is in complete contrast to humans, where extramedullary hematopoiesis (EMH) in the spleen is not seen under normal physiologic conditions. The amount of EMH is generally relatively small and tends to decline with the age of the mouse (Fig. 3.2B). In times of physiologic stress, however, EMH can be extremely prominent, resulting in a marked increase in splenic size. Therefore, a markedly enlarged spleen does not necessarily signify a neoplastic process but may simply be related to high demand for RBCs and/or granulocytes. The limited space for bone marrow

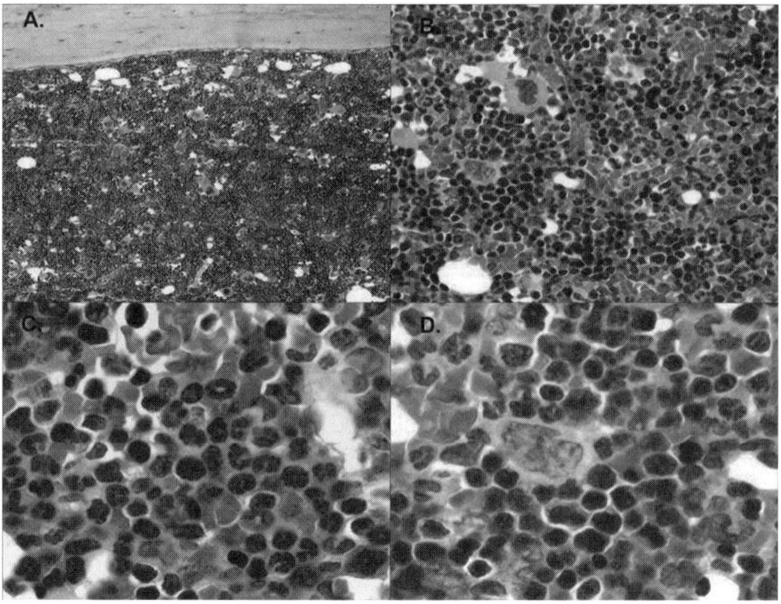

Fig. 3.1 Histology of murine bone marrow. (**A**) Medium (200×) magnification of wild-type adult BALB/c bone marrow demonstrating normal hypercellularity (hematoxylin and eosin stain). (**B**) Higher magnification (400×) of the same marrow, demonstrating trilineage hematopoiesis with open sinuses filled with mature red blood cells and scattered adipocytes (hematoxylin and eosin stain). (**C**) High magnification (1000×) of a myeloid colony within the marrow showing maturing elements including ringed granulocyte precursors (hematoxylin and eosin stain). (**D**) High magnification (1000×) of an erythroid colony with darkly stained round to irregular nuclei surrounding a megakaryocyte (hematoxylin and eosin stain). (See color insert)

expansion is directly related to the increase in splenic hematopoiesis in these circumstances. In neoplastic conditions, bone marrow infiltration by leukemic or lymphomatous cells can lead to expanded reactive hematopoiesis in the spleen, or alternatively, direct expansion of neoplastic hematopoietic elements in the spleen can occur. The white pulp is supported by a network of dendritic and reticular cells organized in several distinct lymphoid zones: the T-lymphocyte-rich central zone, surrounding a central arteriole; adjacent mantle zone of small B lymphocytes; and outer marginal zone of B lymphocytes (Fig. 3.2C). The T-lymphocyte-rich zone is also referred to as the periarteriolar sheath and is composed of a predominance of CD4-positive T cells with fewer CD8-positive cells. The mantle zones contain monomorphic small $IgM^{+}IgD^{+}$ B lymphocytes with little cytoplasm imparting a dark blue appearance to this zone on hematoxylin and eosin staining. The marginal zone also contains small B lymphocytes; however, these cells are $IgM^{+}IgD^{-}$ and have ample cytoplasm imparting a pale appearance to this region. Of note, in contrast to mice, humans have an inner and an outer marginal zone which is surrounded by a large perifollicular zone (Mebius and Kraal 2005). Within the mantle zone region, germinal centers can

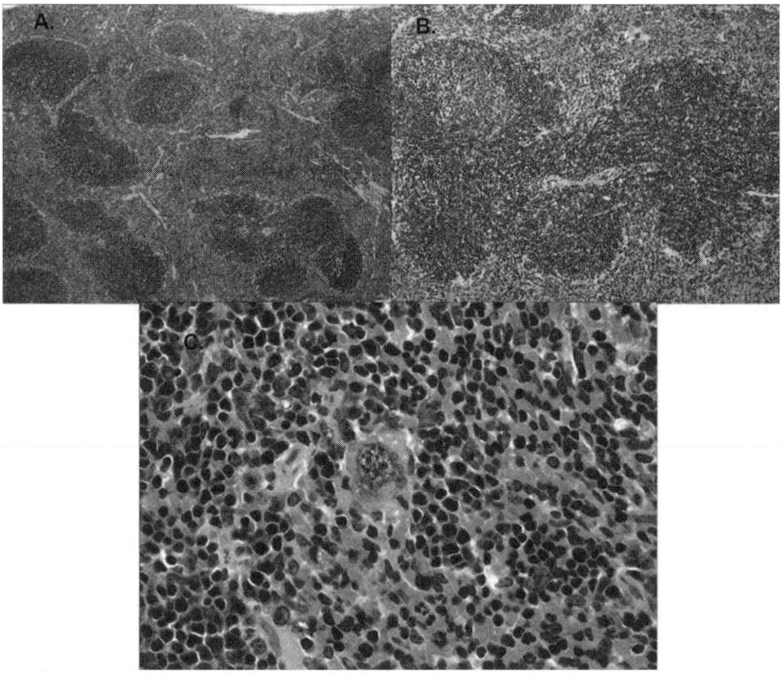

Fig. 3.2 Histology of murine spleen. (**A**) Low power magnification (40×) of an adult wild-type BALB/c mouse showing white pulp nodules surrounded by extramedullary hematopoiesis in the red pulp (hematoxylin and eosin stain). (**B**) Medium power magnification (100×) from the same spleen, demonstrating white pulp lymphoid nodules with a germinal center (upper left) and pale marginal zones (hematoxylin and eosin stain). (**C**) High power magnification (400×) from the same spleen showing red pulp extramedullary hematopoiesis predominantly comprised of darkly staining erythroid elements and a single megakaryocyte (hematoxylin and eosin stain). (See color insert)

occasionally be seen. A so-called dark zone containing proliferating intermediate to large lymphoid cells occupies one area of the germinal center, the other half is designated the light zone, which contains an admixture of centroblasts, centrocytes, and tingible body macrophages. In the nonimmunized animals, germinal centers are small and poorly formed but can become quite prominent with immunization.

Lymph nodes. The lymph nodes contain B-cell follicles in the cortical region that are uniformly distributed within the subcapsular region. The follicles contain a mantle zone and may or may not have a central germinal center. The marginal zones are not visible in the follicles of the lymph node. Within the paracortical regions, between the B-cell follicles, T cells (primarily CD4+) and interdigitating follicular dendritic cells predominate. Deep to this, within the lymph node medulla, plasma cells, immunoblasts, small lymphocytes, and histiocytes can be seen.

Peyer's patch. Peyer's patches are foci of lymphoid tissue located in the wall of the small bowel and, to a lesser extent, in the lower intestinal tract. They are comprised of aggregates of mantle-type B cells most commonly surrounding prominent, reactive germinal centers. Smaller numbers of T cells populate the regions between the follicles, as do scattered immunoblasts and plasma cells. The Peyer's patches are evident macroscopically and are typically infiltrated by neoplastic lymphoid and, occasionally, myeloid cells.

Thymus. Thymic architecture is relatively similar between the mouse and the humans. There is a clear histologic distinction between thymic cortex and medulla due to the decreased density in thymocytes within the medulla. In contrast to human thymic medulla, the Hassall's corpuscles are not as identifiable in the mouse thymus. Infiltration of thymic medulla by thymocytes and expansion of the thymus is typical in precursor T-cell lymphoblastic lymphoma.

3.4 Cytology of Normal Murine Hematopoietic Cells

The cytologic features of murine hematopoietic cells are similar to those of human hematopoietic cells, with the greatest differences observed in the granulocytic series. A brief accounting of the major cytologic features of each cell type is provided below. An outstanding more detailed description can be found elsewhere (Fredrickson and Harris 2000).

Erythroid series. Mature RBCs are biconcave discs with central pallor, as in humans. Reticulocytes are often abundant in peripheral blood smears, comprising 2–4% of the peripheral blood erythrocytes. These newly formed RBCs are larger than mature RBCs and have a basophilic hue with Wright–Giemsa staining secondary to the presence of RNA within the cell. Nucleated RBCs within the bone marrow show a succession from large cells with round nuclei, prominent nucleoli, and deeply basophilic cytoplasm (proerythroblast) to progressively smaller cells with round, hyperchromatic nuclei and paler cytoplasm (polychromatophilic normoblasts). In histologic sections of the spleen showing EMH, nucleated erythroid forms such as polychromatophilic normoblasts are abundant with very dark, somewhat irregular appearing nuclei and scant cytoplasm (Fig. 3.2C).

Neutrophil series. Neutrophils comprise approximately 5–20% of peripheral WBCs, a dramatically lower proportion of WBCs compared to humans where they comprise 40–70%. The nuclei are predominantly band-like and twisted or curled/ringed, and much less frequently are polylobate, as in the human (Fig. 3.3A). To be classified as a neutrophil, some authors suggest that, if ringed, the diameter of center of ring is greater than 50% of the diameter of nucleus or that the nucleus has fully developed segmentation (Kogan et al. 2002). A greater degree of segmentation can be observed in tissue sections of neutrophils in mice than in peripheral blood. The cytoplasm is generally

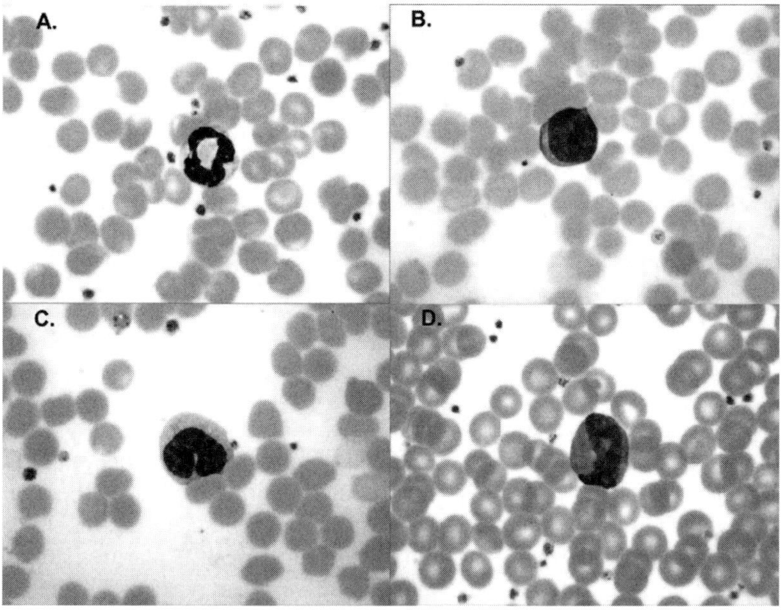

Fig. 3.3 Cytology of murine peripheral blood cells. (**A**) Mature neutrophil from wild-type BALB/c mouse shows a hyperlobate nucleus and very fine azurophilic granules (Wright–Giemsa stain, 1000×). (**B**) Mature lymphocyte from wild-type BALB/c mouse shows a round nucleus and small amounts of basophilic, agranular cytoplasm (Wright–Giemsa stain, 1000×). (**C**) Mature monocyte from wild-type BALB/c mouse shows a kidney-shaped nucleus and pale blue-gray cytoplasm with occasional vaculoes (Wright–Giemsa stain, 1000×). (**D**) Mature eosinophil from wild-type BALB/c mouse shows a hyperlobate nucleus and prominent orange granules (Wright–Giemsa stain, 1000×). (See color insert)

plentiful and pale. In contrast to human neutrophils, the cytoplasmic granules are nearly unidentifiable with Wright–Giemsa staining. Only small violet or eosinophilic granules can be seen. Within the bone marrow, myeloblasts have oval, eccentrically or peripherally placed nuclei, with even chromatin, distinct nucleoli, and basophilic cytoplasm. Only cells with these cytologic features should be considered blasts or immature forms for the purposes of diagnosing leukemias. Promyelocytes are larger, with less prominent nucleoli and a small, central, nuclear clearing that heralds the beginning of the doughnut or ring-shaped nuclei that typify the myelocytes and metamyelocytes. Granules are also difficult to discern in the promyelocyte, particularly in relation to those seen in humans. As mentioned, the characteristic doughnut or ringed nuclei are present within the myelocytes, metamyelocytes, and bands. The earliest forms (myelocytes) have nuclei with a more doughnut-shaped appearance, which progress to a thinner ring-like form in the band cells. As the cells mature, the chromatin becomes more condensed and there are increased small, inconspicuous granules.

Lymphocytes. Mature lymphocytes comprise the majority (80–90%) of the peripheral blood cells, in contrast to humans where only 20–40% of the blood cells are lymphocytes. The morphology of the mature murine lymphocyte is similar to that of the human. The nucleus is dark and round with small amounts pale, agranular cytoplasm (Fig. 3.3B). Within the bone marrow, lymphoblasts are infrequent and difficult to discern from proerythroblasts. Some distinguishing characteristics of lymphoblasts compared to immature erythroid elements include more even or fine chromatin, slightly paler blue cytoplasm, and a more peripherally placed nucleus.

Monocytes. Monocytes are the largest cells in the circulation. They have a round to oval occasionally reniform or bean-shaped nucleus with rope-like chromatin (Fig. 3.3C). Nucleoli are not distinct, and the cytoplasm is slightly basophilic, agranular, and frequently contains vacuoles. In tissue sections stained with hematoxylin and eosin, the nuclei are pale and curved or folded with ample eosinophilic cytoplasm.

Eosinophils and basophils. The eosinophil has similar features to the neutrophilic band; however, the granules are prominent and red-orange in color (Fig. 3.3D). The immature eosinophilic forms have nuclear features similar to their neutrophilic counterparts. Basophils are very rarely seen. They contain large round, darkly basophilic granules throughout the cytoplasm and overlying the nucleus.

3.5 Bethesda Classification Systems of Murine Hematopoietic Disease

As previously mentioned, the necessity to develop a uniform classification system of murine hematopoietic neoplasms was recently recognized by the hematopathology subcommittee of the Mouse Models of Human Cancers Consortium (MMHCC) in order to meaningfully compare and contrast different murine cancer models to one another, as well as to defined human entities (http://emice.nci.nih.gov). Sponsored by the NCI/National Institutes of Health (NIH), the MMHC hematopathology subcommittee reported their consensus proposals for two classification systems in mice: one centered on the classification of nonlymphoid hematopoietic neoplasms (Kogan et al. 2002) and another on the classification of lymphoid neoplasms (Morse et al. 2002). Analogous to the World Health Organization (WHO) classification of human hematopoietic and lymphoid neoplasms (Jaffe et al. 2001), the Bethesda proposals sought to employ a combination of factors, including morphologic, immunophenotypic, genetic, and clinical/biologic characteristics, for the purposes of classification. In addition, they sought to recognize the differences between mouse and human biology and address the existence of gaps in the literature of human diseases that have not been well described or studied in mice. Although this chapter focuses mainly on nonlymphoid hematopoietic

Table 3.1 Bethesda proposals for classification of nonlymphoid and lymphoid hematopoietic neoplasms in mice

Nonlymphoid	Lymphoid
Nonlymphoid leukemias • Myeloid leukemias – Myeloid leukemia without maturation – Myeloid leukemia with maturation – Myeloproliferative disease-like myeloid leukemia – Myelomonocytic leukemia – Monocytic leukemia • Erythroid leukemia • Megakaryocytic leukemia • Biphenotypic leukemia *Nonlymphoid hematopoietic sarcomas* • Granulocytic sarcoma • Histiocytic sarcoma • Mast cell sarcoma *Myeloid dysplasias* • Myelodysplastic syndrome • Cytopenia with increased blasts *Myeloid proliferations (nonreactive)* • Myeloproliferation (genetic) • Myeloproliferative disease	*B-cell neoplasms* • Precursor B-cell neoplasm – Precursor B-cell lymphoblastic lymphoma/ leukemia (pre-B LBL) • Mature B-cell neoplasms – Small B-cell lymphoma (SBL) – Splenic marginal zone B-cell lymphoma – Follicular B-cell lymphoma (FBL) – Diffuse large B-cell lymphoma (DLBCL) – Morphologic variants – Centroblastic (CB) – Immunoblastic (IB) – Histiocyte associated (HA) – Subtypes – Primary mediastinal (thymic) diffuse large B-cell lymphoma – Classical Burkitt lymphoma (BL) – Burkitt-like lymphoma [including mature B-cell lymphomas with lymphoblastic morphology (BLL)] – Plasma cell neoplasm – Plasmacytoma – Extraosseous plasmacytoma (PCT-E) – Anaplastic plasmacytoma (PCT-A) – β-natural killer cell lymphoma (BKNL) *T-cell neoplasms* • Precursor T-cell neoplasm – Precursor T-cell lymphoblastic lymphoma/ leukemia (pre-T LBL) • Mature T-cell neoplasm – Small T-cell lymphoma (STL) – T-natural killer cell lymphoma (TNKL) • T-cell neoplasm, character undetermined – Large cell anaplastic lymphoma (TLCA)

(Adapted from Kogan et al. 2002 and Morse et al. 2002)

malignancies, Table 3.1 summarizes the broad disease categories of the Bethesda classification systems for both murine nonlymphoid and lymphoid hematopoietic neoplasms. Formal guidelines for further defining criteria and subclassification of specific entities in these general categories are contained within the aforementioned references and will be referred to in the discussion of particular disease models below. Finally, as with all classification systems, it should be recognized that while laying a solid foundation for the categorization of murine hematopoietic neoplasms, the Bethesda proposals will undoubtedly be subject to modification as investigators continue to further our understanding of hematopoietic disease in both humans and mice.

3.6 Ancillary Techniques for the Evaluation of Murine Hematopoietic Disease

While morphologic examination of paraffin-embedded mouse tissues, peripheral blood smears, and cytospins of single-cell suspensions is a critical initial step in characterizing hematopoietic neoplasms, valuable additional information may be obtained from a variety of ancillary diagnostic modalities. These include the use of cytochemical and immunohistochemical stains, flow cytometric immunophenotyping for lineage assignment, and less commonly, cytogenetic analysis. Preparation of murine tissues for DNA and RNA for potential molecular genetic analysis should also be considered at time of animal necropsy. It is important to realize that many of these ancillary studies require fresh and/or frozen cells that should, in some instances, be prepared under sterile conditions. For example, although not routinely performed, in vitro methylcellulose colony-forming cell (CFC) assays are often utilized in the evaluation and quantification of multipotential and lineage-restricted myeloid, erythroid, and megakaryocytic progenitors, as well as pre-B-lymphoid cells in murine models, and require sterile preparation of cells to prevent unwanted contamination of these long-term cultures. In addition, similar sterile protocols should also be applied to the preparation of hematopoietic/tumor cells that will undergo transplantation into irradiated recipient animals.

Cytochemistry. Cytochemistry is one of oldest laboratory methodologies used in the diagnosis and classification of human leukemias. Its use dates well before the advent of more sophisticated current diagnostic modalities including flow cytometry and cytogenetics. The application of cytochemical markers to murine samples can provide significant diagnostic information at a relatively inexpensive cost. These assays can be performed from commercially available kits (e.g., Sigma) or alternatively, recipes and protocols can be found in a number of standard hematology laboratory references (Harmening 2002). Commonly used cytochemical stains include Sudan Black B (SBB), which stains myeloid, neutrophilic, eosinophilic, and monocytic cells with variable intensity; Myeloperoxidase (MPO), which stains cells of myeloid and monocytic but not lymphoid lineage; Chloroacetate Esterase (CAE), which stains mast cells (strong), neutrophils, and occasional other cell types and Non-Specific Esterase (NSE), which variably stains cells of monocytic origin. Correlation of these studies with cytologic findings from Wright–Giemsa- or Romanowsky-stained preparations can be extremely useful for evaluating morphologically immature nonlymphoid hematopoietic neoplasms. Of note, because these staining methodologies are enzymatically based, long-term storage of unstained samples may adversely affect staining quality, and thus prompt analysis of freshly prepared samples gives optimal results.

Immunohistochemistry and special stains. The use of immunohistochemistry in the workup of human malignancies (hematopoietic and nonhematopoietic) is standard clinical practice; however, this technique is not commonly employed in the analysis of murine tumors. With the refinement of immunohistochemical techniques and the development of better-characterized antibodies against murine antigens, immunohistochemistry can be invaluable in the workup of hematopoietic tumors. This is particularly true when applied to formalin-fixed tissues that commonly represent the only material that an investigator may have to work with. Prolonged fixation of tissue can adversely affect antigen retrieval with many antibodies, so care should be taken to process fixed samples as quickly as possible. Immunohistochemistry to identify protein tags, such as EGFP, HA, and FLAG, is also highly useful in evaluating the patterns of transgenic protein expression. In addition to standard hematoxylin and eosin (H&E) stains, additional useful histochemical stains can be carried out on tissue sections to evaluate hematological processes. Among these include reticulin or trichrome staining to assess for fibrosis [e.g., chronic idiopathic myelofibrosis (CIMF)], iron stains to examine iron levels (e.g., myelodysplasias), and toluidine blue or Giemsa stains, which can be used to highlight mast cells (e.g., mast cell leukemias or mast cell sarcomas). While many individual investigators are not necessarily equipped to carry out routine immunohistochemistry or special stains on murine tissues, these services are available commercially or through institutional core laboratory facilities. In addition, collaboration with pathologists is critical in the accurate interpretation of immunohistochemical results where it is important to determine appropriate immunoreactivity staining patterns (e.g., nuclear vs. cytoplasmic) and avoid misinterpretation of nonspecific staining.

Flow cytometry. Pathologic diagnosis of hematopoietic malignancies has been greatly facilitated by the advent of flow cytometric analysis. While continuing advances in instrumentation, fluorochromes, and antibodies allow for increasingly sophisticated applications including the isolation and characterization of stem cell and multipotent progenitor subsets, standard three-color analysis is sufficient for most diagnostic immunophenotypic studies. Standard lineage markers are listed in Table 3.2 and can be utilized in a number of combinations for routine immunophenotypic studies. Current and updated recommendations for practical three-color panels for the evaluation of most hematopoietic neoplasms including nonlymphoid hematopoietic tumors are contained within the Bethesda proposals (Kogan et al. 2002; Morse et al. 2002). In addition, the frequent utilization of retroviral expression constructs, which coexpress green fluorescence protein (GFP), as well as other colors (e.g., YFP), allows for specific immunophenotypic evaluation of transduced cells by gating on GFP-positive cell populations in bone marrow transplantation (BMT) models. This makes flow cytometric analysis particularly valuable for the characterization of the transformed cells in these unique murine systems.

Clonality. Methods to identify monoclonality in hematopoietic tumors can be useful, particularly when there is a question of distinguishing a benign reactive process versus a malignant condition. For lymphoid neoplasms, this can be performed by the assessment of either clonal B- or T-cell gene rearrangements of the immunoglobulin heavy chain locus or T-cell receptor loci,

Table 3.2 Commonly used markers for immunophenotypic analysis

Lineage	Antigen	Expression patterns
B cell	CD45R (B220)	B cells, abnormal T cells, NK cells
	CD19	B cells
	IgM	Mature B cells
	IgK	Mature B cells
	CD23(FceR)	Activated B cells
	CD138	Plasma cells
T cell	CD3	T cells
	CD4	Helper T cells
	CD8	Cytotoxic T cells, NK cells
	T-cell receptor (TCR)	T cells
Myeloid/monocytic	Myeloperoxidase (MPO)	Myeloid cells
	Gr-1 (Ly-6 G)	Granulocytes, monocytes
	Mac-1 (CD11b)	Granulocytes, monocytes
	F4/80 (Ly-71)	Monocytes, eosinophils
	Mac-2	Macrophages/histiocytes
	Mac-3	Macrophages/histiocytes
Eythroid	Ter119 (Ly-76)	Erythroid cells (immature to RBC)
	CD71 (transferrin receptor)	Erythroid (immature-to-mid-stage erythroid forms, expression diminishes with maturation)
Megakaryocyte	CD41	Platelets, megakaryoblasts
	CD61	Platelets, megakaryoblasts
	von Willebrand Factor (vWF)	Megakarocytes, megakaryoblasts
Immature/early	CD34	Immature cells, endothelial cells
	Sca-1 (Ly-6A/E)	Immature cells
	c-Kit (CD117)	Immature cells, mast cells
	CD31	Imature cells, endothelial cells
Hematopoietic	CD45 (LCA)	Pan-hematopoietic marker Negative in erythroid cells

respectively, using Southern blot or polymerase chain reaction (PCR) techniques. For nonlymphoid malignancies, analysis of proviral integration sites is often performed where applicable. Less commonly, clonality may be assessed by cytogenetics through conventional G-banded karyotype analysis, fluorescence in situ hybridization (FISH), or the more complex spectral karyotyping (SKY) method, which employs multicolor chromosome-specific paints to differentiate and classify nonhomologous human or murine chromosomes.

3.7 Nonlymphoid Hematopoietic Neoplasms in Mice

The spectrum of hematopoietic malignancies falling under the Bethesda proposals classification system is broad and diverse. It allows for the categorization of neoplastic proliferations of all nonlymphoid hematopoietic cells including myeloid/monocytic, erythroid, megakaryocytic, histiocytic, and mast cell lineages (i.e., leukemias and myeloproliferative processes), as well as stem cell disorders of ineffective hematopoiesis [i.e., myelodysplastic syndromes (MDSs)] (Table 3.1). Nonlymphoid leukemias are often characterized by either cytopenias or leukocytosis with a concurrent increase in nonlymphoid hematopoietic cells in both bone marrow and spleen. The proliferations that are observed may be of immature precursors (i.e., acute leukemia) or mature nonlymphoid cells [i.e., myeloproliferative disorders (MPDs)]. Distinguishing benign reactive processes that result in increases in hematopoietic cells from true neoplastic conditions can be difficult. Reactive abnormalities including leukemoid reactions in the peripheral blood and splenomegaly secondary to EMH can arise from a variety of conditions including infection, drug/toxin exposure, and nutritional deficiencies, all of which should be carefully considered before definitive characterization of a neoplastic condition is made. Useful distinguishing features between benign and neoplastic processes include the presence of monoclonality (see above), transplantability of the hematopoietic process, absence/presence of other inflammatory lesions (e.g., dermatitis), and the persistence/progression of the blood or splenic abnormalities (e.g., via serial nonlethal eye bleeds or physical exam/noninvasive imaging studies).

Representative examples for some disease subcategories are referred to within the Bethesda proposals (Kogan et al. 2002) and can be found in other resources in the literature (Fredrickson and Harris 2000). Our discussion will center on genetic models utilizing both transgenic and BMT platforms that have modeled leukemogenic alleles associated with human hematopoietic disease or genes important for normal hematopoiesis. The illustrations of some of their particular and salient features will serve as a useful reference for investigators as new models are evaluated.

3.7.1 Myeloproliferative Disorders

As the name implies, these proliferative stem cell disorders are characterized by increased bone marrow production of mature nonlymphoid hematopoietic elements manifesting in characteristic peripheral blood and laboratory findings. These disorders classically include chronic myeloid leukemia (CML), polycythemia vera (PV), essential thrombocythemia (ET), and CIMF, and more loosely include chronic eosinophilic leukemia (CEL), chronic myelomonocytic leukemia (CMML), and systemic mastocytosis (SM). Although these entities represent unique clinicopathologic disorders, the identified causative genetic mutations in all MPDs result in constitutive activation of tyrosine kinase (TK) signaling (Bartram et al. 1983; Golub et al. 1994; Longley et al. 1996; Cools et al. 2003a; Levine et al. 2005; Lee et al. 2007). Modeling these disease alleles in mice has been instrumental in understanding their contribution to both normal biology and disease pathogenesis.

BCR–ABL. The BCR–ABL TK fusion oncoprotein is the genetic lesion that defines CML, the prototypic disease for modern molecular oncology. It was the first genetic abnormality identified in human myeloproliferative disease and thus is undoubtedly the most studied and well characterized TK fusion protein. Numerous murine models have demonstrated that BCR–ABL expression is sufficient to initiate the development of a variety of leukemias (e.g., B-ALL, T-ALL, CML, and histiocytic sarcomas), the phenotype of which is dependent upon a number factors including promoter choice, murine strain, oncogenic isoform of BCR–ABL, and experimental conditions [for further review see, Wong and Witte (2001)]. Daley and colleagues were one of the first groups to report a murine bone marrow transplant model capable of faithfully generating a CML-like disease with characteristics of chronic phase human CML (Daley et al. 1990). In these retroviral transplant models, BCR–ABL typically induces an MPD-like myeloid leukemia characterized by leukocytosis with evidence of normal maturation but without significantly increased numbers of immature/blast forms, similar to the peripheral blood findings in human CML. In addition, peripheral basophilia, a distinct feature of human CML, is observed (Daley et al. 1990). As with human CML, marked splenomegaly is typically present. Histopathologic examination of diseased spleen tissue sections reveals effacement of normal splenic architecture with marked expansion of splenic red pulp that is comprised of an infiltrate of maturing granulocytes and concomitant reduction in lymphocytes (Fig. 3.4). This cellular expansion in the murine spleen is often accompanied by a large component of maturing erythroid precursors, which can also be observed as splenic EMH in human BCR–ABL-associated CML. The bone marrow tissue sections show a marked myeloid predominance with normal maturation and are markedly hypercellular with both compression of sinuses and leukemic cells that frequently extend beyond the medullary cavity into surrounding skeletal muscle and soft tissue. The infiltrate extensively involves the liver parenchyma contributing to the invariable hepatomegaly observed (Fig. 3.4). Myeloid infiltrates can also often be found in lymph nodes as well as mucosal-associated lymphoid tissue (e.g., Peyer's patches). Flow cytometric analysis in support of the morphologic findings for a MPD includes a significantly increased Gr1+/Mac1+ population (mature granulocyte population) in both bone marrow and spleen without an increase in the progenitor cell markers CD117 (c-kit) or CD34. As expected, there is a diminution in lymphoid populations as assessed by B- or T-cell markers (e.g., B220 and Thy1.2, respectively). Importantly, however, in time the emergence of acute leukemia (always of lymphoblastic type) is generally noted, equivalent to the blast crisis that is inevitable in human CML (Daley et al. 1990). Interestingly, the CML-like disease cannot be transplanted to secondary recipient mice, whereas the acute lymphoblastic leukemia is transplantable (Daley et al. 1990). This finding suggests that the BCR–ABL-infected stem cell may represent only a minority of stem cells, making transplantation inefficient. It is critical to note that the MPD phenotypes that are observed in these retroviral models are highly dependent on the infection conditions and, largely, the murine genetic background (Elefanty and Cory

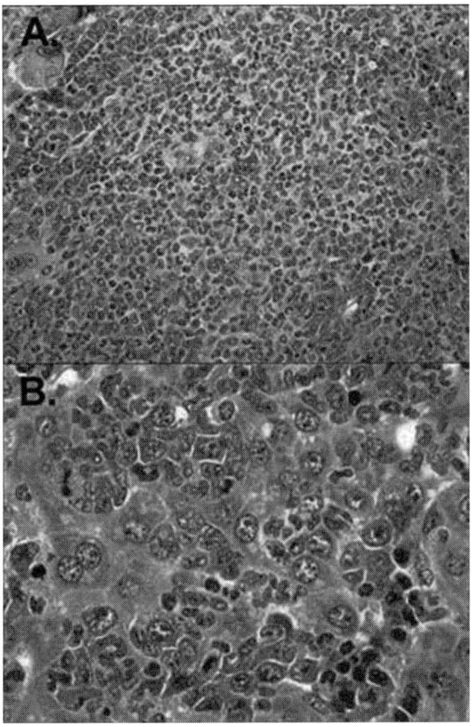

Fig. 3.4 Retroviral transduction of BCR–ABL in a bone marrow transplantation model. (**A**) Spleen from C57BL/6 recipient mouse receiving BCR–ABL transduced marrow showing effacement of the architecture by a diffuse proliferation of maturing myeloid elements. Erythropoiesis is not prominent in this case. Overall, this tumor would be classified as a myeloproliferative disorder-like myeloid leukemia (hematoxylin and eosin stains, 200× magnification). (**B**) Liver parenchyma from the same animal showing an infiltrate of both maturing myeloid and erythroid elements (hematoxylin and eosin stains, 400× magnification). (See color insert)

1992). The same is true of transgenic models of BCR–ABL-induced disease that have resulted in variable phenotypes dependent on the promoters driving BCR–ABL expression. These typically resulted in an immature lymphoid leukemia phenotype; however, transgenic mice expressing $p210^{bcr/abl}$ driven by the promoter of the *tec* gene that is expressed in the hematopoietic stem cell compartment has yielded a disease phenotype that is nearly identical to the MPD seen in the bone marrow transplant models (Honda et al. 1998).

TEL–PDGFRβ. Fusion of the PDGFRβ TK receptor to TEL was originally discovered as a consequence of a t(5;12)(q33;p13) balanced translocation identified in patients with CMML (Golub et al. 1994). Like BCR–ABL, TEL–PDGFRβ is a constitutively activated TK that also causes a fatal MPD-like myeloid leukemia in murine BMT models (Tomasson et al. 1999). This disease is characterized by marked leukocytosis with neutrophilia, splenomegaly, and EMH in hepatic and pulmonary parenchyma. The splenic red pulp is diffusely effaced by maturing myeloid elements, and these animals show a much lesser degree of erythroid hyperplasia than those of the BCR–ABL retrovirally transduced mice. Bone marrow histology reveals marked hypercellularity and a diffuse proliferation of mature myeloid forms, resembling a sea of neutrophilic forms. As with BCR–ABL-induced MPD-like myeloid leukemias, this MPD-like disease is also not transplantable into secondary recipients. Blasts in the bone marrow and spleen are variable from animal to animal, but never comprise >20% of the total cellularity. Although human TEL–PDGFRβ CMML cases are often associated with eosinophilia, this feature is not prominent in the murine transplant models. Similar to BCR–ABL, transgenic models in which TEL–PDGFRβ is driven by a lymphoid-specific immunoglobulin enhancer-promoter induce both T- and B-cell lymphoblastic lymphomas. These animals developed diffuse lymphadenopathy and mediastinal masses, and necroscopic findings supported an immature neoplasm of lymphoid derivation (Tomasson et al. 2001).

FIP1L1–PDGFRα. Hypereosinophilic syndrome (HES)/CEL is a rare hematologic disorder characterized by sustained overproduction of eosinophils in the bone marrow and peripheral eosinophilia resulting in tissue infiltration and organ damage. The genetic etiology of HES/CEL was unclear until the recent discovery of the FIP1L1–PDGFRα TK fusion protein associated with the disease (Cools et al. 2003a). The fusion gene that codes for this oncogenic fusion protein results as a consequence of an interstitial deletion on chromosome 4q12 and causes constitutive activation of the PDGFRα receptor (Cools et al. 2003a). In a murine transplant model, FIP1L1–PDGFRα causes a fatal MPD-like myeloid leukemia, similar to TEL–PDGFRβ-induced myeloproliferative disease (Cools et al. 2003b). Although frequent eosinophils were observed in this model (ranging from 5 to 20% in the peripheral blood), all cells within the granulocytic lineage were increased with the most significant increase in the neutrophils. In a subsequent study, Yamada and colleagues were able to demonstrate that retroviral transduction of FIP1L1–PDGFRα into a transgenic CD2-IL-5 mouse strain is able to induce a MPD-like disease with profound eosinophilia, indicating that FIP1L1–PDGFRα can cooperate with IL-5 to induce murine HES/CEL (Yamada et al. 2006). This study is a reminder that the biological context of these oncogenic fusion genes is critical to recapitulate more faithfully the human disease phenotypes. Of note, ancillary studies used to characterize and quantitate the increased eosinophil population in this report included immunoperoxidase studies for major basic protein (MBP) and flow cytometry identifying $CCR3^{+}/CD11b^{+/low}$ and Siglec-$F^{+}/CD11b^{+/low}$ eosinophil populations. Interestingly, Charcot–Leyden crystals (comprised of MBP), commonly observed in human cases of HES/CEL, were not observed or reported in either study.

JAK2V617F. The recent discovery of a somatic activating mutation in Janus kinase 2 (*JAK2V617F*), which is present in nearly all patients with PV and a large proportion of patients with ET and primary myelofibrosis, has significantly influenced the diagnosis and classification of these similar, but clinicopathologically distinct disorders (Baxter et al. 2005; James et al. 2005; Kralovics et al. 2005; Levine et al. 2005; Levine et al. 2007). PV is a panmyelosis resulting in the accumulation of RBCs but also involves increases in platelets and WBCs and their progenitors. It is the increase in red cell mass that is the clinical hallmark of this disease, an expansion that is independent of the normal pathways that regulate erythropoiesis and not related to other identifiable causes of secondary erythrocytosis. In retroviral bone marrow transplant models, JAK2V617F, but not wild-type JAK2, induces an MPD-like disorder (Bumm et al. 2006; Lacout et al. 2006; Wernig et al. 2006; Zaleskas et al. 2006). Significantly, in contrast to the majority of other constitutively activated TKs implicated in human MPDs that induce a predominantly neutrophilic MPD, a unique and prevailing feature of JAK2V617F expression in murine transplant models is the presence of a marked erythrocytosis, similar to the presentation in the human form of the disease. Although leukocytosis is seen with JAK2V617F expression, data from these models indicate that this feature is primarily observed in the BALB/c but not in the C57Bl/6 background, suggesting that host genetic modifiers likely play a role in disease phenotype (Wernig et al. 2006; Zaleskas et al. 2006). Moreover, while thrombocytosis is commonly observed in both PV and ET, this finding has not been prominently observed in JAK2V617F transplant models. Interestingly, Lacout and colleagues described one subset of animals in their studies with reduced JAK2V617F expression that developed a transient thrombocytosis (Lacout et al. 2006). Although thrombocytosis is not generally observed, these animals exhibit panmyelosis, including megakaryocytic hyperplasia with evidence of a megakaryocytic maturation defect as determined by ploidy analysis (Fig. 3.5A,B) (Wernig et al. 2006). Megakaryocytes from JAK2V617F-transplanted animals are large and dysplastic, frequently occurring singly or in clusters. They display deeply lobulated and hyperlobated nuclei, as well as abnormal patterns of chromatin clumping with emperipolesis of neutrophils in megakaryocyte cytoplasm (Fig. 3.5A,B). These morphologic features are not typically observed in many of the other TK MPD mouse models and appear unique to the JAK2V617F abnormality. Myelofibrosis is a feature of all forms of MPDs in humans but is most prominent in late phase PV and CIMF. Myelofibrosis is also present in the JAK2V617F murine models and is highlighted by reticulin, silver, or trichrome stains (Fig. 3.5C). The degree of myelofibrosis also may be dependent upon the mouse strain employed (e.g., BALB/c vs. C57Bl/6) (Bumm et al. 2006; Lacout et al. 2006; Wernig et al. 2006; Zaleskas et al. 2006). Similar pathologic features from murine transplant models have been observed with other JAK2 mutant alleles including JAK2 exon 12 mutations (e.g., JAK2K539L and JAK2T875N) (Scott et al. 2007). These mutations have been described in patients with PV and idiopathic erythrocytosis, the JAK2T875N mutation being originally identified in an acute megakaryocytic leukemia (AMKL) cell line (Mercher et al. 2006). Finally, murine BMT assays modeling TEL–JAK2 fusions proteins originally observed in human cases of atypical CML, B-ALL, and T-ALL (Lacronique et al. 1997; Peeters et al. 1997) also develop a fatal mixed myeloproliferative and T-cell lymphoproliferative disorder. Interestingly, the features of MPD are more similar to TEL–PDGFRβ and FLT3–ITD (internal tandem duplication) BMT models (see below) with no evidence of polycythemia (Schwaller et al. 1998), suggesting that not all forms of constitutively active JAK2 are the same.

MPLW515L/K. A search for other mutations in cases of JAK2V617F-negative PV, ET, and CIMF revealed novel somatic activating alleles (MPLW515L

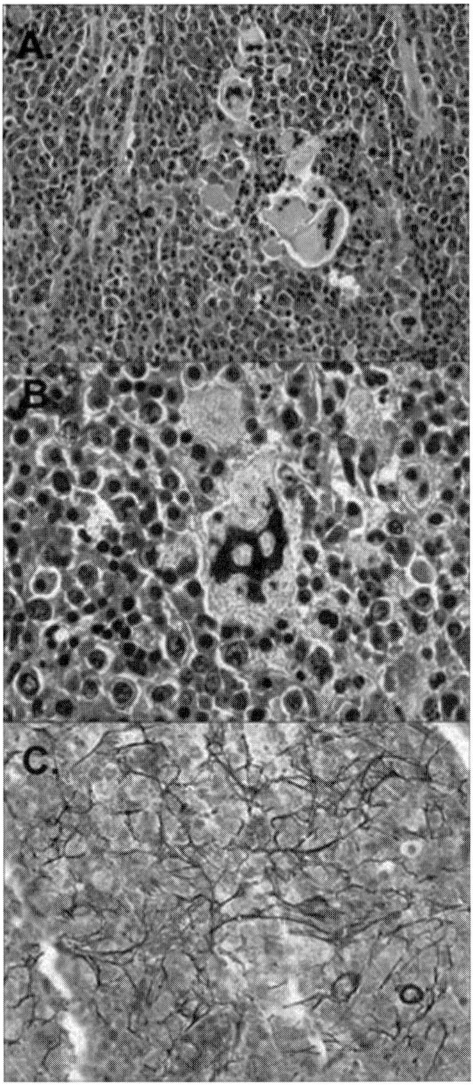

Fig. 3.5 Retroviral transduction of JAK2V617F in a bone marrow transplantation model. (**A**) Histology of Jak2V617F-transduced BALB/c mice showing pathology in representative sections of spleen revealing marked leukocytosis consisting predominantly of maturing myeloid elements and a prominent population of megakaryocytes, including arge, atypical forms occurring in occasional clusters (hematoxylin and eosin stains, 200× magnification). (**B**) Large abnormal megakaryocyte from the same animal showing bizarre nuclear convolutions and emperipolesis of neutrophils in the megakaryocyte cytoplasm. (hematoxylin and eosin stains, 400× magnification). (**C**) Bone marrow from the same animal stained with reticulin stain showing markedly increased numbers of reticulin fibers, indicative of myelofibrosis (400× magnification). (See color insert)

and W515K) in the thrombopoietin TK receptor (Pardanani et al. 2006; Pikman et al. 2006). Like the JAK2V617F mutation, expression of MPLW515L induces a fully penetrant fatal MPD-like myeloid leukemia in a murine bone marrow transplant model. Unlike JAK2V617F, expression of the activated MPL allele induces a marked thrombocytosis (platelet count from 1.9 to 4.0 × 10^{12}/L) but without polycythemia (Pikman et al. 2006). Interestingly, analysis in the MPLW515L model indicated that there was no effect on megakaryocyte ploidy, in contrast to the JAK2V617F allele. Thus, despite sharing similar histopathologic features of JAK2V617F-induced myeloproliferative disease in the BALB/c background, additional investigation will be required to fully understand these phenotypic differences.

RAS mutations. Downstream from many of the TKs described thus far, Ras proteins are a family of guanine nucleotide-binding proteins that cycle between an inactive GDP-bound state and an active GTP-bound state. Oncogenic *ras* alleles are common in myeloid malignancies including acute myeloid leukemia (AML), CMML, and juvenile myelomonocytic leukemia (JMML). As with BCR–ABL and activating FLT3 mutations (see below), the disease phenotype, penetrance, and latency in murine models studying leukemogenic ras mutations can be quite variable (Dunbar et al. 1991; Hawley et al. 1995; Darley et al. 1997; MacKenzie et al. 1999). Conditional activation of an oncogenic K-ras allele (K-Ras^{G12D}) under the control of its endogenous promoter induces a rapidly fatal MPD-like myeloid leukemia characterized by leukocytosis and marked splenomegaly (Braun et al. 2004; Chan et al. 2004). Histopathologic analysis of the marrows revealed a predominantly granulocytic/monocytic proliferation, but with subsets of mice exhibiting a striking erythroid expansion in the spleen (Fig. 3.6A,B) (Braun et al. 2004; Chan et al. 2004). Livers also showed periportal and perivascular infiltration by mature myeloid forms. Overall, the hematopoietic phenotype was comparable to myeloproliferative diseases induced in murine transplant models of BCR–ABL and TEL–PDGFRβ (Braun et al. 2004; Chan et al. 2004). Interestingly, subsets of these mice also developed thymic T-cell lymphoblastic lymphomas and nodal hyperplasia, distinct from the MPD-like leukemia. Other nonhematopoietic pathological findings in this conditional K-ras^{G12D} model included squamous papillomas involving the anal and vulvo-vaginal skin, ear, esophageal, and oral mucosa as well as adenomas of the lung (Chan et al. 2004). Similar to cooperative models with FLT3–ITD and PML–RARα (see below), transgenic animals expressing both endogenous K-ras^{G12D} and PML–RARα induces an acute promyelocytic leukemia (APML) with an incomplete penetrance (Chan et al. 2006). These tumors are characterized by expansion of splenic red pulp and bone marrow by an increased proportion of immature myeloid forms most consistent with features of an acute leukemia. Immunohistochemical analysis of these cells confirmed MPO-expressing myeloid forms, similar to findings in other murine models of APML-like disease (Fig. 3.6C,D).

SHP2 mutations. The SH2-containing tyrosine phosphatase SHP2 (*PTPN11*) is essential for normal activation of the Ras–Erk signaling in most receptor TK and cytokine signaling pathways and is the first protein–tyrosine phosphatase (PTP) implicated in leukemogenesis. Germline mutations in *SHP2* cause the autosomal dominant disorder Noonan syndrome (NS), and *SHP2* mutations have been reported in approximately 35% of JMMLs as well as in smaller percentages of pediatric AML and MDS (Loh et al. 2004; Tartaglia et al. 2004), B-ALL (Tartaglia et al. 2004), and adult AML (Bentires-Alj et al. 2004). The Shp2 mutation *PTPN11*^{D61G}, associated with NS, induces a well-tolerated mild myeloproliferative syndrome in animals heterozygous (*PTPN11*$^{D61G/+}$) for the mutation in a murine knock-in model (Araki et al.

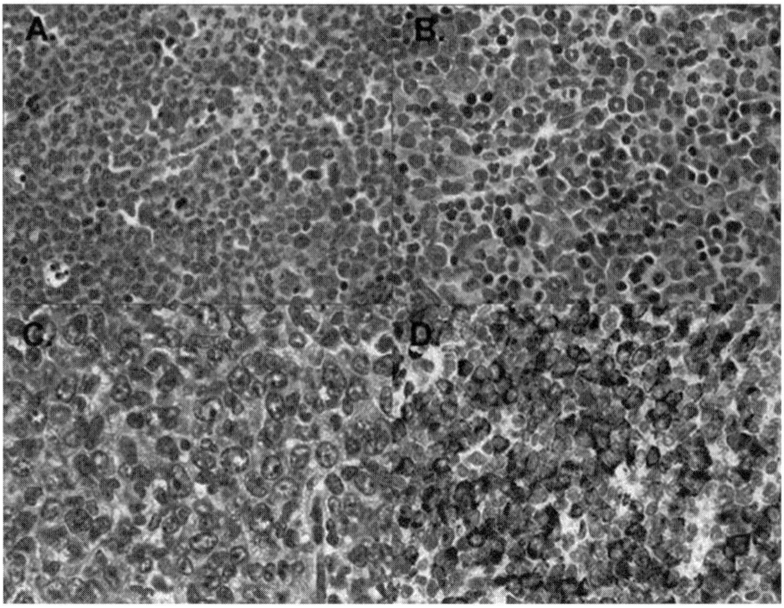

Fig. 3.6 Conditional activation of an oncogenic K-ras allele (K-Ras^{G12D}) in a mixed BALB/c, C57BL/6, and 129 v/Jae genetic background. (**A**) Bone marrow and (**B**) spleen sections reveal a marked maturing myeloid proliferation consistent with a myeloproliferative disorder-like myeloid leukemia (hematoxylin and eosin stains, 400× magnification). (**C**) When a transgenic mouse expressing PML–RARα is crossed with oncogenic K-ras expressing mouse, a short latency, highly penetrant acute promyelocytic leukemia is seen. A representative leukemia within a spleen is pictured here, demonstrating round to irregular nuclei, dispersed chromatin and small amounts of eosinophilic cytoplasm (hematoxylin and eosin stains, 400× magnification). (**D**) Myeloperoxidase immunohistochemistry of the tumor in C is pictured, revealing intense staining for myeloperoxidase consistent with acute promyelocytic leukemia. (See color insert)

2004). BM and spleen tissue sections demonstrated a mild mature myeloid hyperplasia. Also noted in the BM of these animals were frequent pseudo-Gaucher-like cells filled with crystal-like eosinophilic material, which we have also observed in a number of other myeloproliferative mouse models (Fig. 3.7A). In retroviral transplant models, Shp2 mutations primarily associated with JMML and other hematopoietic neoplasms (*PTPN11*^{E76K} or ^{D61Y}) induce a fatal MPD-like myelomonocytic leukemia (similar to that seen in JMML), as well as T-cell acute lymphoblastic leukemia/lymphoma (Mohi et al. 2005) (Fig. 3.7B,C). Importantly, the findings in these oncogenic forms of PTPN11 are similar to those seen in the activated K-ras^{G12D} knock-in mice (Braun et al. 2004; Chan et al. 2004), underscoring the importance of dysregulated RAS signaling in leukemia.

FLT3 mutations. Activating mutations in the FLT3 receptor TK constitute one of the most common genetic lesions in patients with AML and are comprised of two broad classes of mutations, namely ITDs mutations within the

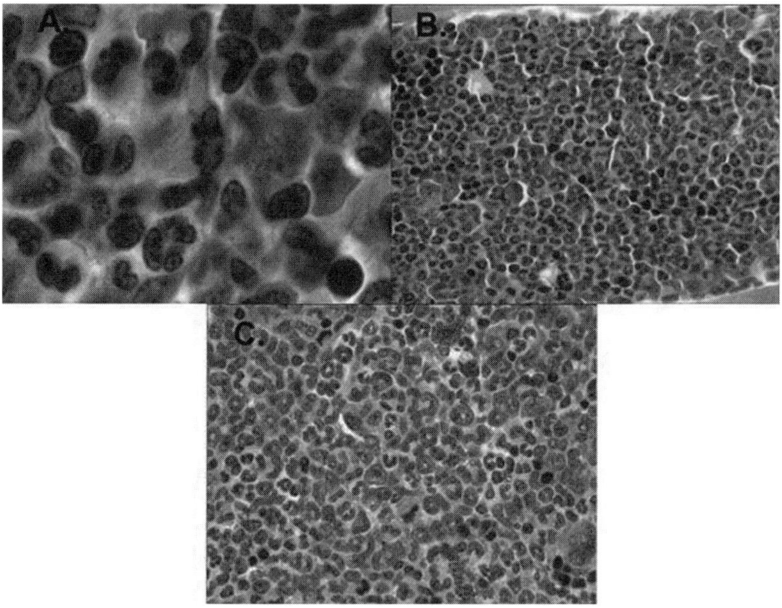

Fig. 3.7 Models of mutant SHP2 disease. (**A**) Marrow from a knock-in mouse model of the mutant SHP2 D61G associated with Noonan syndrome. These mice demonstrate a myeloid proliferation and reactive pseudo-Gaucher cells filled with crystal-like eosinophilic material (hematoxylin and eosin stains, 1000× magnification). (**B**) Marrow and (**C**) spleen from recipient mice transplanted with retrovirally transduced bone marrow expressing the SHP2 mutations D61Y and E76K, found only in juvenile myelomonocytic leukemia (JMML) and other neoplasms. Note the prominent marrow hypercellularity and compression of the sinuses in the bone marrow with a mature myeloid (granulocytic) predominance and massive splenomegaly showing infiltration of spleen with myeloid elements (hematoxylin and eosin stains, 400× magnification). (See color insert)

juxtamembrane domain and activation loop (AL) mutations of the TK domain. FLT3 mutations are commonly present in association with other chromosomal translocations in AML (i.e., PML–RARα and AML–ETO), suggesting the need for cooperativity among genetic lesions for the development of AML. This is supported by murine BMT models in which FLT3–ITD causes a fatal MPD-like myeloid leukemia with marked neutrophilia, similar to other constitutively active TK MPD models (e.g., TEL–PDGFRβ), but not AML (Kelly et al. 2002b). FLT3–ITD also induces a myeloproliferative syndrome with thrombocythemia in transgenic mouse models under the control of the *vav* panhematopoietic promoter (Lee et al. 2005) and myeloproliferative disease with features reminiscent of human CMML when expressed under an endogenous murine *Flt3* promoter (Lee et al. 2007) (Fig. 3.8). Histopathologic sections of spleen in the latter model system shows that the red pulp is expanded largely by maturing myeloid and erythroid elements in both hetero- and homozygous animals but also display a prominent white pulp expansion comprised largely

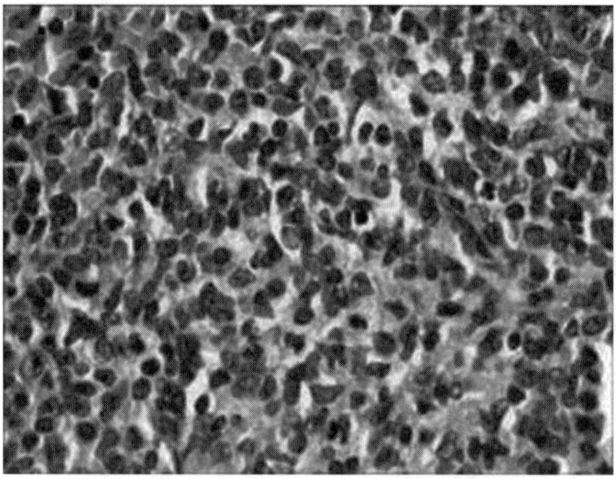

Fig. 3.8 FLT3 model of disease. A myeloproliferative disease with features reminiscent of human chronic myelomonocytic leukemia (CMML) is shown in this model of homozygous FLT3–ITD expressed in C57BL/6 mice under an endogenous murine *Flt3* promoter. In this representative section of spleen, splenic red pulp is expanded by both maturing myeloid and erythroid elements with enlarged white pulp comprised of intermediate-sized mononuclear cell infiltrate with irregular nuclei and ample eosinophilic cytoplasm (pictured here) that have a myelomonocytic phenotype by flow cytometry (hematoxylin and eosin stains, 400× magnification). (See color insert)

of intermediate-sized monocytic cells with moderate amounts of pale cytoplasm. Importantly, neither of these *Flt3* model systems is sufficient to induce acute leukemia. Support for the requirement of additional mutation(s) to induce AML comes from murine models combining both the FLT3–ITD and the PML–RARα fusion proteins, in which transplantation of bone marrow cells transgenic for the PML–RARα fusion protein and transduced with FLT3–ITD are able to induce a short latency fatal disease resembling APML (Kelly et al. 2002a). Interestingly, under comparable BMT conditions in the BALB/c background, FLT3–AL mutations have been shown to induce longer latency acute lymphoid leukemias/lymphomas (T-ALL and B-ALL) (Grundler et al. 2005), a phenotype that has also been seen in the *vav* FLT3–ITD transgenic animal model (Lee et al. 2005), as well as in retroviral models with FLT3–ITD in a mixed B6/C3H murine background (Kelly et al. 2002a). The presence of FLT3-associated lymphoid leukemias in mice is consistent with reports of activating FLT3 mutations in human acute lymphoid malignancies (Armstrong et al. 2003; Armstrong et al. 2004; Paietta et al. 2004).

3.7.2 Acute Myeloid Leukemia

AML is characterized by impaired hematopoietic differentiation, in contrast to MPD where there is normal myeloid maturation. Careful examination of peripheral blood smear, cytologic preparations, and tissue sections is required to discern between these two, often closely related, disease categories. In close parallel with the current WHO classification, the Bethesda proposals employ a percentage cutoff of at least 20% immature forms/blasts (peripheral blood, spleen, or bone marrow) to warrant classification as AML (Kogan et al. 2002). Nonlymphoid immature forms/blasts are typically medium to large in size with basophilic cytoplasm (occasionally with azurophilic granules), round to irregular nuclei with fine chromatin and nucleoli, whereas lymphoblasts will more often be relatively smaller in size with scant amounts of cytoplasm and nucleoli with a more central location. In our experience, Auer rods are never observed in murine myeloblasts, even in APL-like disease. Morphologic determination of immature myeloid blasts is also often aided by the recognition of any accompanying cell populations that are readily recognizable as maturing myeloid forms (e.g. ring granulocytic forms). Ancillary data in support of an acute nonlymphoid leukemia should demonstrate immunophenotypic evidence of myeloid origin (e.g., Mac-1 and MPO), expression of markers typically restricted to immature hematopoietic cells including c-kit, CD34, and Sca-1 and without evidence of lymphoid markers (e.g., B220, CD19, and Thy1.2).

3.7.3 AML Associated with Recurrent Genetic Abnormalities

Recurrent cytogenetic abnormalities associated with human AML include PML–RARα, AML1–ETO, CBFβ–MYH11, and MLL (11q23) rearrangements and currently comprises a distinct category within the WHO classification. While it is clear that these genetic alleles contribute to disease pathogenesis, data from numerous murine systems modeling these mutations suggest that in and of themselves, they are insufficient to induce AML (Brown et al. 1997; Grisolano et al. 1997; Castilla et al. 1999; Rhoades et al. 2000; Higuchi et al. 2002; Westervelt et al. 2003; Kuo et al. 2006). For example, although transgenic models of PML–RARα (e.g., cathespin G-PML–RARα and hMRP8 PML–RARα) induce APL-like disease in mice, this develops after a long latency with incomplete penetrance and is preceded by a pre-leukemic phase characterized by a myeloproliferative syndrome (Brown et al. 1997; Grisolano et al. 1997). Although higher penetrance of APL-like disease is observed in a transgenic cathespin G-PML/RARα knock-in model, the long latency indicates that PML–RARα expression alone is insufficient for APL development and that additional genetic events are required. Moreover, development of AML in CBFβ–MYH11 and AML1–ETO transgenic mice requires the addition of ENU mutagenesis, further supporting this notion (Castilla et al. 1999; Higuchi et al. 2002). Indeed, substantial epidemiologic evidence and data from additional murine models support this "two-hit" model of AML which requires the cooperativity of a constitutive proliferative signal (e.g., FLT3–ITD, K-RAS, and BCR–ABL) and a class of mutations typified by transcription factor mutations or fusion proteins required to impair hematopoietic differentiation (e.g., PML–RARα, MOZ–TIF2, and AML1–ETO) (Deguchi and Gilliland 2002; Kelly and Gilliland 2002). In addition to the FLT3–ITD–PML–RARα (Kelly et al. 2002a) and K-Ras^{G12D}–PML–RARα (Chan et al. 2006) APL models described above, cooperativity has also been demonstrated in murine BMT experiments with BCR–ABL and NUP98–HOXA9 (Dash et al. 2002), TEL–PDGFRβ and AML1–ETO (Grisolano et al. 2003), and FLT3–ITD and AML1–ETO (Schessl et al. 2005).

MOZ–TIF2. The MOZ–TIF2 fusion protein is associated with AML involving the inv(8)(p11q13), a relatively rare cytogenetic abnormality that is frequently associated with acute myelomonocytic leukemias. In a mouse BMT model, retrovirally transduced MOZ–TIF2 is able to induce a fatal and transplantable AML with a relatively long latency (~3–4 months), suggesting that additional cooperating mutations are required for disease development (Deguchi et al. 2003). In addition to hepatosplenomegaly, mice with MOZ–TIF2-induced AML frequently demonstrate other necroscopic findings including generalized lymphadenopathy (axillary, mesenteric, para-aortic, and femoral nodes) and leukemic infiltration into cervical lymph nodes and salivary glands that often spread into the craniofacial region. Left-shifted leukocytosis with immature myeloid and monocytic forms, as well as leukemic blasts in the peripheral blood, can be seen. More homogenous populations of immature myeloid cells and blasts and limited maturation is observed in tissue sections of diseased organs (e.g., spleens, lymph nodes, BM, and liver). Flow cytometric analysis of EGFP-gated cells (a particular advantage of this model which employed the use of an MSCV–MOZ–TIF2–IRES–EGFP retroviral vector) demonstrated that MOZ–TIF2 expressing leukemic cells were Mac-1+, variable-to-low Gr-1+, variable c-kit+, and CD34-negative without B (CD19) or T-cell (Thy1.2) markers. These immunophenotypic features are consistent with the morphologic findings of a prominent immature myeloid population with partial granulocytic differentiation (Deguchi et al. 2003). The overall pathologic features share many in common to those seen in inv(8)(p11q13) human AML.

PU.1. The PU.1 transcription factor is a critical gene essential for normal hematopoietic development. It was first isolated as the product of the *Sfpi1* locus which was overexpressed as a result of a viral insertion leading to murine erythroleukemias (Moreau-Gachelin et al. 1988, 1996). Graded changes in PU.1 concentrations have been shown to have significant effects on hematopoietic lineage fate decisions (DeKoter and Singh 2000; Dahl et al. 2003) and has been examined in a unique PU.1 "knock-down" transgenic murine model. In this model, deletion of an important upstream regulatory element (URE) of the PU.1 gene creates a hypomorphic *Sfpi1* allele such that PU.1 expression is reduced to 20% of normal levels (Rosenbauer et al. 2004). Interestingly, these animals develop a fatal and transplantable AML with marked hepatosplenomegaly and expansion of immature myeloid cells and blasts (c-kit+, Mac1^{low}, Gr1^{low}, MPO positive) (Fig. 3.9) (Rosenbauer et al. 2004). Similar

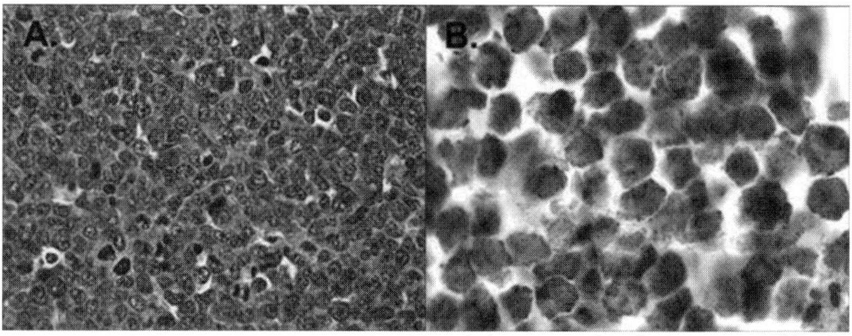

Fig. 3.9 Pu.1 model of acute myeloid leukemia. (**A**) Spleen from PU.1 knock-down C57BL/6 transgenic mouse showing a diffuse infiltrate of immature mononuclear cells with immunophenotypic features of acute myeloid leukemia (hematoxylin and eosin stains, 400× magnification). (**B**) Myeloid derivation confirmed by immunohistochemistry for myeloperoxidase shown in this marrow specimen from the same mouse (1000× magnification). (See color insert)

to PML/RARα transgenic animals, AML in the PU.1 "knock-down" mice is preceded by a pre-leukemic phase characterized by a mature myeloid proliferation. Cytogenetic studies performed by FISH and SKY analysis showed monoclonality, illustrating the utility of these ancillary techniques in this regard. In addition, SKY analysis provides the potential for the identification of recurrent structural abnormalities that might cooperate with PU.1 "knock-down" in the development of AML (Rosenbauer et al. 2004).

C/EBPα. The CCAAT enhancer-binding protein alpha (C/EBPα) is a hematopoietic transcription factor that is critical for the normal differentiation of myeloid progenitors. C/EBPα knockout animals demonstrate a lack of mature granulocytes (Zhang et al. 1997), and mutations within C/EBPα have been found in approximately 9% of AML patient samples (Nerlov 2004). To further highlight its crucial role in myeloid differentiation, a recent mouse transplantation model with expression of BCR–ABL into C/EBPα-null fetal liver cells was able to induce a fatal and transplantable acute erythroleukemia (Fig. 3.10), while BCR–ABL in fetal liver cells wild-type for C/EBPα produced a more typical fatal MPD-like leukemia (Wagner et al. 2006). In keeping with a diagnosis of acute erythroleukemia, the peripheral blood of BCR–ABL–C/EBPα$^{-/-}$animals contained normoblasts and erythroblasts that comprised two-thirds of the nucleated cells with a significant number of proerythroblasts. Identical populations of erythroid precursors were observed in the BM and spleen. In addition to this predominant immature erythroid population, an increase in mast cells was identified and confirmed by immunohistochemistry for mast cell tryptase and toluidine blue stains. Flow cytometric analysis confirmed this diagnosis showing increased expression of the erythroid marker Ter119 and the immaturity marker c-kit and an absence of MPO by immunohistochemistry (Wagner et al. 2006). Erythroid maturation is accompanied by a decrease of CD71 expression (transferrin receptor) in Ter119 cells (Socolovsky

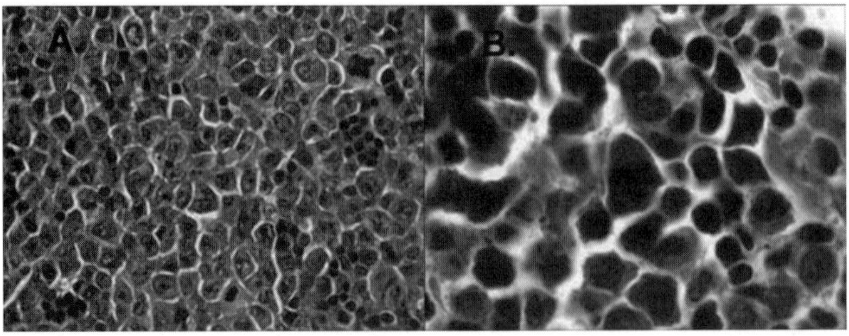

Fig. 3.10 CEBP/α knock-out model of acute erythroleukemia. (**A**) Spleen (400× magnification) and (**B**) bone marrow (1000× magnification) from a C57BL/6 CEBP/α knock-out mouse transplanted with bone marrow retrovirally transduced by BCR–ABL. The infiltrate in both tissues is comprised of an immature population of large blast forms with round to irregular nuclei, containing ample basophilic cytoplasm consistent with proerythroblasts and a diagnosis of acute erythroleukemia. (See color insert)

et al. 2001), and flow cytometric analysis with these two markers demonstrated a marked increase in Ter119^{high}/CD71^{high} cells consistent with morphologic findings. Overall, this model supports the critical role for C/EBPα in driving differentiation down the myeloid pathway.

*CDX2 and CDX4.*The clustered homeobox (*HOX*) genes have been shown to play an important role in normal hematopoiesis, and global *HOX* gene dysregulation is found in both AML and ALL cases in humans (Frohling et al. 2007). As developmental regulators of *HOX* gene expression, the *CDX* family of nonclustered *HOX* genes (e.g., Cdx4 and Cdx1) also appears to play an important role in hematopoiesis during development (Davidson et al. 2003; Davidson and Zon 2006). Recently, the CDX genes have been shown to also be involved in acute leukemia. CDX2 is fused to the *ETV6* (TEL) gene on chromosome 12p13 in a patient with AML and a t(12;13)(p13;q12) translocation (Chase et al. 1999) and more recently has been shown to be expressed in leukemic cells in approximately 90% of patients with AML but not in hematopoietic stem and progenitor cells derived from normal individuals (Scholl et al. 2007). Interestingly, overexpression of full-length CDX2 alone but not the ETV6–CDX2 fusion protein in murine BMT assays induces a long latency, fully penetrant, and transplantable AML (Rawat et al. 2004; Bansal et al. 2006; Scholl et al. 2007). It is characterized by leukocytosis with frequent numbers of immature myeloid cells and blasts in the peripheral blood, BM, spleen, and liver and supported by ancillary flow cytometric findings and immunohistochemistry studies (Rawat et al. 2004; Bansal et al. 2006; Scholl et al. 2007). In a similar series of studies, expression of CDX4 in a murine BMT system also induces a long latency, transplantable, but partially penetrant AML which upon coexpression of the Hox cofactor Meis1a was rendered fully penetrant with a shorter latency of disease (Bansal et al. 2006).

3.8 Hematopoietic Disease Models and Molecularly Targeted Therapy

Modeling human hematopoietic mutations in mice provides invaluable preclinical platforms to assess the therapeutic efficacy of novel molecularly targeted compounds against hematopoietic neoplasms. From a histopathologic perspective, examination of hematopoietic organs (e.g., BM and spleen) from responsive drug-treated animals should reveal morphologic changes that demonstrate a return to more normal histology in these tissues, as well as a reduction/elimination of leukemic infiltrates in other often involved organs (e.g., liver and lungs). As always, additional ancillary diagnostic data including flow cytometric studies should also be employed to support these morphologic changes. Various murine models (including some of aforementioned reports) have been utilized to evaluate the therapeutic efficacy of small molecule compounds for a number of the activated TK alleles associated with human chronic MPDs (Cools et al. 2003b; Weisberg et al. 2005; Peng et al. 2007). In addition, these types of studies are particularly useful in evaluating the therapeutic efficacy of these compounds against drug-resistant alleles. Table 3.3 represents a sampling of reports examining the efficacy of targeted molecular therapeutic agents in nonlymphoid leukemia murine models. While not comprehensive, they provide a useful reference that will undoubtedly grow as novel compounds and new models emerge.

Table 3.3 Murine models of hematopoietic disease and molecularly targeted therapy

Disease allele	Molecular compound(s) (murine disease)	Reference
BCR–ABL	Gleevec (STI571) (MPD)	(Wolff and Ilaria 2001)
	AMN107 (MPD)	(Weisberg et al. 2005)
	IPI-504, Gleevec (STI571) (MPD, B-ALL)	(Peng et al. 2007)
	Gleevec (STI571), Dasatinib (MPD, B-ALL)	(Hu et al. 2006)
FIP1L1–PDGFRα	PKC412 (MPD)	(Cools et al. 2003b)
	AMN107 (MPD)	(Stover et al. 2005)
TEL–PDGFRβ	Gleevec (STI571) (B-ALL)	(Tomasson et al. 1999)
	Gleevec (STI571) (MPD)	(Grisolano et al. 2003)
	AMN107 (MPD)	(Stover et al. 2005)
FLT3–ITD	PKC412 (MPD)	(Weisberg et al. 2002)
	CT53518 (MPD)	(Kelly et al. 2002c)
	PKC412 (B, T-ALL)	(Lee et al. 2005)
ZNF198–FGFR1	PKC412 (MPD)	(Chen et al. 2004)
FGFR3–TDII	PKC412 (B-ALL)	(Chen et al. 2005)
TEL–FGFR3	PKC412 (MPD)	(Chen et al. 2005)
TEL–PDGFRβ/AML1–ETO	Gleevec (STI571), SAHA, TSA (AML)	(Grisolano et al. 2003)
FLT3–ITD/PML–RARα	SU11657, ATRA (APL)	(Sohal et al. 2003)

3.9 Conclusions

Murine models of human hematopoietic neoplasms provide tremendous insights into the pathophysiology underlying these genetic disease alleles. While their expression in mice is frequently able to recapitulate many of the features of their human disease counterparts, it is important to recognize the wide variations in experimental systems that can significantly influence disease phenotype. Comprehensive pathologic evaluation is extremely valuable in making these distinctions and comparisons. While traditional histomorphologic review of diseased tissues and blood smears remains the primary method of evaluation, it is clear that with advances and more prevalent use of ancillary diagnostic techniques, our ability to evaluate murine hematopoietic tumors will continue to expand and, in turn, enhance our understanding of human hematopoietic disease.

References

Araki, T., Mohi, M.G., Ismat, F.A., Bronson, R.T., Williams, I.R., Kutok, J.L., Yang, W., Pao, L.I., Gilliland, D.G., Epstein, J.A., and Neel, B.G. 2004. Mouse model of Noonan syndrome reveals cell type- and gene dosage-dependent effects of Ptpn11 mutation. *Nat Med* **10**(8): 849–857.

Armstrong, S.A., Kung, A.L., Mabon, M.E., Silverman, L.B., Stam, R.W., Den Boer, M.L., Pieters, R., Kersey, J.H., Sallan, S.E., Fletcher, J.A., Golub, T.R., Griffin, J.D., and Korsmeyer, S.J. 2003. Inhibition of FLT3 in MLL. Validation of a therapeutic target identified by gene expression based classification. *Cancer Cell* **3**(2): 173–183.

Armstrong, S.A., Mabon, M.E., Silverman, L.B., Li, A., Gribben, J.G., Fox, E.A., Sallan, S.E., and Korsmeyer, S.J. 2004. FLT3 mutations in childhood acute lymphoblastic leukemia. *Blood* **103**(9): 3544–3546.

Bansal, D., Scholl, C., Frohling, S., McDowell, E., Lee, B.H., Dohner, K., Ernst, P., Davidson, A.J., Daley, G.Q., Zon, L.I., Gilliland, D.G., and Huntly, B.J. 2006. Cdx4 dysregulates Hox gene expression and generates acute myeloid leukemia alone and in cooperation with Meis1a in a murine model. *Proc Natl Acad Sci USA* **103**(45): 16924–16929.

Bartram, C.R., de Klein, A., Hagemeijer, A., van Agthoven, T., Geurts van Kessel, A., Bootsma, D., Grosveld, G., Ferguson-Smith, M.A., Davies, T., Stone, M., and et al. 1983. Translocation of c-abl oncogene correlates with the presence of a Philadelphia chromosome in chronic myelocytic leukaemia. *Nature* **306**(5940): 277–280.

Baxter, E.J., Scott, L.M., Campbell, P.J., East, C., Fourouclas, N., Swanton, S., Vassiliou, G.S., Bench, A.J., Boyd, E.M., Curtin, N., Scott, M.A., Erber, W.N., and Green, A.R. 2005. Acquired mutation of the tyrosine kinase JAK2 in human myeloproliferative disorders. *Lancet* **365**(9464): 1054–1061.

Bentires-Alj, M., Paez, J.G., David, F.S., Keilhack, H., Halmos, B., Naoki, K., Maris, J.M., Richardson, A., Bardelli, A., Sugarbaker, D.J., Richards, W.G., Du, J., Girard, L., Minna, J.D., Loh, M.L., Fisher, D.E., Velculescu, V.E., Vogelstein, B., Meyerson, M., Sellers, W.R., and Neel, B.G. 2004. Activating mutations of the noonan syndrome-associated SHP2/PTPN11 gene in human solid tumors and adult acute myelogenous leukemia. *Cancer Res* **64**(24): 8816–8820.

Bogue, M.A., Grubb, S.C., Maddatu, T.P., and Bult, C.J. 2007. Mouse Phenome Database (MPD). *Nucleic Acids Res* **35**(Database issue): D643–649.

Braun, B.S., Tuveson, D.A., Kong, N., Le, D.T., Kogan, S.C., Rozmus, J., Le Beau, M.M., Jacks, T.E., and Shannon, K.M. 2004. Somatic activation of oncogenic Kras in hematopoietic cells initiates a rapidly fatal myeloproliferative disorder. *Proc Natl Acad Sci USA* **101**(2): 597–602.

Brown, D., Kogan, S., Lagasse, E., Weissman, I., Alcalay, M., Pelicci, P.G., Atwater, S., and Bishop, J.M. 1997. A PMLRARalpha transgene initiates murine acute promyelocytic leukemia. *Proc Natl Acad Sci USA* **94**(6): 2551–2556.

Brunning, R.D., McKenna, R.W.1994. Tumors of the bone marrow. Normal Bone Marrow. In: Atlas of Tumor Pathology. Third series. Washington, D.C.: Armed Forces Institutes of Pathology. pp. 1–18.

Bumm, T.G., Elsea, C., Corbin, A.S., Loriaux, M., Sherbenou, D., Wood, L., Deininger, J., Silver, R.T., Druker, B.J., and Deininger, M.W. 2006. Characterization of murine JAK2V617F- positive myeloproliferative disease. *Cancer Res* **66**(23): 11156–11165.

Castilla, L.H., Garrett, L., Adya, N., Orlic, D., Dutra, A., Anderson, S., Owens, J., Eckhaus, M., Bodine, D., and Liu, P.P. 1999. The fusion gene Cbfb-MYH11 blocks myeloid differentiation and predisposes mice to acute myelomonocytic leukaemia. *Nat Genet* **23**(2): 144–146.

Chan, I.T., Kutok, J.L., Williams, I.R., Cohen, S., Kelly, L., Shigematsu, H., Johnson, L., Akashi, K., Tuveson, D.A., Jacks, T., and Gilliland, D.G. 2004. Conditional expression of oncogenic K-ras from its endogenous promoter induces a myeloproliferative disease. *J Clin Invest* **113**(4): 528–538.

Chan, I.T., Kutok, J.L., Williams, I.R., Cohen, S., Moore, S., Shigematsu, H., Ley, T.J., Akashi, K., Le Beau, M.M., and Gilliland, D.G. 2006. Oncogenic K-ras cooperates with PML-RAR alpha to induce an acute promyelocytic leukemia-like disease. *Blood* **108**(5): 1708–1715.

Chase, A., Reiter, A., Burci, L., Cazzaniga, G., Biondi, A., Pickard, J., Roberts, I.A., Goldman, J.M., and Cross, N.C. 1999. Fusion of ETV6 to the caudal-related homeobox gene CDX2 in acute myeloid leukemia with the t(12;13)(p13;q12). *Blood* **93**(3): 1025–1031.

Chen, J., Deangelo, D.J., Kutok, J.L., Williams, I.R., Lee, B.H., Wadleigh, M., Duclos, N., Cohen, S., Adelsperger, J., Okabe, R., Coburn, A., Galinsky, I., Huntly, B., Cohen, P.S., Meyer, T., Fabbro, D., Roesel, J., Banerji, L., Griffin, J.D., Xiao, S., Fletcher, J.A., Stone, R.M., and Gilliland, D.G. 2004. PKC412 inhibits the zinc finger 198-fibroblast growth factor receptor 1 fusion tyrosine kinase and is active in treatment of stem cell myeloproliferative disorder. *Proc Natl Acad Sci USA* **101**(40): 14479–14484.

Chen, J., Lee, B.H., Williams, I.R., Kutok, J.L., Mitsiades, C.S., Duclos, N., Cohen, S., Adelsperger, J., Okabe, R., Coburn, A., Moore, S., Huntly, B.J., Fabbro, D., Anderson, K.C., Griffin, J.D., and Gilliland, D.G. 2005. FGFR3 as a therapeutic target of the small molecule inhibitor PKC412 in hematopoietic malignancies. *Oncogene* **24**(56): 8259–8267.

Cools, J., DeAngelo, D.J., Gotlib, J., Stover, E.H., Legare, R.D., Cortes, J., Kutok, J., Clark, J., Galinsky, I., Griffin, J.D., Cross, N.C., Tefferi, A., Malone, J., Alam, R., Schrier, S.L., Schmid, J., Rose, M., Vandenberghe, P., Verhoef, G., Boogaerts, M., Wlodarska, I., Kantarjian, H., Marynen, P., Coutre, S.E., Stone, R., and Gilliland, D.G. 2003a. A tyrosine kinase created by fusion of the PDGFRA and FIP1L1 genes as a therapeutic target of imatinib in idiopathic hypereosinophilic syndrome. *N Engl J Med* **348**(13): 1201–1214.

Cools, J., Stover, E.H., Boulton, C.L., Gotlib, J., Legare, R.D., Amaral, S.M., Curley, D.P., Duclos, N., Rowan, R., Kutok, J.L., Lee, B.H., Williams, I.R., Coutre, S.E., Stone, R.M., DeAngelo, D.J., Marynen, P., Manley, P.W., Meyer, T., Fabbro, D., Neuberg, D., Weisberg, E., Griffin, J.D., and Gilliland, D.G. 2003b. PKC412 overcomes resistance to imatinib in a murine model of FIP1L1-PDGFRalpha-induced myeloproliferative disease. *Cancer Cell* **3**(5): 459–469.

Dahl, R., Walsh, J.C., Lancki, D., Laslo, P., Iyer, S.R., Singh, H., and Simon, M.C. 2003. Regulation of macrophage and neutrophil cell fates by the PU.1:C/EBPalpha ratio and granulocyte colony-stimulating factor. *Nature immunology* **4**(10): 1029–1036.

Daley, G.Q., Van Etten, R.A., and Baltimore, D. 1990. Induction of chronic myelogenous leukemia in mice by the P210bcr/abl gene of the Philadelphia chromosome. *Science* **247**(4944): 824–830.

Darley, R.L., Hoy, T.G., Baines, P., Padua, R.A., and Burnett, A.K. 1997. Mutant N- RAS induces erythroid lineage dysplasia in human CD34+ cells. *J Exp Med* **185**(7): 1337–1347.

Dash, A.B., Williams, I.R., Kutok, J.L., Tomasson, M.H., Anastasiadou, E., Lindahl, K., Li, S., Van Etten, R.A., Borrow, J., Housman, D., Druker, B., and Gilliland, D.G. 2002. A murine model of CML blast crisis induced by cooperation between BCR/ABL and NUP98/HOXA9. *Proc Natl Acad Sci USA* **99**(11): 7622–7627.

Davidson, A.J., Ernst, P., Wang, Y., Dekens, M.P., Kingsley, P.D., Palis, J., Korsmeyer, S.J., Daley, G.Q., and Zon, L.I. 2003. cdx4 mutants fail to specify blood progenitors and can be rescued by multiple hox genes. *Nature* **425**(6955): 300–306.

Davidson, A.J. and Zon, L.I. 2006. The caudal-related homeobox genes cdx1a and cdx4 act redundantly to regulate hox gene expression and the formation of putative hematopoietic stem cells during zebrafish embryogenesis. *Developmental biology* **292**(2): 506–518.

Deguchi, K. and Gilliland, D.G. 2002. Cooperativity between mutations in tyrosine kinases and in hematopoietic transcription factors in AML. *Leukemia* **16**(4): 740–744.

Deguchi, K., Ayton, P.M., Carapeti, M., Kutok, J.L., Snyder, C.S., Williams, I.R., Cross, N.C., Glass, C.K., Cleary, M.L., and Gilliland, D.G. 2003. MOZ-TIF2-induced acute myeloid leukemia requires the MOZ nucleosome binding motif and TIF2-mediated recruitment of CBP. *Cancer Cell* **3**(3): 259–271.

DeKoter, R.P. and Singh, H. 2000. Regulation of B lymphocyte and macrophage development by graded expression of PU.1. *Science* **288**(5470): 1439–1441.

Dunbar, C.E., Crosier, P.S., and Nienhuis, A.W. 1991. Introduction of an activated RAS oncogene into murine bone marrow lymphoid progenitors via retroviral gene transfer results in thymic lymphomas. *Oncogene research* **6**(1): 39–51.

Elefanty, A.G. and Cory, S. 1992. Hematologic disease induced in BALB/c mice by a bcr-abl retrovirus is influenced by the infection conditions. *Mol Cell Biol* **12**(4): 1755–1763.

Fredrickson, T.N. and Harris, A.W. 2000. *Atlas of Mouse Hematopathology*. Harwood Academic Publishers, Amsterdam.

Frohling, S., Scholl, C., Bansal, D., and Huntly, B.J.P. 2007. HOX Gene Regulation in Acute Myeloid Leukemia. *Cell Cycle* **6**(18): e1–e5.

Golub, T.R., Barker, G.F., Lovett, M., and Gilliland, D.G. 1994. Fusion of PDGF receptor beta to a novel ets-like gene, tel, in chronic myelomonocytic leukemia with t(5;12) chromosomal translocation. *Cell* **77**(2): 307–316.

Grisolano, J.L., O'Neal, J., Cain, J., and Tomasson, M.H. 2003. An activated receptor tyrosine kinase, TEL/PDGFbetaR, cooperates with AML1/ETO to induce acute myeloid leukemia in mice. *Proc Natl Acad Sci USA* **100**(16): 9506–9511.

Grisolano, J.L., Wesselschmidt, R.L., Pelicci, P.G., and Ley, T.J. 1997. Altered myeloid development and acute leukemia in transgenic mice expressing PML-RAR alpha under control of cathepsin G regulatory sequences. *Blood* **89**(2): 376–387.

Grundler, R., Miething, C., Thiede, C., Peschel, C., and Duyster, J. 2005. FLT3-ITD and tyrosine kinase domain mutants induce 2 distinct phenotypes in a murine bone marrow transplantation model. *Blood* **105**(12): 4792–4799.

Hawley, R.G., Fong, A.Z., Ngan, B.Y., and Hawley, T.S. 1995. Hematopoietic transforming potential of activated ras in chimeric mice. *Oncogene* **11**(6): 1113–1123.

Harmening D.M. 2002. *Clinical Hematology and Fundamentals of Hemostasis*. F.A. Davis Co. Philadelphia, PA

Higuchi, M., O'Brien, D., Kumaravelu, P., Lenny, N., Yeoh, E.J., and Downing, J.R. 2002. Expression of a conditional AML1-ETO oncogene bypasses embryonic lethality and establishes a murine model of human t(8;21) acute myeloid leukemia. *Cancer Cell* **1**(1): 63–74.

Hoff, J. 2000. Methods of blood collection in the mouse. *Lab Animal* **29**(10): 47–53.

Honda, H, Hideaki, O, Suzuki, T, Takahashi, T, Witte, ON, Ozawa, K, Ishikawa, T, Yazaki, Y, Hirai, H. 1998. Development of acute lymphoblastic leukemia and myeloproliferative disorder in transgenic mice expressing p210$^{bcr/abl}$: A novel transgenic model for human Ph^{1}-Positive leukemias. *Blood*, **91**(6) pp. 2067–2075.

Hu, Y., Swerdlow, S., Duffy, T.M., Weinmann, R., Lee, F.Y., and Li, S. 2006. Targeting multiple kinase pathways in leukemic progenitors and stem cells is essential for improved treatment of Ph+ leukemia in mice. *Proc Natl Acad Sci USA* **103**(45): 16870–16875.

Jaffe, E.S., Harris, N.L., Stein, H., and Vardiman, J. 2001. *WHO Classification of Tumours: Pathology and Genetics of Tumours of Haematopoietic and Lymphoid Tissues*. IARC Press, Lyons, France.

James, C., Ugo, V., Le Couedic, J.P., Staerk, J., Delhommeau, F., Lacout, C., Garcon, L., Raslova, H., Berger, R., Bennaceur-Griscelli, A., Villeval, J.L., Constantinescu, S.N., Casadevall, N., and Vainchenker, W. 2005. A unique clonal JAK2 mutation leading to constitutive signalling causes polycythaemia vera. *Nature* **434**(7037): 1144–1148.

Kelly, L.M. and Gilliland, D.G. 2002. Genetics of myeloid leukemias. *Annu Rev Genomics Hum Genet* 3: 179–198.

Kelly, L.M., Kutok, J.L., Williams, I.R., Boulton, C.L., Amaral, S.M., Curley, D.P., Ley, T.J., and Gilliland, D.G. 2002a. PML/RARalpha and FLT3-ITD induce an APL-like disease in a mouse model. *Proc Natl Acad Sci USA* **99**(12): 8283–8288.

Kelly, L.M., Liu, Q., Kutok, J.L., Williams, I.R., Boulton, C.L., and Gilliland, D.G. 2002b. FLT3 internal tandem duplication mutations associated with human acute myeloid leukemias induce myeloproliferative disease in a murine bone marrow transplant model. *Blood* **99**(1): 310–318.

Kelly, L.M., Yu, J.C., Boulton, C.L., Apatira, M., Li, J., Sullivan, C.M., Williams, I., Amaral, S.M., Curley, D.P., Duclos, N., Neuberg, D., Scarborough, R.M., Pandey, A., Hollenbach, S., Abe, K., Lokker, N.A., Gilliland, D.G., and Giese, N.A. 2002c. CT53518, a novel selective FLT3 antagonist for the treatment of acute myelogenous leukemia (AML). *Cancer Cell* **1**(5): 421–432.

Kogan, S.C., Ward, J.M., Anver, M.R., Berman, J.J., Brayton, C., Cardiff, R.D., Carter, J.S., de Coronado, S., Downing, J.R., Fredrickson, T.N., Haines, D.C., Harris, A.W., Harris, N.L., Hiai, H., Jaffe, E.S., MacLennan, I.C., Pandolfi, P.P., Pattengale, P.K., Perkins, A.S., Simpson, R.M., Tuttle, M.S., Wong, J.F., and Morse, H.C., 3rd. 2002. Bethesda proposals for classification of nonlymphoid hematopoietic neoplasms in mice. *Blood* **100**(1): 238–245.

Kralovics, R., Passamonti, F., Buser, A.S., Teo, S.S., Tiedt, R., Passweg, J.R., Tichelli, A., Cazzola, M., and Skoda, R.C. 2005. A gain-of-function mutation of JAK2 in myeloproliferative disorders. *N Engl J Med* **352**(17): 1779–1790.

Kuo, Y.H., Landrette, S.F., Heilman, S.A., Perrat, P.N., Garrett, L., Liu, P.P., Le Beau, M.M., Kogan, S.C., and Castilla, L.H. 2006. Cbf beta-SMMHC induces distinct abnormal myeloid progenitors able to develop acute myeloid leukemia. *Cancer Cell* **9**(1): 57–68.

Lacout, C., Pisani, D.F., Tulliez, M., Gachelin, F.M., Vainchenker, W., and Villeval, J.L. 2006. JAK2V617F expression in murine hematopoietic cells leads to MPD mimicking human PV with secondary myelofibrosis. *Blood* **108**(5): 1652–1660.

Lacronique, V., Boureux, A., Valle, V.D., Poirel, H., Quang, C.T., Mauchauffe, M., Berthou, C., Lessard, M., Berger, R., Ghysdael, J., and Bernard, O.A. 1997. A TEL-JAK2 fusion protein with constitutive kinase activity in human leukemia. *Science* **278**(5341): 1309–1312.

Lee, B.H., Tothova, Z., Levine, R.L., Anderson, K., Buza-Vidas, N., Cullen, D.E., McDowell, E.P., Adelsperger, J., Fröhling, S., Huntly, B.J., Beran, M., Jacobsen, S.E., and Gilliland, D.G. 2007. FLT3 mutations confer enhanced proliferation and survival properties to multipotent progenitors in a murine model of chronic myelomonocytic leukemia. *Cancer Cell* **12**(4): 367–380.

Lee, B.H., Williams, I.R., Anastasiadou, E., Boulton, C.L., Joseph, S.W., Amaral, S.M., Curley, D.P., Duclos, N., Huntly, B.J., Fabbro, D., Griffin, J.D., and Gilliland, D.G.

2005. FLT3 internal tandem duplication mutations induce myeloproliferative or lymphoid disease in a transgenic mouse model. *Oncogene* **24**(53): 7882–7892.

Levine, R.L., Wadleigh, M., Cools, J., Ebert, B.L., Wernig, G., Huntly, B.J., Boggon, T.J., Wlodarska, I., Clark, J.J., Moore, S., Adelsperger, J., Koo, S., Lee, J.C., Gabriel, S., Mercher, T., D'Andrea, A., Frohling, S., Dohner, K., Marynen, P., Vandenberghe, P., Mesa, R.A., Tefferi, A., Griffin, J.D., Eck, M.J., Sellers, W.R., Meyerson, M., Golub, T.R., Lee, S.J., and Gilliland, D.G. 2005. Activating mutation in the tyrosine kinase JAK2 in polycythemia vera, essential thrombocythemia, and myeloid metaplasia with myelofibrosis. *Cancer Cell* **7**(4): 387–397.

Levine, R.L., Pardanani, A., Tefferi, A., and Gilliland, D.G. 2007. Role of JAK2 in the pathogenesis and therapy of myeloproliferative disorders. *Nat Rev Cancer* **7**(9): 673–683.

Liao, A.H., Li, C.H., Li, P.C., and Cheng, W.F. 2005. Non-Invasive Imaging of Small-Animal Tumors: High-Frequency Ultrasound vs. MicroPET. *Conf Proc IEEE Eng Med Biol Soc* 6: 5695–5698.

Loh, M.L., Vattikuti, S., Schubbert, S., Reynolds, M.G., Carlson, E., Lieuw, K.H., Cheng, J.W., Lee, C.M., Stokoe, D., Bonifas, J.M., Curtiss, N.P., Gotlib, J., Meshinchi, S., Le Beau, M.M., Emanuel, P.D., and Shannon, K.M. 2004. Mutations in PTPN11 implicate the SHP-2 phosphatase in leukemogenesis. *Blood* **103**(6): 2325–2331.

Longley, B.J., Tyrrell, L., Lu, S.Z., Ma, Y.S., Langley, K., Ding, T.G., Duffy, T., Jacobs, P., Tang, L.H., and Modlin, I. 1996. Somatic c-KIT activating mutation in urticaria pigmentosa and aggressive mastocytosis: establishment of clonality in a human mast cell neoplasm. *Nat Genet* **12**(3): 312–314.

MacKenzie, K.L., Dolnikov, A., Millington, M., Shounan, Y., and Symonds, G. 1999. Mutant N-ras induces myeloproliferative disorders and apoptosis in bone marrow repopulated mice. *Blood* **93**(6): 2043–2056.

Mebius, R.E. and Kraal, G. 2005. Structure and function of the spleen. *Nat Rev* **5**(8): 606–616.

Mercher, T., Wernig, G., Moore, S.A., Levine, R.L., Gu, T.L., Frohling, S., Cullen, D., Polakiewicz, R.D., Bernard, O.A., Boggon, T.J., Lee, B.H., and Gilliland, D.G. 2006. JAK2T875N is a novel activating mutation that results in myeloproliferative disease with features of megakaryoblastic leukemia in a murine bone marrow transplantation model. *Blood* **108**(8): 2770–2779.

Mohi, M.G., Williams, I.R., Dearolf, C.R., Chan, G., Kutok, J.L., Cohen, S., Morgan, K., Boulton, C., Shigematsu, H., Keilhack, H., Akashi, K., Gilliland, D.G., and Neel, B.G. 2005. Prognostic, therapeutic, and mechanistic implications of a mouse model of leukemia evoked by Shp2 (PTPN11) mutations. *Cancer Cell* **7**(2): 179–191.

Moreau-Gachelin, F., Tavitian, A., and Tambourin, P. 1988. Spi-1 is a putative oncogene in virally induced murine erythroleukaemias. *Nature* **331**(6153): 277–280.

Moreau-Gachelin, F., Wendling, F., Molina, T., Denis, N., Titeux, M., Grimber, G., Briand, P., Vainchenker, W., and Tavitian, A. 1996. Spi-1/PU.1 transgenic mice develop multistep erythroleukemias. *Mol Cell Biol* **16**(5): 2453–2463.

Morse, H.C., 3rd, Anver, M.R., Fredrickson, T.N., Haines, D.C., Harris, A.W., Harris, N.L., Jaffe, E.S., Kogan, S.C., MacLennan, I.C., Pattengale, P.K., and Ward, J.M. 2002. Bethesda proposals for classification of lymphoid neoplasms in mice. *Blood* **100**(1): 246–258.

Nerlov, C. 2004. C/EBPalpha mutations in acute myeloid leukaemias. *Nat Rev Cancer* **4**(5): 394–400.

Paietta, E., Ferrando, A.A., Neuberg, D., Bennett, J.M., Racevskis, J., Lazarus, H., Dewald, G., Rowe, J.M., Wiernik, P.H., Tallman, M.S., and Look, A.T. 2004. Activating FLT3 Mutations in CD117/KIT PositiveT-Cell Acute Lymphoblastic Leukemias. *Blood* **104**(2): 558–60.

Pardanani, A.D., Levine, R.L., Lasho, T., Pikman, Y., Mesa, R.A., Wadleigh, M., Steensma, D.P., Elliott, M.A., Wolanskyj, A.P., Hogan, W.J., McClure, R.F., Litzow, M.R., Gilliland, D.G., and Tefferi, A. 2006. MPL515 mutations in myeloproliferative and other myeloid disorders: a study of 1182 patients. *Blood* **108**(10): 3472–3476.

Peeters, P., Raynaud, S.D., Cools, J., Wlodarska, I., Grosgeorge, J., Philip, P., Monpoux, F., Van Rompaey, L., Baens, M., Van den Berghe, H., and Marynen, P. 1997. Fusion of TEL, the ETS-variant gene 6 (ETV6), to the receptor-associated kinase JAK2 as a result of t(9;12) in a lymphoid and t(9;15;12) in a myeloid leukemia. *Blood* **90**(7): 2535–2540.

Peng, C., Brain, J., Hu, Y., Goodrich, A., Kong, L., Grayzel, D., Pak, R., Read, M., and Li, S. 2007. Inhibition of heat shock protein 90 prolongs survival of mice with BCR-ABL-T315I-induced leukemia and suppresses leukemic stem cells. *Blood* **110**(2): 678–685.

Pikman, Y., Lee, B.H., Mercher, T., McDowell, E., Ebert, B.L., Gozo, M., Cuker, A., Wernig, G., Moore, S., Galinsky, I., Deangelo, D.J., Clark, J.J., Lee, S.J., Golub, T.R., Wadleigh, M., Gilliland, D.G., and Levine, R.L. 2006. MPLW515L Is a Novel Somatic Activating Mutation in Myelofibrosis with Myeloid Metaplasia. *PLoS Med* **3**(7): e270.

Rawat, V.P., Cusan, M., Deshpande, A., Hiddemann, W., Quintanilla-Martinez, L., Humphries, R.K., Bohlander, S.K., Feuring-Buske, M., and Buske, C. 2004. Ectopic expression of the homeobox gene Cdx2 is the transforming event in a mouse model of t(12;13)(p13;q12) acute myeloid leukemia. *Proc Natl Acad Sci USA* **101**(3): 817–822.

Rhoades, K.L., Hetherington, C.J., Harakawa, N., Yergeau, D.A., Zhou, L., Liu, L.Q., Little, M.T., Tenen, D.G., and Zhang, D.E. 2000. Analysis of the role of AML1-ETO in leukemogenesis, using an inducible transgenic mouse model. *Blood* **96**(6): 2108–2115.

Rosenbauer, F., Wagner, K., Kutok, J.L., Iwasaki, H., Le Beau, M.M., Okuno, Y., Akashi, K., Fiering, S., and Tenen, D.G. 2004. Acute myeloid leukemia induced by graded reduction of a lineage-specific transcription factor, PU.1. *Nat Genet* **36**(6): 624–630.

Sakaki K. 1961. Hematological comparison of the mouse blood taken from the eye and the tail. *Exp Anim* 10:14–19.

Schessl, C., Rawat, V.P., Cusan, M., Deshpande, A., Kohl, T.M., Rosten, P.M., Spiekermann, K., Humphries, R.K., Schnittger, S., Kern, W., Hiddemann, W., Quintanilla-Martinez, L., Bohlander, S.K., Feuring-Buske, M., and Buske, C. 2005. The AML1-ETO fusion gene and the FLT3 length mutation collaborate in inducing acute leukemia in mice. *J Clin Invest* **115**(8): 2159–2168.

Scholl, C., Bansal, D., Dohner, K., Eiwen, K., Huntly, B.J., Lee, B.H., Rucker, F.G., Schlenk, R.F., Bullinger, L., Dohner, H., Gilliland, D.G., and Frohling, S. 2007. The homeobox gene CDX2 is aberrantly expressed in most cases of acute myeloid leukemia and promotes leukemogenesis. *J Clin Invest* **117**(4): 1037–1048.

Schwaller, J., Frantsve, J., Aster, J., Williams, I.R., Tomasson, M.H., Ross, T.S., Peeters, P., Van Rompaey, L., Van Etten, R.A., Ilaria, R., Jr., Marynen, P., and Gilliland, D.G. 1998. Transformation of hematopoietic cell lines to growth-factor independence and induction of a fatal myelo- and lymphoproliferative disease in mice by retrovirally transduced TEL/JAK2 fusion genes. *Embo J* **17**(18): 5321–5333.

Scott, L.M., Tong, W., Levine, R.L., Scott, M.A., Beer, P.A., Stratton, M.R., Futreal, P.A., Erber, W.N., McMullin, M.F., Harrison, C.N., Warren, A.J., Gilliland, D.G., Lodish, H.F., and Green, A.R. 2007. JAK2 exon 12 mutations in polycythemia vera and idiopathic erythrocytosis. *N Engl J Med* **356**(5): 459–468.

Socolovsky, M., Nam, H., Fleming, M.D., Haase, V.H., Brugnara, C., and Lodish, H.F. 2001. Ineffective erythropoiesis in Stat5a(–/–)5b(–/–) mice due to decreased survival of early erythroblasts. *Blood* **98**(12): 3261–3273.

Sohal, J., Phan, V.T., Chan, P.V., Davis, E.M., Patel, B., Kelly, L.M., Abrams, T.J., O'Farrell, A.M., Gilliland, D.G., Le Beau, M.M., and Kogan, S.C. 2003. A model of APL with FLT3 mutation is responsive to retinoic acid and a receptor tyrosine kinase inhibitor, SU11657. *Blood* **101**(8): 3188–3197.

Stover, E.H., Chen, J., Lee, B.H., Cools, J., McDowell, E., Adelsperger, J., Cullen, D., Coburn, A., Moore, S.A., Okabe, R., Fabbro, D., Manley, P.W., Griffin, J.D., and Gilliland, D.G. 2005. The small molecule tyrosine kinase inhibitor AMN107 inhibits TEL- PDGFRbeta and FIP1L1-PDGFRalpha in vitro and in vivo. *Blood* **106**(9): 3206–3213.

Tartaglia, M., Martinelli, S., Cazzaniga, G., Cordeddu, V., Iavarone, I., Spinelli, M., Palmi, C., Carta, C., Pession, A., Arico, M., Masera, G., Basso, G., Sorcini, M., Gelb, B.D., and Biondi, A. 2004. Genetic evidence for lineage-related and differentiation stage-related contribution of somatic PTPN11 mutations to leukemogenesis in childhood acute leukemia. *Blood* **104**(2): 307–313.

Tatsumi, T., Huang, J., Gooding, W.E., Gambotto, A., Robbins, P.D., Vujanovic, N.L., Alber, S.M., Watkins, S.C., Okada, H., and Storkus, W.J. 2003. Intratumoral delivery of dendritic cells engineered to secrete both interleukin (IL)-12 and IL-18 effectively treats local and distant disease in association with broadly reactive Tc1-type immunity. *Cancer Res* **63**(19): 6378–6386.

Tomasson, M.H., Williams, I.R., Hasserjian, R., Udomsakdi, C., McGrath, S.M., Schwaller, J., Druker, B., and Gilliland, D.G. 1999. TEL/PDGFbetaR induces hematologic malignancies in mice that respond to a specific tyrosine kinase inhibitor. *Blood* **93**(5): 1707–1714.

Tomasson, M.H., Williams, I.R., Li, S., Kutok, J., Cain, D., Gillessen, S., Dranoff, G., Van Etten, R.A., and Gilliland, D.G. 2001. Induction of myeloproliferative disease in mice by tyrosine kinase fusion oncogenes does not require granulocyte-macrophage colony-stimulating factor or interleukin-3. *Blood* **97**(5): 1435–1441.

Wagner, K., Zhang, P., Rosenbauer, F., Drescher, B., Kobayashi, S., Radomska, H.S., Kutok, J.L., Gilliland, D.G., Krauter, J., and Tenen, D.G. 2006. Absence of the transcription factor CCAAT enhancer binding protein alpha results in loss of myeloid identity in bcr/abl-induced malignancy. *Proc Natl Acad Sci USA* **103**(16): 6338–6343.

Weisberg, E., Boulton, C., Kelly, L.M., Manley, P., Fabbro, D., Meyer, T., Gilliland, D.G., and Griffin, J.D. 2002. Inhibition of mutant FLT3 receptors in leukemia cells by the small molecule tyrosine kinase inhibitor PKC412. *Cancer Cell* **1**(5): 433–443.

Weisberg, E., Manley, P.W., Breitenstein, W., Bruggen, J., Cowan-Jacob, S.W., Ray, A., Huntly, B., Fabbro, D., Fendrich, G., Hall-Meyers, E., Kung, A.L., Mestan, J., Daley, G.Q., Callahan, L., Catley, L., Cavazza, C., Azam, M., Neuberg, D., Wright, R.D., Gilliland, D.G., and Griffin, J.D. 2005. Characterization of AMN107, a selective inhibitor of native and mutant Bcr-Abl. *Cancer Cell* **7**(2): 129–141.

Wernig, G., Mercher, T., Okabe, R., Levine, R.L., Lee, B.H., and Gilliland, D.G. 2006. Expression of Jak2V617F causes a polycythemia vera-like disease with associated myelofibrosis in a murine bone marrow transplant model. *Blood* **107**(11): 4274–4281.

Westervelt, P., Lane, A.A., Pollock, J.L., Oldfather, K., Holt, M.S., Zimonjic, D.B., Popescu, N.C., DiPersio, J.F., and Ley, T.J. 2003. High-penetrance mouse model of acute promyelocytic leukemia with very low levels of PML-RARalpha expression. *Blood* **102**(5): 1857–1865.

Wolff, N.C. and Ilaria, R.L., Jr. 2001. Establishment of a murine model for therapy-treated chronic myelogenous leukemia using the tyrosine kinase inhibitor STI571. *Blood* **98**(9): 2808–2816.

Wong, S. and Witte, O.N. 2001. Modeling Philadelphia chromosome positive leukemias. *Oncogene* **20**(40): 5644–5659.

Yamada, Y., Rothenberg, M.E., Lee, A.W., Akei, H.S., Brandt, E.B., Williams, D.A., and Cancelas, J.A. 2006. The FIP1L1-PDGFRA fusion gene cooperates with IL-5 to induce murine hypereosinophilic syndrome (HES)/chronic eosinophilic leukemia (CEL)-like disease. *Blood* **107**(10): 4071–4079.

Zaleskas, V.M., Krause, D.S., Lazarides, K., Patel, N., Hu, Y., Li, S., and Van Etten, R.A. 2006. Molecular pathogenesis and therapy of polycythemia induced in mice by JAK2 V617F. *PLoS ONE* 1: e18.

Zhang, D.E., Zhang, P., Wang, N.D., Hetherington, C.J., Darlington, G.J., and Tenen, D.G. 1997. Absence of granulocyte colony-stimulating factor signaling and neutrophil development in CCAAT enhancer binding protein alpha-deficient mice. *Proc Natl Acad Sci USA* **94**(2): 569–574.

Chapter 4
Mechanisms of DNA Double-Strand Break Repair in Hematopoietic Homeostasis and Oncogenesis

Sarah A. Maas, Lura Brianna Caddle, and Kevin D. Mills

Contents

List of Abbreviations

AID	Activation-induced cytidine deaminase
ALL	Acute lymphoblastic leukemia
AML	Acute myeloid leukemia
ART	Artemis
AT	Ataxia telangiectasia
ATM	Ataxia telangiectasia mutated

S.A. Maas and K.D. Mills
The Jackson Laboratory, Bar Harbor, ME 04609, USA
sarah.maas@jax.org, kevin.mills@jax.org

S. Li (ed.), *Mouse Models of Human Blood Cancers*,
DOI: 10.1007/978-0-387-69132-9_4, © Springer Science+Business Media, LLC 2008

ATR	ATM and Rad3 related
B-ALL	B-cell acute lymphoblastic leukemia
BFB	Breakage–fusion–bridge
CHO	Chinese hamster ovary
CML	Chronic myelogenous leukemia
CSR	Class switch recombination
DNA–PKcs	DNA-dependent protein kinase catalytic subunit
DSB	DNA double-strand break
FA	Fanconi anemia
GC	Gene conversion
H2AX	Histone H2A variant X
HR	Homologous recombination
ICL	Interstrand crosslinking
Ig	Immunoglobulin
IgH	Immunoglobulin heavy chain
IR	Ionizing radiation
Lig4	Ligase IV
MDS	Myelodysplastic syndrome
MEF	Mouse embryonic fibroblast
MMC	Mitomycin-C
MRN	Mre11-Rad50-Nbs1 complex
NHEJ	Nonhomologous end joining
Ph	Philadelphia
Pre-T LBL	Pre-T cell lymphoblastic leukemia
RAG	Recombination-activating gene
RPA	Replication protein A
RS	Recombination signal sequences
RS-SCID	Radiation-sensitive SCID
SCE	Sister chromatid exchange
SCID	Severe combined immunodeficiency
SDSA	Synthesis-dependent strand annealing
SHM	Somatic hypermutation
SSA	Single-strand annealing
ssDNA	Single-stranded DNA
T-ALL	T-cell acute lymphoblastic leukemia or lymphoma
TCR	T-cell receptor
TOPOIII	Topoisomerase III
XLF	XRCC4-like factor

4.1 Introduction

Chromosomal instability is a hallmark of cancer associated with many, if not all, tumor types (reviewed in Aplan, 2006; Ferguson and Alt, 2001; Mills et al., 2003) (Fig. 4.1). Structural and numerical chromosomal abnormalities often

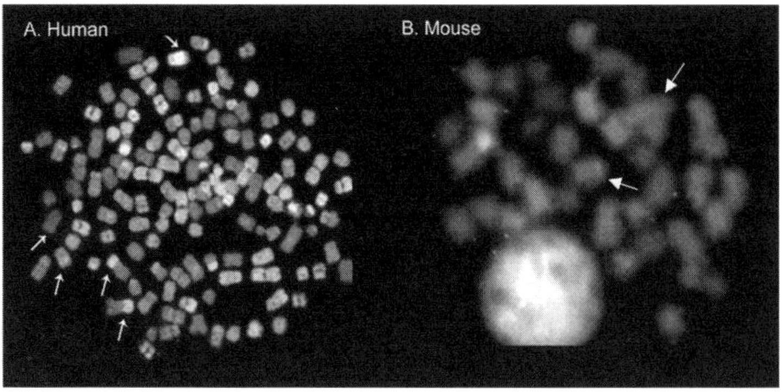

Fig. 4.1 Genomic instability observed in human and mouse tumor cells. (**A**) Spectral karyotype analysis of a human bladder cancer cell line. The aneuploid J82 cell line contains multiple chromosomal aberrations. White arrows indicate translocations. Adapted from Padilla-Nash et al. (2006). (**B**) Spectral karyotype analysis of a mouse pro-B cell lymphoma deficient for *Dclre1c* and *Trp53*. White arrows indicate translocations. (See color insert)

play key roles in tumorigenesis and can occur as principle lesions in tumor precursor cells. These molecular alterations to the genome occur as a consequence of various exogenous or endogenous insults, producing chromosomal translocations, interstitial deletions, gene amplifications, and other aberrations. While extensive and nonrecurrent chromosomal lesions are associated with many different cancer types, specific characteristic lesions are often associated with given tumors, especially those of hematologic origin (Agarwal et al., 2006; Aplan, 2006; Ferguson and Alt, 2001).

Hematologic malignancies, affecting lymphoid, myeloid, and erythroid cells, frequently occur with characteristic chromosomal rearrangements. By contrast with solid tumors, hematologic malignancies frequently, but not invariably, incur simple, reciprocal translocations, which are often recognized for their diagnostic and prognostic value. In the past two decades, a vast body of research has shown that many of these chromosomal rearrangements, especially those occurring in hematologic malignancies, lead either to the deregulation of a specific cellular proto-oncogene or to the formation of a novel fusion oncogene (reviewed in Aplan, 2006). Analysis of karyotypic instability in malignant hematological cells and tissues has, in some cases, directly led to the identification of new oncogenes and more recently opened the possibility of developing better and more highly specific therapeutic modalities targeting tumor-specific genetic alterations.

The catalogue of recognized chromosomal translocations that characterize specific tumor types continues to grow. The prototypical example of such a characteristic rearrangement is the Philadelphia (Ph) chromosome, associated with chronic myelogenous leukemia (CML) and acute lymphoblastic leukemia (ALL) (de Klein et al., 1982). The Ph chromosome encodes for a chimeric protein comprising part of the breakpoint cluster region (*BCR*) gene, located on chromosome (Chr) 22 (region q11), and the Abelson gene (*ABL*) on Chr 9 (region q34). This chimeric BCR–ABL protein acts as a constitutive tyrosine kinase that increases cellular proliferation, eventually resulting in tumorigenesis.

Subsequent to the identification of the Ph chromosome, it has become clear that hematologic cancers can arise with a broad range of analogous reciprocal chromosomal translocations. In neoplasias derived from B or T lymphocytes, these translocations often result from mistakes or failures in V(D)J recombination, immunoglobulin (Ig) class switch recombination (CSR), or somatic hypermutation (SHM), processes of somatic rearrangement in developing/maturing Ig or T-cell receptor (*TCR*) genes (reviewed in Aplan, 2006; Chaudhuri and Alt, 2004; Jung and Alt, 2004; Kuppers and Dalla-Favera, 2001; Mills et al., 2003; Weinstock et al., 2006b). Burkitt's lymphoma is typically characterized by a marker t(8;14) translocation. This chromosomal aberration juxtaposes the potent oncogene *Myc* with strong regional enhancers within the Ig heavy chain (IgH) locus. Other lymphoid malignancies, such as B-cell acute lymphoblastic leukemia (B-ALL) and pre-T lymphoblastic leukemia (pre-T LBL), typically show characteristic translocations involving the Ig loci, and it has become apparent that these genomic regions are especially prone to translocation due to gene rearrangements that occur as a necessary step in the developmental program of lymphoid maturation. Lymphoid translocations typically result in oncogene amplification due to potent enhancer elements within the Ig and TCR loci rather than fusion proteins (Table 4.1).

While such translocations, usually afflicting the Ig or TCR loci, characterize numerous lymphoid malignancies, myeloid neoplasias can incur a variety of specific translocations that do not appear to be the direct consequence of DNA double-strand breaks (DSBs) introduced during a developmental program. Instead, myeloid malignancies often exhibit a different type of chromosomal translocation. Although recurrent, balanced translocations are also observed in myeloid malignancies, these translocations typically create fusion genes that encode for constitutively active chimeric proteins (Table 4.1).

Recurrent translocations observed in leukemias and lymphomas often produce novel gene products that are candidate targets for highly specific drugs. For example, the highly effective small molecule tyrosine kinase inhibitor imatinib, which targets the BCR–ABL fusion protein, has proven one of the most effective therapies now available to Ph+ CML patients (Druker et al., 2001). Molecular analysis of the BCR–ABL fusion protein exemplifies how knowledge of recurrent translocations and their gene products can be used both to understand and improve upon current chemotherapeutic mechanisms and, potentially, to develop effective new therapeutic modalities. Importantly, molecular characterization of recurrent chromosomal abnormalities associated with specific types of hematologic malignancies may also facilitate better assignment of patients into particular risk categories, permitting specifically targeted customized therapeutic regimes.

Patients with the same gross cancer diagnosis often respond dramatically differently to the same chemotherapy regimen, a likely consequence of both

Table 4.1 Some commonly observed recurrent translocations associated with lymphoid and myeloid leukemias

Diagnosis	Translocation	Activated genes	Mechanism of activation	References
ALL–Burkitts lymphoma	t(8;14)(q24;q32)	*MYC, IGH*	Translocation to *IGH*	Aplan (2006), Mitelman Database
ALL	t(8;22)(q24;q11)	*MYC*	Translocation to *IGL*	Aplan (2006)
ALL	t(2;8)(p12;q24)	*MYC*	Translocation to *IGK*	Aplan (2006)
ALL	t(12;21)(p12;q22)	*TEL–AML*	Gene fusion	Aplan (2006)
ALL	t(1;19)(q21;p13)	*E2A–PBX1*	Gene fusion	Aplan (2006)
ALL	t(17;19)(q22;p13)	*E2A–HLF*	Gene fusion	Aplan (2006)
ALL	t(1:11)(p32;q23)	*MLL, MLL/EPS15*	Gene fusion	Hashimoto et al., (2001), Mitelman Database
ALL	inv(7)(p15;q34)	*TRB@/HOXA*	Gene fusion	Mitelman Database
ALL	t(11;19)(q23;p13)	*MLL, MLL/MLLT1*	Gene fusion	Mitelman Database
ALL—Ph + chromosome	t(9;22)(q34;q11)	*BCR-ABL*	Gene fusion	Mitelman Database
ALL	t(12;21)(p13,q22)	*ETV6/RUNX1 (TEL/AML1)*	Gene fusion	Frost et al. (2004), Mitelman Database
ALL	inv(14)(q11;q32)	*IGH/TRA@, TCL1A*	Gene fusion	Sugimoto et al. (1999)
ALL	t(4;11)(q21;q23)	*MLL–AF4*	Gene fusion	Aplan (2006)
ALCL	t(2;5)(p23;q35)	*NPM–ALK*	Gene fusion	Aplan (2006)
ALCL	t(8;14)(q24;q11)	*MYC*	Translocation to *TRA@/D@*	Aplan (2006)
ALCL	t(7;19)(q35;p13)	*LYL1*	Translocation to *TRB@*	Aplan (2006)
ALCL	t(1;14)(p32;q11)	*SCL*	Translocation to *TRA@/D@*	Aplan (2006)
ALCL	t(14;21)(q11;q22)	*OLIG2*	Translocation to *TRA@/D@*	Aplan (2006)
ALCL	t(11;14)(p15;q11)	*LMO1(RBTN1)*	Translocation to *TRA@/D@*	Aplan (2006)
ALCL	t(11;14)(p13;q11)	*LMO2(RBTN2)*	Translocation to *TRA@/D@*	Aplan (2006)
ALCL	t(10;14)(q24;q11)	*HOX11*	Translocation to *TRA@/D@*	Aplan (2006)
ALCL	t(5;14)(q35;q32)	*HOX11L2 (TLX3)*	unknown	Aplan (2006) and Nagel et al. (2003)
ALCL	t(10;11)(p13;q21)	*CALM-AF10*	Gene fusion	Aplan (2006)
ALCL	t(4;11)(q21;p15)	*NUP98-RAP1GDS1*	Gene fusion	Aplan (2006)

Table 4.1 (continued)

Diagnosis	Translocation	Activated genes	Mechanism of activation	References
ALCL	t(14;18)(q32;q21)	*IGH/BCL2*	Translocation to *IGH*	Mitelman Database
CLL	t(14;19)(q32;q13)	*IGH/CEBPA*	Translocation to *IGH*	Frost et al. (2004)
CML—Ph + chromosome	t(9;22)(q34;q11)	*BCR–ABL*	Gene fusion	Aplan (2006), Mitelman Database
CML	t(9;11)(p22q23)	*AF9–MLL*	Gene fusion	Aplan (2006)
APL	t(15;17)(q21;q21)	*PML–RARA*	Gene fusion	Aplan (2006)
APL	t(11;17)(q23;q21)	*PLZF–RARA*	Gene fusion	Aplan (2006)
AML	t(4;11)(q21;q23)	*HRAS–MLL*	Gene fusion	Aplan (2006)
AML	t(11;v)(q23;v)	*MLL*	Gene fusion	Aplan (2006)
AML or CMML	t(12;v)(p13;v)	*ETV6*	Gene fusion	Aplan (2006)
AML	t(11;v)(p15;v)	*NUP98*	Gene fusion	Aplan (2006)
AML	t(8;21)(q22;q22)	*AML1–ETO*	Gene fusion	Aplan (2006)
AML	inv(16)(p13;q22)	*CBFB–MYH11*	Gene fusion	Aplan (2006)
AML	t(16;21)(p11;q22)	*FUS-ERG*	Gene fusion	Aplan (2006)
AML	t(5;14)(q33;q32)	*CEV14–PDGFRB*	Gene fusion	Aplan (2006)
AML	t(8;22)(p11;q13)	*P300-MOZ*	Gene fusion	Aplan (2006)
AML	t(6;9)(p23;q34)	*DEK,NUP214*	Gene fusion	Aplan (2006)
AMKL	t(1;22)(p13;q13)	*RBM15,MKL*	Gene fusion	Aplan (2006)
AML	t(3;21)(q26;q22)	*AML1–EV11*	Gene fusion	Aplan (2006)

Mitelman Database of Chromosome Aberrations in Cancer (Cancer Genome Anatomy Project), http://cgap.nci.nih.gov/Chromosomes/Mitelman. It is important to note that the revised nomenclature for T-cell receptor A–D loci (formerly known as *TCRA-D*; now known as *TRA-D@*) has been used in creating this table.

individual genetic variation and tumor-specific properties. Therefore, better knowledge of characteristic chromosomal abnormalities, and their pathologic effects, will permit the use of more individualized treatment strategies that provide maximal therapeutic effect with minimal side effects. For example, acute myeloid leukemia (AML) patients exhibiting either an inverted Chr 16 or t(8;21) translocation generally respond well to high doses of the drug cytarabine, while AML patients with other cytogenetic abnormalities do not (Bloomfield et al., 1998). Similarly, Ph+ CML patients respond favorably to imatinib, showing high rates of remission, while Ph– CML patients, who present with similar symptoms, generally respond poorly (Druker et al., 2001). Characterization of such molecular anomalies will not only permit the design of highly specific therapeutics that have fewer widespread side effects but will also allow customization of treatment regimens specifically tailored to individual patients' particular needs.

Understanding the mechanisms of recurrent chromosomal abnormalities could also aid in better understanding particular risk factors associated with specific types of lymphoid and other hematologic malignancies and could help in designing better diagnostic and prognostic tests. Exposure to environmental clastogens likely results in DNA damage that can, in turn, drive the development of hematologic malignancies (Takahashi and Ohnishi, 2005 and references therein). The extent and types of DNA damage have been, in many cases, extensively analyzed at the molecular level, and results from these exhaustive molecular studies have suggested that different toxins may produce unique DNA damage profiles that could potentially be exploited for diagnostic or therapeutic effect, if the precise series of downstream consequences of such chromosomal damage can be ascertained in sufficient detail. In these cases, understanding the contributions of individual toxins to specific recurrent genome instability and mutations could be a key facet in the development of early detection schemes, individualized treatment methods, and most importantly, effective prevention strategies.

Genomic instability and translocations that lead to tumorigenesis can result from a variety of sources. One type of genomic insult, which leads to such instability, is the misrepair of DSBs (Agarwal et al., 2006; Helleday et al., 2007; Sonoda et al., 2006; Valerie and Povirk, 2003; Weinstock et al., 2006b). Both exogenous and endogenous sources can contribute to the introduction of DSBs throughout the genome. To effectively and efficiently repair damage from varied internal and external sources, mammalian cells appear to rely on two major DSB repair pathways: homologous recombination (HR) and nonhomologous end joining (NHEJ). Misregulation of either pathway can result in unrepaired DSBs, and these can produce chromosomal translocations with the potential for subsequent tumorigenesis. Molecular characterization of recurrent translocations and other genomic instability present in these mouse models is the underpinning for further dissection of the mechanisms that lead to genome instability, translocations, and ultimately, tumorigenesis in humans. In this chapter, the roles of HR and NHEJ both in normal cellular function and as contributing factors to hematologic malignancies in both humans and mouse models will be discussed.

4.2 Sources of DNA Double-Strand Breaks

4.2.1 Endogenous Sources of DNA Breakage

While DSBs can arise in B and T lymphocytes as a result of the developmentally programmed Ig and *TCR* gene rearrangement (discussed in detail in Section 3.2.), nonprogrammed DSBs can also occur, in many cell types, either randomly or in genomic regions that are especially prone to breakage, as the result of normal cellular processes. In some cases, single-strand DNA nicks, as consequences of base excision repair, chemical or radiation damage, or other means, can produce DSBs, especially when a replication fork encounters and attempts to replicate past the nick (reviewed in Mills et al., 2003; Sonoda et al., 2006; Valerie and Povirk, 2003).

Unprogrammed DSBs can occur throughout the genome but may be especially likely in regions with particularly unstable sequence or chromatin structures, such as chromosomal fragile sites (Arlt et al., 2006). Fragile sites are generally classified as regions of DNA that exhibit gaps or breaks on metaphase chromosomes after partial inhibition of DNA synthesis. Common fragile sites are found throughout the genome and are stable in normal cells. These regions are generally A and T rich, which is thought to contribute to increased DNA flexibility, leading to lower resistance to mechanical stress. Breakage at fragile sites is associated with chromosomal rearrangements and translocations that contribute to oncogenesis (reviewed in Arlt et al., 2006). The breakage at fragile sites that leads to such rearrangements is hypothesized to result from the stalling of replication forks at the repetitive sequence of these regions.

4.2.2 Exogenous Sources of DNA Breakage

DSBs can also result from exogenous sources of damage (Migliore and Coppede, 2002; Pages and Fuchs, 2002). One of the most common types of exogenous insults is damage that results from ionizing radiation (IR). IR induces a large range of types of DNA lesions, and it is hypothesized that multiple pathways cooperate to repair the damage resulting from exposure to IR, including the DSB repair mechanisms discussed below. In addition, DNA damage can result from exposure to a wide range of environmental toxins. Many toxins found in the environment, such as heavy metals and components of tobacco smoke, have been shown to induce damage that results in DSB formation (reviewed in Migliore and Coppede, 2002; Pages and Fuchs, 2002; Takahashi and Ohnishi, 2005). DSBs resulting from such exogenous damage may also contribute, in as yet poorly defined ways, to lesions that lead to hematopoietic cancers.

4.3 DNA Double-Strand Break Repair Pathways

4.3.1 Homologous Recombination

The first major pathway of DSB repair is HR [for detailed reviews of HR and DSB repair see Dudas and Chovanec (2004), Helleday et al. (2007), Karran (2000), Pastink et al. (2001)]. HR catalyzes the conservative, usually error-free, repair of DSBs using an undamaged template DNA double-strand as a donor for sequence replication and replacement. Homology-mediated DSB repair can occur either in an error-free fashion, when recombination uses an undamaged sister chromatid template, or can result in nucleotide changes following repair, when recombination from a nonidentical template occurs.

Homology-mediated DSB repair is first initiated by 5′- to 3′-resection of double-stranded DNA ends by the action of the Mre11/Rad50/Nbs1 complex [(Bannister and Schimenti, 2004; Farah et al., 2005; Kobayashi et al., 2004; Krishna et al., 2007; Szostak et al., 1983); reviewed in (Dudas and Chovanec, 2004) and (Helleday et al., 2007)]. This produces a 3′-overhanging single DNA strand that becomes inserted into the undamaged homologous template to form a nucleoprotein filament containing heteroduplex DNA. This heteroduplex formation results in the displacement of a single DNA strand, termed a D-loop, at the site of the donor invasion, and a cruciform Holliday junction at the transition between the heteroduplex and the homoduplex DNA (Helleday et al., 2007). The annealed 3′-end in the heteroduplex is then used as a primer for de novo DNA synthesis to replace missing sequences. At this point, HR can be divided into distinct subpathways depending on the details in resolution of the Holliday junction and replication intermediates. Major subtypes of HR include gene conversion (GC) without crossing over, GC with an associated crossover event, and synthesis-dependent strand annealing (SDSA) (Dudas and Chovanec, 2004; Helleday et al., 2007). Another distinct mode of homology-driven break repair that does not involve DNA synthesis or Holliday junction formation, termed single-strand annealing (SSA), leads to deletion of DNA sequences flanking the DSB (Helleday et al., 2007; Karran, 2000; Pastink et al., 2001).

4.3.1.1 Gene Conversion

A favored mode of HR-mediated DSB repair in mammalian cells is conservative, homology-mediated repair from an undamaged sister chromatid template. This process can result in GC either with or without sister chromatid exchange (SCE) (Fig. 4.2). GC from a sister chromatid can occur in the late-S or G2 phase

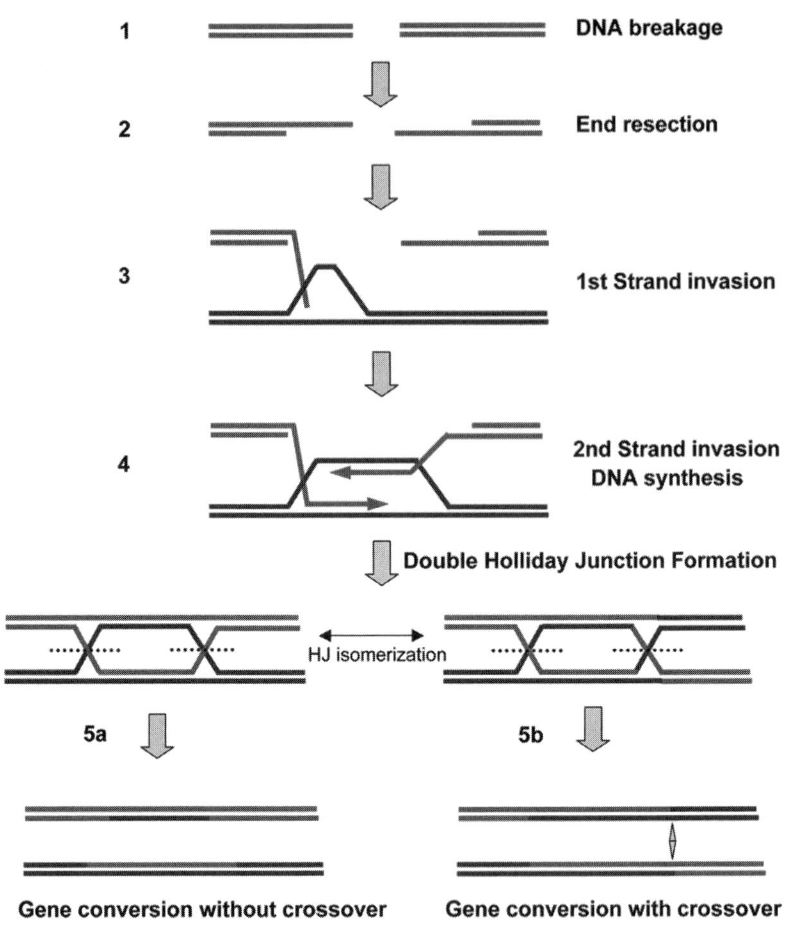

Fig. 4.2 Schematic of gene conversion (GC). Following DNA double-strand breakage (**1**), single-strand end resection in the $3' \rightarrow 5'$-direction produces single-stranded 3′-overhanging ends (**2**). These then serve as donors for strand invasion and heteroduplex formation, resulting in D-loop intermediates (**3**). Second-strand invasion and DNA synthesis leads to bi-directional replication and migration of the resultant Holliday junctions (**4**). Finally, isomerization of the Holliday junction, followed by cleavage and re-ligation of the Holliday junction joint molecules, produces a gene conversion product, either with (**5b**) or without (**5a**) crossing-over

of the cell cycle when a replicate DNA double strand is present and available. This results in restoration of the DNA double strand without the loss or alteration of DNA sequences in the vicinity of the DSB. This mode of HR repair is thought to occur through the formation of a double Holliday junction intermediate (Helleday et al., 2007; Szostak et al., 1983). By this mechanism, both DNA ends resulting from the DSB invade the undamaged homologous template to form two cruciform Holliday junctions connecting the donor and target strands. Each strand invasion then primes new DNA synthesis and, through the activities of an incompletely understood group of proteins which likely includes RecQ family helicases and topoisomerase III (TOPOIII), the Holliday junctions can be translated away from the point of initial branch formation (Bachrati et al., 2006; Cheok et al., 2005; Hickson, 2003; Plank et al., 2006).

In addition to linear translation along the length of the two-participant DNA strands, Holliday junctions may also isomerize to produce either of two structurally equivalent structures. Finally, the double Holliday junction becomes resolved via nucleolytic cleavage, by an as yet unidentified resolvase, to produce the intact, repaired DNA double strands (Sharples, 2001). Depending on the isomerization state of the Holliday junction at the time of resolution, this can generate either a noncrossover product or a recombinant crossover product (reviewed in Helleday et al., 2007). Because the Holliday junction isomers are energetically equivalent and should thus both occur at the same frequency, it is expected that crossover and noncrossover events should be detected at the same rate (reviewed in Helleday et al., 2007). Curiously, however, crossover events of DSB repair appear to occur less frequently than noncrossover events, at least in some experimental contexts (reviewed in Helleday et al., 2007). Thus, it is possible that additional factors influence the asymmetric resolution of double Holliday junction intermediates. Indeed, there is some evidence that the *BLM* gene product, a member of the RecQ helicase family, functions to prevent crossover events (Cheok et al., 2005; Hickson, 2003; Khakhar et al., 2003; Raynard et al., 2006; Wu and Hickson, 2003).

4.3.1.2 Synthesis-Dependent Strand Annealing

Another conservative HR-mediated repair pathway is SDSA (Fig. 4.3). As with GC, SDSA is initiated by DNA resection, strand invasion, and D-loop formation. In this mode of HR repair, a single Holliday junction, rather than a double Holliday junction, is produced (Fig. 4.3; see also Helleday et al., 2007). Branch migration then occurs in the direction of DNA synthesis, probably by the same mechanism as double Holliday junction branch migration leading to GC. Continued sliding of the junction beyond the end of the newly synthesized single strand results in its release from the heteroduplex, re-formation of the target homoduplex DNA, and production of a 3′-single strand that can be annealed to its complementary sequence in the originally broken duplex. SDSA is completed when any overhanging single-stranded flaps are removed by endonucleolytic cleavage, and the staggered DNA nicks are ligated to restore the intact double strand.

4.3.1.3 Single-Strand Annealing

SSA is a distinct, nonconservative subtype of homology-mediated DSB repair that does not lead to recombination but results in the deletion of nucleotides flanking the DSB (Agarwal et al., 2006; Helleday et al., 2007) (Fig. 4.4). SSA

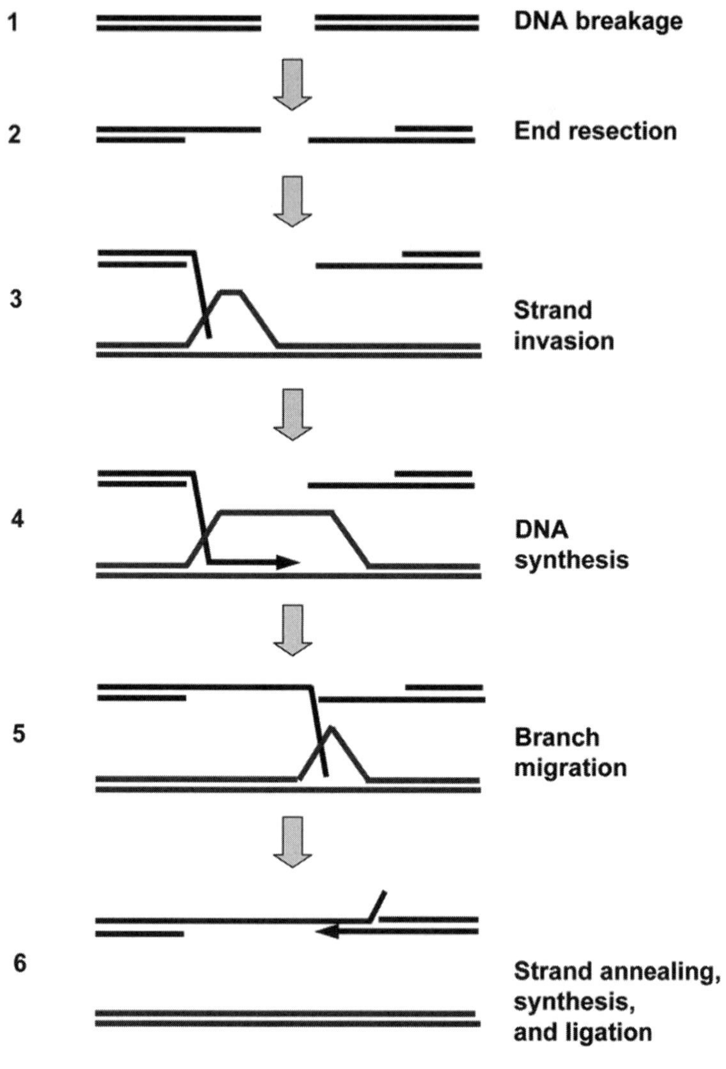

Fig. 4.3 Schematic of synthesis-dependent strand annealing (SDSA). Following DNA breakage (**1**), $3' \rightarrow 5'$-end resection (**2**), and first-strand invasion (**3**), as depicted for gene conversion in Fig. 4.2, unidirectional DNA synthesis (**4**) and branch migration (**5**) generates a newly replicated stretch of DNA terminated by sequence complementary to a portion of DNA adjacent to the original break (**5**). D-loop melting and annealing of complementary DNA ends (**6**) then promotes fill-in synthesis and re-ligation to restore the intact DNA double strand

occurs between short, directly repeated sequences located on either side of the DSB. Helicase-dependent DNA unwinding and exonucleolytic degradation produce complementary single-DNA strands that are subsequently annealed via RAD52 activity (Bachrati and Hickson, 2003; Hickson, 2003; Khakhar et al., 2003; Sharma et al., 2004). The resulting double-stranded DNA product

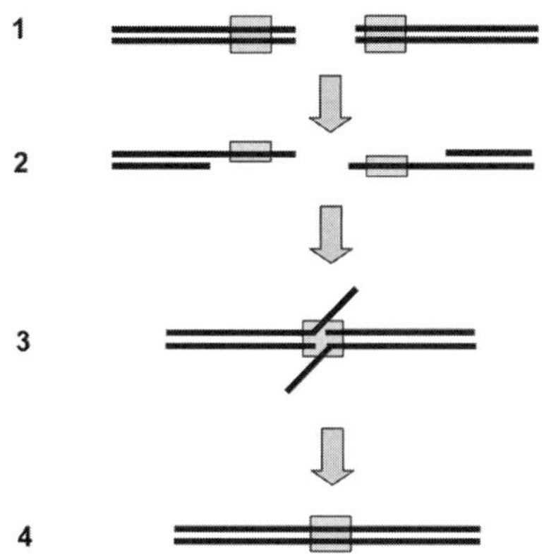

Fig. 4.4 Schematic of single-strand annealing (SSA). Following DNA breakage at a position flanked by short stretches of homologous sequence shown as shaded boxes (**1**), $3' \rightarrow 5'$-end resection exposes single-stranded 3′-overhangs with embedded complementary DNA sequence (**2**). Annealing of complementary sequences produces unpaired "flaps" of noncomplementary single-stranded DNA (**3**). These are trimmed by a flap endonuclease, and ligation of the DNA double-strand break (DSB) or staggered single-strand nicks restores the DNA double strand, accompanied by loss of a single repeat and flanking DNA sequence (**4**)

contains two staggered single-strand nicks and may also include overhanging, noncomplementary single-stranded DNA (ssDNA). The overhanging ends are removed by endonucleolytic cleavage directed against the junction of the double-stranded and ssDNA, and the nick is sealed via ligation (Gottlich et al., 1998). The end product of SSA is repair of the DSB with loss of a variable amount of flanking sequence (Fig. 4.4).

4.3.1.4 Homologous Recombination and Genomic Instability

Chromosomal rearrangements can result when a DNA break fails to rejoin with its cognate end and instead mis-joins with another target chromosome. This is generally prevented because homology-driven repair using an undamaged sister chromatid template is strongly favored in post-replication cells, resulting both in conservative repair of the DSB without sequence alteration and averting recombination with ectopic targets. However, DSBs may occasionally become repaired using templates other than the identical sister chromatid. When HR targets the homologous chromosome rather than the identical chromatid, GC leading to loss of the original sequence and replacement with the sequence from the recombination target may occur. Loss of heterozygosity can result from targeting of the two nonidentical sequences that can, in turn, act as the molecular basis for tumor formation when a tumor suppressor gene is affected.

Alternatively, HR may target homologous sequences resident on nonhomologous chromosomes (Elliott and Jasin, 2002; Weinstock et al., 2006a, b). Most mammalian genomes are replete with highly repetitive DNA sequence elements, such as LINEs, SINEs, or Alu sequences, that may serve as HR substrates between nonhomologous chromosomes (reviewed in Agarwal et al., 2006). Indeed, instability within, and possibly recombination between, Alu sequences located within the major breakpoint cluster region of the *BCR* and *ABL* genes has been implicated in the formation of the *BCR–ABL* fusion tyrosine kinase gene driving Ph+ leukemias and lymphomas (Chissoe et al., 1995; Jeffs et al., 1998; 2001; Papadopoulos et al., 1990; Zhang et al., 1995). Moreover, elegant work by Maria Jasin and colleagues has shown that even limited homologous sequence may be sufficient to promote interchromosomal HR resulting in translocations (Richardson and Jasin, 2000; Richardson et al., 1998; 1999; Tremblay et al., 2000). Given that translocations appear to frequently produce novel fusion genes, this latter mechanism may constitute a major mode of chromosomal instability leading to cancer, especially in blood cancers where reciprocal translocations are common.

4.3.1.5 Homologous Recombination Genes and Proteins

The eukaryotic HR machinery includes a number of DNA damage sensor and early response genes, such as members of the *Rad51* gene family, the *Rad52* epistasis group, *RecQ* family helicases, and the breast cancer susceptibility genes *Brca1* and *Brca2*, as well as numerous other accessory factors.

Damage Sensing

The first step in DSB repair, by either DSB repair pathway, is DNA damage sensing and signal transduction. The earliest steps of DNA break response initiate a signal through the MRE11–RAD50–NBS1 (MRN) complex and the ataxia telangiectasia-mutated (ATM) protein. The MRN complex likely plays several crucial roles in DNA break repair, including structural bridging of DNA ends to permit rejoining of cognate ends by NHEJ machinery, upstream activation of ATM, and execution of ATM-dependent downstream effector functions (Dudas and Chovanec, 2004). Both *Rad50* and *Nbs1* are essential genes in mammals, and thus genetic manipulation of these genes has proven difficult although specific mutant alleles of each gene have provided information as to their molecular function (Dudas and Chovanec, 2004). Introduction of hypomorphic alleles of *Rad50* or *Nbs* results in decreased ATM kinase activity, implicating the MRN complex in full ATM activation in response to damage. However, the precise mechanism for this activity upstream of ATM remains unclear.

ATM represents another key factor involved in early DNA damage response and the coordination of downstream pathways. ATM, together with the *Atm- and Rad3-related* gene product ATR, and the DNA-dependent protein kinase catalytic subunit, DNA–PKcs, defines a family of PI3-kinase-related kinases that are critical for responding to and repairing genotoxic stress of many types. ATM is thought to exist as a homodimer that can undergo autophosphorylation and subsequent dissociation following damage recognition (McGowan and Russell, 2004). The dissociated, active monomers then target additional downstream effectors, likely including MRN components, p53, and histone H2A variant X (H2AX). In mammalian cells, ATM is activated in this fashion early in the response to as few as two DNA DSBs. One key piece of evidence implicating ATM as a regulator of HR is the observation that mice doubly deficient for *Atm* and for the HR gene *Rad52* exhibit a mild protection from cancer (Treuner et al., 2004). This intriguing finding suggests that, in the absence of *Atm*, a compensatory HR-mediated DSB repair pathway may carry the risk of oncogenic translocations. Moreover, it has been recently shown that NHEJ and HR cooperate to maintain post-replicative genome stability (Couedel et al., 2004; Mills et al., 2004). Such cooperative DSB repair may be under the control or coordination of ATM. Interestingly, one recent study also found that the ATM protein plays a direct role in stabilizing the DNA DSBs that are an obligate predecessor of V(D)J recombination (Bredemeyer et al., 2006). It was suggested that the combined cell cycle checkpoint, pro-apoptotic, and DSB repair functions of ATM collaborate to ensure efficient and correct V(D)J recombination and to eliminate those cells that fail in this process.

ATR, together with its binding partner ATRIP, appears to be key checkpoint factor responsive to stalled or collapsed replication forks, as well as other damage incurred during the replicative or post-replicative phases of the cell cycle (Cortez et al., 2001; Costanzo et al., 2003; McGowan and Russell, 2004; Shechter et al., 2004; Zou et al., 2002). While the precise mode of ATR activation is not fully elucidated, it is likely stimulated upon binding, through ATRIP, to replication protein A (RPA) complexed to ssDNA. Such RPA–ssDNA complexes are both replication-associated and HR-associated, in the latter case forming at an early stage of the recombination reaction. Although ATR is an essential factor, thus precluding the analysis of knockout mice, cells containing hypomorphic alleles or siRNA-mediated knockdown of ATR exhibit significant defects in cellular proliferation and are uniquely susceptible to replication stress or stalling. Cells with impaired ATR function are highly prone to spontaneous breakage of common chromosomal fragile sites and show a hyper-response to the replication inhibitor aphidicolin, a DNA polymerase inhibitor (Casper et al., 2002).

Rad51 Family

In vertebrates, RAD51 is an essential HR factor constituting the core factor in most, if not all, HR reactions. In mammals, the *Rad51* gene family comprises at least six members: *Rad51*, *Rad51L1*, *Rad51L2*, *Rad51L3*, *Xrcc2*, and *Xrcc3*. *Rad51* encodes a single-strand DNA-binding factor that forms a nucleoprotein filament with HR donor sequences necessary for heteroduplex formation. In the initial phase of an HR reaction, RPA binds 3′-resected DNA ends (see above) to form a precursor nucleoprotein filament. In the second phase of the reaction, RPA is displaced by RAD51, and the newly formed RAD51–DNA filament then promotes DNA strand transfer and heteroduplex formation with the complementary target sequence, producing a D-loop. RAD51 is thus essential for initiation and probably for completion of HR. In mice, null alleles of *Rad51* result in very early embryonic lethality (Lim and Hasty, 1996; Tsuzuki et al., 1996). In the chicken DT40 cell line, deficiency for *Rad51* results in profound defects in HR, accompanied by decreased proliferation, spontaneous chromosomal instability, and dramatic sensitivity to a range of DNA-damaging agents, including DSB-inducing agents (Sonoda et al., 1998).

The precise roles of the other *Rad51* family members in HR are less certain. All family members show single-strand DNA binding and DNA-stimulated ATPase activities (Braybrooke et al., 2000; Lio et al., 2003; Masson et al., 2001a, b; Sigurdsson et al., 2001), but these activities are, in some cases, dispensable for HR function. Data from numerous in vitro experiments have suggested that various complexes, comprising subsets of the *Rad51* family members, can stimulate RAD51-dependent strand pairing/transfer, and at least RAD51L2 may also facilitate dissociation of double-stranded DNA (Kurumizaka et al., 2001; 2002; Lio et al., 2003; Liu et al., 1998; 2002; 2007; Masson et al., 2001a; Sigurdsson et al., 2001). Finally, some evidence has implicated the RAD51-like proteins in Holliday junction resolution although this role remains controversial [for example, see Liu et al. (2004)].

The Rad52 Epistasis Group

Rad52, the archetypal member of the *Rad52* epistasis group, is a centrally important HR factor in yeast, but does not appear to play a critical function in HR reactions in higher eukaryotes (Dudas and Chovanec, 2004). The basis for this difference is not yet understood, but one possibility, for which there is some evidence, is the existence of additional, as yet unidentified, *Rad52* homologs that are more closely functionally related to the yeast *Rad52*. Other members of the *Rad52* epistasis group include *Rad54*, *Rad55*, and *Rad59* (reviewed in Heyer et al., 2006). RAD52 functions to promote annealing of complementary stretches of ssDNA and apparently acts as an accessory factor mediating RAD51-dependent heteroduplex formation by promoting the loading of RAD51 onto DNA at the target recombination site (Benson et al., 1998; New et al., 1998; Shinohara and Ogawa, 1998; Sung, 1997). It has also been suggested, largely based on analysis of yeast mutants, that RAD52 antagonizes the HR-repressive effects of RPA at sites of damage and stabilizes RAD51 nucleoprotein complexes, thereby shifting the DNA-binding equilibrium toward RAD51 and away from RPA.

A second member of the *Rad52* epistasis group, *Rad54*, encodes a *Snf2* family chromatin remodeling factor central to the *Rad52* epistasis group of proteins, with DNA-dependent ATPase activity (Heyer et al., 2006). Upon binding to DNA, RAD54 translocates along the double strand, via ATP hydrolysis. During the presynapsis phase of an HR reaction, RAD54 appears to promote the replacement of RPA with RAD51 in the presynaptic nucleoprotein filament.

Next, during synapsis, RAD54 interacts with RAD51 to stimulate joint molecule formation critical for D-loop formation and strand exchange. Finally, RAD54 appears to participate in branch migration and may also function to disassemble the RAD51 nucleoprotein filament although this latter role is somewhat controversial (Heyer et al., 2006). Despite RAD54 being a central player in RAD51-dependent HR, *Rad54* knockout mice are viable and are not, on their own, especially cancer prone. Cells derived from *Rad54* null mice proliferate nearly as well as their normal counterparts but exhibit substantial sensitivity to DNA-damaging agents such as IR or mitomycin-C (MMC)-induced interstrand cross linking. In the latter case, *Rad54*-deficient cells show normal rates of spontaneous SCE but are severely compromised in MMC-induced SCE. For a comprehensive review of *Rad54* function, see Heyer et al. (2006).

RecQ Helicase Family

The *RecQ* helicase family constitutes a highly conserved set of DNA-directed helicases that may be found in prokaryotes and eukaryotes. The human genome contains at least five genes encoding *RecQ* family members: *BLM*, *RECQ1*, *RECQ4*, *RECQ5*, and *WRN*. Mutations in *BLM, RECQ4,* and *WRN* have been associated with Bloom's, Rothmund–Thompson, and Werner's syndromes, respectively. Each of these disorders exhibits a dramatic cancer predisposition and some aspects of premature aging. This latter feature has generated tremendous interest in the RecQ helicase family as a potential link between cancer and aging.

BLM

The BLM helicase, which interacts with TOPOIII, is capable of unwinding short stretches of naked duplex DNA but is highly stimulated by association with RPA. A number of potential roles in HR have been ascribed to the BLM helicase, but the details of its in vivo molecular functions still remain unclear. It is thought that BLM suppresses hyper-SCE perhaps by disruption of D-loop recombination intermediates. Indeed, BLM appears to favor specific structures, including D-loops and Holliday junctions, and has been shown to promote Holliday junction branch migration. As noted above, crossing over appears to be generally suppressed during homology-mediated recombination, and BLM may participate in this suppression. In this context, another possible function for BLM is to modulate the outcome of Holliday junction resolution. This is likely accomplished by BLM-dependent processing of double Holliday junctions to catenated structures that can be fully resolved via TOPOIIIα. BLM-mediated crossover suppression may also involve SDSA. Recent data have suggested that in addition to disrupting recombination by D-loop binding, BLM can also channel these HR intermediates into the SDSA pathway by dissolution of the heteroduplex to permit re-annealing of the newly synthesized strand with its original complementary strand, at least in *Drosophila* (Weinert and Rio, 2007).

WRN

Unlike other members of the RecQ helicase family, WRN contains both the classical helicase activity and a 3′- to 5′-exonuclease activity that target multiple DNA or RNA–DNA hybrid structures (see Dudas and Chovanec, 2004; Helleday et al., 2007; Hickson, 2003). Like BLM, the helicase activity of WRN appears to also be highly structure specific. The observation that cells from Werner's syndrome patients show defects in recombination intermediate resolution suggests that WRN functions in HR, probably by influencing DSB repair pathway choice. In this context, WRN can bind to NBS1, a member of the MRN complex, and to the Ku70/Ku80 heterodimer, a core NHEJ complex.

In addition to its role in HR, WRN is thought to function in a nonessential fashion in DNA replication. Such a role is suggested by WRN association with a series of replication factors, including PCNA and RPA. Moreover, WRN appears to stimulate the replication-associated flap endonuclease activity of FEN1 and may thus promote the processing of normal Okazaki fragments. Finally, some evidence indicates that WRN also plays a specialized role in telomere replication by disruption of G-quadruplex stretches (Dudas and Chovanec, 2004; Helleday et al., 2007; Hickson, 2003).

4.3.1.6 Homologous Recombination and Cancer

Ataxia Telangiectasia

AT is a rare autosomal recessive disorder caused by defects in *Atm* (described above) that produces progressive cerebellar degeneration with a characteristic ataxic gait, stereotypical oculocutaneous telangiectasia, and several growth and developmental abnormalities (reviewed in Matei et al., 2006; Taylor and Byrd, 2005). Another signature feature of AT is a marked, but variable, immunodeficiency, leading to frequent upper respiratory infections. AT is also associated with a severe sensitivity to IR and a very high risk of cancers, especially of lymphoid origin (reviewed in Matei et al., 2006; Taylor and Byrd, 2005).

The immunological defects associated with AT result from a range of both cellular and humoral immune defects that produce a variable, sometimes severe, lymphopenia (Waldmann et al., 1983). AT produces marked thymic hypoplasia and a shift in the representation of specific T-cell subsets (reviewed in Matei et al., 2006). It has been suggested that the low peripheral T-cell numbers are the combined result of low thymic output, perhaps as a result of the hypoplastic state, and a gross T-cell survival defect in the periphery (Matei et al., 2006). AT patients also exhibit humoral immunity defects, presenting as reductions in specific Ig isotypes. Initial models attributed the humoral defect principally to a failure of T-cell help, but more recent studies have also implicated *Atm* in IgH CSR (Lumsden et al., 2004; Reina-San-Martin et al., 2004).

In addition to the T cell, and to a lesser extent, associated B-cell developmental defects, AT patients also show a dramatic predisposition to T-cell malignancies, suggesting, perhaps, a common molecular origin for both features. Relative to nonaffected individuals, AT patients exhibit a roughly 200-fold higher risk of lymphoid cancers, especially early in life. Consistent with the immunological defects, T-cell tumors in AT patients are approximately four-fold more frequent than B-cell tumors. During childhood, the major AT-associated tumor type is T-cell acute lymphoblastic leukemia or lymphoma (T-ALL), with a shift toward pro-lymphocytic leukemia as patients enter adulthood (Taylor et al., 1996). These disease features, together with the observation that leukemias arising in adult AT patients tend to have a more mature T-cell phenotype, suggest that ATM acts as a lymphoid tumor suppressor at many thymic and post-thymic stages of T-cell development (reviewed in Matei et al., 2006).

ATM and Sporadic Cancers

Fanconi Anemia

Fanconi anemia (FA) is a rare cancer predisposition syndrome that features a progressive anemia, chromosomal instability, and developmental abnormalities (reviewed in Tischkowitz and Dokal, 2004). FA has been associated with genes defining at least 12 FA complementation groups: A, B, C, D1, D2, E, F, G, I, J, L, and M (FANCA–FANCM) (Dokal, 2000). These genes have been identified largely through functional cloning in FA cell lines but also by candidate gene screening and positional cloning approaches. Cells from FA patients, like other HR-deficient cells, show dramatic hypersensitivity to DNA interstrand cross-linking (ICL) agents like MMC, but the precise role of FA gene products in mediating ICL repair is, as yet, unclear (Tischkowitz and Dokal, 2004). *FANCD1* is allelic with the breast cancer susceptibility gene *BRCA2*, and the FANCD2 protein interacts with DNA damage sensor/checkpoint factors ATM and ATR, suggesting that the FA pathway may intersect multiple modes of DNA DSB repair, including HR.

Clinically, FA results in early aplastic anemia with a propensity for total bone marrow failure, skeletal abnormalities, skin pigmentation defects, and a host of less frequent developmental deficiencies. FA patients also show a dramatic predisposition to cancers, mainly of hematopoietic origin. One study found that 23% of FA patients develop some type of blood-related malignancy, with nearly 70% of these malignancies being either myelodysplastic syndrome (MDS) or AML (Mathew, 2006). Less frequently, FA patients may develop solid tumors of the liver, head and neck, vulva, or cervix. Some studies have also investigated somatic inactivation or mutation of FA genes in sporadic AML cases, finding monoallelic mutations in approximately 5–10% of sporadic cases.

Variant Alleles of Rad51-Family Genes

Given the apparently central roles that RAD51 and RAD51-like proteins play in the maintenance of genome integrity via HR-mediated DSB repair, it is reasonable to expect that the *Rad51*-family genes should also act as tumor suppressors. While there has thus far been a paucity of evidence for a tumor-suppressive role in model systems, there is some indication that naturally occurring variants of *Rad51*-like genes can modulate cancer susceptibility (Auranen et al., 2005; Figueiredo et al., 2004; Han, et al., 2004; Kuschel et al., 2002; Rafii et al., 2002; Rodriguez-Lopez et al., 2004; Thacker, 2005; Wang et al., 2001). However, in most cases, a relatively small sample size has precluded a definitive evaluation of the cancer risk conferred by the variant allele. A number of studies have identified a variant allele of *Xrcc2*, in which Arg188 is converted to His (*Xrcc2*^{R188H}), as potentially increasing the susceptibility to breast cancer (Kuschel et al., 2002; Rafii et al., 2002). Similarly, a variant of *Rad51L3* (*Rad51L3*^{E233G}) may be weakly associated with increased breast cancer risk (Rodriguez-Lopez et al., 2004). Although the *Xrcc3*^{T241M} variant was initially reported to correlate with increased melanoma risk, this association remains controversial (Araujo et al., 2002; Rafii et al., 2002). Thus far, none of the variant alleles of *Rad51*-like genes have been reported to increase the risk or susceptibility to hematologic malignancies.

Xrcc2 Deletions

In addition to potentially deleterious alleles of *Xrcc2* that may predispose to some cancers, somatic rearrangements such as deletion or translocation may alter or inactivate *Xrcc2* specifically in cancer cells. The human *Xrcc2* gene is located on chromosome 7q36, a genomic location frequently affected by structural lesions in a broad range of cancers. A survey of Recurrent Aberrations in the Mitelman Database of Chromosome Aberrations in Cancer (Cancer Genome Anatomy Project; http://cgap.nci.nih.gov/Chromosomes/Mitelman) reveals 84 case reports of copy number gains at 7q36, with 51 of these occurring in hematopoietic malignancies, and 80 case reports of deletions affecting 7q36, with 76 of these occurring in hematopoietic malignancies. While these lesions are likely to encompass numerous genes and the specifically relevant gene(s) have not been definitively identified, it is possible that either gains or losses of *Xrcc2* could contribute to oncogenic genome instability by altering the stoichiometry of HR complexes.

4.3.2 Nonhomologous End Joining

The second DSB repair pathway, NHEJ, is a pathway that repairs DSBs irrespective of DNA end sequence. Unlike homology-mediated repair pathways, NHEJ does not rely on DNA homology to repair DSBs; therefore, DSBs repaired by the NHEJ pathway may contain errors. It is generally believed that NHEJ is the repair pathway utilized most during G1 in mammalian cells, likely due to the lack of homologous sister chromatids during this phase of the cell cycle (reviewed in Mills et al., 2003; Valerie and Povirk, 2003). In addition, NHEJ is the major repair pathway of DSBs introduced through a variety of endogenous sources and also contributes to the repair of a vast number of DSBs that occur as a result of exogenous insults. DSBs that escape repair by NHEJ, whether they are introduced as part of a developmental program or through exposure to endogenous or exogenous insults, can often lead to translocations and subsequent oncogenesis. We discuss these mechanisms in the context of hematopoietic cancers below.

4.3.2.1 V(D)J Recombination

V(D)J recombination is the process by which antigen receptors in maturing B and T lymphocytes are assembled (reviewed in Bassing et al., 2002; Jung and Alt, 2004) (see Fig. 4.5 for overview). Somatic DNA rearrangements of variable (V), diversity (D), and joining (J) gene segments within the Ig or TCR loci generate mature, functional antibody receptors. An initial step in antibody receptor gene rearrangement is the obligatory introduction of DSBs at specific locations within these genes to allow in frame recombination of these different antibody receptor segments. Targeted recombination of V(D)J component parts occurs in a precisely ordered fashion through recognition of specific recombination signal (RS) sequences that flank the constituent gene segments by the recombination-activating gene (RAG) endonuclease.

The RS elements are comprised of conserved palindromic heptamer (CACAGTG) and nonamer (ACAAAAACC) consensus sequences. These are separated by nonconserved spacers of either 12 or 23 base pairs, referred to as 12RS or 23RS sequences (Max et al., 1979; Sakano et al., 1979). Importantly, recombination strongly favors usage of a 12RS sequence and a 23RS sequence, with 12/12 or 23/23 recombination events generally prevented (this phenomenon is referred to as 12/23 restriction). In developing B cells, *IgH* genes are assembled via a highly organized process where D to J rearrangements occur first (DJ), followed by V to DJ joining (VDJ). The IgH locus is arranged such that the J and V segments are flanked by 23RS sequences, while the D segments are flanked by 12RS sequences (Early et al., 1980). This arrangement permits ordered D to J followed by V to DJ recombination, since this recombination pattern follows the 12/23 restriction.

Functional IgH rearrangement then prompts a signal for progenitor B cells to proceed in the B-lymphoid differentiation pathway. Processes that lead to differentiation include allelic exclusion, proliferative expansion, and differentiation to the pre-B-cell stage. In pre-B cells, the Ig light chain loci, Igκ? and Igλ, also undergo functional gene rearrangements through 12RS/23RS recombination. Functional light chain rearrangements generated through proper recombination events permit further B-cell differentiation. Similar to B-lineage development, the proper joining of TCR locus gene segments through 12RS/23RS recombination permits progression of pre-T cells to mature T lymphocytes.

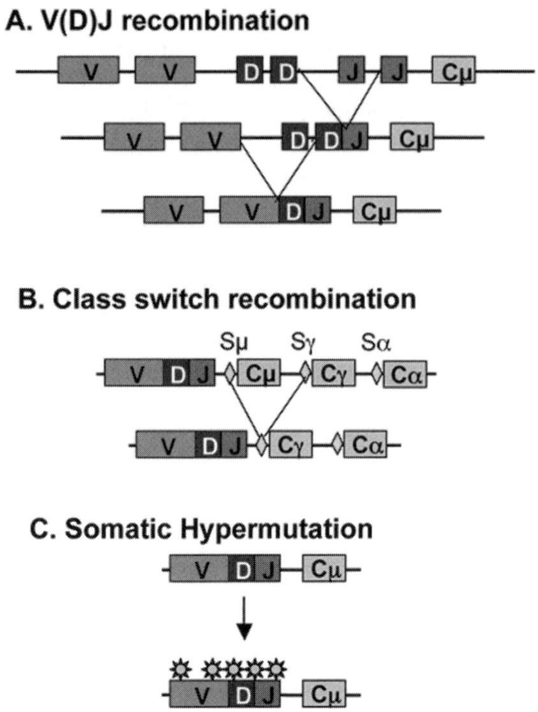

Fig. 4.5 Schematic of types of somatic alterations that occur during lymphocyte development. (**A**) During V(D)J recombination, rearrangements between V (*green rectangles*), D (*blue rectangles*), and J (*pink rectangles*) gene segments create mature, functional antibody receptors in B and T cells. These rearrangements occur in a precise order, with D to J joins occurring first followed by V to DJ joins. (**B**) Class switch recombination changes the isotype of the immunoglobulin constant region through constant region (*light blue rectangle*) rearrangements. Small sequence elements known as switch regions (*yellow diamonds*) permit recombination between different constant gene segments. (**C**) In somatic hypermutation, single or multiple mutations are introduced throughout the recombined V(D)J segment (*blue sunbursts*) to change antibody affinity of a functional receptor. Adapted from Kuppers and Dalla-Favera (2001). (See color insert)

4.3.2.2 RAG Endonuclease

The RAG endonuclease consists of an obligate heterodimeric protein complex encoded by two extremely tightly linked genes, *Rag1* and *Rag2* (Oettinger et al., 1990; Schatz et al., 1989). The genes encoding RAG1/2 are expressed in early progenitor lymphocytes, and expression levels oscillate throughout lymphocyte differentiation and maturation, as RAG1/2 activity is necessary for V(D)J recombination at different stages of B- and T-lineage cell development. It was further shown that another round of RAG expression may occur in mature germinal center B lymphocytes following antigen stimulation (Hikida et al., 1996). It is thought that expression of RAG1/2 in mature lymphocytes contributes to altered antibody specificity through a process termed receptor editing. RAG2 activity is restricted to cells in G0/G1 phases of the cell cycle through phosphorylation-mediated degradation (Lee and Desiderio, 1999). Mice deficient in either RAG1 or RAG2 show a complete block in lymphocyte development at the progenitor stage with no other apparent physical or morphological defects, illustrating the specificity of RAG1/2 in lymphocyte development (Mombaerts et al., 1992; Shinkai et al., 1992).

RAG1/2 recognizes and binds to recombining 12RS and 23RS sequences and introduces a nick adjacent to the RS sequences to initiate coordinated cleavage. The 3′-hydroxyl group, exposed by the nick, catalyzes a transesterification reaction on an adjacent DNA strand through nucleophilic attack, generating two blunt, 5′-phosphorylated RS ends, which can be ligated, and two covalently sealed hairpin coding ends, which must be opened before joining can occur (McBlane et al., 1995). Interestingly, these two types of ends have distinct features. The RS ends become precisely fused due to the exact sequence homology in the ligated ends, while the ends of the coding segments result in imprecise joining once ligation occurs. Asymmetric nicking by RAG in the coding joins can result in the addition of palindromic nucleotide extensions called P-nucleotides (McCormack et al., 1989). The RAG complex remains stably bound to the four free DNA ends in a post-cleavage synaptic complex (Fugmann et al., 2000). It has subsequently been shown that a catalytic DDE amino acid triad in RAG1 is necessary for the formation of hairpins through direct transesterification (Landree et al., 1999; Swanson, 2001). Mice containing an engineered mutation that deletes the C-terminal portion of RAG2, leaving only the highly conserved core region, exhibit a partial arrest in lymphocyte development with decreased overall numbers of B and T cells (Akamatsu et al., 2003). The specificity of sequence sites recognized by the RAG1/2 endonuclease complex, combined with the spatial and temporal expression pattern, contributes to the infrequency of aberrant cleavage by RAG and, therefore, the precise regulation of V(D)J recombination.

4.3.2.3 Class Switch Recombination and Somatic Hypermutation

Once mature B cells have been stimulated by antigen, two additional somatic alterations to Ig loci may occur to modify antigen-binding affinity and antibody effector function (summarized in Fig. 4.5). Differentiating B lymphocytes first express one IgH constant region (Cμ). However, upon antigen stimulation, CSR can occur as the mature B-cell exchanges the Cμ constant region exon for one of seven alternate downstream exons. This switching, in turn, allows the production of antibodies of a different class and effector function.

Each of the C genes in the IgH locus is preceded by specific DNA sequence elements termed switch regions, consisting of highly repetitive, G-rich, non-template DNA. There is no known consensus target for switch regions. CSR occurs through a deletional recombination mechanism that occurs between two switch regions. CSR differs from V(D)J recombination in that the RAG endonuclease is not required for recombination of switch regions. SHM, on the other hand, introduces mutations in the V region of both heavy and light chain loci, and these mutations act to increase antigen-binding affinity to enable selection of B cells that produce higher affinity antibodies.

Although the exact mechanism of transcription of switch regions during CSR is not well characterized, it is hypothesized that the switch regions, which exhibit G-rich sequences on the nontemplate strand, are susceptible to unique chromatin conformations that permit transcription of these regions (reviewed in Chaudhuri and Alt, 2004). Interestingly, the switch region transcripts remain stably associated with the template DNA strand, forming a DNA–RNA hybrid, while the displaced nontemplate DNA strand exists as a ssDNA loop. This entire structure is called an R-loop (Reaban and Griffin, 1990; Reaban et al., 1994; Tian and Alt, 2000).

CSR and SHM both require the expression and activity of activation-induced cytidine deaminase (AID) (reviewed in Chaudhuri and Alt, 2004; Longerich et al., 2006). AID is expressed in activated mature B-lymphocytes and specifically targets *Ig* genes. AID deaminates cytosine residues within the Ig loci, converting them to uracils. These uracils are either replicated to introduce corresponding single-nucleotide mutations (in SHM) or are removed (in CSR). Removal of uracil mismatches creates nicks in the DNA strand which, when in close proximity to other nicks in switch regions, leads to DSBs and subsequent recombination between switch regions. On the other hand, in SHM, single mutations can lead to changes in antibody affinity or specificity. At least in SHM, AID requires the cooperative activity of RPA for proper targeting to Ig regions undergoing SHM (Chaudhuri et al., 2004). Mice deficient in AID and humans with hypomorphic AID mutations show no apparent phenotypes except the inability for B cells to undergo CSR and SHM. Mice engineered to overexpress AID were predicted to show increased rates of tumorigenesis because of increased cytosine deamination and subsequent DSB induction; however, thymic lymphomas and epithelial tumors isolated from these mice did not show identifiable chromosomal translocations. Instead, oncogenic transformation in these tumors was found to be due to somatic mutation.

4.3.2.4 Mechanics of Nonhomologous End Joining

The molecular components required for DSB repair by the NHEJ pathway were first identified through analysis of yeast and mammalian cell lines deficient in DNA repair. Analysis of IR-sensitive Chinese hamster ovary (CHO) cell lines led to the identification of several complementation groups (Taccioli et al., 1998; 1994). Furthermore, examination of V(D)J recombination in these cells determined that RAG-induced DSBs introduced during V(D)J recombination were likely repaired by components of the NHEJ pathway.

Conserved core NHEJ components are found in both yeast and vertebrates, while noncore components are found only in vertebrates. Known core NHEJ factors include Ku70 and Ku80, DNA Ligase IV (LIG4), and XRCC4 while noncore components include Artemis (ART), DNA–PKcs, and a recently identified factor, Cernunnos. It is important to note that these factors are required for both V(D)J recombination in B- and T-lymphocyte development as well as for repair of DSBs that occur throughout the genome as a result of endogenous damage or clastogenic insult.

4.3.2.5 Nonhomologous End Joining Genes and Proteins

The core components conserved in all eukaryotes are required for both RS join formation subsequent to DSB initiation by RAG as well as for repair of randomly occurring DSBs throughout the genome, while the nonconserved proteins may play additional roles independent of NHEJ (reviewed in Mills et al., 2003; see Fig. 4.6). Further experimentation with IR-sensitive CHO lines led to the characterization of the roles of each NHEJ protein in DSB repair. In vertebrates, Ku70 and Ku80 are predicted, based on the crystal structure, to form a ring-shaped complex that can encompass and shield the broken DNA end until other NHEJ components are recruited to facilitate repair. Binding of the Ku complex to DNA–PKcs permits activation of DNA–PKcs through autophosphorylation, and this heterotrimeric complex is then called the DNA–PK holoenzyme. The activated DNA–PK complex is the first NHEJ component to respond to a DSB, but the precise role this protein complex plays in joining broken DNA ends has not been completely characterized. Possible roles for DNA–PK include protecting broken ends from aberrant enzymatic or endonuclease activity, keeping broken ends close together until ligation and acting as a scaffold to allow other NHEJ factors to bind to and complete DSB repair. However, Ku-deficient ES cells show different joining impairment and IR sensitivity as compared with DNA–PKcs-deficient ES cells, illustrating a DNA–PKcs-independent function for Ku proteins (Gao et al., 1998a).

DNA–PKcs is thought to be important in other cellular applications beyond NHEJ although these functions are not well understood. One of the important roles of DNA–PKcs in NHEJ repair is to recruit and bind to the ART protein. ART was first identified through analysis of two types of human severe combined immunodeficiency (SCID) disorders, SCIDA and RS SCID. ART is homologous to β-lactamases, proteins that repair interstrand DNA crosslinks and is thought to be necessary for end processing of DSBs, including the opening of hairpins that form during the process of NHEJ repair. Both DNA–PK and ART are primarily required for coding, and not RS, joining during V(D)J recombination (Callebaut et al., 2002).

XRCC4 and DNA LIG4 form a heterodimeric complex that is required for ligation of repaired ends. Deficiencies in either protein result in identical phenotypes, including the inability to form coding and RS joins during V(D)J recombination, illustrating the indispensable NHEJ-specific functions of these proteins.

Recently, a seventh component of the NHEJ pathway, Cernunnos (also known as XLF for XRCC4-like factor), was identified independently by two groups (Ahnesorg et al., 2006; Buck et al., 2006). Knockdown of the gene encoding the

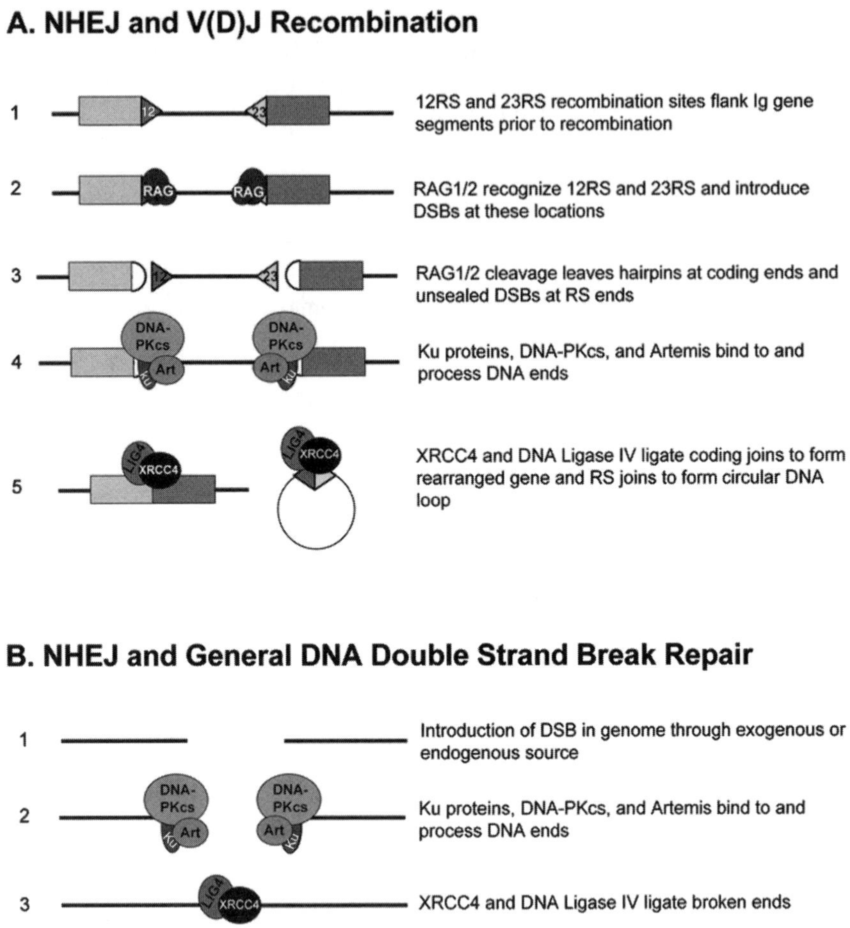

A. NHEJ and V(D)J Recombination
1
12
23
12RS and 23RS recombination sites flank Ig gene segments prior to recombination
2
RAG
RAG
RAG1/2 recognize 12RS and 23RS and introduce DSBs at these locations
3
12
23
RAG1/2 cleavage leaves hairpins at coding ends and unsealed DSBs at RS ends
4
DNA-PKcs
Art
Ku
DNA-PKcs
Art
Ku
Ku proteins, DNA-PKcs, and Artemis bind to and process DNA ends
5
LIG4
XRCC4
LIG4
XRCC4
XRCC4 and DNA Ligase IV ligate coding joins to form rearranged gene and RS joins to form circular DNA loop
B. NHEJ and General DNA Double Strand Break Repair
1
Introduction of DSB in genome through exogenous or endogenous source
2
DNA-PKcs
Art
Ku
DNA-PKcs
Art
Ku
Ku proteins, DNA-PKcs, and Artemis bind to and process DNA ends
3
LIG4
XRCC4
XRCC4 and DNA Ligase IV ligate broken ends

Fig. 4.6 Roles of nonhomologous end joining (NHEJ) in repair of programmed and unprogrammed exogenously induced DNA double-strand breaks (DSBs). **(A)** NHEJ is required for gene rearrangements that occur during V(D)J recombination. The RAG1/2 endonuclease complex recognizes recombination signal (RS) sequences that flank *Ig* gene segments to be recombined (steps 1 and 2). RAG cleavage induces covalently sealed hairpin formation at the DNA ends of the coding segments and leaves the DNA fragments containing RS sequence ends unsealed (step 3). DNA–PKcs, the Ku70/Ku80 complex (Ku), and Artemis (Art) recognize the DSB and process the coding hairpin ends to prepare for ligation (step 4). In the last step, both coding joins and RS sequence end joins are ligated separately, leaving a rearranged coding gene segment and a circular loop containing the RS sequences and intervening DNA (step 5). **(B)** NHEJ is also required to repair DSBs throughout the genome that occurs as a result of unprogrammed endogenous or exogenous insults (step 1). The NHEJ factors and mechanism of DSB repair for unprogrammed DSBs are identical to those utilized in programmed DSB repair (steps 2 and 3)

Cernunnos protein, *NHEJ1*, in human cell lines leads to radiosensitivity and impaired NHEJ-mediated DSB repair similarly to that observed in other NHEJ-deficient cell lines (Ahnesorg et al., 2006). In addition, murine ES cells engineered to lack Cernunnos activity do not undergo V(D)J recombination and show defects in forming both coding joins and RS joins (Zha et al., 2007). Furthermore, Cernunnos-deficient ES cells show increased IR sensitivity and have intrinsic defects in DSB repair, providing further evidence that Cernunnos/XLF is an important component of NHEJ-mediated DSB repair (Zha et al., 2007). Immunoprecipitation experiments have since established that Cernunnos interacts directly with the XRCC4/LIG4 complex (Callebaut et al., 2006).

Nonhomologous End Joining Deficient Mouse Models

Mice deficient for each of the NHEJ components, with the exception of Cernunnos, have been identified or engineered. These mouse models have proved valuable tools in understanding the role of NHEJ in different cell types and how similar NHEJ deficiencies can result in human disease. Mice deficient in DNA–PKcs, Ku70, Ku80, or ART show severe immune deficiencies due to the lack of NHEJ during V(D)J recombination that results in the absence of mature B- and T-cell lymphocytes and show increased sensitivity to IR (Bosma and Carroll, 1991; Gao et al., 1998a; Gu et al., 1997; Kurimasa et al., 1999; Nussenzweig et al., 1996; Ouyang et al., 1997; Rooney et al., 2002; Taccioli et al., 1998). In addition, it was found that classical SCID mice have a mutation within DNA–PKcs (Bosma and Carroll, 1991). A deficiency in either Ku70 or Ku80 results in small mice with additional defects, including cell proliferation defects, premature senescence, and increased neuronal apoptosis, although mice deficient in either Ku protein are viable (Gu et al., 1997; Nussenzweig et al., 1996; Ouyang et al., 1997). Embryos null for *Lig4* or *Xrcc4*, which exhibit late embryonic lethality, show more severe phenotypes, including impaired lymphocyte development (as determined in cells or by in vitro analysis of fetal liver cultures isolated from null embryos) and severe neuronal apoptosis (Barnes et al., 1998; Frank et al., 1998; Gao et al., 1998b). Mouse embryonic fibroblasts (MEFs) isolated from *Xrcc4–/–* or *Lig4–/–* embryos show marked genomic instability, including increased sensitivity to irradiation and chromosomal translocations.

Cells containing unrepaired DSBs normally undergo apoptosis mediated by the checkpoint protein p53, encoded by the *Trp53* gene in mice and *TP53* gene in humans. Interestingly, *Trp53* deficiency rescues viability in *Lig4*- and *Xrcc4*-deficient mice and prevents the neuronal apoptosis observed in the single mutant mice, suggesting that the neurodevelopmental failure and the embryonic lethality may be linked. However, NHEJ repair in developing lymphocytes in these doubly deficient mice is still compromised, producing a SCID phenotype and eventually leading to the development of progenitor (pro) B-cell lymphomas through translocations involving the IgH locus and the oncogene *c-myc*. Similarly, mice doubly null for the gene encoding ART, *Dclre1c*, and

Trp53 also develop pro-B-cell lymphomas (Rooney et al., 2004). Interestingly, mice doubly null for both *Ku80* and *Lig4* are viable (Karanjawala et al., 2002). This unexpected result suggests that loss of Ku80 function may initiate other DSB repair pathways, since the embryonic lethality observed in the NHEJ-specific factor *Lig4* single-deficient mice is rescued when combined with *Ku80* deficiency.

As described, deficiencies in NHEJ proteins often result in B-lineage lymphomagenesis, since the DSBs introduced during V(D)J recombination cannot be properly repaired and often act as substrates for translocations that contribute to oncogenesis. Based on this outcome, NHEJ factors have been proposed to function as tumor suppressors in developing lymphocytes. However, recent work has established that one NHEJ component, ART, plays an important tumor suppressor role in additional somatic tissues beyond developing lymphocytes, at least in a *Trp53* compromised context (Woo et al., 2007). This result provides convincing evidence to support a role for NHEJ in widespread tumor suppression, independent of its role in V(D)J recombination.

4.3.2.6 Nonhomologous End Joining and Telomere Maintenance

Eukaryotic cells, which contain linear chromosomes, have developed a process to readily distinguish the ends of normal chromosomes from DSBs within the genome that require repair. Telomeres are structural components comprised of short repeated DNA elements and scaffolding proteins, such as shelterin and TRF2, which terminate the ends of linear chromosomes and protect against structural abnormalities such as chromosome fusion and attrition (reviewed in Murnane and Sabatier, 2004). Telomeres are established and maintained through the activity of telomerase, a specialized reverse transcriptase required for replication of the highly repetitive telomere sequences that cap eukaryotic chromosomes. In normal cells, expression and activity of telomerase diminishes over time. However, transfection of normal human cells with telomerase results in cessation of telomere shortening and immortalization, providing evidence that telomere shortening and attrition directly correlate with cell aging and senescence (Bodnar et al., 1998). Although normal hematopoietic stem cells exhibit typical telomere shortening, they are one of the few somatic cell types to exhibit prolonged telomerase activity, and the significance of this finding is not well understood.

Surprisingly, mice engineered to lack telomerase activity are viable. However, each subsequent generation of telomerase-deficient mice shows progressively severe defects in chromosome maintenance, apparent as increased genome instability in cells, which could confer tumorigenesis when transplanted into nude mice (Blasco et al., 1997). When a telomerase deficiency is combined with *Trp53* deficiency, normally unstable DNA intermediates and structures such as chromosome end-to-end fusions and breakage–fusion–bridge (BFB) cycles are maintained through subsequent cell cycles. Although at early stages a p53 deficiency rescues the adverse effects observed in telomere-deficient mice,

mice doubly deficient for these genes subsequently show increased rates of genome instability that result in tumorigenesis (Chin et al., 1999).

Chromosome ends that lack proper telomeres can become a substrate for NHEJ repair. Although the exact roles NHEJ factors may play in telomere maintenance remain to be fully determined, recent work has established that at least two NHEJ components play important roles in protecting telomere structure and function. During NHEJ repair, the ring-shaped Ku70/Ku80 complex binds to free DNA ends (Walker et al., 2001). Apparently contradictory evidence suggests that this complex also binds to telomere components and can either promote normal telomere maintenance and prevent end-to-end fusions (Hsu et al., 1999; 2000; Samper et al., 2000) or can facilitate fusion of dysfunctional telomeres (Celli et al., 2006). In a further paradox, binding of the Ku70/Ku80 complex to telomeres appears to protect chromosome ends with dysfunctional telomeres from being repaired by other DNA repair mechanisms such as homology-mediated recombination (Celli et al., 2006). LIG4, another NHEJ-specific factor, prevents end-to-end chromosome fusions in mice with dysfunctional telomeres. Together, these results implicate NHEJ factors in normal telomere maintenance although the precise mechanism by which this occurs remains elusive.

4.3.2.7 Nonhomologous End Joining and Cancer

Several human disorders are associated with hypomorphic or null alleles of different *NHEJ* genes. Many such alleles result in human SCID phenotypes as a consequence of improper V(D)J function. Mutant alleles of the human *DCLRE1C* gene, encoding the ART protein, cause SCID-A and RS-SCID, and there is some evidence to suggest that hypomorphic *DCLRE1C* alleles are correlated with increased predisposition to lymphoma (Ege et al., 2005; Moshous et al., 2001; 2003a, b; Nicolas et al., 1998). Another condition commonly associated with mutant alleles of both *DCLRE1C* and *RAG1/2* is Omenn syndrome. Hypomorphic missense mutations in the *RAG* genes have been identified in several families and were found to severely restrict, but not entirely eliminate, RAG function, permitting some lymphocyte development and subsequent activity in Omenn syndrome patients (Villa et al., 1998). However, the severity of SCID-like symptoms varies between patients, and it is unclear whether these differences can be attributed directly to RAG function or whether some of this variability is a result of other polymorphic modifier genes. A subset of Omenn syndrome patients do not have mutations within the *RAG* genes, indicating that mutations in other genes, including *DCLRE1C*, may cause Omenn-like symptoms (Gennery et al., 2005).

Mutations in core NHEJ components resulting in human disorders are far less common. LIG4 syndrome, an extremely rare autosomal recessive disorder caused by mutations within the *LIG4* gene, is characterized by immunodeficiency and associated microcephaly, growth retardation, and developmental delay (O'Driscoll et al., 2001). However, only a few cases of LIG4 syndrome have been reported. Of note, not all of the patients who exhibit these symptoms have mutations within any known NHEJ factor, hinting at the possibility of as yet unidentified factors required for this pathway. Finally, the gene encoding for Cernunnos was originally identified in patients who exhibited phenotypes reminiscent of the ones observed in other NHEJ- or DSB repair-deficient disorders, including microcephaly, mild to severe SCID phenotypes, and radiosensitivity (Buck et al., 2006).

In addition to SCID phenotypes, many other lymphocyte disorders in humans have been attributed to genomic lesions similar to those observed in NHEJ-deficient mouse models (reviewed in Franco et al., 2006). In both *Dclre1c/Trp53*-and *Lig4/Trp53*-deficient mice, progenitor B-cell lymphomas develop with characteristic fusions between *Igh* and *Myc* loci as a result of the inability to properly undergo V(D)J recombination (Rooney et al., 2002; 2004; Zhu et al., 2002). Similarly, many human lymphoid tumors carry translocations involving the fusion of Ig or TCR loci to proto-oncogenes. In addition, lesions that lead to hematopoietic malignancies have been identified in the chromosomal locations associated with each gene encoding a member of the NHEJ pathway, suggesting that mutations or translocations in these genes may cause hematologic malignancies. Analysis of mice deficient in various NHEJ components could provide insight into similar malignancies in humans.

Susceptibility of Tumorigenesis During V(D)J Recombination and CSR

DSBs are intermediate products of both V(D)J and CSR reactions, which can serve as substrates for chromosomal rearrangements and translocations if left unrepaired (reviewed in Aplan, 2006; Weinstock et al., 2006b). Hematopoietic malignant transformations resulting from these processes are likely due to the high frequency of specific gene alterations and rearrangements that occur throughout development and maturation of these cell types. Translocations that occur in human hematopoietic malignancies are usually simple reciprocal translocations, often involving either the *Ig* or the *TCR* loci, which bring the translocated proto-oncogene in close proximity to strong enhancers within these loci. This process makes oncogenic transformation a rapid step that does not result in high levels of general genome instability in these tumors.

Burkitt's lymphoma is characterized by a recurrent t(8;14) translocation. As in the mouse models of NHEJ deficiency, the translocation breakpoint brings regions of the *IgH* locus on Chr 14 in close proximity with Chr 8, containing the *Myc* locus. The initial breaks within *IgH* likely result from mistakes during V(D)J recombination. Sequencing of translocation junctions of human patients diagnosed with endemic Burkitt's lymphoma revealed that many of these tumors contain breakpoints within V or J regions of *IgH*, indicating the translocation occurred in the initial steps of V(D)J recombination.

Translocation data retrieved from the Mitelman breakpoint database identified 90 human patients diagnosed with mature B-cell neoplasms and 40 diagnosed with ALLs that showed a characteristic translocation containing

IgH and the potent oncogene *BCL2*. Analysis of tumors from patients diagnosed with follicular lymphoma, a type of tumor arising in mature B cells, also showed translocation breakpoints between *IgH* and *BCL2* (reviewed in Kuppers and Dalla-Favera, 2001; Mills et al., 2003). Molecular examination of the breakpoint sequences of these tumors revealed that many of these joins are often within an RS sequence near a D region. Furthermore, these joins show germline sequence at the 5′-end of the D region involved in the breakpoint, suggesting that these breaks were introduced during de novo V(D)J formation and not mediated through DSBs introduced at already rearranged V(D)J joins. There is some evidence to suggest that the oncogene partner chosen in translocations involving *IgH* may be dependent on the developmental stage of B-cell development. Mantle-zone lymphomas, which typically show t(11;14) (*BCL1*/*IgH*) translocations, show J joins similar to those in normal B cells, while follicular lymphomas with t(14;18) translocations and *BCL2* amplifications show preferential usage of the most downstream J and D genes, indicating that the cells may have been undergoing a secondary D to J rearrangement (Jager et al., 2000; Welzel et al., 2001).

Another type of Burkitt's lymphoma, sporadic Burkitt's lymphoma, is associated with a similar t(8;14) translocation. However, in this case, the translocation breakpoint maps to a different region of the *IgH* locus, often occurring within the switch regions. This finding indicates that these tumors generally develop from RAG-induced DSBs that are introduced during CSR. Many different lymphoid tumor types, including B-cell chronic lymphocytic leukemia, diffuse large cell lymphoma, extranodal lymphoma, and multiple myeloma, have translocation breakpoints within the switch regions on Chr 14 (reviewed in Kuppers and Dalla-Favera, 2001). Together, these results indicate that misrepair of DSBs introduced at any stage of lymphoid development can lead to the development of lymphoid tumors.

4.4 Perspective

The genome is at nearly constant risk of damage from a barrage of internal and external insults. Such damage is a substantial threat to genetic integrity, carrying the risk of gene loss, mutation, or chromosomal rearrangements including translocations. Each of these events can lead to cell death or neoplastic transformation. To preserve genomic integrity and resist the potentially deleterious downstream effects of DNA damage, eukaryotic cells employ a wide range of efficient and highly coordinated DNA damage response and repair mechanisms. To effect the repair of DSBs, mammalian cells rely on two predominant, complementary pathways: HR and NHEJ. The combined, and sometimes overlapping, action of these two pathways generally ensures the rapid resolution of DSBs and the restoration of the intact genome. The apparent importance of these pathways in repairing broken DNA suggested that such repair should thus be critical to prevent the kinds of chromosomal abnormalities so frequently noted in a broad range of cancers. Indeed, there is rapidly burgeoning evidence, garnered to a large extent from highly valuable mouse models, pointing to a tumor-suppressive role for various DSB repair factors. In this context, development of new and better models of DNA damage response and repair defects, and particularly those that faithfully recapitulate human cancer phenotypes, will significantly impact our mechanistic understanding of neoplasia. To date, many of the mouse models of DSB response/repair have relied on gene-targeted inactivation of the gene of interest. While this approach has been highly informative and provided key insights into the function of specific genes, another important avenue for modeling cancer, including blood cancers, will be the identification or generation of mice that reflect tumor-specific alleles, naturally occurring allelic variants, specific polymorphisms, and complex multi-gene interactions. With the rapidly expanding molecular, genetic, and informatic tools that can be brought to bear on cancer models of all types, these challenges become increasingly tractable to solve. With this perspective in mind, important new discoveries concerning the roles of DSB repair in preventing or promoting blood cancers hold the promise of significant clinical impacts, now and in the future.

Acknowledgments We thank Dr. Sophie La Salle for critical review of this manuscript.

References

Agarwal S, Tafel AA, Kanaar R (2006). DNA double-strand break repair and chromosome translocations. *DNA Repair (Amst)* 5: 1075–81.

Ahnesorg P, Smith P, Jackson SP (2006). XLF interacts with the XRCC4-DNA ligase IV complex to promote DNA nonhomologous end-joining. *Cell* 124: 301–13.

Akamatsu Y, Monroe R, Dudley DD, Elkin SK, Gartner F, Talukder SR et al. (2003). Deletion of the RAG2 C terminus leads to impaired lymphoid development in mice. *Proc Natl Acad Sci U S A* 100: 1209–14.

Aplan PD (2006). Causes of oncogenic chromosomal translocation. *Trends Genet* 22: 46–55.

Araujo FD, Pierce AJ, Stark JM, Jasin M (2002). Variant XRCC3 implicated in cancer is functional in homology-directed repair of double-strand breaks. *Oncogene* 21: 4176–80.

Arlt MF, Durkin SG, Ragland RL, Glover TW (2006). Common fragile sites as targets for chromosome rearrangements. *DNA Repair (Amst)* 5: 1126–35.

Auranen A, Song H, Waterfall C, Dicioccio RA, Kuschel B, Kjaer SK et al. (2005). Polymorphisms in DNA repair genes and epithelial ovarian cancer risk. *Int J Cancer* 117: 611–8.

Bachrati CZ, Borts RH, Hickson ID (2006). Mobile D-loops are a preferred substrate for the Bloom's syndrome helicase. *Nucleic Acids Res* 34: 2269–79.

Bachrati CZ, Hickson ID (2003). RecQ helicases: suppressors of tumorigenesis and premature aging. *Biochem J* 374: 577–606.

Bannister LA, Schimenti JC (2004). Homologous recombinational repair proteins in mouse meiosis. *Cytogenet Genome Res* 107: 191–200.

Barnes DE, Stamp G, Rosewell I, Denzel A, Lindahl T (1998). Targeted disruption of the gene encoding DNA ligase IV leads to lethality in embryonic mice. *Curr Biol* 8: 1395–8.

Bassing CH, Swat W, Alt FW (2002). The mechanism and regulation of chromosomal V(D)J recombination. *Cell* 109 Suppl: S45–55.

Benson FE, Baumann P, West SC (1998). Synergistic actions of Rad51 and Rad52 in recombination and DNA repair. *Nature* 391: 401–4.

Blasco MA, Lee HW, Hande MP, Samper E, Lansdorp PM, DePinho RA et al. (1997). Telomere shortening and tumor formation by mouse cells lacking telomerase RNA. *Cell* 91: 25–34.

Bloomfield CD, Lawrence D, Byrd JC, Carroll A, Pettenati MJ, Tantravahi R et al. (1998). Frequency of prolonged remission duration after high-dose cytarabine intensification in acute myeloid leukemia varies by cytogenetic subtype. *Cancer Res* 58: 4173–9.

Bodnar AG, Ouellette M, Frolkis M, Holt SE, Chiu CP, Morin GB et al. (1998). Extension of life-span by introduction of telomerase into normal human cells. *Science* 279: 349–52.

Bosma MJ, Carroll AM (1991). The SCID mouse mutant: definition, characterization, and potential uses. *Annu Rev Immunol* 9: 323–50.

Braybrooke JP, Spink KG, Thacker J, Hickson ID (2000). The RAD51 family member, RAD51L3, is a DNA-stimulated ATPase that forms a complex with XRCC2. *J Biol Chem* 275: 29100–6.

Bredemeyer AL, Sharma GG, Huang CY, Helmink BA, Walker LM, Khor KC et al. (2006). ATM stabilizes DNA double-strand-break complexes during V(D)J recombination. *Nature* 442: 466–70.

Buck D, Malivert L, de Chasseval R, Barraud A, Fondaneche MC, Sanal O et al. (2006). Cernunnos, a novel nonhomologous end-joining factor, is mutated in human immunodeficiency with microcephaly. *Cell* 124: 287–99.

Callebaut I, Malivert L, Fischer A, Mornon JP, Revy P, de Villartay JP (2006). Cernunnos interacts with the XRCC4 x DNA-ligase IV complex and is homologous to the yeast nonhomologous end-joining factor Nej1. *J Biol Chem* 281: 13857–60.

Callebaut I, Moshous D, Mornon JP, de Villartay JP (2002). Metallo-beta-lactamase fold within nucleic acids processing enzymes: the beta-CASP family. *Nucleic Acids Res* 30: 3592–601.

Casper AM, Nghiem P, Arlt MF, Glover TW (2002). ATR regulates fragile site stability. *Cell* 111: 779–89.

Celli GB, Denchi EL, de Lange T (2006). Ku70 stimulates fusion of dysfunctional telomeres yet protects chromosome ends from homologous recombination. *Nat Cell Biol* 8: 885–90.

Chaudhuri J, Alt FW (2004). Class-switch recombination: interplay of transcription, DNA deamination and DNA repair. *Nat Rev Immunol* 4: 541–52.

Chaudhuri J, Khuong C, Alt FW (2004). Replication protein A interacts with AID to promote deamination of somatic hypermutation targets. *Nature* 430: 992–8.

Cheok CF, Bachrati CZ, Chan KL, Ralf C, Wu L, Hickson ID (2005). Roles of the Bloom's syndrome helicase in the maintenance of genome stability. *Biochem Soc Trans* 33: 1456–9.

Chin L, Artandi SE, Shen Q, Tam A, Lee SL, Gottlieb GJ et al. (1999). p53 deficiency rescues the adverse effects of telomere loss and cooperates with telomere dysfunction to accelerate carcinogenesis. *Cell* 97: 527–38.

Chissoe SL, Bodenteich A, Wang YF, Wang YP, Burian D, Clifton SW et al. (1995). Sequence and analysis of the human ABL gene, the BCR gene, and regions involved in the Philadelphia chromosomal translocation. *Genomics* 27: 67–82.

Cortez D, Guntuku S, Qin J, Elledge SJ (2001). ATR and ATRIP: partners in checkpoint signaling. *Science* 294: 1713–6.

Costanzo V, Shechter D, Lupardus PJ, Cimprich KA, Gottesman M, Gautier J (2003). An ATR- and Cdc7-dependent DNA damage checkpoint that inhibits initiation of DNA replication. *Mol Cell* 11: 203–13.

Couedel C, Mills KD, Barchi M, Shen L, Olshen A, Johnson RD et al. (2004). Collaboration of homologous recombination and nonhomologous end-joining factors for the survival and integrity of mice and cells. *Genes Dev* 18: 1293–304.

de Klein A, van Kessel AG, Grosveld G, Bartram CR, Hagemeijer A, Bootsma D et al. (1982). A cellular oncogene is translocated to the Philadelphia chromosome in chronic myelocytic leukaemia. *Nature* 300: 765–7.
Dokal I (2000). The genetics of Fanconi's anaemia. *Baillieres Best Pract Res Clin Haematol* 13: 407–25.
Druker BJ, Talpaz M, Resta DJ, Peng B, Buchdunger E, Ford JM et al. (2001). Efficacy and safety of a specific inhibitor of the BCR-ABL tyrosine kinase in chronic myeloid leukemia. *N Engl J Med* 344: 1031–7.
Dudas A, Chovanec M (2004). DNA double-strand break repair by homologous recombination. *Mutat Res* 566: 131–67.
Early P, Huang H, Davis M, Calame K, Hood L (1980). An immunoglobulin heavy chain variable region gene is generated from three segments of DNA: VH, D and JH. *Cell* 19: 981–92.
Ege M, Ma Y, Manfras B, Kalwak K, Lu H, Lieber MR et al. (2005). Omenn syndrome due to ARTEMIS mutations. *Blood* 105: 4179–86.
Elliott B, Jasin M (2002). Double-strand breaks and translocations in cancer. *Cell Mol Life Sci* 59: 373–85.
Farah JA, Cromie G, Steiner WW, Smith GR (2005). A novel recombination pathway initiated by the Mre11/Rad50/Nbs1 complex eliminates palindromes during meiosis in Schizosaccharomyces pombe. *Genetics* 169: 1261–74.
Ferguson DO, Alt FW (2001). DNA double strand break repair and chromosomal translocation: lessons from animal models. *Oncogene* 20: 5572–9.
Figueiredo JC, Knight JA, Briollais L, Andrulis IL, Ozcelik H (2004). Polymorphisms XRCC1-R399Q and XRCC3-T241M and the risk of breast cancer at the Ontario site of the Breast Cancer Family Registry. *Cancer Epidemiol Biomarkers Prev* 13: 583–91.
Franco S, Alt FW, Manis JP (2006). Pathways that suppress programmed DNA breaks from progressing to chromosomal breaks and translocations. *DNA Repair (Amst)* 5: 1030–41.
Frank KM, Sekiguchi JM, Seidl KJ, Swat W, Rathbun GA, Cheng HL et al. (1998). Late embryonic lethality and impaired V(D)J recombination in mice lacking DNA ligase IV. *Nature* 396: 173–7.
Frost BM, Forestier E, Gustafsson G, Nygren P, Hellebostad M, Jonsson OG et al. (2004). Translocation t(12;21) is related to in vitro cellular drug sensitivity to doxorubicin and etoposide in childhood acute lymphoblastic leukemia. *Blood* 104: 2452–7.
Fugmann SD, Lee AI, Shockett PE, Villey IJ, Schatz DG (2000). The RAG proteins and V(D)J recombination: complexes, ends, and transposition. *Annu Rev Immunol* 18: 495–527.
Gao Y, Chaudhuri J, Zhu C, Davidson L, Weaver DT, Alt FW (1998a). A targeted DNA-PKcs-null mutation reveals DNA-PK-independent functions for KU in V(D)J recombination. *Immunity* 9: 367–76.
Gao Y, Sun Y, Frank KM, Dikkes P, Fujiwara Y, Seidl KJ et al. (1998b). A critical role for DNA end-joining proteins in both lymphogenesis and neurogenesis. *Cell* 95: 891–902.
Gennery AR, Hodges E, Williams AP, Harris S, Villa A, Angus B et al. (2005). Omenn's syndrome occurring in patients without mutations in recombination activating genes. *Clin Immunol* 116: 246–56.
Gottlich B, Reichenberger S, Feldmann E, Pfeiffer P (1998). Rejoining of DNA double-strand breaks in vitro by single-strand annealing. *Eur J Biochem* 258: 387–95.
Gu Y, Seidl KJ, Rathbun GA, Zhu C, Manis JP, van der Stoep N et al. (1997). Growth retardation and leaky SCID phenotype of Ku70-deficient mice. *Immunity* 7: 653–65.
Han J, Colditz GA, Samson LD, Hunter DJ (2004). Polymorphisms in DNA double-strand break repair genes and skin cancer risk. *Cancer Res* 64: 3009–13.
Hashimoto K, Nakagawa Y, Morikawa H, Niki M, Egashira Y, Hirata I et al. (2001). Co-overexpression of DEAD box protein rck/p54 and c-myc protein in human colorectal adenomas and the relevance of their expression in cultured cell lines. *Carcinogenesis* 22: 1965–70.

Helleday T, Lo J, van Gent DC, Engelward BP (2007). DNA double-strand break repair: From mechanistic understanding to cancer treatment. *DNA Repair (Amst)* 6: 923–35.

Heyer WD, Li X, Rolfsmeier M, Zhang XP (2006). Rad54: the Swiss Army knife of homologous recombination? *Nucleic Acids Res* 34: 4115–25.

Hickson ID (2003). RecQ helicases: caretakers of the genome. *Nat Rev Cancer* 3: 169–78.

Hikida M, Mori M, Takai T, Tomochika K, Hamatani K, Ohmori H (1996). Reexpression of RAG-1 and RAG-2 genes in activated mature mouse B cells. *Science* 274: 2092–4.

Hsu HL, Gilley D, Blackburn EH, Chen DJ (1999). Ku is associated with the telomere in mammals. *Proc Natl Acad Sci U S A* 96: 12454–8.

Hsu HL, Gilley D, Galande SA, Hande MP, Allen B, Kim SH et al. (2000). Ku acts in a unique way at the mammalian telomere to prevent end joining. *Genes Dev* 14: 2807–12.

Jager U, Bocskor S, Le T, Mitterbauer G, Bolz I, Chott A et al. (2000). Follicular lymphomas' BCL-2/IgH junctions contain templated nucleotide insertions: novel insights into the mechanism of t(14;18) translocation. *Blood* 95: 3520–9.

Jeffs AR, Benjes SM, Smith TL, Sowerby SJ, Morris CM (1998). The BCR gene recombines preferentially with Alu elements in complex BCR-ABL translocations of chronic myeloid leukaemia. *Hum Mol Genet* 7: 767–76.

Jeffs AR, Wells E, Morris CM (2001). Nonrandom distribution of interspersed repeat elements in the BCR and ABL1 genes and its relation to breakpoint cluster regions. *Genes Chromosomes Cancer* 32: 144–54.

Jung D, Alt FW (2004). Unraveling V(D)J recombination; insights into gene regulation. *Cell* 116: 299–311.

Karanjawala ZE, Adachi N, Irvine RA, Oh EK, Shibata D, Schwarz K et al. (2002). The embryonic lethality in DNA ligase IV-deficient mice is rescued by deletion of Ku: implications for unifying the heterogeneous phenotypes of NHEJ mutants. *DNA Repair (Amst)* 1: 1017–26.

Karran P (2000). DNA double strand break repair in mammalian cells. *Curr Opin Genet Dev* 10: 144–50.

Khakhar RR, Cobb JA, Bjergbaek L, Hickson ID, Gasser SM (2003). RecQ helicases: multiple roles in genome maintenance. *Trends Cell Biol* 13: 493–501.

Kobayashi J, Antoccia A, Tauchi H, Matsuura S, Komatsu K (2004). NBS1 and its functional role in the DNA damage response. *DNA Repair (Amst)* 3: 855–61.

Krishna S, Wagener BM, Liu HP, Lo YC, Sterk R, Petrini JH et al. (2007). Mre11 and Ku regulation of double-strand break repair by gene conversion and break-induced replication. *DNA Repair (Amst)* 6: 797–808.

Kuppers R, Dalla-Favera R (2001). Mechanisms of chromosomal translocations in B cell lymphomas. *Oncogene* 20: 5580–94.

Kurimasa A, Kumano S, Boubnov NV, Story MD, Tung CS, Peterson SR et al. (1999). Requirement for the kinase activity of human DNA-dependent protein kinase catalytic subunit in DNA strand break rejoining. *Mol Cell Biol* 19: 3877–84.

Kurumizaka H, Ikawa S, Nakada M, Eda K, Kagawa W, Takata M et al. (2001). Homologous-pairing activity of the human DNA-repair proteins Xrcc3.Rad51C. *Proc Natl Acad Sci U S A* 98: 5538–43.

Kurumizaka H, Ikawa S, Nakada M, Enomoto R, Kagawa W, Kinebuchi T et al. (2002). Homologous pairing and ring and filament structure formation activities of the human Xrcc2*Rad51D complex. *J Biol Chem* 277: 14315–20.

Kuschel B, Auranen A, McBride S, Novik KL, Antoniou A, Lipscombe JM et al. (2002). Variants in DNA double-strand break repair genes and breast cancer susceptibility. *Hum Mol Genet* 11: 1399–407.

Landree MA, Wibbenmeyer JA, Roth DB (1999). Mutational analysis of RAG1 and RAG2 identifies three catalytic amino acids in RAG1 critical for both cleavage steps of V(D)J recombination. *Genes Dev* 13: 3059–69.

Lee J, Desiderio S (1999). Cyclin A/CDK2 regulates V(D)J recombination by coordinating RAG-2 accumulation and DNA repair. *Immunity* 11: 771–81.
Lim DS, Hasty P (1996). A mutation in mouse rad51 results in an early embryonic lethal that is suppressed by a mutation in p53. *Mol Cell Biol* 16: 7133–43.
Lio YC, Mazin AV, Kowalczykowski SC, Chen DJ (2003). Complex formation by the human Rad51B and Rad51C DNA repair proteins and their activities in vitro. *J Biol Chem* 278: 2469–78.
Liu N, Lamerdin JE, Tebbs RS, Schild D, Tucker JD, Shen MR et al. (1998). XRCC2 and XRCC3, new human Rad51-family members, promote chromosome stability and protect against DNA cross-links and other damages. *Mol Cell* 1: 783–93.
Liu N, Schild D, Thelen MP, Thompson LH (2002). Involvement of Rad51C in two distinct protein complexes of Rad51 paralogs in human cells. *Nucleic Acids Res* 30: 1009–15.
Liu Y, Masson JY, Shah R, O'Regan P, West SC (2004). RAD51C is required for Holliday junction processing in mammalian cells. *Science* 303: 243–6.
Liu Y, Tarsounas M, O'Regan P, West SC (2007). Role of RAD51C and XRCC3 in genetic recombination and DNA repair. *J Biol Chem* 282: 1973–9.
Longerich S, Basu U, Alt F, Storb U (2006). AID in somatic hypermutation and class switch recombination. *Curr Opin Immunol* 18: 164–74.
Lumsden JM, McCarty T, Petiniot LK, Shen R, Barlow C, Wynn TA et al. (2004). Immunoglobulin class switch recombination is impaired in Atm-deficient mice. *J Exp Med* 200: 1111–21.
Masson JY, Stasiak AZ, Stasiak A, Benson FE, West SC (2001a). Complex formation by the human RAD51C and XRCC3 recombination repair proteins. *Proc Natl Acad Sci U S A* 98: 8440–6.
Masson JY, Tarsounas MC, Stasiak AZ, Stasiak A, Shah R, McIlwraith MJ et al. (2001b). Identification and purification of two distinct complexes containing the five RAD51 paralogs. *Genes Dev* 15: 3296–307.
Matei IR, Guidos CJ, Danska JS (2006). ATM-dependent DNA damage surveillance in T-cell development and leukemogenesis: the DSB connection. *Immunol Rev* 209: 142–58.
Mathew CG (2006). Fanconi anaemia genes and susceptibility to cancer. *Oncogene* 25: 5875–84.
Max EE, Seidman JG, Leder P (1979). Sequences of five potential recombination sites encoded close to an immunoglobulin kappa constant region gene. *Proc Natl Acad Sci U S A* 76: 3450–4.
McBlane JF, van Gent DC, Ramsden DA, Romeo C, Cuomo CA, Gellert M et al. (1995). Cleavage at a V(D)J recombination signal requires only RAG1 and RAG2 proteins and occurs in two steps. *Cell* 83: 387–95.
McCormack WT, Tjoelker LW, Carlson LM, Petryniak B, Barth CF, Humphries EH et al. (1989). Chicken IgL gene rearrangement involves deletion of a circular episome and addition of single nonrandom nucleotides to both coding segments. *Cell* 56: 785–91.
McGowan CH, Russell P (2004). The DNA damage response: sensing and signaling. *Curr Opin Cell Biol* 16: 629–33.
Migliore L, Coppede F (2002). Genetic and environmental factors in cancer and neurodegenerative diseases. *Mutat Res* 512: 135–53.
Mills KD, Ferguson DO, Alt FW (2003). The role of DNA breaks in genomic instability and tumorigenesis. *Immunol Rev* 194: 77–95.
Mills KD, Ferguson DO, Essers J, Eckersdorff M, Kanaar R, Alt FW (2004). Rad54 and DNA Ligase IV cooperate to maintain mammalian chromatid stability. *Genes Dev* 18: 1283–92.
Mombaerts P, Iacomini J, Johnson RS, Herrup K, Tonegawa S, Papaioannou VE (1992). RAG-1-deficient mice have no mature B and T lymphocytes. *Cell* 68: 869–77.
Moshous D, Callebaut I, de Chasseval R, Corneo B, Cavazzana-Calvo M, Le Deist F et al. (2001). Artemis, a novel DNA double-strand break repair/V(D)J recombination protein, is mutated in human severe combined immune deficiency. *Cell* 105: 177–86.

Moshous D, Callebaut I, de Chasseval R, Poinsignon C, Villey I, Fischer A et al. (2003a). The V(D)J recombination/DNA repair factor artemis belongs to the metallo-beta-lactamase family and constitutes a critical developmental checkpoint of the lymphoid system. *Ann N Y Acad Sci* 987: 150–7.

Moshous D, Pannetier C, Chasseval Rd R, Deist Fl F, Cavazzana-Calvo M, Romana S et al. (2003b). Partial T and B lymphocyte immunodeficiency and predisposition to lymphoma in patients with hypomorphic mutations in Artemis. *J Clin Invest* 111: 381–7.

Murnane JP, Sabatier L (2004). Chromosome rearrangements resulting from telomere dysfunction and their role in cancer. *Bioessays* 26: 1164–74.

Nagel S, Kaufmann M, Drexler HG, MacLeod RA (2003). The cardiac homeobox gene NKX2-5 is deregulated by juxtaposition with BCL11B in pediatric T-ALL cell lines via a novel t(5;14)(q35.1;q32.2). *Cancer Res* 63: 5329–34.

New JH, Sugiyama T, Zaitseva E, Kowalczykowski SC (1998). Rad52 protein stimulates DNA strand exchange by Rad51 and replication protein A. *Nature* 391: 407–10.

Nicolas N, Moshous D, Cavazzana-Calvo M, Papadopoulo D, de Chasseval R, Le Deist F et al. (1998). A human severe combined immunodeficiency (SCID) condition with increased sensitivity to ionizing radiations and impaired V(D)J rearrangements defines a new DNA recombination/repair deficiency. *J Exp Med* 188: 627–34.

Nussenzweig A, Chen C, da Costa Soares V, Sanchez M, Sokol K, Nussenzweig MC et al. (1996). Requirement for Ku80 in growth and immunoglobulin V(D)J recombination. *Nature* 382: 551–5.

O'Driscoll M, Cerosaletti KM, Girard PM, Dai Y, Stumm M, Kysela B et al. (2001). DNA ligase IV mutations identified in patients exhibiting developmental delay and immunodeficiency. *Mol Cell* 8: 1175–85.

Oettinger MA, Schatz DG, Gorka C, Baltimore D (1990). RAG-1 and RAG-2, adjacent genes that synergistically activate V(D)J recombination. *Science* 248: 1517–23.

Ouyang H, Nussenzweig A, Kurimasa A, Soares VC, Li X, Cordon-Cardo C et al. (1997). Ku70 is required for DNA repair but not for T cell antigen receptor gene recombination in vivo. *J Exp Med* 186: 921–9.

Padilla-Nash HM, Barenboim-Stapleton L, Difilippantonio MJ, Ried T (2006). Spectral karyotyping analysis of human and mouse chromosomes. *Nat Protoc* 1: 3129–42.

Pages V, Fuchs RP (2002). How DNA lesions are turned into mutations within cells? *Oncogene* 21: 8957–66.

Papadopoulos PC, Greenstein AM, Gaffney RA, Westbrook CA, Wiedemann LM (1990). Characterization of the translocation breakpoint sequences in Philadelphia-positive acute lymphoblastic leukemia. *Genes Chromosomes Cancer* 1: 233–9.

Pastink A, Eeken JC, Lohman PH (2001). Genomic integrity and the repair of double-strand DNA breaks. *Mutat Res* 480–481: 37–50.

Plank JL, Wu J, Hsieh TS (2006). Topoisomerase IIIalpha and Bloom's helicase can resolve a mobile double Holliday junction substrate through convergent branch migration. *Proc Natl Acad Sci U S A* 103: 11118–23.

Rafii S, O'Regan P, Xinarianos G, Azmy I, Stephenson T, Reed M et al. (2002). A potential role for the XRCC2 R188H polymorphic site in DNA-damage repair and breast cancer. *Hum Mol Genet* 11: 1433–8.

Raynard S, Bussen W, Sung P (2006). A double Holliday junction dissolvasome comprising BLM, topoisomerase IIIalpha, and BLAP75. *J Biol Chem* 281: 13861–4.

Reaban ME, Griffin JA (1990). Induction of RNA-stabilized DNA conformers by transcription of an immunoglobulin switch region. *Nature* 348: 342–4.

Reaban ME, Lebowitz J, Griffin JA (1994). Transcription induces the formation of a stable RNA.DNA hybrid in the immunoglobulin alpha switch region. *J Biol Chem* 269: 21850–7.

Reina-San-Martin B, Chen HT, Nussenzweig A, Nussenzweig MC (2004). ATM is required for efficient recombination between immunoglobulin switch regions. *J Exp Med* 200: 1103–10.

Richardson C, Jasin M (2000). Frequent chromosomal translocations induced by DNA double-strand breaks. *Nature* 405: 697–700.
Richardson C, Moynahan ME, Jasin M (1998). Double-strand break repair by interchromosomal recombination: suppression of chromosomal translocations. *Genes Dev* 12: 3831–42.
Richardson C, Moynahan ME, Jasin M (1999). Homologous recombination between heterologs during repair of a double-strand break. Suppression of translocations in normal cells. *Ann N Y Acad Sci* 886: 183–6.
Rodriguez-Lopez R, Osorio A, Ribas G, Pollan M, Sanchez-Pulido L, de la Hoya M et al. (2004). The variant E233G of the RAD51D gene could be a low-penetrance allele in high-risk breast cancer families without BRCA1/2 mutations. *Int J Cancer* 110: 845–9.
Rooney S, Sekiguchi J, Whitlow S, Eckersdorff M, Manis JP, Lee C et al. (2004). Artemis and p53 cooperate to suppress oncogenic N-myc amplification in progenitor B cells. *Proc Natl Acad Sci U S A* 101: 2410–5.
Rooney S, Sekiguchi J, Zhu C, Cheng HL, Manis J, Whitlow S et al. (2002). Leaky Scid phenotype associated with defective V(D)J coding end processing in Artemis-deficient mice. *Mol Cell* 10: 1379–90.
Sakano H, Huppi K, Heinrich G, Tonegawa S (1979). Sequences at the somatic recombination sites of immunoglobulin light-chain genes. *Nature* 280: 288–94.
Samper E, Goytisolo FA, Slijepcevic P, van Buul PP, Blasco MA (2000). Mammalian Ku86 protein prevents telomeric fusions independently of the length of TTAGGG repeats and the G-strand overhang. *EMBO Rep* 1: 244–52.
Schatz DG, Oettinger MA, Baltimore D (1989). The V(D)J recombination activating gene, RAG-1. *Cell* 59: 1035–48.
Sharma S, Sommers JA, Wu L, Bohr VA, Hickson ID, Brosh RM, Jr. (2004). Stimulation of flap endonuclease-1 by the Bloom's syndrome protein. *J Biol Chem* 279: 9847–56.
Sharples GJ (2001). The X philes: structure-specific endonucleases that resolve Holliday junctions. *Mol Microbiol* 39: 823–34.
Shechter D, Costanzo V, Gautier J (2004). ATR and ATM regulate the timing of DNA replication origin firing. *Nat Cell Biol* 6: 648–55.
Shinkai Y, Rathbun G, Lam KP, Oltz EM, Stewart V, Mendelsohn M et al. (1992). RAG-2-deficient mice lack mature lymphocytes owing to inability to initiate V(D)J rearrangement. *Cell* 68: 855–67.
Shinohara A, Ogawa T (1998). Stimulation by Rad52 of yeast Rad51-mediated recombination. *Nature* 391: 404–7.
Sigurdsson S, Van Komen S, Bussen W, Schild D, Albala JS, Sung P (2001). Mediator function of the human Rad51B-Rad51C complex in Rad51/RPA-catalyzed DNA strand exchange. *Genes Dev* 15: 3308–18.
Sonoda E, Hochegger H, Saberi A, Taniguchi Y, Takeda S (2006). Differential usage of non-homologous end-joining and homologous recombination in double strand break repair. *DNA Repair (Amst)* 5: 1021–9.
Sonoda E, Sasaki MS, Buerstedde JM, Bezzubova O, Shinohara A, Ogawa H et al. (1998). Rad51-deficient vertebrate cells accumulate chromosomal breaks prior to cell death. *Embo J* 17: 598–608.
Sugimoto J, Hatakeyama T, Narducci MG, Russo G, Isobe M (1999). Identification of the TCL1/MTCP1-like 1 (TML1) gene from the region next to the TCL1 locus. *Cancer Res* 59: 2313–7.
Sung P (1997). Function of yeast Rad52 protein as a mediator between replication protein A and the Rad51 recombinase. *J Biol Chem* 272: 28194–7.
Swanson PC (2001). The DDE motif in RAG-1 is contributed in trans to a single active site that catalyzes the nicking and transesterification steps of V(D)J recombination. *Mol Cell Biol* 21: 449–58.
Szostak JW, Orr-Weaver TL, Rothstein RJ, Stahl FW (1983). The double-strand-break repair model for recombination. *Cell* 33: 25–35.

Color Plates

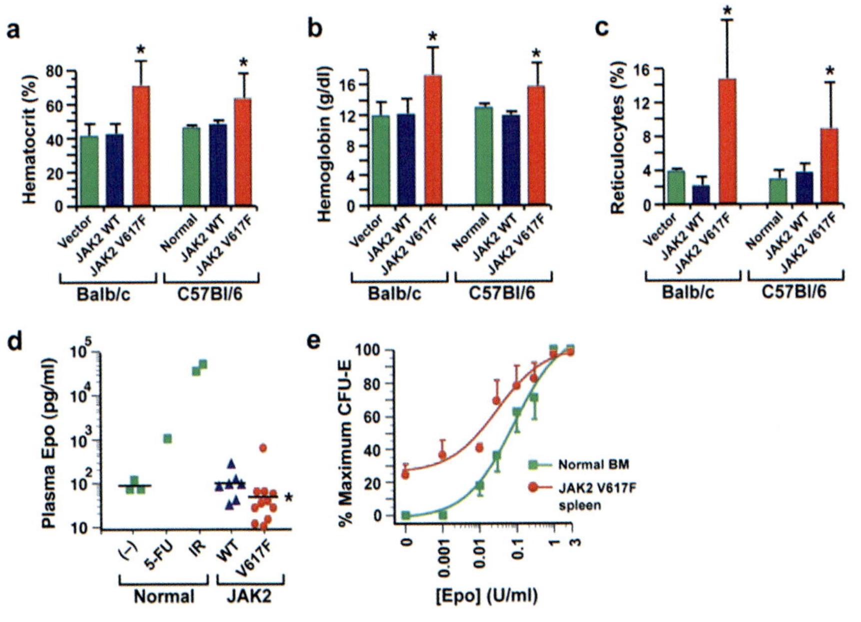

Fig. 1.4 JAK2-V617F induces polycythemia through autonomous overproduction of erythrocytes. (**a**) Hematocrit, (**b**) blood hemoglobin, and (**c**) reticulocyte counts from cohorts of Balb/c or B6 mice transplanted with syngeneic BM cells transduced with empty vector (*green*), or retrovirus expressing murine JAK2 WT (*blue*) or JAK2-V617F (*red*). In the case of the B6 cohorts, untransplanted mice ("normal") were used as controls. (**d**) Plasma Epo levels for the three groups (B6 background). (**e**) Percent maximal CFU-E from normal BM (*green*) or spleen of JAK2-V617F recipients (*red*). Adapted from Zaleskas et al. (2006)

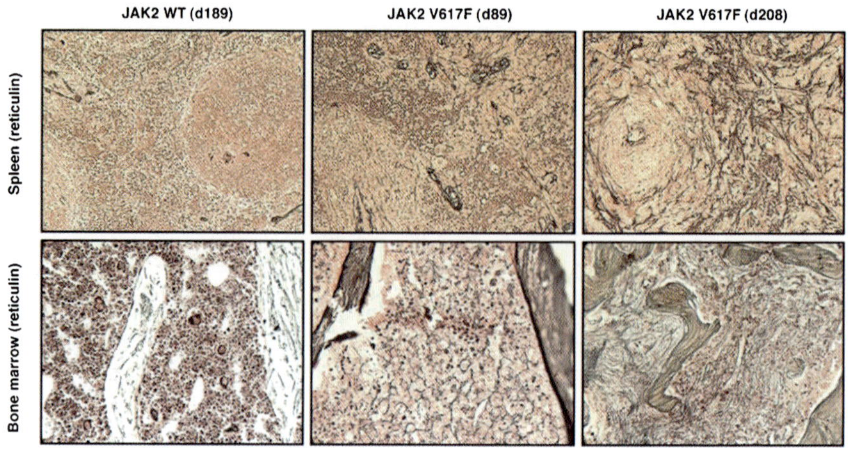

Fig. 1.5 Development of myelofibrosis in JAK2-V617F recipient mice. Increasing fibrosis (demonstrated by reticulin staining) in spleen (*top panels*) and bone marrow (BM) (*bottom panels*) of representative JAK2-V617F recipients at about 3 (middle panels) and 7 months (*right panels*) after transplantation. Note the marked increase in reticulin staining at 7 months in the JAK2-V617F recipients, but not in recipients of JAK2 wild-type (WT)-transduced BM (*left panels*). Adapted from Zaleskas et al. (2006)

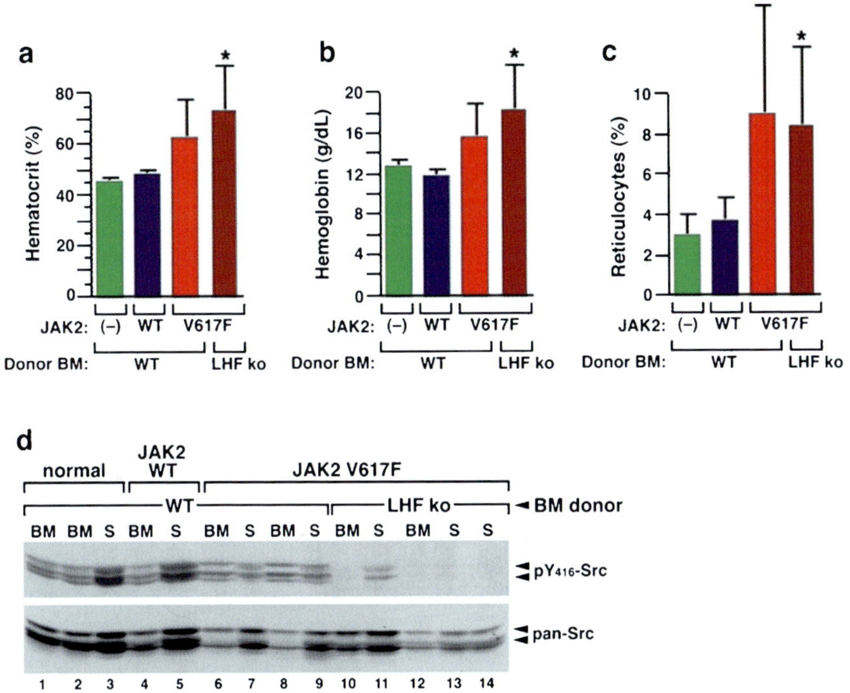

Fig. 1.6 Polycythemia induced by JAK2-V617F is independent of Src family kinases. (**a**) Hematocrit, (**b**) blood hemoglobin, and (**c**) reticulocyte counts from normal (–) B6 mice (*green*), B6 recipients of B6 wild-type (WT) bone marrow (BM) transduced with retrovirus expressing murine JAK2 WT (*blue*) or JAK2-V617F (*red*), and B6 $Lyn^{-/-}Hck^{-/-}Fgr^{-/-}$ BM transduced with retrovirus expressing JAK2-V617F (*orange*). (**d**) Western blot analysis of extracts of primary myeloerythroid cells from individual normal (lanes 1–3) B6 mice, recipients of WT BM transduced with JAK2 WT retrovirus (lanes 4–5), recipients of WT BM transduced with JAK2-V617F retrovirus (lanes 6–9), and recipients of $Lyn^{-/-}Hck^{-/-}Fgr^{-/-}$ BM transduced with JAK2-V617F retrovirus (lanes 10–14). The membrane was blotted with antibody recognizing the phosphorylated activation loop tyrosine (Y146 homolog) of c-Src, Lyn, Hck, Fyn, Lck, and Yes (*top panel*) and subsequently with antibody against total c-Src, Fyn, Yes, and Fgr (*bottom panel*). Adapted from Zaleskas et al. (2006)

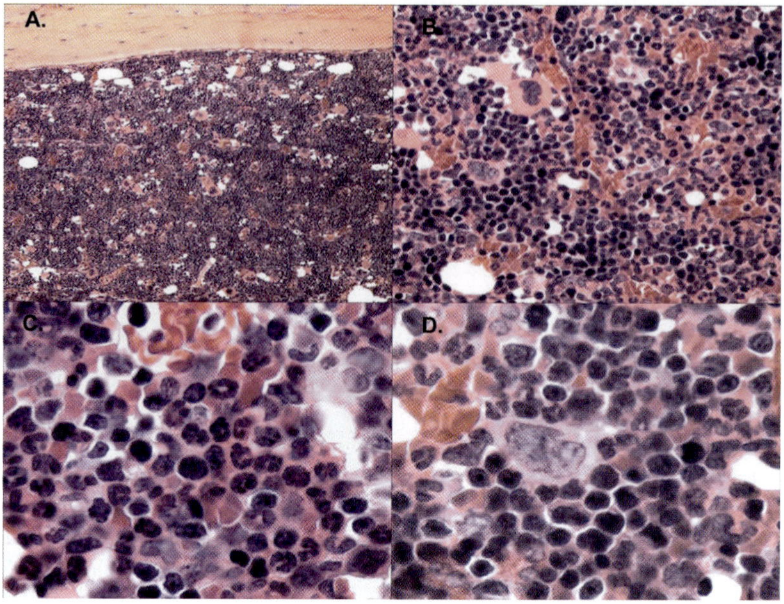

Fig. 3.1 Histology of murine bone marrow. (**A**) Medium (200×) magnification of wild-type adult BALB/c bone marrow demonstrating normal hypercellularity (hematoxylin and eosin stain). (**B**) Higher magnification (400×) of the same marrow, demonstrating tri-lineage hematopoiesis with open sinuses filled with mature red blood cells and scattered adipocytes (hematoxylin and eosin stain). (**C**) High magnification (1000×) of a myeloid colony within the marrow showing maturing elements including ringed granulocyte precursors (hematoxylin and eosin stain). (**D**) High magnification (1000×) of an erythroid colony with darkly stained round to irregular nuclei surrounding a megakaryocyte (hematoxylin and eosin stain)

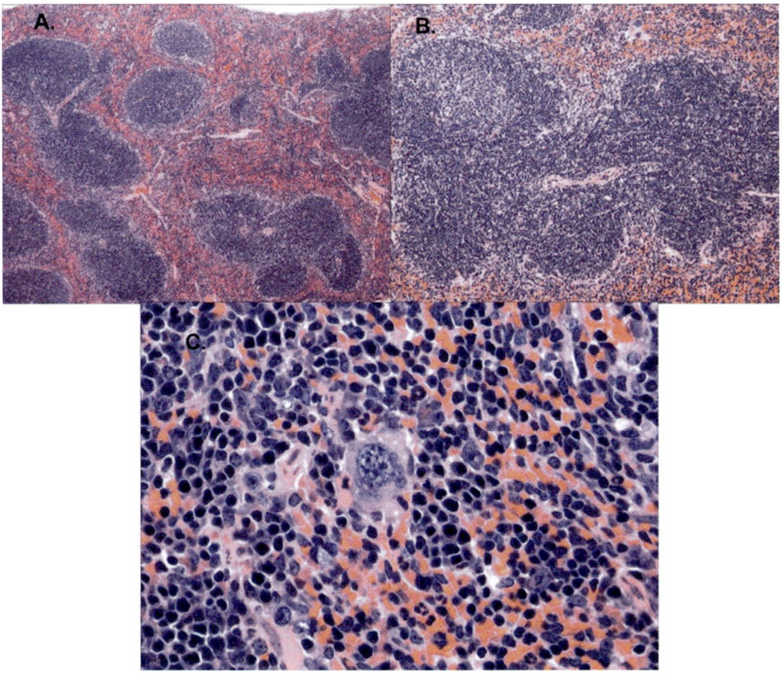

Fig. 3.2 Histology of murine spleen. (**A**) Low power magnification (40×) of an adult wild-type BALB/c mouse showing white pulp nodules surrounded by extramedullary hematopoiesis in the red pulp (hematoxylin and eosin stain). (**B**) Medium power magnification (100×) from the same spleen, demonstrating white pulp lymphoid nodules with a germinal center (upper left) and pale marginal zones (hematoxylin and eosin stain). (**C**) High power magnification (400×) from the same spleen showing red pulp extramedullary hematopoiesis predominantly comprised of darkly staining erythroid elements and a single megakaryocyte (hematoxylin and eosin stain)

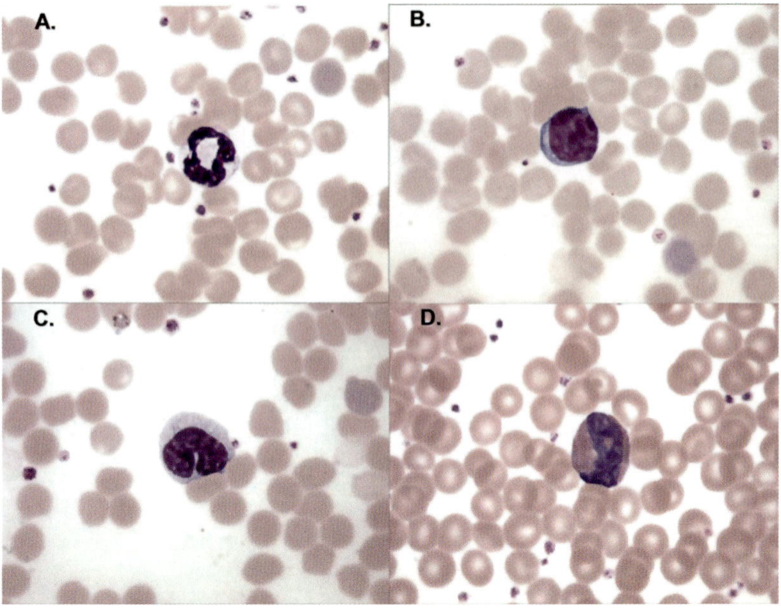

Fig. 3.3 Cytology of murine peripheral blood cells. (**A**) Mature neutrophil from wild-type BALB/c mouse shows a hyperlobate nucleus and very fine azurophilic granules (Wright–Giemsa stain, 1000×). (**B**) Mature lymphocyte from wild-type BALB/c mouse shows a round nucleus and small amounts of basophilic, agranular cytoplasm (Wright–Giemsa stain, 1000×). (**C**) Mature monocyte from wild-type BALB/c mouse shows a kidney-shaped nucleus and pale blue-gray cytoplasm with occasional vaculoes (Wright–Giemsa stain, 1000×). (**D**) Mature eosinophil from wild-type BALB/c mouse shows a hyperlobate nucleus and prominent orange granules (Wright–Giemsa stain, 1000×)

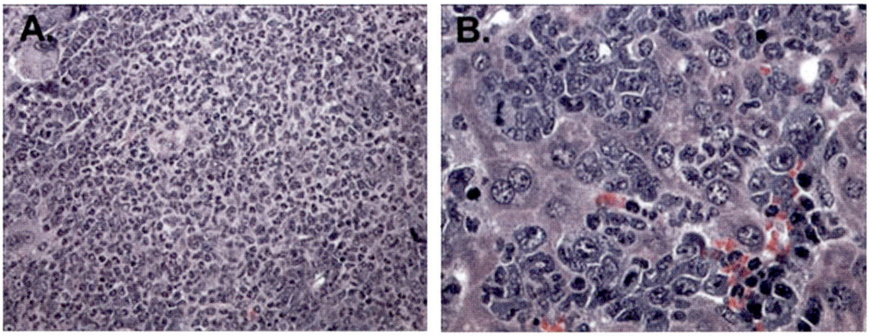

Fig. 3.4 Retroviral transduction of BCR–ABL in a bone marrow transplantation model. (**A**) Spleen from C57BL/6 recipient mouse receiving BCR–ABL transduced marrow showing effacement of the architecture by a diffuse proliferation of maturing myeloid elements. Erythropoiesis is not prominent in this case. Overall, this tumor would be classified as a myeloproliferative disorder-like myeloid leukemia (hematoxylin and eosin stains, 200× magnification). (**B**) Liver parenchyma from the same animal showing an infiltrate of both maturing myeloid and erythroid elements (hematoxylin and eosin stains, 400× magnification)

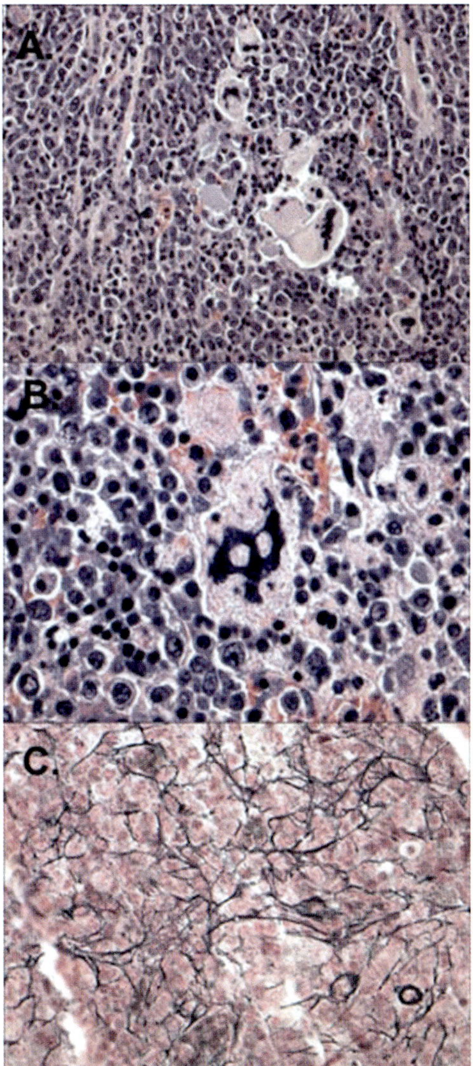

Fig. 3.5 Retroviral transduction of JAK2V617F in a bone marrow transplantation model. (**A**) Histology of Jak2V617F-transduced BALB/c mice showing pathology in representative sections of spleen revealing marked leukocytosis consisting predominantly of maturing myeloid elements and a prominent population of megakaryocytes, including arge, atypical forms occurring in occasional clusters (hematoxylin and eosin stains, 200× magnification). (**B**) Large abnormal megakaryocyte from the same animal showing bizarre nuclear convolutions and emperipolesis of neutrophils in the megakaryocyte cytoplasm. (hematoxylin and eosin stains, 400× magnification). (**C**) Bone marrow from the same animal stained with reticulin stain showing markedly increased numbers of reticulin fibers, indicative of myelofibrosis (400× magnification)

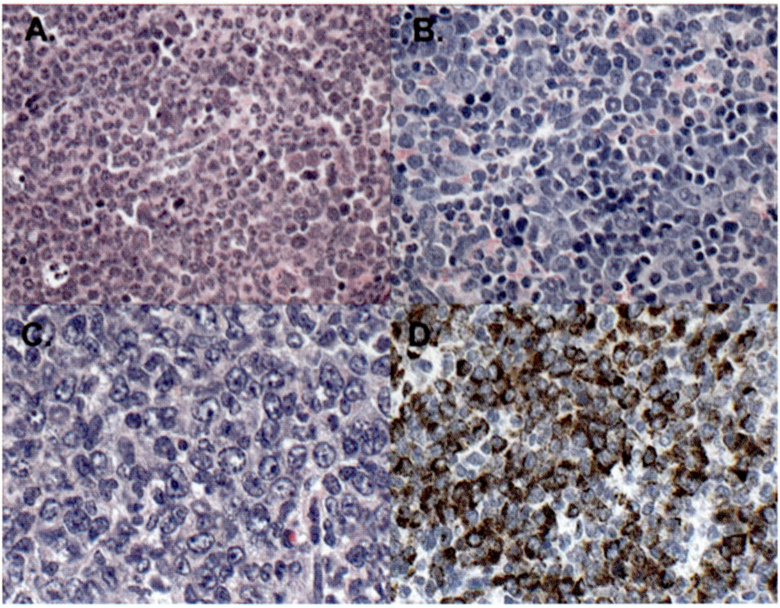

Fig. 3.6 Conditional activation of an oncogenic K-ras allele (K-Ras^{G12D}) in a mixed BALB/c, C57BL/6, and 129 v/Jae genetic background. (**A**) Bone marrow and (**B**) spleen sections reveal a marked maturing myeloid proliferation consistent with a myeloproliferative disorder-like myeloid leukemia (hematoxylin and eosin stains, 400× magnification). (**C**) When a transgenic mouse expressing PML–RARα is crossed with oncogenic K-ras expressing mouse, a short latency, highly penetrant acute promyelocytic leukemia is seen. A representative leukemia within a spleen is pictured here, demonstrating round to irregular nuclei, dispersed chromatin and small amounts of eosinophilic cytoplasm (hematoxylin and eosin stains, 400× magnification). (**D**) Myeloperoxidase immunohistochemistry of the tumor in C is pictured, revealing intense staining for myeloperoxidase consistent with acute promyelocytic leukemia

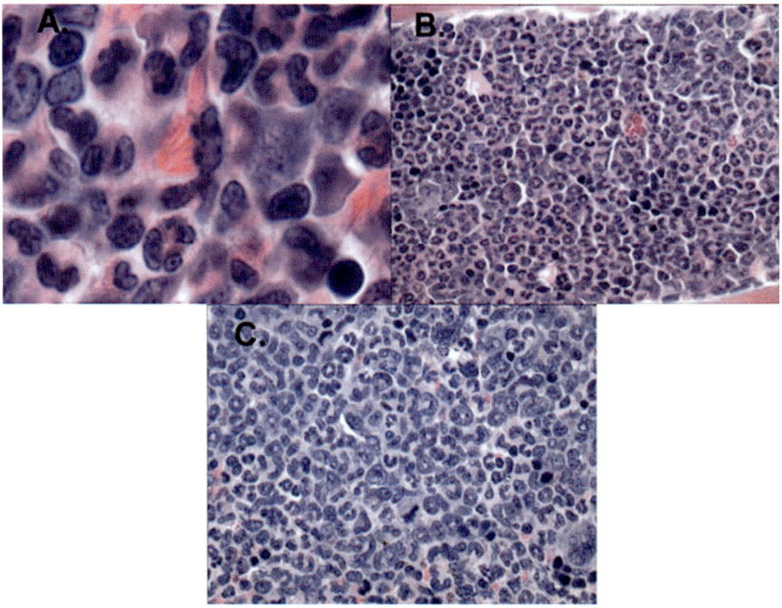

Fig. 3.7 Models of mutant SHP2 disease. (**A**) Marrow from a knock-in mouse model of the mutant SHP2 D61G associated with Noonan syndrome. These mice demonstrate a myeloid proliferation and reactive pseudo-Gaucher cells filled with crystal-like eosinophilic material (hematoxylin and eosin stains, 1000× magnification). (**B**) Marrow and (**C**) spleen from recipient mice transplanted with retrovirally transduced bone marrow expressing the SHP2 mutations D61Y and E76K, found only in juvenile myelomonocytic leukemia (JMML) and other neoplasms. Note the prominent marrow hypercellularity and compression of the sinuses in the bone marrow with a mature myeloid (granulocytic) predominance and massive splenomegaly showing infiltration of spleen with myeloid elements (hematoxylin and eosin stains, 400× magnification)

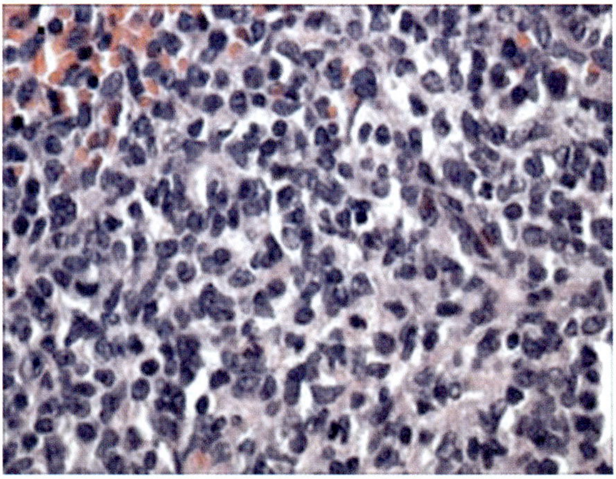

Fig. 3.8 FLT3 model of disease. A myeloproliferative disease with features reminiscent of human chronic myelomonocytic leukemia (CMML) is shown in this model of homozygous

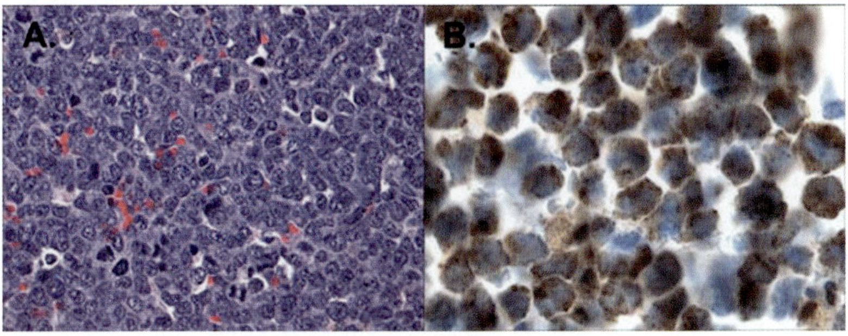

Fig. 3.9 Pu.1 model of acute myeloid leukemia. (**A**) Spleen from PU.1 knock-down C57BL/6 transgenic mouse showing a diffuse infiltrate of immature mononuclear cells with immunophenotypic features of acute myeloid leukemia (hematoxylin and eosin stains, 400× magnification). (**B**) Myeloid derivation confirmed by immunohistochemistry for myeloperoxidase shown in this marrow specimen from the same mouse (1000× magnification)

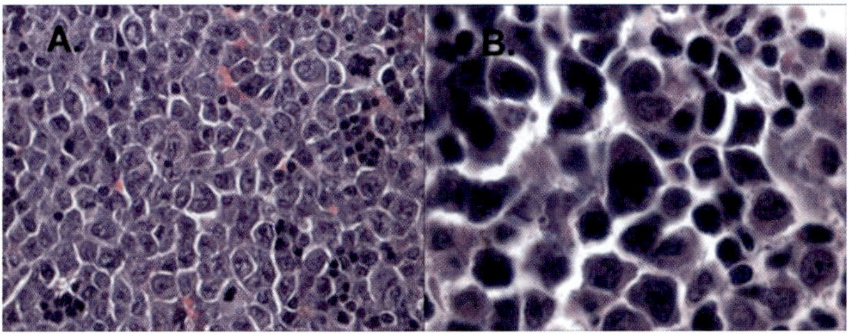

Fig. 3.10 CEBP/α knock-out model of acute erythroleukemia. (**A**) Spleen (400× magnification) and (**B**) bone marrow (1000× magnification) from a C57BL/6 CEBP/α knock-out mouse transplanted with bone marrow retrovirally transduced by BCR–ABL. The infiltrate in both tissues is comprised of an immature population of large blast forms with round to irregular nuclei, containing ample basophilic cytoplasm consistent with proerythroblasts and a diagnosis of acute erythroleukemia

Fig. 3.8 *(continued)* FLT3–ITD expressed in C57BL/6 mice under an endogenous murine *Flt3*promoter. In this representative section of spleen, splenic red pulp is expanded by both maturing myeloid and erythroid elements with enlarged white pulp comprised of intermediate-sized mononuclear cell infiltrate with irregular nuclei and ample eosinophilic cytoplasm (pictured here) that have a myelomonocytic phenotype by flow cytometry (hematoxylin and eosin stains, 400× magnification)

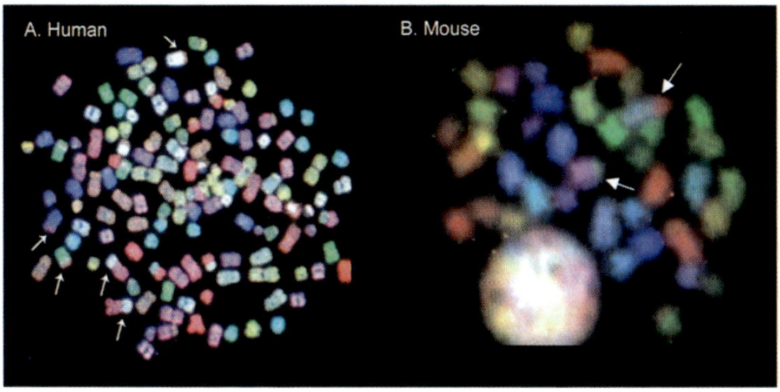

Fig. 4.1 Genomic instability observed in human and mouse tumor cells. (**A**) Spectral karyotype analysis of a human bladder cancer cell line. The aneuploid J82 cell line contains multiple chromosomal aberrations. White arrows indicate translocations. Adapted from Padilla-Nash et al. (2006). (**B**) Spectral karyotype analysis of a mouse pro-B cell lymphoma deficient for *Dclre1c* and *Trp53*. White arrows indicate translocations

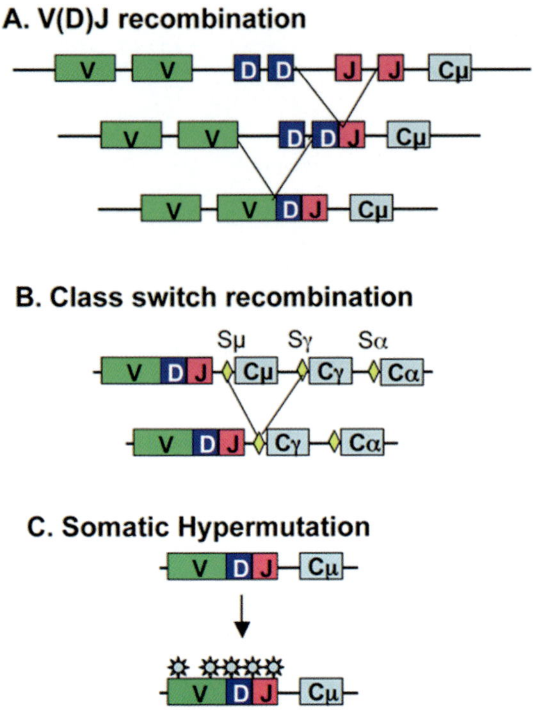

Fig. 4.5 Schematic of types of somatic alterations that occur during lymphocyte development. **(A)** During V(D)J recombination, rearrangements between V (*green rectangles*), D (*blue rectangles*), and J (*pink rectangles*) gene segments create mature, functional antibody receptors in B and T cells. These rearrangements occur in a precise order, with D to J joins occurring first followed by V to DJ joins. (**B**) Class switch recombination changes the isotype of the immunoglobulin constant region through constant region (*light blue rectangle*) rearrangements. Small sequence elements known as switch regions (*yellow diamonds*) permit recombination between different constant gene segments. (**C**) In somatic hypermutation, single or multiple mutations are introduced throughout the recombined V(D)J segment (*blue sunbursts*) to change antibody affinity of a functional receptor. Adapted from Kuppers and Dalla-Favera (2001)

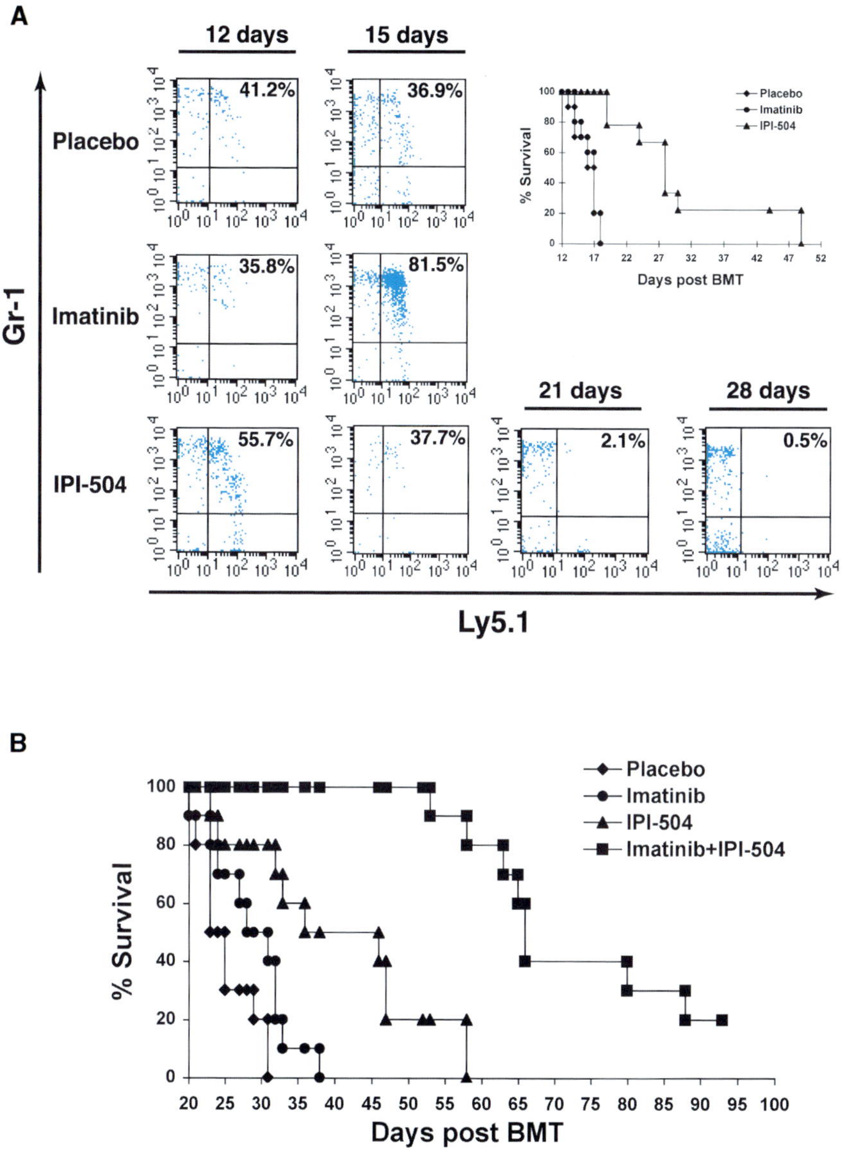

Fig. 7.1 Inhibition of heat shock protein 90 (Hsp90) by IPI-504 preferentially reduces growth of myeloid leukemic cells harboring the BCR–ABL–T315I mutant. (**A**) Bone marrow cells from C57BL/6-Ly5.2 mice were transduced by BCR–ABL–WT, and bone marrow cells from C57BL/6-Ly5.1 mice were transduced by BCR–ABL–T315I. The transduced cells were 1:1 mixed, and 0.5×10^6 mixed cells were injected into each recipient mouse (C57BL/6-Ly5.2). The mice were treated with placebo ($n = 10$), imatinib (100 mg/kg, twice a day) ($n = 10$), and IPI-504 (50 mg/kg, once every 2 days) ($n = 10$), respectively, beginning at 8 days post-BMT. At days 12 and 15 post-BMT, GFP^+ cells viable cells in peripheral blood of the mice were analyzed for $Gr\text{-}1^+Ly5.1^+$ cells that represented BCR–ABL–T315I-expressing myeloid cells. $Gr\text{-}1^+Ly5.1^-$ cells represented BCR–ABL–WT-expressing myeloid cells. Percentages of BCR–ABL–T315I-expressing myeloid cells in peripheral blood of IPI-504-treated chronic

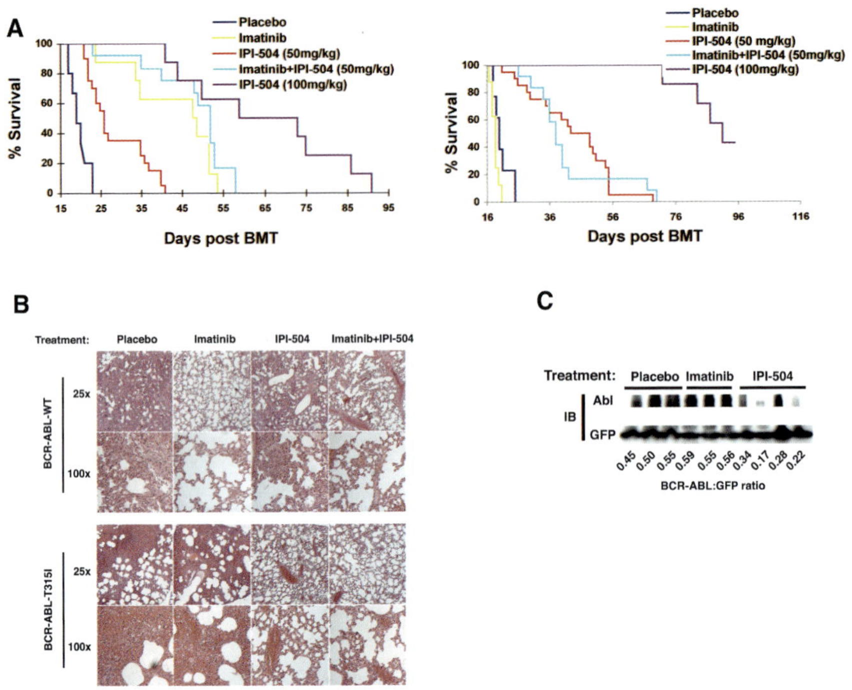

Fig. 7.2 Heat shock protein 90 (Hsp90) is a therapeutic target for chronic myeloid leukemia (CML) induced by either BCR–ABL–WT or BCR–ABL–T315I. (**A**) Treatment with the Hsp90 inhibitor IPI-504 prolonged the survival of CML mice. Mice with BCR–ABL–WT (*left panel*)- or BCR–ABL–T315I (*right panel*)-induced CML were treated with placebo ($n = 15$ for BCR–ABL–WT; $n = 13$ for BCR–ABL–T315I), imatinib(100 mg/kg, twice a day by gavage) ($n = 8$ for both BCR–ABL–WT and BCR–ABL–T315I), IPI-504 (50 mg/kg, once every 2 days by gavage) ($n = 20$ for both BCR–ABL–WT and BCR–ABL–T315I), IPI-504 (100 mg/kg, once every 2 days by gavage) ($n = 8$ for both BCR–ABL–WT; $n = 7$ for BCR–ABL–T315I), and imatinib+IPI-504 ($n = 12$ for both BCR–ABL–WT and BCR–ABL–T315I), respectively, beginning at day 8 post-transplantation. The IPI-504-treated mice with BCR–ABL–T315I-induced CML lived longer than those with BCR–ABL–WT-induced CML (comparing between *left* and *right panels*) (**B**) Photomicrographs of hematoxylin- and eosin-stained lung sections from drug-treated mice at day 14 post-transplantation. (**C**) Western blot analysis of spleen cell lysates for degradation of BCR–ABL in IPI-504-treated CML mice. IB, immunoblot. Adapted from [90]

Fig. 7.1 *(continued)* myeloid leukemia (CML) mice were further analyzed at days 21 and 28 post-BMT. The FACS results for one representative mouse from each treatment group were shown. IPI-504 but not imatinib significantly prolonged survival of the CML mice. (**B**) Simultaneous inhibition of Hsp90 and BCR–ABL kinase activity with IPI-504 and imatinib significantly prolongs survival of CML mice carrying both T315-expressing and WT–BCR–ABL leukemia cells. BALB/c mice were used to induce CML, and each treatment group had 10 mice. Adapted from [90]

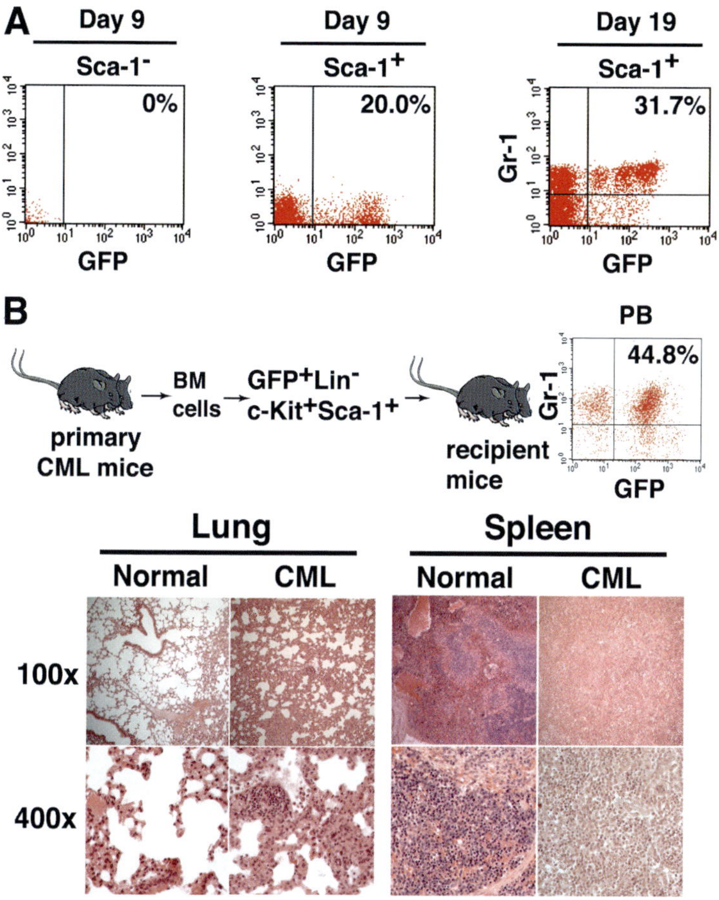

Fig. 7.3 Identification of bone marrow cell populations that function as chronic myeloid leukemia (CML) stem cells. (**A**) BCR–ABL-transduced BM cells from B6 mice were sorted by Sca-1 MACS columns (Miltenyi Biotec), followed by transferring Sca-1$^-$ or Sca-1$^+$ population into B6 mice (1×10^5 cells/mouse; 4 mice per cell population group) to induce CML. GFP$^+$ myeloid cells (Gr-1$^+$) in peripheral blood (PB) of the mice were examined at days 9 and 19 after the induction of leukemia. All mice receiving Sca-1$^+$ population died of CML by day 42. (**B**) BCR–ABL-expressing HSCs function as CML stem cells. BM cells from CML mice in B6 background were sorted by FACS for BCR–ABL-expressing HSCs (GFP$^+$Lin$^-$c-kit$^+$Sca-1$^+$), followed by transferring into lethally irradiated B6 mice (2×10^4 cells/mouse). GFP$^+$ myeloid cells (Gr-1$^+$) were detected in peripheral blood. In contrast to the normal control mice, CML mice showed complete infiltration of the lungs with myeloid leukemic cells and complete disruption of follicular architecture of the spleen by infiltrating leukemic cells. Adapted from [18]

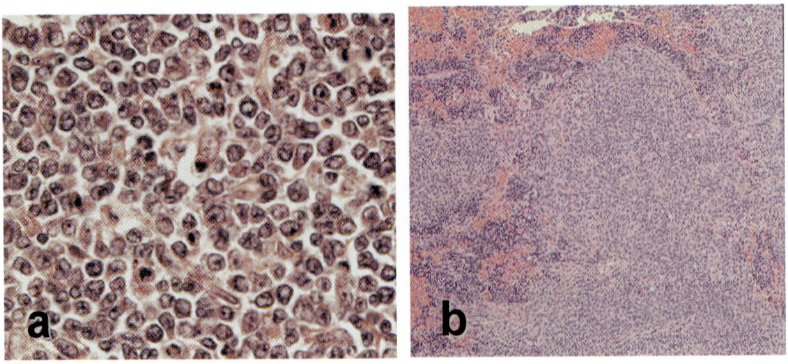

Fig. 9.2 (**a**) Histopathology of a major type pre-B lymphoma in a SL/Kh mouse. ×400, H.E. (**b**) Follicular center cell lymphoma in a (SL/Kh × NFS)F1 × NFS mouse [8]. ×100, H.E.

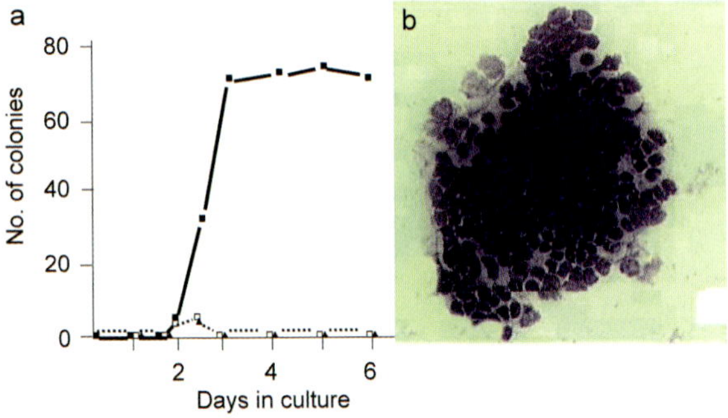

Fig. 9.8 (**a**) Kinetics of colony formation by pre-B cells after transfection of SL/Kh BM cells with constitutively activated mutant Stat5a cDNA [36]. Closed square, transfected with mutant Stat5a cDNA; open square, with wild type Stat5a cDNA; closed triangle, mock transfection. (**b**) A colony of pre-B cells in semisold medium [36]

Taccioli GE, Amatucci AG, Beamish HJ, Gell D, Xiang XH, Torres Arzayus MI et al. (1998). Targeted disruption of the catalytic subunit of the DNA-PK gene in mice confers severe combined immunodeficiency and radiosensitivity. *Immunity* 9: 355–66.
Taccioli GE, Cheng HL, Varghese AJ, Whitmore G, Alt FW (1994). A DNA repair defect in Chinese hamster ovary cells affects V(D)J recombination similarly to the murine scid mutation. *J Biol Chem* 269: 7439–42.
Takahashi A, Ohnishi T (2005). Does gammaH2AX foci formation depend on the presence of DNA double strand breaks? *Cancer Lett* 229: 171–9.
Taylor AM, Byrd PJ (2005). Molecular pathology of ataxia telangiectasia. *J Clin Pathol* 58: 1009–15.
Taylor AM, Metcalfe JA, Thick J, Mak YF (1996). Leukemia and lymphoma in ataxia telangiectasia. *Blood* 87: 423–38.
Thacker J (2005). The RAD51 gene family, genetic instability and cancer. *Cancer Lett* 219: 125–35.
Tian M, Alt FW (2000). Transcription-induced cleavage of immunoglobulin switch regions by nucleotide excision repair nucleases in vitro. *J Biol Chem* 275: 24163–72.
Tischkowitz M, Dokal I (2004). Fanconi anaemia and leukaemia – clinical and molecular aspects. *Br J Haematol* 126: 176–91.
Tremblay A, Jasin M, Chartrand P (2000). A double-strand break in a chromosomal LINE element can be repaired by gene conversion with various endogenous LINE elements in mouse cells. *Mol Cell Biol* 20: 54–60.
Treuner K, Helton R, Barlow C (2004). Loss of Rad52 partially rescues tumorigenesis and T-cell maturation in Atm-deficient mice. *Oncogene* 23: 4655–61.
Tsuzuki T, Fujii Y, Sakumi K, Tominaga Y, Nakao K, Sekiguchi M et al. (1996). Targeted disruption of the Rad51 gene leads to lethality in embryonic mice. *Proc Natl Acad Sci U S A* 93: 6236–40.
Valerie K, Povirk LF (2003). Regulation and mechanisms of mammalian double-strand break repair. *Oncogene* 22: 5792–812.
Villa A, Santagata S, Bozzi F, Giliani S, Frattini A, Imberti L et al. (1998). Partial V(D)J recombination activity leads to Omenn syndrome. *Cell* 93: 885–96.
Waldmann TA, Broder S, Goldman CK, Frost K, Korsmeyer SJ, Medici MA (1983). Disorders of B cells and helper T cells in the pathogenesis of the immunoglobulin deficiency of patients with ataxia telangiectasia. *J Clin Invest* 71: 282–95.
Walker JR, Corpina RA, Goldberg J (2001). Structure of the Ku heterodimer bound to DNA and its implications for double-strand break repair. *Nature* 412: 607–14.
Wang WW, Spurdle AB, Kolachana P, Bove B, Modan B, Ebbers SM et al. (2001). A single nucleotide polymorphism in the 5́ untranslated region of RAD51 and risk of cancer among BRCA1/2 mutation carriers. *Cancer Epidemiol Biomarkers Prev* 10: 955–60.
Weinert BT, Rio DC (2007). DNA strand displacement, strand annealing and strand swapping by the Drosophila Bloom's syndrome helicase. *Nucleic Acids Res* 35: 1367–76.
Weinstock DM, Elliott B, Jasin M (2006a). A model of oncogenic rearrangements: differences between chromosomal translocation mechanisms and simple double-strand break repair. *Blood* 107: 777–80.
Weinstock DM, Richardson CA, Elliott B, Jasin M (2006b). Modeling oncogenic translocations: distinct roles for double-strand break repair pathways in translocation formation in mammalian cells. *DNA Repair (Amst)* 5: 1065–74.
Welzel N, Le T, Marculescu R, Mitterbauer G, Chott A, Pott C et al. (2001). Templated nucleotide addition and immunoglobulin JH-gene utilization in t(11;14) junctions: implications for the mechanism of translocation and the origin of mantle cell lymphoma. *Cancer Res* 61: 1629–36.
Woo Y, Wright SM, Maas SA, Alley TL, Caddle LB, Kamdar S et al. (2007). The nonhomologous end joining factor Artemis suppresses multi-tissue tumor formation and prevents loss of heterozygosity. *Oncogene*.

Wu L, Hickson ID (2003). The Bloom's syndrome helicase suppresses crossing over during homologous recombination. *Nature* 426: 870–4.

Zha S, Alt FW, Cheng HL, Brush JW, Li G (2007). Defective DNA repair and increased genomic instability in Cernunnos-XLF-deficient murine ES cells. *Proc Natl Acad Sci U S A* 104: 4518–23.

Zhang JG, Goldman JM, Cross NC (1995). Characterization of genomic BCR-ABL breakpoints in chronic myeloid leukaemia by PCR. *Br J Haematol* 90: 138–46.

Zhu C, Mills KD, Ferguson DO, Lee C, Manis J, Fleming J et al. (2002). Unrepaired DNA breaks in p53-deficient cells lead to oncogenic gene amplification subsequent to translocations. *Cell* 109: 811–21.

Zou L, Cortez D, Elledge SJ (2002). Regulation of ATR substrate selection by Rad17-dependent loading of Rad9 complexes onto chromatin. *Genes Dev* 16: 198–208.

Chapter 5
Modeling Human Leukemia Using Immune-Compromised Mice

Fumihiko Ishikawa, Yariko Saito, and Leonard D. Shultz

Contents

5.1 Introduction

Various mutations have been found to cause leukemia, myeloid proliferative disorders, or lymphoid proliferative disorders in mice when directly introduced as transgenes or by transplantation of mouse hematopoietic cells expressing these genes through targeted vectors. These mouse models of hematological malignancies have provided important insights into leukemogenesis. However, models that facilitate studies of human leukemia cells in vivo are required to understand the biology of human leukemia. Studies of human leukemia cells that engraft in immunodeficient mouse models permit analyses of the mechanisms underlying human leukemic cell proliferation within the bone marrow, migration from the bone marrow into peripheral circulation, identification of specific microenvironmental niches for human leukemic cells, and the functional interactions of human leukemic cells with the elements of such niches. Such in vivo human leukemia models can also be used to simulate therapy

F. Ishikawa
Research Unit for Human Disease Models, RIKEN Research Center for Allergy and Immunology, Yokohama 230-0045, Japan
f_ishika@rcai.riken.jp

S. Li (ed.), *Mouse Models of Human Blood Cancers*,
DOI: 10.1007/978-0-387-69132-9_5, © Springer Science+Business Media, LLC 2008

targeting human leukemic cells. To accomplish these goals, xenogeneic transplantation of human leukemia cells into various strains of immunodeficient mouse recipients has been attempted. This chapter reviews the history of xenotransplantation for primary human leukemia and discusses new generations of xenotransplantation models for human leukemia.

5.2 Development of Immune-Compromised Mice and Humanized Mice

To allow the engraftment of human normal or leukemic cells in the mouse microenvironment, immunodeficient mouse strains have been used as recipients to prevent rejection of human cells. Immunodeficient strains that support engraftment of primary human cells resulted from the discovery of the protein kinase, DNA-activated, catalytic polypeptide (*Prkdc*); severe combined immunodeficiency ($Prkdc^{scid}$) mutation in CB17 mice [1]. However, the engraftment levels of human hematopoietic cells were unacceptably low due to the age-dependent appearance of mouse T and B cells (leakiness) and the high levels of host innate immune function. In contrast to CB17-*scid* mice, targeted mutations in either of the recombination activating genes (*Rag*) *1* and *Rag2* resulted in the development of mouse strains with improved depletion of acquired immunity without age-dependent leakiness [2, 3]. In these mice, as with CB17-*scid* mice, the high activity of residual innate immunity limited the engraftment of human cells.

These limitations in the engraftment of human cells were partially overcome by backcrossing the *scid* mutation onto the non-obese diabetic (NOD) strain, which are utilized as a model for type I diabetes mellitus. The advantage of NOD-*scid* (NOD/SCID) mice over CB17-*scid* mice is the lower NK cell activity and impaired complement activity conferred by the NOD strain background [4]. Additional defects in the innate immunity in NOD/SCID mice have led to heightened levels of human hematopoietic cell engraftment.

Further systematic introductions of mutations into NOD or NOD/SCID backgrounds resulted in the development of NOD-$Rag1^{null}$ [5], NOD-$Rag1^{null}$ $Prf1^{null}$ [6], and NOD-$scid\beta 2m^{null}$ mice [7] with incremental improvements in human hematopoietic cell engraftment. However, the relatively short life spans of these mouse strains and poor engraftment of the human T-lymphoid compartment continued to pose significant obstacles in development of the xenotransplantation model with a fully humanized immuno-hematopoietic system.

Targeted mutations at the interleukin-2 receptor (IL-2R) gamma-chain locus (*Il2rg*) were found to result not only in severe impairments in B- and T-cell development and function but also in complete prevention of NK cell development [8, 9]. Several strains with targeted mutations in the *Il2rg* locus were developed independently, using various genetic modifications to this locus backcrossed onto a number of diverse strain backgrounds including the

NOD/SCID [10, 11], BALB/c-*Rag2*^{null}, and *H2*^{d}-*Rag2*^{null}. The strain developed by backcrossing a targeted mutation leading to the complete absence of the γ-chain into the NOD/SCID strain is the NOD/LtSz-*scid Il2rg*^{null}, referred to as NOD/SCID/IL2rγ^{null} mice in this chapter. The NOD/SCID/IL2rγ^{null} mice, especially when used as neonatal recipients, proved to be superior in terms of the efficiency of normal human hematopoietic stem cell (HSC) engraftment compared to the NOD/SCID/β2m^{null} recipients [12]. The transplantation of purified human HSCs into the NOD/SCID/IL2rγ^{null} newborns resulted in long-term engraftment of normal human hematopoiesis, leading to the propagation of not only differentiated myeloid progeny but also lymphoid (T, B, NK) progeny, dendritic cells, erythrocytes, and platelets. These findings suggest that the NOD/SCID/IL2rγ^{null} recipients may be useful for the establishment of the in vivo mouse models of human leukemia.

5.3 Engraftment Studies of Hematological Malignancies

5.3.1 In Vivo Models of Human AML

Acute myelogenous leukemia (AML) is the most common leukemia in adults. While there are subtypes of AML that carry favorable prognoses, overall survival in AML is quite poor, even with current treatment protocols that include combined chemotherapy and stem cell transplantation. In vivo animal models for human AML are crucial in understanding leukemogenesis and in developing therapeutic modalities. While immortalized human leukemic cell lines have been shown to engraft in CB17-*scid* mice, the engraftment of primary AML cells in CB17-*scid* mice has been hindered presumably due to high residual NK cell activity [13–16].

The limitation in primary AML engraftment was partially overcome by using NOD/SCID mice as recipients, due to the attenuation of NK cell activity in these mice [17]. Ailles et al. reported the successful engraftment of four different subtypes (M1, M2, M4, and M5) of primary AML cells [18]. Two other groups reported that the engraftment levels of primary AML cells correlate with disease severity in patients [19, 20]. The observation that primary AML cells from AML M3 (acute promyelocytic leukemia) patients carrying a relatively good prognosis do not engraft well in NOD/SCID mice is consistent with these findings.

Using AML-engrafted NOD/SCID mice, an in vivo chemotherapy model has been developed to predict or simulate sensitivity/resistance of patient-derived AML cells against various anti-cancer drugs [21]. Although the decrease in leukemic cell burden and leukemia cell apoptosis in the engrafted mice after treatment with various chemotherapeutic drugs has been reported, whether therapeutic response in the mouse model correlates with that in patients is undetermined. Transplantation of leukemic cells derived from patients at different stages of disease, such as initial diagnosis and relapse, will provide information that may help predict sensitivity and resistance of leukemic cells in the patients. To answer these questions, however, the efficiency of AML engraftment needs to be improved, to achieve consistent levels of long-term engraftment using limited patient material available.

To achieve higher levels of AML engraftment, researchers have taken two approaches. First, induction of myeloid cell proliferation and differentiation using exogenous cytokine administration or endogenous production of cytokines by transgenes has been attempted. Second, residual innate immunity in recipient mice has been further depleted by backcrossing mutations in major histocompatibility complex (MHC) class I light chain (β2m) or common cytokine gamma chain (γc) onto the *scid*, *Rag-1^{null}*, or *Rag2^{null}* backgrounds. Both NOD/SCID/cytokine transgenic and NOD/SCID/β2m^{null} mice supported higher levels of AML engraftment compared with NOD/SCID mice [22]. However, the improvement of AML chimerism in the recipients by exogenous cytokine administration varied among investigators. Development of innate immunity-depleted NOD/SCID mouse strains enables us to obtain more efficient engraftment of primary AML cells. When NOD/SCID/β2m^{null} and NOD/SCID/IL2rγ^{null} recipients were compared, AML engraftment levels as well as normal HSC engraftment levels were significantly higher in the NOD/SCID/IL-2rγ^{null} mice [23]. NOG mice [24] and Rag2^{null}/γc^{null} mice carrying truncated form of *IL2rg* gene also supported efficient engraftment of primary AML mononuclear cells (MNCs). The suppression of innate immunity by blocking IL2rγ-mediated signaling is considered essential to inhibit the rejection of primary human AML cells in xenogeneic microenvironment.

5.3.2 In Vivo Models of Human ALL

Acute lymphocytic leukemia (ALL) is the most common hematological malignancy in childhood. Based on ontogenic classification, pediatric ALL is divided into T-ALL, B-precursor ALL, and mature B-ALL. B-precursor ALL accounts for 80–85% of total pediatric ALL cases. B-ALL can be further classified into subgroups based on the presence of chromosome abnormalities such as t(9;22) generating the Philadelphia (Ph) chromosome, t(12;21) generating the *TEL–AML1* fusion gene, and t(4;11) and other rearrangements involving the *MLL* gene at 11q23. Xenogeneic transplantation has been performed using subgroups of B-precursor ALL carrying the MLL rearrangements or the Ph+ abnormality. In the long-term observation of ALL engraftment in NOD/SCID mice, the chromosomal abnormalities or Ig gene arrangements identified in the primary ALL cells are largely retained in the ALL cells that have engrafted in NOD/SCID recipients, suggesting that these ALL engraftment models reproduce ALL disease present in the patients [25, 26]. As in human primary AML engraftment models, in vivo chemosensitivity and chemoresistance of engrafted ALL cells to anti-cancer drugs, including vincristine, dexamethasone, methotrexate, and L-arginine, have been examined [25, 27]. In these models, both single-drug treatment and combined chemotherapy resulted in the decrease of ALL cells in vivo and prolonged the survival of ALL-engrafted mice. Furthermore, immunotherapeutic modalities such as induction of anti-minor antigen cytotoxic T lymphocytes (CTL) and donor lymphocyte infusion have been tested using ALL-engrafted SCID models [28, 29]. In the future, the reconstitution of immunity from normal HSCs along with leukemia derived from individual patients may allow direct and precise examination of immunotherapy against various types of leukemic cells in vivo.

5.3.3 In Vivo Models of Human CML

Chronic myeloid leukemia (CML) is a clonal multilineage myeloproliferative disorder caused by the constitutive activation of the ABL tyrosine kinase through the *BCR–ABL* oncogene. The *BCR–ABL* oncogene and the chimeric 210-kDa BCR–ABL protein is the product of the Ph chromosome 22q, created by the translocation of the *c-abl* proto-oncogene on human chromosome 9 to chromosome 22, almost invariably in CML. An alternative translocation breakpoint in the *BCR* gene, resulting in a 190-kDa BCR–ABL protein, also occurs in Ph-positive (Ph+) ALL. The presence of the Ph chromosome in multiple lineages, including the granulocytic, monocytic, megakaryocytic, erythroid, and B-lymphoid lineages, suggests that the malignant clone in CML originates in the HSC compartment. Recently, the presence of leukemic colony-forming, in vitro self-renewing granulocyte-macrophage progenitors (GMPs) were reported in patients with CML in blast crisis [30], and similar findings have been reported in mouse models of CML [31], suggesting complex multistep processes in the pathogenesis of this disorder. An animal model of human primary CML that can recapitulate these processes in vivo is required. Some of the first such in vivo models used the SCID and SCID-hu mice as recipient [32–35]. While the infusion of blast crisis CML cell lines such as K562, EM-2, BV173, and KBM-5 [34, 36, 37] into SCID recipients led to disseminated leukemia, similar attempts using primary patient samples resulted in low levels of engraftment even at very high graft doses (up to 1.4×10^8 cells) in the case of chronic phase CML [34, 35]. Similarly, intraperitoneal or subrenal capsule injection of blast crisis CML cells into the human fetal bone implants resulted in poor dissemination of CML to the recipient BM [33, 34]. With the availability of the NOD/SCID strain, multiple groups reported improved levels of long-term engraftment of both chronic phase and blast crisis primary human CML cells [38–41]. Using this system, it was possible to phenotypically restrict CML-initiating cells into the CD34+ fraction. In one study, preselection of patient samples with high frequencies of Ph+ long-term culture-initiating cells (LTC-ICs) was used to improve engraftment efficiencies in both NOD/SCID and

NOD/SCID/β2m^{null} recipients [42]. While these models represent significant progress in the development of in vivo models of primary human CML, xenotransplantation systems that allow the demonstration of self-renewing long-term engrafting CML-initiating cells are required to further characterize CML pathogenesis. The clarification of the complex cellular evolution in which CML disease develops over multiple lineages would require efficient engraftment of highly purified primary CML populations. Development of such models will also allow in vivo examination of therapeutic responses and drug resistance, for instance in the case of imatinib-resistant CML.

5.3.4 In Vivo Models of Human MM

Multiple myeloma (MM) is an aggressive clonal B-cell malignancy originating from the plasma cell. It is characterized by BM plasmacytosis accompanied by lytic bone lesions and excess production of monoclonal immunoglobulin production detectable in serum and/or urine. With currently available treatment modalities including high-dose therapies, the prognosis is dismal, with a median survival of 4 years. The development of in vivo models for MM is crucial for basic understanding of MM pathogenesis as well as for preclinical evaluation of novel therapies. However, an efficient and reproducible engraftment of primary human MM cells has been difficult to achieve. Currently available in vivo models for MM include the injection of pre-established human MM cell lines into NOD/SCID recipients subcutaneously or intravenously [43–45] and the SCID-hu model in which human MM cell lines or primary MM cells are injected into subcutaneous human fetal bone implants in the SCID recipients [46, 47]. In one study, the intravenous injection of KMS-11 MM cell line into NOD/SCID recipients resulted in progressive BM infiltration, hind-leg paralysis due to central nervous system involvement, and the production of monoclonal kappa light chain of human type into the recipient sera [43]. Using this xenograft model, the authors tested the in vivo efficacy of alemtuzumab. In another study, the RPMI8226 human MM cell line was injected subcutaneously into NOD/SCID recipients, resulting in subcutaneous tumor formation [44]. This system was used to test the effects of 1ʹ-acetoxychavicol acetate, a nuclear factor kappa B (NF-κB) inhibitor in vivo. Mitsiades et al. transplanted RPMI8226/S human MM cell line stably expressing green fluorescent protein (GFP), allowing visualization of MM cell infiltration by whole-body fluorescence imaging [45]. Yaccoby et al. first reported the transplantation of primary human MM cells in the SCID-hu system, where MM cells from 12 out of 15 patients were found to engraft [47]. On the other hand, Tassone et al. used the SCID-hu system to monitor the growth and response to chemotherapy of GFP-transduced INA-6 human MM cell line [46]. While these systems represent the currently available in vivo models of MM, they are certainly not the optimal system to study primary human MM engraftment. The majority of studies use cell lines, rather than primary cells, and the engraftment of primary cells requires injection of a large number (1×10^6–1×10^7) of cells. Successful serial transplantation demonstrating the presence of a self-renewing MM stem cell population has not been reported to date. Therefore, a more sensitive xenotransplantation system is required to establish a human primary MM model that recapitulates human MM disease in vivo. NOG mice have been used as recipients of KMM-1 and U-266 MM cell lines [48]. While this has resulted in engraftment of the cell lines, cell doses required were still high (2×10^6–1×10^7). Development of a more sensitive and efficient xenotransplantation model that allows not only the in vivo recapitulation of primary human MM disease but also the examination of MM stem cells by the engraftment of purified primary MM cell populations in limiting dilutions and serial transplantations is needed in the future.

5.4 Human Leukemia Stem Cells (LSCs)

Past paradigms of leukemia development have focused on malignant clones that result in disease due to their highly proliferative nature. However, the presence of developmental hierarchy in leukemia, which parallels that of normal hematopoiesis, has been suggested by clonality studies such as those using specific chromosomal translocations found in certain types of leukemia. These studies have suggested the presence of leukemia stem cells (LSCs) analogous to normal HSCs. The development of xenotransplantation systems with significant levels of human leukemia engraftment has provided the in vivo assay systems required for the identification of putative LSCs prospectively and functionally.

5.4.1 LSCs in Human AML

Bonnet and Dick reported that CD34+CD38– AML cells, not CD34+CD38+ or CD34–AML cells, initiate leukemia after transplantation into NOD/SCID recipients [49]. These findings have been confirmed by other investigators using SCID-repopulating models [50, 51]. In some models, CD34+CD38– AML cells seem to meet all the criteria for stem cells, that is, multilineage development capacity, long-term engraftment capacity, and self-renewal capacity. Especially, transplantation into *scid*-, *Rag1*^{null}-, and *Rag2*^{null}-deficient strains that are also γc^{null} result in efficient engraftment, allowing the examination of the self-renewal capacity of purified candidate LSCs [24]. Currently, one of the most promising approaches is the identification of antigens that can discriminate AML stem cells from normal HSCs. CD123 (IL3-Ra) and CD90 are antigens differentially expressed in AML stem cells and normal HSCs [52, 53]. Hosen et al. reported CD96 as a potential marker specifically expressed in LSCs (CD34+CD38-CD90– cells) but not in normal

HSCs (CD34+CD38–CD90+ cells) [54]. Jordan and colleagues have been studying agents that can selectively eradicate leukemic cells including LSCs (CD34+CD38–CD123+ cells) but spare normal HSCs (CD34+CD38–CD123– cells) [55, 56]. CD44, a physiological E-selectin ligand, is expressed on the surface of LSCs, and LSCs adhere to their niche via CD44-hyaluronic acid binding. Neutralizing antibody against CD44 prevented homing and engraftment of human primary LSCs [57]. Intriguingly, blocking of CD44 signal resulted in the induction of differentiation/maturation of leukemic blasts. Similar findings were confirmed using mouse leukemia model where *Bcr–abl*-transduced CD44$^{-/-}$ murine hematopoietic stem progenitors exhibited defective homing capacity resulting in decreased engraftment [58].

Although the microenvironment including osteoblasts, endothelial cells, or fibroblasts are of mouse origin, xenograft models using *scid* mice enabled investigators to analyze the interaction between stem cells and their niche. The pioneer work by Lapidot and colleagues clarified the role of SDF-1 and CXCR-4 in mobilization and homing of normal HSCs and leukemic cells using a scid-repopulating assay [59, 60]. Although human AML cells express lower and heterogenous level CXCR-4 on their surface, the blockade of signaling between these two molecules by neutralizing antibody against CXCR-4 and SDF-1 inhibited the growth of AML in NOD/SCID mice. As LSCs retain their quiescence and self-renewal capacity in the mouse microenvironment, further studies would be expected to identify other molecular mechanism underlying stem–niche interaction.

5.4.2 LSCs in Human ALL

In contrast to AML stem cells, LSCs and stem cell hierarchy of pediatric B-ALL have not been clarified. Within B-precursor ALL, LSCs with distinct chromosomal abnormalities might exhibit different biology or might have different origins of leukemogenesis. LSCs need to be determined not only based on ontogenic classification but also on genetic subtypes.

Using in vitro colony assay and fluorescence in situ hybridization (FISH) analysis, Hotfilder et al. reported that LSCs are present in CD34+CD19– fraction in Ph+ ALL and MLL-AF4 ALL [61]. FISH analyses revealed that 50–60% CD34+CD19– cells derived from ALL patient BM possess these leukemic translocations. In the MEC assay, CD34+CD19– cells generate G, M, GM, E, and mixed colonies, while CD34+CD19+ cells could not differentiate into myeloid lineage.

Castor et al. investigated the functional heterogeneity within three distinct genetic subtypes of B-ALL: p210 Ph+ ALL, p190 Ph+ ALL, and ETV6/RUNX1 ALL [62]. The frequency of translocation in CD34+CD38–CD19+ and CD34+CD38–CD19– cells is different among three different subtypes. The vast majority of CD34+CD38–CD19+ cells carry the t(12;21) translocation generating the *ETV6/RUNX1* (*TEL/AML1*) fusion gene, while CD34+CD38–CD19– cells do not. These findings suggest that the expression of CD19 determines the functional characteristics of primitive B-ALL cells.

Consistent with these observations, B-ALL patient BM CD34+CD38– cell populations have been found to contain cells with clonogenic leukemic T-cell receptor rearrangement [63]. Therefore, CD19 may serve as an antigen allowing the discrimination between LSCs and normal HSCs, allowing successful purging of LSCs from autologous grafts. At the same time, the significance of CD38 expression within CD34+CD19+ and CD34+CD19– populations in primary B-ALL must be further clarified using highly purified cells in sensitive xenotransplantation systems.

5.5 Summary

The development of in vivo models of human hematopoietic malignancies has occurred concomitantly with that of highly immunodeficient mouse strains that act as xenotransplantation recipients. The establishment of sensitive and reproducible xenotransplantation assays has allowed the in vivo examination of human leukemia biology and the identification and characterization of LSCs. Technical advances such as intrafacial vein injection in newborn recipients and intrafemoral injection in adults have also facilitated successful engraftment of highly purified primary human cells. These models of human hematopoietic malignancies are expected to provide new insights into leukemia biology and pathophysiology and contribute to the development of novel therapies, bridging the gap between the bench and the bedside.

References

1. Bosma, G.C., Custer, R.P. & Bosma, M.J. A severe combined immunodeficiency mutation in the mouse. *Nature* **301**, 527–530 (1983).
2. Mombaerts, P. et al. RAG-1-deficient mice have no mature B and T lymphocytes. *Cell* **68**, 869–877 (1992).
3. Shinkai, Y. et al. RAG-2-deficient mice lack mature lymphocytes owing to inability to initiate V(D)J rearrangement. *Cell* **68**, 855–867 (1992).
4. Shultz, L.D. et al. Multiple defects in innate and adaptive immunologic function in NOD/LtSz-scid mice. *J Immunol* **154**, 180–191 (1995).
5. Shultz, L.D. et al. NOD/LtSz-Rag1null mice: an immunodeficient and radioresistant model for engraftment of human hematolymphoid cells, HIV infection, and adoptive transfer of NOD mouse diabetogenic T cells. *J Immunol* **164**, 2496–2507 (2000).
6. Shultz, L.D. et al. NOD/LtSz-Rag1nullPfpnull mice: a new model system with increased levels of human peripheral leukocyte and hematopoietic stem-cell engraftment. *Transplantation* **76**, 1036–1042 (2003).
7. Christianson, S.W. et al. Enhanced human CD4+ T cell engraftment in beta2-microglobulin-deficient NOD-scid mice. *J Immunol* **158**, 3578–3586 (1997).

8. Cao, X. et al. Defective lymphoid development in mice lacking expression of the common cytokine receptor gamma chain. *Immunity* **2**, 223–238 (1995).
9. Sugamura, K. et al. The interleukin-2 receptor gamma chain: its role in the multiple cytokine receptor complexes and T cell development in XSCID. *Annu Rev Immunol* **14**, 179–205 (1996).
10. Ito, M. et al. NOD/SCID/gamma(c)(null) mouse: an excellent recipient mouse model for engraftment of human cells. *Blood* **100**, 3175–3182 (2002).
11. Shultz, L.D. et al. Human lymphoid and myeloid cell development in NOD/LtSz-scid IL2R gamma null mice engrafted with mobilized human hemopoietic stem cells. *J Immunol* **174**, 6477–6489 (2005).
12. Ishikawa, F. et al. Development of functional human blood and immune systems in NOD/SCID/IL2 receptor {gamma} chain(null) mice. *Blood* **106**, 1565–1573 (2005).
13. Honma, Y., Ishii, Y., Sassa, T. & Asahi, K. Treatment of human promyelocytic leukemia in the SCID mouse model with cotylenin A, an inducer of myelomonocytic differentiation of leukemia cells. *Leuk Res* **27**, 1019–1025 (2003).
14. Kiser, M. et al. Oncogene-dependent engraftment of human myeloid leukemia cells in immunosuppressed mice. *Leukemia* **15**, 814–818 (2001).
15. Pirruccello, S.J. et al. OMA-AML-1: a leukemic myeloid cell line with CD34+ progenitor and CD15+ spontaneously differentiating cell compartments. *Blood* **80**, 1026–1032 (1992).
16. Terpstra, W. et al. Conditions for engraftment of human acute myeloid leukemia (AML) in SCID mice. *Leukemia* **9**, 1573–1577 (1995).
17. Lapidot, T. et al. A cell initiating human acute myeloid leukaemia after transplantation into SCID mice. *Nature* **367**, 645–648 (1994).
18. Ailles, L.E., Gerhard, B., Kawagoe, H. & Hogge, D.E. Growth characteristics of acute myelogenous leukemia progenitors that initiate malignant hematopoiesis in nonobese diabetic/severe combined immunodeficient mice. *Blood* **94**, 1761–1772 (1999).
19. Pearce, D.J. et al. AML engraftment in the NOD/SCID assay reflects the outcome of AML: implications for our understanding of the heterogeneity of AML. *Blood* **107**, 1166–1173 (2006).
20. Lumkul, R. et al. Human AML cells in NOD/SCID mice: engraftment potential and gene expression. *Leukemia* **16**, 1818–1826 (2002).
21. Yalcintepe, L., Frankel, A.E. & Hogge, D.E. Expression of interleukin-3 receptor subunits on defined subpopulations of acute myeloid leukemia blasts predicts the cytotoxicity of diphtheria toxin interleukin-3 fusion protein against malignant progenitors that engraft in immunodeficient mice. *Blood* **108**, 3530–3537 (2006).
22. Feuring-Buske, M. et al. Improved engraftment of human acute myeloid leukemia progenitor cells in beta 2-microglobulin-deficient NOD/SCID mice and in NOD/SCID mice transgenic for human growth factors. *Leukemia* **17**, 760–763 (2003).
23. Ishikawa, fF. et al. Chemotherapy-resistant human AML stem cells home to and engraft within the bone marrow endosteal region. *Nature Biotechnology* **25**, 1315–1321 (2007).
24. Ninomiya, M. et al. Homing, proliferation and survival sites of human leukemia cells in vivo in immunodeficient mice. *Leukemia* **21**, 136–142 (2007).
25. Liem, N.L. et al. Characterization of childhood acute lymphoblastic leukemia xenograft models for the preclinical evaluation of new therapies. *Blood* **103**, 3905–3914 (2004).
26. Nijmeijer, B.A. et al. Monitoring of engraftment and progression of acute lymphoblastic leukemia in individual NOD/SCID mice. *Experimental Hematology* **29**, 322–329 (2001).
27. Schimmel, K.J., Nijmeijer, B.A., van Schie, M.L., Falkenburg, J.H. & Guchelaar, H.J. Limited antitumor-effect associated with toxicity of the experimental cytotoxic drug cyclopentenyl cytosine in NOD/scid mice with acute lymphoblastic leukemia. *Leuk Res* (2007).
28. Nijmeijer, B.A., van Schie, M.L., Verzaal, P., Willemze, R. & Falkenburg, J.H. Responses to donor lymphocyte infusion for acute lymphoblastic leukemia may be determined by both

qualitative and quantitative limitations of antileukemic T-cell responses as observed in an animal model for human leukemia. *Exp Hematol* **33**, 1172–1181 (2005).
29. Nijmeijer, B.A., Willemze, R. & Falkenburg, J.H. An animal model for human cellular immunotherapy: specific eradication of human acute lymphoblastic leukemia by cytotoxic T lymphocytes in NOD/scid mice. *Blood* **100**, 654–660 (2002).
30. Jamieson, C.H. et al. Granulocyte-macrophage progenitors as candidate leukemic stem cells in blast-crisis CML. *N Engl J Med* **351**, 657–667 (2004).
31. Jaiswal, S. et al. Expression of BCR/ABL and BCL-2 in myeloid progenitors leads to myeloid leukemias. *Proc Natl Acad Sci U S A* **100**, 10002–10007 (2003).
32. Hoyle, C.F. & Negrin, R.S. Engraftment of chronic myeloid leukemia in SCID mice. *Hematol Oncol* **16**, 87–100 (1998).
33. Namikawa, R., Ueda, R. & Kyoizumi, S. Growth of human myeloid leukemias in the human marrow environment of SCID-hu mice. *Blood* **82**, 2526–2536 (1993).
34. Sawyers, C.L., Gishizky, M.L., Quan, S., Golde, D.W. & Witte, O.N. Propagation of human blastic myeloid leukemias in the SCID mouse. *Blood* **79**, 2089–2098 (1992).
35. Sirard, C. et al. Normal and leukemic SCID-repopulating cells (SRC) coexist in the bone marrow and peripheral blood from CML patients in chronic phase, whereas leukemic SRC are detected in blast crisis. *Blood* **87**, 1539–1548 (1996).
36. Beran, M. et al. Biological properties and growth in SCID mice of a new myelogenous leukemia cell line (KBM-5) derived from chronic myelogenous leukemia cells in the blastic phase. *Cancer Res* **53**, 3603–3610 (1993).
37. Skorski, T., Nieborowska-Skorska, M. & Calabretta, B. A model of Ph' positive chronic myeloid leukemia-blast crisis cell line growth in immunodeficient SCID mice. *Folia Histochem Cytobiol* **30**, 91–96 (1992).
38. Dazzi, F. et al. The kinetics and extent of engraftment of chronic myelogenous leukemia cells in non-obese diabetic/severe combined immunodeficiency mice reflect the phase of the donor's disease: an in vivo model of chronic myelogenous leukemia biology. *Blood* **92**, 1390–1396 (1998).
39. Lewis, I.D., McDiarmid, L.A., Samels, L.M., To, L.B. & Hughes, T.P. Establishment of a reproducible model of chronic-phase chronic myeloid leukemia in NOD/SCID mice using blood-derived mononuclear or CD34+ cells. *Blood* **91**, 630–640 (1998).
40. Verstegen, M.M., Cornelissen, J.J., Terpstra, W., Wagemaker, G. & Wognum, A.W. Multilineage outgrowth of both malignant and normal hemopoietic progenitor cells from individual chronic myeloid leukemia patients in immunodeficient mice. *Leukemia* **13**, 618–628 (1999).
41. Wang, J.C. et al. High level engraftment of NOD/SCID mice by primitive normal and leukemic hematopoietic cells from patients with chronic myeloid leukemia in chronic phase. *Blood* **91**, 2406–2414 (1998).
42. Eisterer, W. et al. Different subsets of primary chronic myeloid leukemia stem cells engraft immunodeficient mice and produce a model of the human disease. *Leukemia* **19**, 435–441 (2005).
43. Carlo-Stella, C. et al. CD52 antigen expressed by malignant plasma cells can be targeted by alemtuzumab in vivo in NOD/SCID mice. *Exp Hematol* **34**, 721–727 (2006).
44. Ito, K. et al. 1′-acetoxychavicol acetate is a novel nuclear factor kappaB inhibitor with significant activity against multiple myeloma in vitro and in vivo. *Cancer Res* **65**, 4417–4424 (2005).
45. Mitsiades, C.S. et al. Fluorescence imaging of multiple myeloma cells in a clinically relevant SCID/NOD in vivo model: biologic and clinical implications. *Cancer Res* **63**, 6689–6696 (2003).
46. Tassone, P. et al. A clinically relevant SCID-hu in vivo model of human multiple myeloma. *Blood* **106**, 713–716 (2005).
47. Yaccoby, S., Barlogie, B. & Epstein, J. Primary myeloma cells growing in SCID-hu mice: a model for studying the biology and treatment of myeloma and its manifestations. *Blood* **92**, 2908–2913 (1998).

48. Dewan, M.Z. et al. Prompt tumor formation and maintenance of constitutive NF-kappaB activity of multiple myeloma cells in NOD/SCID/gammacnull mice. *Cancer Sci* **95**, 564–568 (2004).
49. Bonnet, D. & Dick, J.E. Human acute myeloid leukemia is organized as a hierarchy that originates from a primitive hematopoietic cell. *Nat Med* **3**, 730–737 (1997).
50. Feuring-Buske, M. & Hogge, D.E. Hoechst 33342 efflux identifies a subpopulation of cytogenetically normal CD34(+)CD38(–) progenitor cells from patients with acute myeloid leukemia. *Blood* **97**, 3882–3889 (2001).
51. Sperr, W.R. et al. Human leukaemic stem cells: a novel target of therapy. *European journal of clinical investigation* **34 Suppl 2**, 31–40 (2004).
52. Buccisano, F. et al. CD90/Thy-1 is preferentially expressed on blast cells of high risk acute myeloid leukaemias. *Br J Haematol* **125**, 203–212 (2004).
53. Jordan, C.T. et al. The interleukin-3 receptor alpha chain is a unique marker for human acute myelogenous leukemia stem cells. *Leukemia* **14**, 1777–1784 (2000).
54. Hosen, N. et al. CD96 is a leukemic stem cell-specific marker in human acute myeloid leukemia. *Proc Natl Acad Sci U S A* **104**, 11008–11013 (2007).
55. Guzman, M.L. et al. The sesquiterpene lactone parthenolide induces apoptosis of human acute myelogenous leukemia stem and progenitor cells. *Blood* **105**, 4163–4169 (2005).
56. Guzman, M.L. et al. Preferential induction of apoptosis for primary human leukemic stem cells. *Proc Natl Acad Sci U S A* **99**, 16220–16225 (2002).
57. Jin, L., Hope, K.J., Zhai, Q., Smadja-Joffe, F. & Dick, J.E. Targeting of CD44 eradicates human acute myeloid leukemic stem cells. *Nat Med* **12**, 1167–1174 (2006).
58. Krause, D.S., Lazarides, K., von Andrian, U.H. & Van Etten, R.A. Requirement for CD44 in homing and engraftment of BCR-ABL-expressing leukemic stem cells. *Nat Med* **12**, 1175–1180 (2006).
59. Dar, A., Kollet, O. & Lapidot, T. Mutual, reciprocal SDF-1/CXCR4 interactions between hematopoietic and bone marrow stromal cells regulate human stem cell migration and development in NOD/SCID chimeric mice. *Exp Hematol* **34**, 967–975 (2006).
60. Tavor, S. et al. CXCR4 regulates migration and development of human acute myelogenous leukemia stem cells in transplanted NOD/SCID mice. *Cancer Res* **64**, 2817–2824 (2004).
61. Hotfilder, M. et al. Leukemic stem cells in childhood high-risk ALL/t(9;22) and t(4;11) are present in primitive lymphoid-restricted CD34+CD19- cells. *Cancer Res* **65**, 1442–1449 (2005).
62. Castor, A. et al. Distinct patterns of hematopoietic stem cell involvement in acute lymphoblastic leukemia. *Nat Med* **11**, 630–637 (2005).
63. George, A.A. et al. Detection of leukemic cells in the CD34(+)CD38(-) bone marrow progenitor population in children with acute lymphoblastic leukemia. *Blood* **97**, 3925–3930 (2001).

Chapter 6
Dietary Restriction: A Model System Probing the Cell Fate Decision Between Cancer and Senescence

Robin P. Ertl and David E. Harrison

Contents

6.1 Introduction

A major aspect of cancer is unregulated cell proliferation. Yet, in general as organisms age, their cells lose the ability to proliferate, which leads to cellular senescence (Hayflick 1965; Smith and Pereira-Smith 1996). It is important to remember that the ability of stem cells to repopulate a tissue in vivo requires more than just proliferation. It requires a coordinated pattern of homing, engraftment, self-renewal, differentiation, and proliferation. In this chapter, all of these necessary functions are referred to collectively as repopulating ability (RA). The loss of RA can cause severe clinical problems with age, such as anemia (Robinson 2003; Guralnik et al. 2004; Penninx et al. 2004). There are treatments that can increase RA and delay senescence. Unfortunately, most of

---

D.E. Harrison
The Jackson Laboratory, Bar Harbor, ME 04609, USA
david.harrison@jax.org

S. Li (ed.), *Mouse Models of Human Blood Cancers*,
DOI: 10.1007/978-0-387-69132-9_6, © Springer Science+Business Media, LLC 2008

these treatments also increase the risk of cancer (Campisi 2003; Pardal et al. 2005; Beausejour and Campisi 2006). The maximal potential lifespan of an organism, therefore, seems to depend on balancing the need to maintain the RA versus the potential risk that cells will transform.

The exact mechanisms of aging are largely unknown. However, we do know that the balance of these two cell fates—cell senescence versus cancer—depends, in part, on the type of cellular damage present. General cellular damage can be a marker for cellular turnover or apoptosis, and accumulated genetic damage may lead to cellular senescence or cancer. To avoid the lineage of genetically damaged cells from having systemic consequences, the organism can either repair the damage or minimize the effect by shutting down the cell (Fig. 6.1). DNA repair is a major field and a topic for other reviews. The focus of this chapter is the cellular response when DNA repair is insufficient and damaged cells must try to minimize deleterious effects by balancing risks.

The central role of stem cells in cancer has come under increasing scrutiny. Krivtsov et al. (2006) showed that it is possible to generate cancerous cells from definitive hematopoietic cells by a single transposition. In general, though, more than a single mutation is needed to transform a cell line (Pardal, Clarke and Morrison 2003; Pardal et al. 2005; Krivtsov et al. 2006; Giordano et al. 2007). It is unlikely that all the requisite mutations will occur within the lifespan of a single cell. Thus, to acquire the several mutations necessary for transformation into a carcinoma, mutations must occur in cells that have a self-renewal capacity, such as, stem cells.

Tumor suppressors may be the mechanism by which this cell fate decision is regulated. Recent studies have shown that in hematopoietic stem cells (HSCs) (Janzen et al. 2006), pancreatic islets (Krishnamurthy et al. 2006), and neural stem cells (Molofsky et al. 2005, 2006), a decrease in the tumor suppressor $p16^{INK4a}$ results in an increase in stem cell/precursor cell RA. Conversely, as $p16^{INK4a}$ increases with age, there is a decrease in RA. The tumor suppressor p53 also exhibits a similar inverse relationship between a tissue's RA and gene

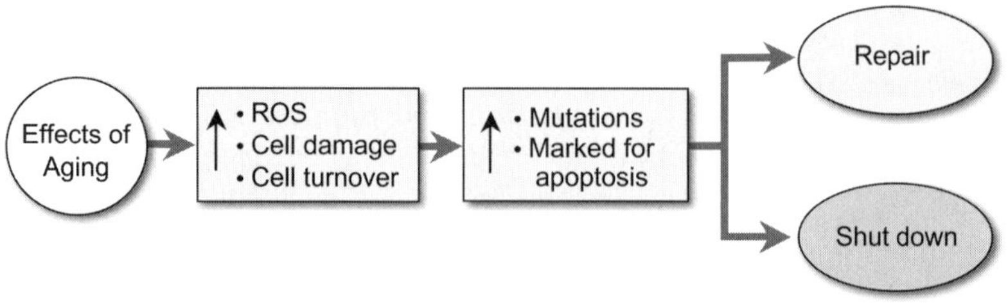

Fig. 6.1 Cell fate decision imposed by damage. Effects of aging result from lifelong exposure to damaging conditions such as reactive oxygen species (ROS) leading to mutations and apoptosis. This damage forces a cell fate decision: to avoid cancer, cells must either repair the damage or, if the damage is irreparable, shut down

expression (Tyner et al. 2002; TeKippe, Harrison and Chen 2003; Maier et al. 2004; Dumble et al. 2007; Gatza et al. 2007).

Recent studies of $p16^{INK4a}$ expression in stem cells indicate that its highest levels occur in the most primitive precursors and that expression of tumor suppressors increases with age (Molofsky et al. 2005, 2006; Janzen et al. 2006; Krishnamurthy et al. 2006). This is consistent with the hypothesis that most cancerous cell lines are derived from stem cells acquiring multiple mutations and that induction of tumor suppressors with age is necessary to obviate the effects of accumulated, spontaneous mutations. The lack of induction of $p16^{INK4a}$ in less primitive progenitors is potentially explained by the fact that they exist in the body for a shorter period of time, acquire fewer mutations, and are ultimately replaced by new lineages derived from differentiation of the most primitive precursors.

Mice are an ideal organism in which to study the relationships between senescence and cancer. With age, they exhibit an increased incidence of spontaneous cancers, a general decrease in RA, and altered stem cell functions. The fact that they have a short lifespan—aging 30 times faster than humans—and are relatively small makes longitudinal studies of mammalian aging practical in a modest space. In addition, the full genomic sequence is known for several strains of mice, many antibodies and other reagents are available, cell surface markers to identify specific cell types are known, and many assays and techniques have been worked out in detail (Information available through The Jackson Laboratory public website, www.jax.org). In this chapter, we will examine stem cell aging in several mouse models and discuss possible mechanisms regulating the balance between cancer and senescence.

6.2 Current Paradigm

The recent studies that utilized $p16^{INK4a}$ knockouts (KOs) caused Beausejour and Campisi (2006), Janzen et al. (2006), Krishnamurthy et al. (2006), and Molofsky et al. (2006) to propose a model governing the cell fate decision which, in part, determines the maximal lifespan of an organism; their similar models are summarized in Fig. 6.2. These models relate the regulation of stem cell proliferative ability by $p16^{INK4a}$ to the intricate balance between cancer risk and cellular senescence. This bimodal fate can be envisioned as walking down a path that runs along a mountain ridge. To each side there is a steep chasm, and as we go along, the path narrows. To reach our maximal lifespan, we try to balance the two fates: If we loose our balance and go to the right, we fall off the path and die due to lack of proliferation leading to senescence. If we lose our balance in the other direction, while we increase proliferation, we fall off the path and die from cancer. Thus, to reach the maximal lifespan, we need to allow just enough proliferation to avoid senescence, yet the least proliferation possible to avoid cancer. The longer we live, though, the narrower the path becomes

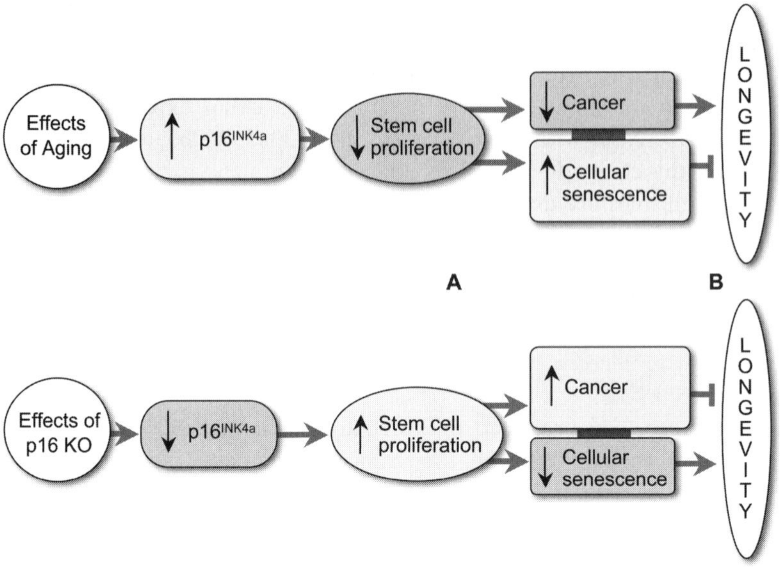

Fig. 6.2 Current paradigm. The recent articles of Beausejour and Campisi (2006), Janzen et al. (2006), Krishnamurthy et al. (2006), and Molofsky et al. (2006) have proposed a model governing the cell fate decision that balances the consequences of cancer risk and cellular senescence as a function of cell proliferation (**A**) regulated by P16. This balance, in part, determines the longevity (**B**)

and the more difficult it is to avoid either senescence or cancer due to the accumulation of spontaneous mutations.

6.3 Cancer, Senescence, and Evolution

For any theoretical relationship between cancer and senescence to be more than a laboratory artifact created by random chance in a particular species, the relationship must have evolved as a result of positive selective pressure or pleiotropy via an evolutionary stable strategy. Aranda-Anzaldo and Dent (2007) suggested that cancer and senescence are not viable targets of selective pressures because, through evolutionary history, these events usually occur post-reproduction. They cite, as an example, feral mice with 90% mortality by 40 weeks of age, yet with little or no evidence of cancer at that age. That does not mean that the feral mice cannot get cancer; however, it occurs so late in life that it does not exert enough selective pressure to overcome genetic drift. Aranda-Anzaldo and Dent (2007) suggest that tumor suppressors such as p53 and p16^{INK4a} in the Campisi model (Fig. 6.2) are primarily required during development to eliminate cells that have mutated, failed to replicate properly, or are not required for later stages of development. Their conclusions depend in part on two factors: (1) the occurrence of cancer in juvenile or reproducing animals was rare in evolutionary history and (2) prior to the industrial revolution, there were no cancer-causing environmental factors that required tumor suppressors for the survival of young adults.

In fact, these questions are far from settled. The data indicating that cancer is rare in juvenile and reproducing animals are based on organisms that have already evolved intricate systems of DNA repair, tumor suppression, and apoptosis. The deletion of only one of these pathways (e.g., p53) dramatically reduces lifespan, with cancers that develop by 6 months of age or less, an age at which it would significantly decrease reproductive fitness.

While the biological burden of cancer-causing mutagens is commonly associated with discharge of pollutants starting with the industrial revolution, in fact, the greatest burden is from the environmental factors and the food we consume (Ames and Gold 1998), with the most potent mutagens occurring naturally. These mutagens are thought to have evolved by what is referred to as plant–animal warfare (Gonzalez and Nebert 1990). Plants, to expand their habitat, developed natural defense mechanisms to limit predation. Animals, to continue to occupy that niche, then evolved detoxification pathways to these compounds, thus causing plants to generate ever more potent mutagens, in a cycle of adaptation and evolution that continues.

Compared to many animals, mammals mature and reproduce slowly. Through evolutionary history, maturing and reproducing mammals were faced with the normal background mutation rate and the consequences of naturally occurring mutagens. These could have provided the selective pressure required to develop the complex pathways of tumor suppression and DNA repair needed to maintain genomic stability and postpone cancers until after the necessary reproductive period.

The mutation rate and the incidence of cancer are, therefore, reasonable targets upon which evolutionary forces can act. In fact, the mutation rate is thought to be highly regulated: a certain number of mutations must occur, prior to reproductive fitness, to provide natural selection with the needed genetic diversity in subsequent generations. However, excessive mutations will have deleterious, if not lethal, effects.

Research into the age when senescence occurs, and whether senescence is a valid target of evolutionary selective pressure, has similarly been considered in species that have already undergone significant evolutionary selection to determine their lifespans. The selective pressure that determined the age at which cellular senescence occurs may have been the pressure to ensure fitness during reproduction—that is to say senescence is caused by exhaustion or decline of mechanisms evolved to be present until the age-specific force of selection approaches zero. In the mouse, this age would be near the end of the female reproductive lifespan. The feral mouse, for example, must avoid predators during its reproductive period, so diseases of aging, such as muscular atrophy, are not expressed until reproductive fitness declines. In the case of cellular senescence, a number of cellular characteristics may be functionally linked. The forces of evolution may exert pressure so that all processes in the linked pathways are functional until an age just prior to the end of reproductive fitness. Such linkages may explain, for instance, why HSCs can be transplanted and repopulate the marrow far more than would be needed in several mouse lifetimes.

Some post-mitotic organisms do not appear to develop cancer, having neither the opportunity, with no adult cell turnover, nor the time, given their short lifespan. Yet, they express p53. This indicates, as Aranda-Anzaldo and Dent (2007) suggest, that p53 arose due to developmental requirements. However, in mammals, cancer and senescence are in an equilibrium determined by evolutionarily selective pressures. P53 may have been altered through evolutionary history to regulate the proliferative ability in response to mutations throughout the entire lifecycle, just as p53 regulates proliferative ability and apoptosis during development of post-mitotic organisms. As organisms evolved, the need for continuous cell turnover throughout their life cycles, there arose the need to mitigate the vulnerabilities to cancers caused by cell turnover. If, in fact, there was no natural selection on the balance between cancers and senescence, then this relationship should vary with the strain examined as a function of genetic drift. The rates of both cancer and senescence, however, correlate closely in many species, suggesting evolution directly by natural selection or indirectly by pleiotropy, not random drift.

Cancer and senescence are both linked by the proliferative ability upon which both depend. As we propose below, the cell fate decision may not be black and white, but rather a gray scale of possibilities where the balance between cancer and senescence exists throughout an organism's lifespan: As the organism ages, there are fewer options, forcing a cell fate decision, similar to the metaphor given earlier where the path along the precipice narrows the further you progress down the path. In this model, it is useful to think of both cancer and senescence as outcomes of processes continually altered over the lifetime of the organism—that cellular senescence is the exhaustion of a lineage of proliferating cells and that cancer results from the accumulation of mutations which short-circuit the normal mechanisms halting proliferation. The accumulation of mutations leading to cancer may occur throughout the lifespan of the organism. The need to have sufficient proliferation to avoid senescence, but at the same time defend against the increased mutations associated with that proliferation, may be the selective pressure responsible for the development of cancer defense systems. The breakdown of these systems, post-reproduction, leads to diseases of aging.

6.4 The Role of p16 in Mice

The current data from p16^{INK4a} studies in mice are consistent with the model proposed in Fig. 6.2 for regulating the balance between cancer and senescence. Janzen et al. (2006), Krishnamurthy et al. (2006), and Molofsky et al. (2006)

found that, with age, $p16^{INK4a}$ levels increased in precursor/stem cell subpopulations to a greater extent than in differentiated cells. This increase correlated with a decrease in RA while RA increased in $p16^{INK4a}$ KO mice. The decrease in $p16^{INK4a}$ and increase in RA in KO mice was accompanied by an increase in cancer incidence. These results suggest that the increase in $p16^{INK4a}$ with age is a preprogrammed response decreasing proliferative ability to mitigate the increase in cancer risk that occurs with age.

Janzen et al. (2006) examined these trends in the primitive precursors of hematopoiesis in C57BL/6 (B6) mice, long-term HSCs (LT-HSCs). Using the BrdU assay, they observed a decrease in the turnover of LT-HSCs with age commensurate with the increase in $p16^{INK4a}$. In B6 KO $p16^{INK4a}$ mice, where there is a decrease in $p16^{INK4a}$ levels, they found a significant increase in HSC turnover. This measure of cell proliferation is a composite of both differentiation into definitive cell types and self-renewal. The increase in Hes-1, a downstream effector of Notch signaling associated with self-renewal, combined with the increase in the number of LT-HSCs present in the KO mice, indicates that part of the observed increase in proliferation is because of the increase in self-renewal. These data are consistent with the concept that increased $p16^{INK4a}$ expression is a preprogrammed response to age post-reproduction. However, this concept contradicts the idea that such responses cannot evolve in the life cycle during a period with little or no selective pressure. Is the increase in $p16^{INK4a}$ then a response to other changes with age that occur earlier in the lifecycle?

In an especially rigorous measure of RA, transplanting bone marrow (BM) serially into successive recipients causes a tremendous stress on precursor cells due to increased demand for proliferation and self-renewal. A single serial transplantation causes a decline in HSC functional abilities in B6 mice that is far greater than a lifetime of normal function (Harrison, Astle and Stone 1989; Harrison et al. 1993; Chen, Astle and Harrison 2000; Yuan et al. 2005). After three successive serial transplantations, Janzen et al. (2006) found an increase in the $p16^{INK4a}$ expression along with a decrease in the number of leukocytes. In the $p16^{INK4a}$ KO mice under the same serial transplant conditions, leukocytes numbers were increased compared to similarly aged controls (Janzen et al. 2006). These data support the contention that $p16^{INK4a}$ is, in fact, suppressing both the proliferation and the risk of cancer in these serially transplanted HSCs. This tumor suppressor is not the entire answer, though, as the number of leukocytes also decreases after serial transplantation in $p16^{INK4a}$ KO mice, albeit to a lesser extent, suggesting that p53 and/or other factors are involved in this cell fate decision.

This increase in RA, caused by the decrease in $p16^{INK4a}$ in the KO mice, is thought to be a contributing factor to the decrease in apoptosis and the subsequent increase in survival after serial transplantation. Two fundamental questions remain: (1) What causes the increase in $p16^{INK4a}$ levels? The observed increase in $p16^{INK4a}$ levels may be a consequence of normal aging; however, if this increase occurs only at an age with little or no evolutionary forces at work, how did this increase evolve? It also may be a response to the partial exhaustion of proliferative ability or a response to the mutation rate and the risk of cancer. Are these processes active during earlier stages of the life history and thus under evolutionary selective pressures? The observed increase in p16^{INK4a} after serial transplantation may be a response to the mutation rate rather than the aging of the cell lineage. (2) If these processes are active during other parts of our life cycle, do we spend our entire life balancing this cell fate decision or can this decision be delayed in order to lengthen lifespan?

Thus far, all studies that examined p16^{INK4a} in precursors/stem cells in a variety of organs suggest that aspects of RA are regulated by p16^{INK4a}. However, while the reported measures of B6 HSC RA (discussed above) are consistent with this theory, not all measures of HSC RA decrease at times when p16^{INK4a} levels are known to increase. Unlike other strains, in B6 mice, the RA of total marrow goes up with age (Chen, Astle and Harrison 2000) while RA per HSC remains fairly constant (Rossi et al. 2005; Ertl et al. 2008). This occurs at an age when Janzen et al. reported that p16^{INK4a} levels were increasing in B6 mice (Janzen et al. 2006). We do know that there is an increase in lifespan in B6 mice compared to most other strains. Thus, the increase in RA of total marrow with age might be the result of a compensatory mechanism. Combined, these data suggest that the regulation of this pathway must be more complex than shown in Fig. 6.2.

6.5 The Role of p53 in Mice

The tumor suppressor p53 is thought to cause apoptosis, leading to a decreased RA with age at the tissue level, thus bringing about organ or organismal senescence. Similar to p16^{INK4a}, p53 concentration showed an inverse relationship to RA at the organ level. Reduced p53 activity in p53$^{-/-}$mutants was associated with twice as many LT-HSCs that gave rise to 37% more 9-day spleen colony forming units (CFU-S), along with an increase in the number of proliferating HSCs and hematopoietic progenitors (TeKippe, Harrison and Chen 2003; Dumble et al. 2007; Gatza et al. 2007; Table 6.1). The RA of transplanted BM from p53-deficient mice is two- to four-fold greater than for controls, an advantage that increased with the time after transplant. This was in part due to the two- to three-fold increase in the number of donor LT-HSCs present in the recipient BM (TeKippe, Harrison and Chen 2003). Importantly, decreasing the p53 expression to increase HSC function has a severe cost—only half of transplant recipients survive after 4 months, and they are all dead by 8 months, time points at which HSC recipients usually survive. In the genetic mutant p53$^{+/m}$, which has greater in vivo concentrations of p53 than wild-type mice, there was reduced marrow cellularity and atrophy (Dumble et al. 2007). At these higher levels of p53, the numbers of HSCs in old mice were reduced when compared to wild-type controls. When these p53$^{+/m}$ HSCs were transplanted into lethally

Table 6.1 Relationships among p53 dosage, longevity, cancer, and hematopoietic stem cell (HSC) function

	Donor marrow composition*			Recipient marrow composition†		Effects of genotype on donor marrow function				
p53 genotype	BMC 10^6	CFU-S, day 9	LT-HSC‡	Percent survival	LT-HSC‡	Median longevity (weeks)§	Cancer incidence (%)Δ	Aged HSC no. (%)**	Aged HSC proliferation (%)††	Aged HSC reconstitution (%)‡‡
p53 −/−	231	20.2	0.010%	44%	0.018%	18	100	ND	ND	ND
p53 +/−	ND	ND	ND	ND	ND	52	90	0.22	0.070	80
p53 +/+	296	14.7	0.004%	92%	0.006%	118	45	0.15	0.029	59
p53 +/m	ND	ND	ND	ND	ND	96	6	0.08	0.019	31

CFU-S, colony forming units; LT-HSCs, long-term HSCs.
The first six columns are data from TeKippe, Harrison and Chen (2003). Five-month data represents result of a competitive repopulation study. The next five columns are from Dumble et al. (2007).
*4–6 males at 2–5 months.
†5 months post-transplantation.
‡Lin^-, Sca^+, $cKit^+$, $CD34^-$.
§Age in weeks at which 50% of a p53 cohort died.
ΔPercentage of mice in a p53 cohort that develop cancer in a lifespan.
**Percentage of HSCs (lin^-, Sca^+, $cKit^+$, $Flk\text{-}2^+$) in total marrow cells from aged (18 to 20-months old) mice.
†Percentage of proliferating HSCs in total marrow cells.
‡‡Percentage of hematopoietic system reconstituted by 500 aged HSCs from donors of a given p53 genotype 12 weeks after transplantation.

irradiated recipients, they exhibited reduced homing and engraftment (Dumble et al. 2007).

As mentioned in the previous section, the p16^{INK4a} data indicate that it is not the sole regulator of the balance between cancer and senescence. The inverse correlation between p53 and apoptosis, another regulator of cell proliferation, suggests that there may be several critical regulators of this cell fate decision.

6.6 Does Dietary Restriction Break the Paradigm?

Insights into the regulation of cell proliferation are found in mice treated with lifelong diet restriction (DR). DR is a treatment that reduces food intake to about 70% of the normal diet. Even at these reduced levels, the NIH-31 (4% fat) diet provides all the essential nutrients without the need for dietary supplements. With lifelong DR, there is a significant increase in lifespan concurrent with a reduction in the incidence of cancer (Bronson and Lipman 1991; Blackwell et al. 1995; Turturro et al. 2002) and many other markers of aging (Miller and Harrison 1985; Effros et al. 1991; Masoro 1993; Luan et al. 1995; Chen, Astle and Harrison 1998, 2003). For the paradigm in Fig. 6.2 to hold, the risk of cancer and cellular senescence must be inversely correlated as the organism balances the risks to achieve maximal fitness. The question then is whether the resulting increase in lifespan due to the decrease in cancer is concomitant with a substantial decrease in cell proliferative abilities. At least with HSCs, this is not the case. As detailed below, there is no increase in senescence shown as a reduction of HSC RA with DR. In fact, both the risk of cancer and cell senescence are simultaneously reduced (Ertl et al. 2008). However, DR may not necessarily break the paradigm but instead delay this cell fate decision.

6.7 Model Systems to Examine Effects of DR

If we are to examine the underlying mechanism regulating this cell fate decision, we need a model that distinguishes the epigenetic health changes caused by under-eating from the phenotypes of aging that are genetically regulated. As noted above, recent studies of the role of tumor suppressors p53 and p16^{INK4a}, combined with the necessary role of self-renewal needed to transform cell lines, make adult stem cells ideal candidates for study. The role of these primitive cells is to replace tissue after it becomes defective. Of the adult stem cells, for which phenotypes can be directly measured, HSCs are by far the best characterized. The lineages of cells produced from differentiation of HSCs are defined, and quantitative assays of HSC function in vivo have been worked out in detail (Harrison, Astle and Stone 1989; Van Zant et al. 1990; Harrison and Zhong 1992; Harrison et al. 1993; Morrison et al. 1996; Chen, Astle and Harrison 2000;

Sudo et al. 2000; Liang, Van Zant and Szilvassy 2005; Sharma et al. 2005; Yuan et al. 2005; Min, Montecino-Rodriguez and Dorshkind 2006). In addition, well-defined cell surface markers can identify and be used to separate both the primitive precursors and the definitive cell types (Spangrude, Heimfeld and Weissman 1988; Spangrude and Brooks 1993; Morrison and Weissman 1994; Goodell et al. 1996; Christensen and Weissman 2001; Ishida, Zeng and Ogawa 2002; Bryder, Rossi and Weissman 2006; Lin and Goodell 2006; Pearce et al. 2007; Rossi, Bryder and Weissman 2007).

Mice are ideal models in which to investigate the effects of lifelong DR and the accumulation of spontaneous mutations that lead to cancer (The Jackson Laboratory 1997). They age rapidly (30 times faster than humans), and the use of inbred strains allows the investigation of such phenomena without the confounding effects of genetic variability (Flurkey, Currer and Harrison 2007). Thus, studying HSCs in DR inbred mice is an ideal platform from which to probe the paradigm in Fig. 6.2 and determine how cells make a fate decision amongst normal function, cancer, and senescence.

Both BALB/cByJ (BALB) and B6 mice exhibit the same overt response to DR. Upon autopsy, old DR mice, compared to similarly aged ad libitum (AL) controls, exhibit lower incidences of most cancers, less brittle bones, less heart calcification, and a younger morphology of internal organs, all culminating in a longer lifespan (Miller and Harrison 1985; Bronson and Lipman 1991; Effros et al. 1991; Masoro 1993; Blackwell et al. 1995; Luan et al. 1995; Chen, Astle and Harrison 1998, 2003; Turturro et al. 2002). These two strains of mice, though, differ dramatically in the effect of DR on the RA of LT-HSCs, as discussed in detail below (Ertl et al. 2008).

6.8 Competitive Repopulation

The crux of the proposed paradigm in Fig. 6.2 depends on the relationship between cancer and proliferation. A highly sensitive assay that measures both proliferation and differentiation of HSCs is the competitive repopulation assay (CRA), given in detail elsewhere (Harrison, Astle and Stone 1989; Harrison and Zhong 1992; Harrison et al. 1993; Chen, Astle and Harrison 2000, 2003; Sharma et al. 2005; Yuan et al. 2005; Ertl et al. 2008). The CRA is an ex vivo assay that takes advantage of the standard BM transplant. The marrow to be tested (donor) is mixed with an aliquot of a standard pool of marrow obtained from genetically identifiable young mice (competitor). The mixture is injected into lethally irradiated recipient mice, where all mice—donor, competitor and recipients—are strain matched. The result is that HSCs from both the competitor and the donor repopulate the recipient. RA of each donor in an experiment are expressed in repopulating units (RUs) relative to the marrow of the standard competitor pool.

The standard dosages of irradiation used in such experiments (usually about 1000 mGy) kill or disable the host HSCs and their descendent precursor cells so they are replaced by donor and competitor cells over the next few weeks (Harrison and Zhong 1992) and for the rest of their lives, usually about 1 year. Initially after transplantation, host cells are replaced by descendants of the multipotent progenitors (MPPs) in the transplanted marrow. During the first month post-transplantation, the MPP cells and their descendants are replaced by cells differentiated from the short-term HSCs (ST-HSCs). By 4 months post-transplantation, the ST-HSCs, MPPs, and definitive cells present are due to the action of only LT-HSCs, because the other, more differentiated, cells have been exhausted.

Comparing the contributions of the donor and competitor to the definitive cells present in peripheral blood 4–6 months post-transplantation gives the RA of a given donor's LT-HSCs. The quantitative advantage of using a competitor pool as a standard to which all donors can be compared is obvious. In addition, this combination of donor and competitor cells minimizes the stress to the mouse. It assures rescue from lethal irradiation, regardless of the RA of the donor cells, because the competitor cells alone are sufficient to maintain recipient health (Harrison, Astle and Stone 1989; Harrison et al. 1993; Chen, Astle and Harrison 2000).

While the CRA has been well utilized in examining HSCs, this technique can be, in theory, extended to the measurement of RA of any transplantable adult stem cell line. A wide variety of genetic markers are available to distinguish cells descended from donor and competitor stem cells. For non-HSCs, a major difficulty is removing endogenous stem cells from the recipient while avoiding harm that might prevent growth of donor stem cells. Another difficulty is separating cells based on their stage of differentiation—from adult stem cells to definitive somatic cells.

6.9 DR in BALB Mice

The BALB strain of mice is an important model system because, unlike B6 mice, their BM shows a significant loss in RA with age (Miller and Harrison 1985; Chen, Astle and Harrison 2000; Ertl et al. 2008). Lifelong DR of BALB mice prevents the age-related loss in the RA, producing levels greater than found in young controls (Miller and Harrison 1985; Ertl et al. 2008). When the RA is expressed per HSC, there is a 20- to 50-fold loss with age, which is also greatly alleviated by DR (Ertl et al. 2008). Thus, by altering the function per stem cell and the number of stem cells present, DR delays the effects of aging and maintains the overall RA of BALB BM.

HSC markers. The combined concentration of LT- and ST-HSCs can be determined by flow cytometry of cells expressing the cell surface marker, cKit, that also have a high drug efflux capacity defined by the double negative, linear segment of the Hoechst-staining profile. The linear segment is defined as the side population (SP) (Goodell et al. 1996, 1997; Goodell 1999; Lin and Goodell 2006; Pearce et al. 2007). While this segment contains multiple cell types, the tip is known to be enriched for LT-HSCs (Goodell et al. 1996; Lin and Goodell 2006). This method of determination (SP+Kit) shows a slight increase in the number of HSCs present in BALB mice with lifelong DR compared to young mice and a RA per stem cell that is equivalent to the young. Combined, these account for the slight increase with age in overall RA of the BM from mice on DR (SP+Kit criterion, Table 6.2).

The flow criterion historically used to enrich subpopulations for LT-HSCs in B6 mice (Spangrude, Heimfeld and Weissman 1988; Spangrude and Brooks 1993; Morrison and Weissman 1994; Christensen and Weissman 2001; Ishida, Zeng and Ogawa 2002; Bryder, Rossi and Weissman 2006; Rossi, Bryder and Weissman 2007) uses the markers lineage$^-$, Sca$^+$, cKit$^+$, CD34$^-$, and CD135$^-$ (mKSL). The expression of Sca, however, is lower in BALB marrow than in B6 marrow. While the expression is lower, initial data suggest that cells expressing these cell surface markers are still proportional to the total subpopulation of LT-HSCs (Spangrude and Brooks 1993; Ertl et al. 2008). Using this criterion in BALB mice, we see a nearly eight-fold increase in LT-HSCs after lifelong DR, compared to young controls. This is concomitant with a five-fold decrease in the RA per LT-HSC; however, even with this loss, the RA is 10-fold greater than similarly aged

Table 6.2 Hematopoietic stem cell (HSC) frequency and function in BALB mice utilizing different flow criteria

	Young AL	Old AL	Old DR
mKSL criterion			
LT-HSC/10^6 viable BMC	99 ± 19	1847 ± 341***	752 ± 145***
RU/10^6 viable BMC	10 ± 2	6 ± 3	15 ± 4
RU/10^3 LT-HSC	107 ± 29	2 ± 1**	21 ± 2*
SP + Kit criterion			
HSC/10^6 viable BMC	261 ± 48	199 ± 68	336 ± 56
RU/10^6 viable BMC	11 ± 3	0.3 ± 0.1**	17 ± 7
RU/10^3 HSC	47 ± 21	2 ± 1**	54 ± 26

AL, ad libitum; DR, diet restriction; LT-HSC, long-term HSC.
For each flow criterion, the frequency of HSCs and RA [in repopulating units (RUs)] were determined in separate groups of BALB BMC donors (young = 2–7 months; old = 2–25 months). The mKSL flow criterion (Min, Montecino-Rodriguez and Dorshkind 2006) used lineage$^-$, Sca-1$^+$, c-kit$^+$, CD34$^-$, flk2$^-$, while the SP + Kit criterion used the Hoescht effluxing, double negative side population (Goodell et al. 1996, 1997; Goodell 1999; Lin and Goodell 2006), plus cKit$^+$. Because HSCs were defined per viable BMC and RA (RU) per total BMCs, the ratio is a lower limit. However, flow cytometry viabilities were about the same in both experiments, so relative ratios are correct. Within any given determination and criterion, measurements are compared to young AL controls where $^*P < 0.05$, $^{**}P < 0.01$, $^{***}P < 0.001$. (This research was originally published in *Blood.* Ertl, R. P., Chen, J., Astle, C. M., Duffy, T. M. and Harrison, D. E. Effects of dietary restriction on hematopoietic stem-cell aging are genetically regulated. *Blood.* 2008; 111:1709–1716. © the American Society of Hematology

AL controls. Thus, this flow criterion (mKSL criterion, Table 6.2) likewise supports the previous finding that lifelong DR prevents most of the loss of RA per stem cell with age (Ertl et al. 2008). This, combined with the increase in the number of stem cells present in the marrow, explains the slight increase in the overall RA of the BM with DR compared to young controls.

The results from the two different flow criteria are not directly comparable because they enrich different subpopulations, and in our studies, were done with different cohorts of mice. There are similarities in the overall trends. A notable exception is the trend in AL-fed aged mice, which varied greatly in total RA and number of HSCs, likely due to variations in health status of aged mice (Table 6.2). The robustness of the decline with age is seen with both flow criteria when RA is expressed per stem cell: marrow from old AL-fed donors compared to young AL-fed donors showed enormous losses of RA per LT-HSC (53-fold loss with mKSL criterion, 23-fold loss with SP+Kit criterion; Table 6.2). Also robust is the effect of DR on aged marrow, with both criteria the RA per HSC was greatly improved (10-fold improvement with mKSL criterion, 27-fold improvement with SP+Kit criterion; Table 6.2).

These studies suggest that, while DR reduces the risk of cancer and increases lifespan compared to AL controls, in BALB mice it also reduces or eliminates the loss of RA per HSC with age (Ertl et al. 2008). Because both cancer and senescence are decreased at the same time, these data appear to contradict the paradigm proposed by Campisi (Fig. 6.2). However, all of the results observed in both DR and tumor suppressor studies can be explained if DR is, in fact, *delaying* the cell fate decision between cancer and senescence, as proposed in Fig. 6.3 and discussed in detail latter in this chapter.

Clonal stability. One of the measures of the stem cell exhaustion in BM is whether HSCs have a stable production of all the lineages of definitive hematopoiesis. Young mice exhibit this characteristic, referred to as clonal stability, producing the different types of hematopoietic cells in the same ratios over extended periods of time (Harrison, Astle and Stone 1989; Harrison and Zhong 1992; Harrison et al. 1993). Experimentally, clonal stability is determined by setting up a CRA in which the numbers of genetically distinguishable donor and competitor cells are under limiting conditions—1–4 $\times$ 10^5 cells of each per mouse. With the average number of engrafting LT-HSCs present in mouse BM at around one per 10^5 cells, this means that, given normal random distribution, very few LT-HSCs are present. Under these conditions, once the transplanted LT-HSCs are responsible for the entire production of definitive hematopoietic cells (after 4 months), the percent of donor-derived cells from the different lineages should be correlated. In addition, the ratios should be correlated over time, showing they are derived proportionally over time from the same few LT-HSCs (Harrison, Astle and Stone 1989; Harrison and Zhong 1992; Harrison et al. 1993). With this assay, young BALB mice exhibit clonal stability between 5 and 8 months, with a high correlation coefficient (r = 0.97), explaining 90% of the variance (Table 6.3). With age, HSCs exhibit a loss of clonal stability, giving an insignificant correlation coefficient

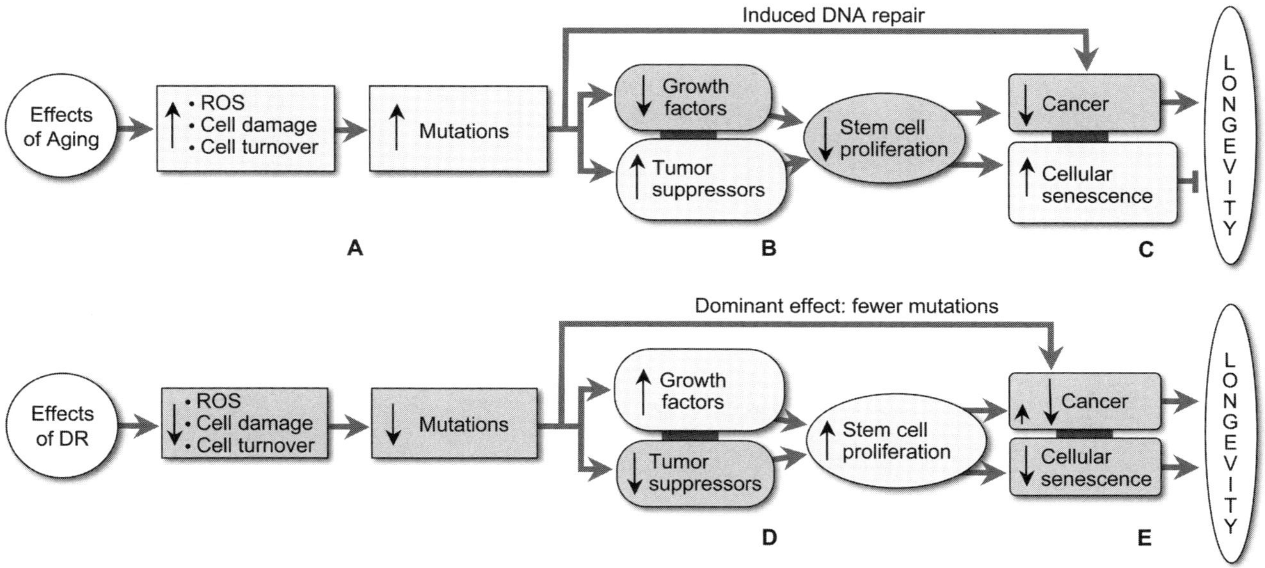

Fig. 6.3 Proposed model. The modification of Fig. 6.2 considers both the accumulation of age-related damage (**A**, see Fig. 6.1) and the subsequent response: initiating repair and/or preventing the spread of deleterious mutations by inhibiting proliferation (**B**). Alterations in the equilibrium between cancer and cellular senescence (**C**), in part, determine the longevity. Like other factors that decrease mutations, diet restriction (DR) increases stem cell proliferation (**D**), thus decreasing cellular senescence. However, the decrease in mutations also decreases cancer (**E**), thus explaining the increase in stem cell function and longevity and the decrease in cancer observed with DR

Table 6.3 Effects of age and diet restriction (DR) on hematopoietic stem cell (HSC) pluripotentially and clonal stability in BALB mice

	Young AL	Old AL	Old DR
HSC pluripotentiality (correlation coefficients between percentages donor erythrocytes and lymphocytes)			
L : E at 1.5 months	0.31 (NS)	0.003 (NS)	0.55 ($P < 0.05$)
L : E at 5 months	0.90 ($P < 0.01$)	0.91 ($P < 0.01$)	0.96 ($P < 0.01$)
L : E at 8 months	0.91 ($P < 0.01$)	0.89 ($P < 0.01$)	0.92 ($P < 0.01$)
HSC clonal stability (correlation coefficients between average donor percentages at two time points)			
1.5:5 months	0.29 (NS)	0.24 (NS)	0.35 (NS)
1.5:8 months	0.33 (NS)	0.43 (NS)	0.20 (NS)
5:8 months	0.97 ($P < 0.01$)	0.48 (NS)	0.95 ($P < 0.01$)

AL, ad libitum.
To estimate HSC pluriponentiality, data were analyzed for correlations between percentages of donor lymphocytes (L) and erythrocytes (E) within each recipient at each of the three time points for each donor group (young = 3 months; old = 25 months). To estimate clonal stability during reconstitution, correlation coefficients were also calculated on average donor contributions between each set of two time points. NS means not significant ($P > 0.05$). (This table was published in *Exp Hematol*, 31, Chen, J., Astle, C. M., and Harrison, D. E., Hematopoietic senescence is postponed and hematopoietic stem cell function is enhanced by dietary restriction, 1097–1103, Copyright Elsevier (2003)).

($r = 0.48$), explaining only 23% of the variance. This demonstrates that BALB HSCs are slowly exhausted with age, leading toward senescence. DR prevents the loss of clonal stability with age, giving high correlation coefficients over time, approaching those of the young ($r = 0.95$), again explaining nearly 90% of the variance. This independent measure verifies that DR can both delay senescence and reduce the risk of cancer (Miller and Harrison 1985).

6.10 DR in B6 Mice

While DR in B6 mice is also known to increase lifespan and decrease the risk of cancer (Bronson and Lipman 1991; Blackwell et al. 1995; Turturro et al. 2002), alterations in HSC function are vastly different from those seen in BALB mice. In B6 mice, the overall RA of BM increases three-fold with age (Harrison, Astle and Stone 1989; Chen, Astle and Harrison 2000). The increase with age results from a three-fold increase in the number of LT-HSCs present in BM (Ertl et al. 2008). Thus, with age, the RA per HSC remains fairly constant while the overall function of BM actually increases. This is not to say that B6 mice do not age, because they do exhibit many of the overt signs of aging, including a decrease in HSC homing and engraftment, alterations in the ability to produce different hematopoietic lineages, and earlier stem cell exhaustion after serial transplantation (Chen, Astle and Harrison 2000; Sudo et al. 2000; Liang, Van Zant and

Szilvassy 2005; Rossi et al. 2005; Min, Montecino-Rodriguez and Dorshkind 2006; Rossi, Bryder and Weissman 2007). However, the effects are far less severe than in BALB mice. The increase in overall marrow RA with a constant RA per LT-HSC is unaltered by lifelong DR (Ertl et al. 2008).

Overall, data on HSC aging in AL- and DR-treated B6 and BALB mice suggest that Fig. 6.2 needs to be modified, as the original model proposed by Campisi (Campisi 2003; Beausejour and Campisi 2006) does not explain all of the observed results. While the data from B6 mice do not contradict the concept that DR delays the cell fate decision between cancer and senescence, in this strain, DR is not the causative agent increasing the marrow RA. The lack of effect of DR is likely due to the elevated levels of repopulating function present in old B6 mice, which eliminate the need for further enhancement.

6.11 The need to Examine Multiple Strains

The greatest advantage of using mice as research models, besides the shorter lifespan, is the fact that inbred mice are genetically identical (The Jackson Laboratory 1997; Flurkey, Currer and Harrison 2007). Being genetically identical permits us to tease apart effects of specific genes. Also, the lack of genetic variance within a given strain reduces the biological variability caused by multiple alleles and recombination. The reduced biological variability gives us greater sensitivity with which to examine the contribution of different factors, each of which may only have a small effect.

The combination of alleles at different loci within a single inbred strain may not, however, give a good indication of in vivo conditions in wild mice on a segregating background, such as found in the human population. The process of inbreeding mice has removed the interactions created by heterozygosity and hybrid vigor. Examining different strains, though, allows us to examine the interactions of different allelic combinations. Thus, to understand the organismal relationships in complex systems involving multiple loci and pathways, such as cancer or aging, the treatments or models should be tested in multiple strains (Flurkey, Currer and Harrison 2007). This assures us that observed results are not anomalies associated with specific alleles or specific combinations of alleles whose homozygous occurrence may be selected against in a wild segregating population and thus, rarely found in nature.

Our DR studies in BALB and B6 mice illustrate the value of examining multiple strains. If the effect of cancer versus senescence had been examined in only the standard B6 mouse, we could have constructed a simpler model and missed the importance of the DR effect on retarding or preventing the dramatic changes in HSC number and RA caused by aging of BALB mice. DR effects on hematopoeisis in BALB and B6 mice have been consistently and significantly different. However, in all animals examined, DR has decreased the overt signs of aging, decreased the incidence of cancer, and increased lifespan.

6.12 Problems with Comparisons Between Strains

While, in principle, the various techniques successful in one strain of mice should be directly applicable to all strains of mice, in practice, minor obstacles need to be worked out. As stated above, the comparison of HSC RA between BALB and B6 mice is hampered by the strain-dependent expression of Sca-1. This cell surface marker is used to differentiate between progenitors and definitive cells. In B6 mice, 99% of the ability to repopulate marrow comes from cells expressing Sca. However, in BALB mice, only 25% of the cells responsible for repopulating the marrow express Sca (Spangrude and Brooks 1993). While expression is lower in BALB, all the cells that do express Sca-1 have the same RA as cells isolated from B6 marrow. Thus, the concentration of LT-HSCs determined by the mKSL criterion in BALB still has utility. Although the actual number is underestimated, it should be proportional to the pool of LT-HSCs as a whole and thus give a valid comparison amongst the young, old, and old DR BALB mice.

The altered expression of cell surface markers between strains of mice calls into question the exact composition of HSC subpopulations and prevents direct comparisons. Validating trends using multiple flow criteria is one approach to overcome this problem. While each flow criterion identifies different subpopulations, a robust trend will be observable regardless of the criterion used. This approach, however, may miss minor but important trends. As an alternative, Morrison's group recently developed the Slam marker system, which appears to give valid HSC numbers in a wider variety of strains and conditions than previous marker systems (Kiel et al. 2005; Yilmaz, Kiel and Morrison 2006). This flow criterion of lineage-, $CD150^+$, and $CD48^-$ identifies a subpopulation highly enriched for both ST^- and LT-HSC. When transplanted into lethally irradiated recipients, they are capable of repopulating the BM. This subpopulation can be further gated for CD34 to separate ST-HSCs ($CD34^+$) from LT-HSC ($CD34^-$), as detailed elsewhere (Rossi, Bryder and Weissman 2007). Our laboratory has recently tried this set of cell surface markers on both BALB and B6 mice. Our preliminary data indicate a significant, but not complete, overlap between the different flow criteria, consistent with the observations of Morrison's group.

With the aid of a new flow cytometer with a greater number of colors, we will verify degrees of overlap between the different flow criteria in marrow cells from different strains of mice at different ages. Transplanting a limited number of cells into lethally irradiated recipients, with a genetically identifiable standard competitor, will assess the RA of HSCs sorted by the different flow criteria.

These experiments should markedly improve our ability to compare hematopoietic precursor concentrations among mouse strains.

6.13 Proposed Model

The current model in Fig. 6.2 does not explain how DR can decrease the incidence of both cancer and senescence (Ertl et al. 2008). We therefore propose a modification of this model that considers both the accumulation of age-related damage (Fig. 6.3A) and the subsequent response (Fig. 6.3B–E). In this new model, aging and DR are modifiers of cellular functions that alter the accumulation rate and the overall number of mutations. Other modifiers may also have these effects; however, we focus on aging and DR because they have been well studied. In our model, as organisms age, they accumulate damage (Fig. 6.3A) from a variety of sources, such as reactive oxygen species (ROS). This damage will directly or indirectly increase cell turnover and the incidence of mutations. The amount and rate of damage can, however, be altered by DR. The ability of DR to decrease tumor incidence along with other age-related damage is well documented (Bronson and Lipman 1991; Blackwell et al. 1995; Turturro et al. 2002).

As shown in Fig. 6.3b,c, cells respond to damage by initiating repair or by preventing the spread of deleterious mutations by inhibiting proliferation or both. Tumor suppressors have been shown to play an essential role in regulating proliferation (Tyner et al. 2002; TeKippe, Harrison and Chen 2003; Maier et al. 2004; Dumble et al. 2007; Gatza et al. 2007). It is, however, equally likely that the cytokines, such as growth factors, could be down regulated in order to inhibit stem cell proliferation. Thus, an increase in age-related damage will induce DNA repair along with decreasing stem cell proliferation by increasing tumor suppressors or by decreasing growth factors. This will alter the equilibrium between cancer and cellular senescence. The induced DNA repair and decrease in stem cell proliferation will decrease the risk of cancer. The decrease in proliferation, though, has the negative consequence of increasing cellular senescence. It is this balance between cancer and senescence that, in part, determines the maximal lifespan obtainable.

As shown in Fig. 6.3d,e, a decrease from the normal level of spontaneous mutations that occur with age would lead to lower levels of tumor suppressor expression and possibly an increase in growth factors. The net result is a relative stimulation of stem cell RA compared to controls, thus decreasing cellular senescence. The previous model (Fig. 6.2) suggested that the cellular senescence and cancer were in a tight equilibrium. Here, we suggest that while they are still in an equilibrium, which is a key element in determining lifespan, they can be altered independently. In this model, DR decreases damage (including mutations) and thus decreases the need for tumor suppression. This removes inhibition of stem cell proliferation and decreases cellular senescence. The increase in proliferation will increase the risk of cancer, but the overall reduction of mutations is the predominant effect. Thus, it is possible for DR to both decrease cellular senescence and cancer at the same time, as found in BALB in vivo. This model (Fig. 6.3) predicts that DR diminishes genomic damage in BALB but not B6 HSCs, a unique and testable prediction.

6.14 Future Research

While the linkage between tumor suppressors and RA has been established, many parts of our model are speculative. However, there are a number of specific testable predictions that will determine whether the model has value. The Campisi model (Fig. 6.2) suggests that $p16^{INK4a}$ expression increases with age. Our model (Fig. 6.3) predicts that the $p16^{INK4a}$ expression will correlate with the mutation rate. This correlation could explain the previous age relationship of $p16^{INK4a}$, if under the same conditions, the numbers of mutations also increased with age. Independent measures of tumor suppressor expression and spontaneous mutation rates with age in different strains will test whether our model is valid.

It also remains to be established whether the mechanism by which DR retards aging is by a reduction of cellular damage leading to a decrease in the mutation rate. Furthermore, it is important to distinguish whether this is a transitory effect that requires a lifetime of treatment to significantly alter stem cell aging or a set-point mechanism that improves stem cell function within a few months. Initial data suggest that lifelong DR is required (Chen, Astle and Harrison 2003). It is known that ROS damage goes up with age and that ROS will directly cause mutations when it comes into contact with DNA (Wiesner, Zsurka and Kunz 2006; Dröge and Schipper 2007; Mallette and Ferbeyre 2007; Muller et al. 2007). However, in vivo the vast majority of naturally occurring oxygen radicals are found close to the mitochondria and the smooth endoplasmic reticulum. Oxygen radicals, by definition, are charged and very reactive and thus will travel only angstroms before donating the extra electron to another molecule. Thus, it is possible for ROS to directly damage mitochondrial DNA but less apt to directly damage genomic DNA leading to cancer. To date, researchers have searched without success for a carrier allowing a reactive species to cross the nuclear envelope and provide a direct mechanism of ROS-induced mutations. However, ROS can damage the cell in many other ways that mark the cell for turnover. This rapid turnover of cells under high-stress conditions may cause the increased mutation rate observed with elevated ROS in vivo. DR retards much of the damage and degradation associated with aging. If our model is valid, DR should decrease ROS and cellular turnover, resulting in a decrease in the mutations observed.

If DR decreases mutation rates, this should have two consequences: (1) It should decrease the need to shut down cell proliferation to obviate the risk of cancer and thus increase stem cell RA. (2) It should simultaneously decrease the risk of cancer. While the latter is not surprising, it is important because most mechanisms that enhance a cell's RA also increase the incidence of cancer.

6.15 Conclusion

To achieve a maximal healthy lifespan, a balance must exist between increasing stem cell senescence in order to decrease cancer versus decreasing stem cell senescence at the risk of increasing cancer. Tumor suppressors such as p53 and $p16^{INK4a}$ may play a major role in regulating this cell fate decision as we age.

While the need to make this decision is inevitable, it can be delayed. DR demonstrates that the two cellular fates are not inexplicably linked in an inverse relationship. In fact, with DR treatment, a decrease in HSC senescence combines with a simultaneous decrease in the risk of cancer to increase lifespan. The ability of DR in aged BALB mice to improve HSC RA without increasing the risk of cancer may result from a decreased mutation rate intrinsic to the HSC.

Establishing the effects of DR on tumor suppressors, ROS and mutation rates are the first steps in verifying or disproving our proposed model. Details of the underlying mechanism are still largely unknown. Is the maximal potential lifespan determined by epigenetic conditions, is it determined by inherited genes, or is it determined by a combination? Do hormones, which regulate other pathways, such as the insulin/IGF-1 pathway, drive the effect or is it driven by a stress response to DNA damage or lipid peroxidation? If the response depends on damage, is it linked to the type and amount of damage?

Understanding the various mechanisms that regulate aging, in particular how stem cell senescence decisions are made and how they can be delayed, has important health implications. In the clinic, it might be possible for DR mimics to delay stem cell senescence without increasing cancer. A better understanding of ROS may make it possible to reduce the effective oxygen radical burden. Elucidating stem cell senescence pathways in different strains of inbred mice may help us explain the large differences in cancer susceptibility and suggest new avenues for preventative therapy.

References

Ames, B. N., and Gold, L. S. 1998. The causes and prevention of cancer: the role of environment. Biotherapy. 11:205–220.

Aranda-Anzaldo, A., and Dent, M. A. R. 2007. Reassessing the role of p53 in cancer and ageing from an evolutionary perspective. Mech Ageing Dev. 128:293–302.

Beausejour, C. M., and Campisi, J. 2006. Ageing: balancing regeneration and cancer. Nature. 443:404–405.

Blackwell, B. N., Bucci, T. J., Hart, R. W., et al. 1995. A. Longevity, body weight, and neoplasia in ad libitum-fed and diet-restricted C57BL6 mice fed NIH-31 open formula diet. Toxicol Pathol. 23:570–582.

Bronson, R. T., and Lipman, R. D. 1991. Reduction in rate of occurrence of age related lesions in dietary restricted laboratory mice. Growth Dev Aging. 55:169–184.
Bryder, D., Rossi, D. J., and Weissman, I. L. 2006. Hematopoietic stem cells: the paradigmatic tissue-specific stem cell. Am J Pathol. 169:338–346.
Campisi, J. Cancer and ageing: rival demons? 2003. Nat Rev Cancer. 3:339–349.
Chen, J., Astle, C. M., and Harrison, D. E. 1998. Delayed immune aging in diet-restricted B6CBAT6F1 mice is associated with preservation of naive T cells. J Gerontol A Biol Sci Med Sci. 53:B330–B337.
Chen, J., Astle, C. M., and Harrison, D. E. 2000. Genetic regulation of primitive hematopoietic stem cell senescence. Exp Hematol. 28:442–450.
Chen, J., Astle, C. M., and Harrison, D. E. 2003. Hematopoietic senescence is postponed and hematopoietic stem cell function is enhanced by dietary restriction. Exp Hematol. 31:1097–1103.
Christensen, J. L., and Weissman, I. L. 2001. Flk-2 is a marker in hematopoietic stem cell differentiation: A simple method to isolate long-term stem cells. Proc Natl Acad Sci USA. 98:14541–14546.
Dröge, W., and Schipper, H. M. 2007. Oxidative stress and aberrant signaling in aging and cognitive decline. Aging Cell. 6:361–370.
Dumble, M., Moore, L., Chambers, S. M., et al. 2007. The impact of altered p53 dosage on hematopoietic stem cell dynamics during aging. Blood. 109:1736–1742.
Effros, R. B., Walford, R. L., Weindruch, R., et al. 1991. Influences of dietary restriction on immunity to influenza in aged mice. J Gerontol. 46:B142–B147.
Ertl, R. P., Chen, J., Astle, C. M., et al. (2008). Effects of dietary restriction on hematopoietic stem cell aging are genetically regulated. Blood. 111:1709–1716.
Flurkey, K., Currer, J. M., and Harrison, D. E. 2007. The Mouse in Aging Research. In: The Mouse in Biomedical Research, 2nd Edition, Vol III, Normative Biology, Husbandry, and Models. Fox J. G. et al., (eds). American College of Laboratory Animal Medicine (Elsevier), Burlington, MA. pp. 637–672.
Gatza, C., Moore, L., Dumble, M., et al. 2007. Tumor suppressor dosage regulates stem cell dynamics during aging. Cell Cycle. 6:52–55.
Giordano, A., Fucito, A., Romano, G., et al. 2007. Carcinogenesis and environment: the cancer stem cell hypothesis and implications for the development of novel therapeutics and diagnostics. Front Biosci. 12:3475–3482.
Gonzalez, F. J., and Nebert, D. W. 1990. Evolution of the P450 gene superfamily: animal-plant 'warfare', molecular drive and human genetic differences in drug oxidation. Trends Genet. 6:182–186.
Goodell, M. A. 1999. Introduction: Focus on hematology. CD34(+) or CD34(−): does it really matter? Blood. 94:2545–2547.
Goodell, M. A., Brose, K., Paradis, G., et al. C. 1996. Isolation and functional properties of murine hematopoietic stem cells that are replicating in vivo. J Exp Med. 183:1797–1806.
Goodell, M. A., Rosenzweig, M., Kim, H., et al. 1997. Dye efflux studies suggest that hematopoietic stem cells expressing low or undetectable levels of CD34 antigen exist in multiple species. Nat Med. 3:1337–1345.
Guralnik, J. M., Eisenstaedt, R. S., Ferrucci, L., et al. 2004. Prevalence of anemia in persons 65 years and older in the United States: evidence for a high rate of unexplained anemia. Blood. 104:2263–2268.
Harrison, D. E., Astle, C. M., and Stone, M. 1989. Numbers and functions of transplantable primitive immunohematopoietic stem cells. Effects of age. J Immunol. 142:3833–3840.
Harrison, D. E., and Zhong, R. K. 1992. The same exhaustible multilineage precursor produces both myeloid and lymphoid cells as early as 3–4 weeks after marrow transplantation. Proc Nat Acad Sci USA. 89:10134–10138.
Harrison, D. E., Jordan, C. T., Zhong, R. K., et al. 1993. Primitive hematopoietic stem cells: direct assay of most productive populations by competitive repopulation with simple binomial, correlation and covariance calculations. Exp Hematol. 21:206–219.

Hayflick, L. 1965. The limited in vitro lifetime of human diploid cell strains. Exp Cell Res. 37:614–636.
Ishida, A., Zeng, H., and Ogawa, M. 2002. Expression of lineage markers by CD34+ hematopoietic stem cells of adult mice. Exp Hematol. 30:361–365.
Janzen, V., Forkert, R., Fleming, H. E., et al. 2006. Stem-cell ageing modified by the cyclin-dependent kinase inhibitor p16INK4a. Nature. 443:421–426.
Kiel, M. J., Yilmaz, O. H., Iwashita, T., et al. 2005. SLAM family receptors distinguish hematopoietic stem and progenitor cells and reveal endothelial niches for stem cells. 2005;121:1109–1121.
Krishnamurthy, J., Ramsey, M. R., Ligon, K. L., et al. 2006. p16INK4a induces an age-dependent decline in islet regenerative potential. Nature. 443:453–457.
Krivtsov, A. V., Twomey, D., Feng, Z., et al. 2006. Transformation from committed progenitor to leukaemia stem cell initiated by MLL-AF9. Nature. 442:818–822.
Liang, Y., Van Zant, G., and Szilvassy, S. J. 2005. Effects of aging on the homing and engraftment of murine hematopoietic stem and progenitor cells. Blood. 106:1479–1487.
Lin, K. K., and Goodell, M. A. 2006. Purification of hematopoietic stem cells using the side population. Methods Enzymol. 420:255–264.
Luan. X., Zhao, W., Chandrasekar, B., et al. 1995. G. Calorie restriction modulates lymphocyte subset phenotype and increases apoptosis in MRL/lpr mice. Immunol Lett. 47:181–186.
Maier, B., Gluba, W., Bernier, B., et al. 2004. Modulation of mammalian life span by the short isoform of p53. Genes Dev. 18:306–319.
Mallette, F.A., and Ferbeyre, G. 2007. The DNA damage signaling pathway connects oncogenic stress to cellular senescence. Cell Cycle. 6:1831–1836.
Masoro, E. J. 1993. Dietary restriction and aging. J Am Geriatr Soc. 41:994–999.
Miller, R. A., and Harrison, D. E. 1985. Delayed reduction in T cell precursor frequencies accompanies diet-induced lifespan extension. J Immunol. 134:1426–1429.
Min, H., Montecino-Rodriguez, E., and Dorshkind, K. 2006. Effects of aging on the common lymphoid progenitor to pro-B cell transition. J Immunol. 176:1007–1012.
Molofsky, A. V., He, S., Bydon, M., et al. 2005. Bmi-1 promotes neural stem cell self-renewal and neural development but not mouse growth and survival by repressing the p16Ink4a and p19Arf senescence pathways. Genes Dev. 19:1432–1437.
Molofsky, A. V., Slutsky, S. G., Joseph, N. M., et al. 2006. Increasing p16INK4a expression decreases forebrain progenitors and neurogenesis during ageing. Nature. 443:448–452.
Morrison, S. J., and Weissman, I. L. 1994. The long-term repopulating subset of hematopoietic stem cells is deterministic and isolatable by phenotype. Immunity. 1:661–673.
Morrison, S. J., Wandycz, A. M., Akashi, K., et al. 1996. The aging of hematopoietic stem cells. Nat Med. 2:1011–1016.
Muller, F. L., Lustgarten, M. S., Jang, Y., et al. 2007. Trends in oxidative aging theories. Free Radic Biol Med. 43:477–503.
Pardal, R., Clarke, M. F., and Morrison, S. J. 2003. Applying the principles of stem-cell biology to cancer. Nat Rev Cancer. 3:895–902.
Pardal, R., Molofsky, A. V., He, S., et al. 2005. Stem cell self-renewal and cancer cell proliferation are regulated by common networks that balance the activation of proto-oncogenes and tumor suppressors. Cold Spring Harb Symp Quant Biol. 70:177–185.
Pearce, D. J., Anjos-Afonso, F., Ridler, C. M., et al. 2007. Age dependent increase in SP distribution within Hematopoiesis: implications for our understanding of the mechanism of aging. Stem Cells. 25:828–835.
Penninx, B.W., Pahor, M., Cesari, M., et al. 2004. Anemia is associated with disability and decreased physical performance and muscle strength in the elderly. J Am Geriatr Soc. 52:719–724.
Robinson, B. 2003. Cost of anemia in the elderly. J Am Geriatr Soc. 51:S14–S17.
Rossi, D. J., Bryder, D., Zahn, J. M., et al. 2005. Cell intrinsic alterations underlie hematopoietic stem cell aging. Proc Nat Acad Sci USA. 102:9194–9199.

Rossi, D. J., Bryder, D., and Weissman, I. L. 2007. Hematopoeitic stem cell aging: Mechanism and consequence. Exp Gerontol. 42:385–390.

Sharma, Y., Flurkey, K., Astle, C. M., et al. 2005. Mice severely deficient in growth hormone have normal hemaotopoiesis. Exp Hematol. 33:776–783.

Smith, J. R., and Pereira-Smith, O.M. 1996. Replicative senescence: implications for in vivo aging and tumor suppression. Science. 273:63–67.

Spangrude, G.J., and Brooks, D. M. 1993. Mouse strain variability in the expression of the hematopoietic stem cell antigen Ly-6A/E by bone marrow cells. Blood. 82:3327–3332.

Spangrude, G. J., Heimfeld, S., and Weissman, I. L. 1988. Purification and characterization of mouse hematopoietic stem cells. Science. 241:58–62. [Erratum in Science. 1989;244:1030].

The Staff of The Jackson Laboratory. 1997. Handbook on Genetically Standardized JAX® Mice. Bar Harbor, ME: The Jackson Laboratory.

Sudo, K., Ema, H., Morita, Y., et al. 2000. Age-associated characteristics of murine hematopoietic stem cells. J Exp Med. 192:1273–1280.

TeKippe, M., Harrison, D. E., and Chen, J. 2003. Expansion of hematopoietic stem cell phenotype and activity in *Trp53*-null mice. Exp Hematol. 31:521–527.

Turturro, A., Duffy, P., Hass, B., et al. 2002. Survival characteristics and age-adjusted disease incidences in C57BL/6 mice fed a commonly used cereal-based diet modulated by dietary restriction. J Gerontol A Biol Sci Med Sci. 57:B379–B389.

Tyner, S. D., Venkatachalam, S., Choi, J., et al. 2002. p53 mutant mice that display early ageing-associated phenotypes. Nature. 415:45–53.

Van Zant, G., Holland, B. P., Eldridge, P. W., et al. 1990. Genotype-restricted growth and aging patterns in hematopoietic stem cell populations of allophenic mice. J Exp Med. 171:1547–1565.

Wiesner, R. J., Zsurka, G., and Kunz, W. S. 2006. Mitochondrial DNA damage and the aging process: facts and imaginations. Free Radic Res. 40:1284–1294.

Yilmaz, O. H., Kiel, M. J., and Morrison, S. J. 2006. SLAM family markers are conserved among hematopoietic stem cells from old and reconstituted mice and markedly increase their purity. Blood. 107:924–930.

Yuan, R., Astle, C. M., Chen, J., et al. 2005. Genetic regulation of hematopoietic stem cell exhaustion during development and growth. Exp Hematol. 33:243–250.

Chapter 7
Modeling Human Philadelphia Chromosome-Positive Leukemia in Mice

Shaoguang Li

Contents

Abstract The BCR-ABL oncogene tranforms cells through sustained activation of signal transduction pathways in the cells. Identification of signaling pathways that play critical roles in leukemogenesis is the key to developing effective therapies against these targets. The success of this approach relies on establishment and use of physiological disease models to determine and evaluate potential therapeutic targets. Mouse models provide a powerful tool for studying signaling pathways in leukemic cells and for developing new therapeutic strategies for treating leukemia patients.

7.1 Introduction

Human Philadelphia chromosome-positive (Ph^+) leukemias induced by the *BCR–ABL* oncogene are among the most common hematologic malignancies and include chronic myeloid leukemia (CML) and B-cell acute lymphoblastic leukemia (B-ALL). CML has a triphasic clinical course: a chronic phase, in which BCR–ABL-expressing pluripotent stem cells massively expand but undergo normal differentiation to form mature neutrophils; an accelerated phase, in which neutrophil differentiation becomes progressively impaired

S. Li
Division of Hematology/Oncology, Department of Medicine, University of Massachusetts Medical School, Worcester, MA 01605, USA
Shaoguang.Li@umassmed.edu

S. Li (ed.), *Mouse Models of Human Blood Cancers*,

DOI: 10.1007/978-0-387-69132-9_7, © Springer Science+Business Media, LLC 2008

and the cells become less sensitive to myelosuppressive medications; and blast crisis, a condition resembling acute leukemia in which myeloid or lymphoid blasts fail to differentiate. The transition from chronic phase to blast crisis results from additional genetic alterations, and this process is not well understood. CML and Ph^+ B-ALL have a common stem cell origin [1] and often coexist in a patient [2, 3]. This suggests that these two diseases are closely related and may represent two different stages or forms of the same disease. Curative therapy for CML requires management of both CML (chronic phase and myeloid/lymphoid blast crisis) and Ph^+ B-ALL.

The Abl tyrosine kinase inhibitor imatinib mesylate (Gleevec, STI571) has become the most effective drug for leukemia therapy and has been shown to induce a complete hematologic response in the majority of chronic phase CML patients [4]. However, imatinib was unable to abrogate BCR–ABL-expressing leukemic cells [5] and induced cellular and clinical drug resistance [6–12], suggesting that use of imatinib as a single agent may not prevent eventual disease progression to terminal blast crisis or cure CML. Moreover, imatinib is much less effective in treating CML blast crisis patients [13, 14]. Recently, a newly developed Abl kinase inhibitor (termed dasatinib or BMS-354825 and produced by Bristol-Myers Squibb) has been shown to have an inhibitory effect on almost all imatinib-resistant BCR–ABL mutants [15], offering some hope for overcoming imatinib resistance. However, the BCR–ABL–T315I mutant, which frequently appears in patients resistant to imatinib therapy, is still resistant to dasatinib [15]. Two other novel Abl kinase inhibitors, termed AP23464 and AMN107 (nilotinib), have also been effective against several frequently observed imatinib-resistant BCR–ABL mutants but ineffective against the BCR–ABL–T315I mutant [16, 17]. While clinical trials are ongoing to determine the long-term effectiveness of these drugs in treating imatinib-resistant Ph^+ leukemia patients, it has been shown that imatinib does not completely eradicate CML stem cells [18]. It is critical to develop anti-stem cell therapies that are synergistic with available treatment strategies. The success of this approach requires understanding the signaling pathways utilized by BCR–ABL to induce Ph^+ leukemias and active in leukemic stem cells. Investigation of signaling pathways active in leukemic stem cells is critical to developing curative therapeutic strategies for Ph^+ leukemia.

7.2 Molecular Mechanisms of Ph^+ Leukemia

The molecular basis of Philadelphia chromosome is the *BCR–ABL* oncogene. The *BCR* gene, on chromosome 22, breaks at either exon 1, exon 12/13, or exon 19 and fuses to the *c-ABL* gene on chromosome 9 to form, respectively, three types of *BCR–ABL*: P190, P210, or P230. In humans, each of the three forms of the *BCR–ABL* oncogene is associated with a distinct type of leukemia [19]. The P190 form is most often present in B-ALL but only rarely in CML. However, P190-induced B-ALL may proceed from a transient chronic phase CML

[20, 21]. P210 is the predominate form in CML and in some acute lymphoid and myeloid leukemias in CML blast crisis. P230 was recently found in a very mild form of CML [22]. Lymphoid blast crisis of CML and Ph^+ B-ALL are pathologically similar and account for 20% of adults and 5% of children with acute lymphoblastic leukemia. Among those patients, 50% of adults and 20% of children carry P210BCR–ABL and the rest carry P190BCR–ABL [13, 23]. In addition, Ph^+ B-ALL is pathologically similar to CML diagnosed in lymphoid blast crisis (which is derived from chronic phase CML) [24], effective therapies for acute lymphoid leukemia are still not available.

CML transition from chronic phase to blast crisis is a devastating process in Ph^+ leukemia. Although the mechanism underlying the disease progression remains unclear, additional genetic changes are believed to play a role in this process. Mutations of tumor suppressor genes, including the retinoblastoma gene (Rb), p16, and p53, have been found to be associated with CML blast crisis patients [25–27]. However, it is still not known how BCR–ABL-expressing cells acquire these additional genetic lesions. A plausible mechanism is an increase in genetic instability caused by BCR–ABL. Several studies have shown that BCR–ABL deregulates the functions of DNA repair-related genes. For example, BCR–ABL down-regulates expression of the DNA repair enzyme DNA–PKcs [28]. P210BCR–ABL may interact with the xeroderma pigmentosum group B protein, which could lead to the impairment of DNA repair function [29]. Expression of two other genes related to genetic stability, *BRCA-1* and *RAD51*, is also deregulated by BCR–ABL [30, 31]. BCR–ABL can also cause over-expression and increased activity of the error-prone polymerase ß, leading to an increased mutagenesis [30]. A recent study showed that BCR–ABL associates with rad 3-related protein (ATR), which is involved in DNA repair, and inhibits the activation of ATR following DNA damage, leading to alteration of cellular responses to DNA damage [32]. Although BCR–ABL is a primary growth stimulator for leukemic cells [33], it is generally accepted that the concomitant effect of BCR–ABL on cell survival and DNA double strand break repair may lead to the acquisition of secondary genetic abnormalities contributing to CML disease progression [34]. The above examples providing evidence that BCR–ABL can cause disruption of DNA repair mechanisms indicate that this effect of BCR–ABL may play a major role in progression of chronic phase CML.

7.3 BCR–ABL Signaling

BCR–ABL has been shown to activate multiple signaling molecules/pathways, including Ras, MAPK, STAT, JNK/SAPK, PI-3 kinase, NF-kB, and c-MYC [35], as well as cytokine production [36, 37]. Studies also link BCR–ABL to apoptotic pathways [38–49] and to activation of Src family kinases in cultured cells [50–52] and in mice [53]. It is not known what signaling pathways are active in leukemic stem cells that are insensitive to almost all anti-leukemia drugs.

Importantly, the role of a particular signaling pathway in BCR–ABL leukemogenesis could be cell-content dependent.

Different signaling pathways are required for proliferation of myeloid or lymphoid leukemic cells. As described above, P190 and P210 forms of BCR–ABL are associated with distinct leukemia: B-ALL for P190 and CML for P210 although P210 also induces acute lymphoid leukemia in CML blast crisis. A simple explanation for the induction of different type leukemia by P190 and P210 is that this could be caused by structural differences between these two forms of the *BCR–ABL* oncogene. Different forms of *BCR–ABL* (P190, P210, and P230) contain the same portion of the *c-ABL* gene but different lengths of the *BCR* gene. BCR in BCR–ABL comprises three functional domains: a coiled-coil domain, serine-rich sequences, and the C-terminal domain. P190 contains the first two domains of BCR, and P210 and P230 also contain some and the majority of the C-terminal domain of BCR, respectively. The C-terminal domain that is lacking in the P190 BCR protein comprises the *dbl*-like domain (present in both P210 and P230) and the GAP^{rac} domain (present only in P230). Both *dbl*-like domain and GAP^{rac} domain are homologous to regulators of small, Ras-related GTP-binding proteins. Despite the structural differences in P190 and P210BCR–ABL proteins, there is little evidence showing that these two kinases may stimulate different signaling pathways in cells, which lead to induction of different type of leukemia. In fact, P190 can induce CML in mice, as efficiently as P210 can [54], suggesting that distinct leukemia induced by P190 and P210 does not reflect the structural differences between the two kinases. An alternative explanation for induction of either CML or B-ALL is that different cell types (myeloid or lymphoid) require different signaling networks for malignant transformation. This cell-content-dependent signaling in leukemia induction is supported by the finding that three Src kinases (Lyn, Hck, and Fgr) are required for proliferation of leukemic cells in B-ALL but not CML induced by BCR–ABL [53] although these Src kinases are activated by BCR–ABL in both myeloid and lymphoid leukemic cells. This suggests that these three Src kinases are potential targets for B-ALL but not for chronic phase CML although this study does not exclude a role for other Src family kinases in the induction of CML by BCR–ABL. These results indicate that BCR–ABL utilizes different signaling network to induce B-ALL or CML, suggesting different therapeutic strategies for treating these two diseases. This idea about different signaling network used by BCR–ABL to induce B-ALL or CML is supported by the observation that the BCR–ABL SH2 domain is required for efficient induction of CML-like disease but not of B-ALL [55]. The cell type-specific signaling may represent a common mechanism in cancer development, and identification of unique signaling network involved in the induction of each type of cancer is critical to developing effective therapies.

Src kinases in BCR–ABL signaling. Src kinases activated by BCR–ABL are key signaling molecules in B-ALL development [53]. It is important to identify signaling pathways downstream of Src kinases in Ph$^+$ leukemia. Hck has been shown to phosphorylate and activate STAT5 in BCR–ABL-expressing myeloid cells [56]. However, a cell culture study using a mutant form of BCR–ABL that is resistant to the BCR–ABL kinase inhibitor imatinib shows that inhibition of Src kinases with CGP76030 does not affect activation of STAT5, and instead, activation of Akt is impaired by this drug [57]. A study using SHP-1 (SH2-containing tyrosine phosphotase-1)-deficient mice shows that SHP-1 interacts with Lyn in myeloid [58] and lymphoid [59] cells; BCR–ABL forms complex with SHP-1 [60]. Several lines of evidence also implicate relationship between cytokines and activation of Src kinases. Fyn, Hck, and Lyn are activated following IL-3 stimulation, and growth of progenitor cells induced by stem cell factor (SCF) is reduced in the absence of Lyn that is activated by SCF [61]. On the other hand, BCR–ABL can render cells independent of cytokines such as IL-3 [37, 62, 63]. These results indicate that the signaling pathways stimulated by BCR–ABL overlap at least partially with those activated by these cytokines.

Src kinases directly interact with BCR–ABL [50, 51] through its SH3, SH2, and SH1 domains and through the distal portion of the C-terminal tail, which is required for transformation of the myeloid leukemia cell line to IL-3 independency by BCR–ABL [52]. Src kinases are also involved in BCR–ABL function indirectly through other signaling molecules or pathways. BCR–ABL forms a stable complex with protein tyrosine phosphatases [60, 64], which could be regulated by Src kinases [58, 65]. Src kinases are also functionally associated with Btk (Bruton's tyrosine kinase). Btk activation has been shown to induce cell transformation [66], and Lyn phosphorylates and activates Btk [66, 67].

7.4 Mouse Models of Ph^+ Leukemia

Transgenic model. Since more than two decades ago, attempts have been made to generate transgenic mice expressing different forms (P190, P210, or P230) of BCR–ABL oncogene. In these different strains of transgenic mice, variable types of promoters are used to drive BCR–ABL transgenes. These promoters include Eμ [68], MPSV–LTR [68], metallothionein [69–71], BCR [72, 73], tec [74], and MSCV–LTR [75]. The BCR–ABL transgenic models show evidence that BCR–ABL is important in the initiation of leukemia and provide useful tools for studying molecular mechanisms by which the BCR–ABL oncogene induces the disease. However, there are two general problems related to these transgenic models. First, the P210 BCR–ABL transgene driven by the BCR promoter causes embryonic lethality [73]. Second, in the mice that develop leukemia, the disease type is mainly lymphoid (B-ALL or T-ALL) but not myeloid [68–71] although some degree of myeloproliferative disorder develops when the promoter of the *tec* gene is used [74]. In addition, disease latency in these mice is relatively long, making it difficult to use these models for developing therapeutic strategies.

Inducible tet-off model. Although the BCR–ABL transgenic models show the requirement of BCR–ABL in the initiation of leukemia, they do not indicate whether expression of BCR–ABL is necessary to maintain leukemia phenotype. The first animal model to address this concern is the inducible tet-off system in transgenic mice [33], in which the induction of BCR–ABL expression is induced by withdrawal of tetracycline from drinking water of the mice. Upon tetracycline withdrawal, all mice develop lethal B-ALL. Importantly, the leukemic phenotype is reversibly dependent on the continuous expression of BCR–ABL, even after multiple rounds of induction and reversion of BCR–ABL expression. These results demonstrate that BCR–ABL is required for both induction and maintenance of leukemia. Because the MMTV–LTR promoter is used in this transgenic strain to control expression of tTA (tetracycline transactivator), BCR–ABL is turned on only in $B220^+$ B-lymphoid cells but not in hematopoietic stem cells (HSCs), explaining the lack of the induction of CML-like disease in these mice. Subsequently, the inducible tet-off BCR–ABL transgenic mouse is generated using human CD34 regulatory element [76]. In this model, the *cre* responder gene is expressed in HSCs, common myeloid progenitor cells, and megakaryocytic/erythroid progenitor cells. However, the mice did not display an increase in granulopoiesis, a characteristic of CML, although megakaryocytic lineage is affected in the mice. A better model that mimics human CML is developed using the murine stem cell leukemia (*SCL*) gene 3′-enhancer [77]. In these SCLtTA/BCR–ABL mice, BCR–ABL causes neutrophilia, leukocytosis, and organ invasion by myeloid cells, closely resembling CML-like disease although white blood cell counts in the mice are relatively lower compared to human CML. It is surprising that CML in these mice are not transplantable in NOD/SCID recipient mice, and this needs to be explained mechanistically in the future, as human CML is viewed as a stem cell disease. In addition, the SCLtTA/BCR–ABL mice are of mixed-strain background, resulting in variable life span ranging from 4 weeks to 17 weeks. Although this model is very useful in studying molecular mechanisms of BCR–ABL leukemogenesis, variable survival and mixed genetic background of the mice may not favor drug-testing experiments.

Xenotransplantation model. CML is a stem cell disorder. When leukemic cells from bone marrow and peripheral blood of CML patients are intravenously injected into irradiated severe combined immunodeficient (SCID) mice, the mice are repopulated with neoplastic Ph^+ $CD34^+$ cells [78, 79]. This model provides a powerful tool for studying disease mechanisms of Ph^+ leukemia. However, mice with engrafted human CML cells do not develop lethal leukemia although leukemic cells proliferate in the mice. This could be caused by many reasons. First, the latency of leukemia is longer than the lifespan of immune-deficient recipient mice. Second, residual immunity of recipient mice may reduce engraftment of human CML cells. Third, it is possible that technically the number of leukemic stem cells in intravenously injected human CML cells is not high enough to allow development of leukemia in recipient mice. Recently, a better NOD/SCID strain with less immune resistance and longer lifespan has been developed [80], and this NOD/SCID model will significantly improve engraftment of human CML cells.

Retroviral transduction/transplantation model. The initial efforts in establishing a BCR–ABL retroviral mouse model were taken about two decades ago [81], but at that time the system was hampered by low efficiency of disease induction. For example, in the originally described mouse retroviral bone marrow transduction/transplantation system, only about 25% of the recipients of BCR–ABL-transduced bone marrow cells developed CML-like leukemia [82–84], and some mice did not develop any disease, probably due to low viral titer and inefficient viral transduction. To overcome these deficiencies, during last 10 years efforts have been made to significantly improve the existing systems to develop an efficient and accurate mouse model of human CML and B-ALL. These improvements include modifications of the retroviral vector backbone, use of a transient retroviral packaging system, and change of viral transduction conditions [54, 85, 86]. After retrovirally expressing the *BCR–ABL* oncogene in bone marrow cells, which are derived from donor BALB/c mice pretreated with 5-fluorouracil (5-FU), 100% of syngeneic recipients develop CML-like leukemia within 4–6 weeks. The same CML-like disease can also be induced in C57BL/6 [53] and other inbred strains (unpublished results). The control retroviral construct does not induce leukemia in mice. Mouse CML-like disease is characterized by leukocytosis with greatly elevated numbers of maturing neutrophils, organ infiltration, and splenomegaly (Table 7.1). The target cells for BCR–ABL are primitive multipotential HSCs [54], precisely mimicking most of the pathological characteristics of human CML. Myeloid cells transduced by the *BCR–ABL* oncogene express BCR–ABL protein [54].

In addition to inducing human CML, BCR–ABL is also associated with a subset of human B-ALL as described above. To induce B-ALL, effort has been made to express BCR–ABL in the progenitor cells that give rise to the lymphoid cell lineage. The target cells for Abelson virus-induced pre-B leukemia, which is phenotypically similar to BCR–ABL-induced B-ALL, are fairly abundant in normal bone marrow from BALB/c mice. Hence, bone marrow cells from

Table 7.1 Pathological characteristics of leukemias induced by BCR–ABL

	CML-like disease		B-ALL	
	BALB/c	C57BL/6	BALB/c	C57BL/6
WEC ($\times 10^3/\mu l$)	295±59	105±38	68±21	45±17
% of neutrophils in PB	>60	>50	<2	<1
% of B-lymphocyte in PB	<7	<9	>90	>80
Spleen wt. (g)	0.91±0.11	0.46±0.09	0.43±0.07	0.29±0.04
Liver enlargement	↑↑↑↑	↑↑↑	↑↑	↑
Lung hemorrhage	+	+	–	–
Pleural effusion	–	–	+	+

B-ALL, B-cell acute lymphoblastic leukemia; CML, chronic myeloid leukemia.
Note that normal white blood cell count should be less than $10\times 10^3/\mu l$.

non-5-FU-treated donor mice were used to induce B-ALL in recipient mice. In doing so, the recipient mice develop B-ALL, and Southern blot analysis of these mice shows that the BCR–ABL provirus exists only in the malignant B cells [54, 55]. The leukemic cells express the B-cell markers CD19, B220 (CD45R), BP1, CD24, and CD43 and show rearrangement of immunoglobulin heavy chain genes, suggesting that these leukemic cells are pro- or pre-B cells and are phenotypically similar to human Ph^+ B-ALL. Diseased mice developed lymphadenopathy, moderate splenomegaly (Table 7.1), and bone marrow involvement with leukemic cells. In addition, these mice developed hemorrhagic pleural effusion (Table 7.1), which was a major cause of death. Furthermore, B-leukemic cells also cause the same leukemia in secondary recipients and can grow in culture. This efficient retroviral transduction/transplantation system provides a powerful tool for elucidating the common and distinct signaling pathways contributing to the diseases.

7.5 Translational Research Using Ph^+ Leukemia Mouse Models

The retroviral tranduction/transplantation model of BCR–ABL-induced leukemia has been successfully used in studying BCR–ABL domain functions and *BCR–ABL* cooperative genes [87]. More importantly, the model has been used widely in studying BCR–ABL-activated downstream signaling pathways and developing new therapeutic strategies as described below.

Identification of crucial signaling pathways. Because the retroviral tranduction/transplantation model produces efficient and accurate leukemia induced by BCR–ABL, this model provides a powerful system in exploring molecular mechanisms and testing therapeutic strategies. One of earliest examples of utilizing this model to genetically determine contribution of a particular signaling pathway in leukemogenesis is to test the role of interleukin-3 (IL-3) and granulocyte–macrophage colony-stimulating factor (GM-CSF) in the development of BCR–ABL-induced CML. In this study, mice deficient for IL-3 and GM-CSF were used to investigate whether induction of CML by BCR–ABL is affected in the absence of these two cytokine genes. The results show that IL-3 and GM-CSF are not required for induction of CML by BCR–ABL [88] although some studies suggest a role of these two genes in BCR–ABL transformation. Other examples for using this model in exploring signaling pathways activated by BCR–ABL include studies of STAT5, Ras, Grb-2, JNK, Cbl, ICSBP [87], and Src family kinases [53].

Testing of new therapeutic targets and strategies. For the reasons described above, retroviral transduction/transplantation mouse model of Ph^+ leukemia provides an excellent system for identifying novel therapeutic targets and evaluating efficacy of therapeutic agents. Effectiveness of imatinib in treating CML or B-ALL induced by BCR–ABL has been tested in this leukemia mouse model. The results show that imatinib significantly prolongs survival of CML

[53, 89] or ALL [53] mice but does not cure the diseases, suggesting that imatinib cannot eradicate leukemic stem cells. Another good example of testing therapeutic drugs using the leukemia model is to test heat shock protein 90 (Hsp90) as a therapeutic target for the treatment of Ph^+ leukemia [90]. Treatment with an Hsp90 inhibitor (termed IPI-504) results in BCR–ABL protein degradation, decreased numbers of CML stem cells, and prolonged survival of CML mice bearing wild-type or mutant BCR–ABL T315I. Hsp90 inhibition more potently suppresses BCR–ABL–T315I-expressing leukemia clones relative to the wild-type clones in mice (Fig. 7.1). Combination treatment with IPI-504 and imatinib is more effective than either treatment alone in prolonging survival of mice simultaneously bearing both wild-type and T315I leukemic cells (Fig. 7.2). Together, these results provide a rationale for use of an Hsp90 inhibitor as a first-line treatment in CML by inhibiting leukemia stem cells and preventing the emergence of imatinib-resistant clones in patients. Although current therapeutic drugs such as BCR–ABL kinase inhibitors and Hsp90 inhibitors are effective in treating leukemia mice and patients, none of available drugs is curative for Ph^+ leukemia, likely due to the inability of these drugs to completely kill leukemic stem cells. Study of biology of leukemic stem cells and identification of effective targets in these cells will provide better therapeutic strategies for Ph^+ leukemia.

Identification of leukemic stem cells. Study of biology of leukemic stem cells requires having a reliable in vivo model system, and the development of anti-stem cells therapy depends on the understanding of differences between normal and leukemic stem cells. An important characteristic of stem cells is the ability for self-renewal, and only long- and short-term self-renewing HSCs have this capability [91] although other cell lineages in the hematopoietic system may have an effect on HSCs. However, in abnormal situation, some hematopoietic progenitors that do not normally self-renew can aberrantly acquire self-renewing capacity during leukemogenesis to become leukemic stem cells. For example, granulocyte–macrophage progenitors have been found to acquire stem cell property in human CML myeloid blast crisis through activation of ß-catenin [92], which is also involved in self-renewal of normal HSCs [93, 94]. It is still an open question whether cancer stem cells exist in all types of tumors; however, it is convincing that leukemic stem cells and normal HSCs share mechanisms for regulation of self-renewal. For example, the cells capable of initiating human

Fig. 7.1 represented BCR–ABL–WT-expressing myeloid cells. Percentages of BCR–ABL–T315I-expressing myeloid cells in peripheral blood of IPI-504-treated CML mice were further analyzed at days 21 and 28 post-BMT. The FACS results for one representative mouse from each treatment group were shown. IPI-504 but not imatinib significantly prolonged survival of the CML mice. (**B**) Simultaneous inhibition of Hsp90 and BCR–ABL kinase activity with IPI-504 and imatinib significantly prolongs survival of CML mice carrying both T315-expressing and WT–BCR–ABL leukemia cells. BALB/c mice were used to induce CML, and each treatment group had 10 mice. Adapted from [90]. (See color insert)

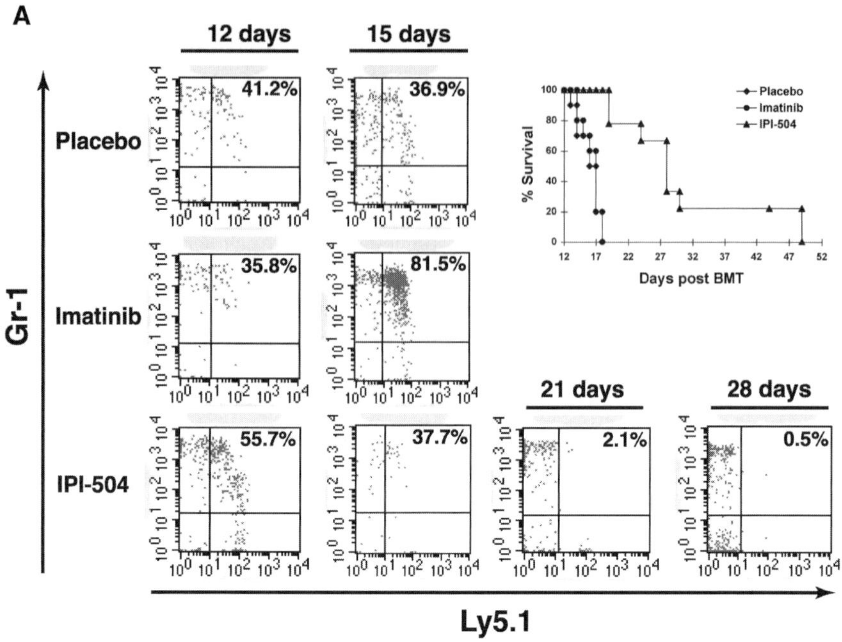

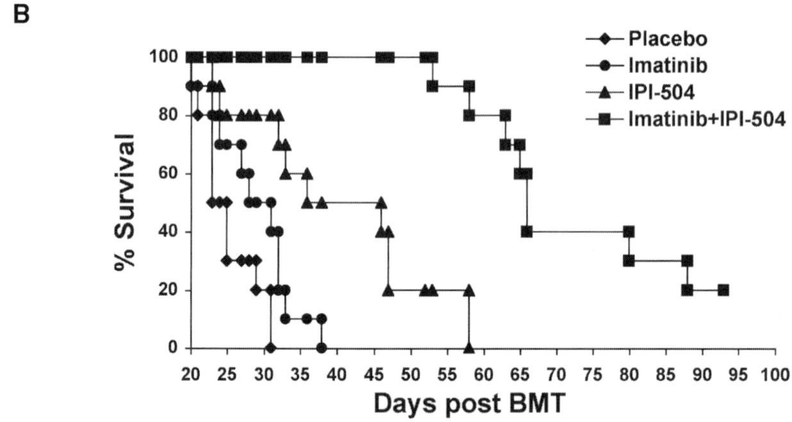

Fig. 7.1 (*continued*) **Inhibition of Hsp90 by IPI-504 preferentially reduces growth of myeloid leukemic cells harboring the BCR–ABL–T315I mutant.** (**A**) Bone marrow cells from C57BL/6-Ly5.2 mice were transduced by BCR–ABL–WT, and bone marrow cells from C57BL/6-Ly5.1 mice were transduced by BCR–ABL–T315I. The transduced cells were 1:1 mixed, and 0.5 $\times$ 10^6 mixed cells were injected into each recipient mouse (C57BL/6-Ly5.2). The mice were treated with placebo ($n = 10$), imatinib (100 mg/kg, twice a day) ($n = 10$), and IPI-504 (50 mg/kg, once every 2 days) ($n = 10$), respectively, beginning at 8 days post BMT. At days 12 and 15 post BMT, GFP^+ cells viable cells in peripheral blood of the mice were analyzed for $Gr\text{-}1^+Ly5.1^+$ cells that represented BCR–ABL–T315I-expressing myeloid cells. $Gr\text{-}1^+Ly5.1^-$ cells

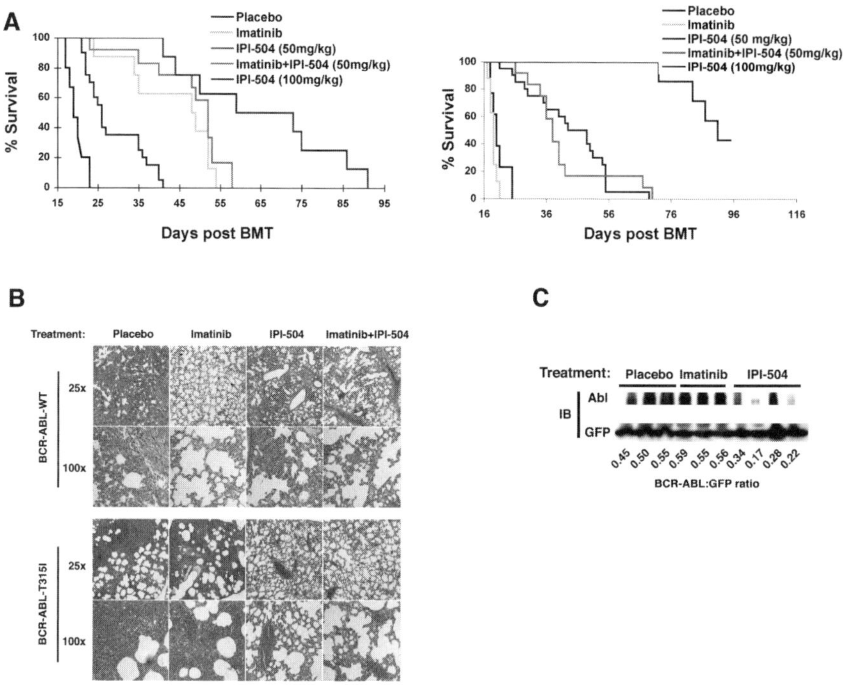

Fig. 7.2 Hsp90 is a therapeutic target for CML induced by either BCR–ABL–WT or BCR–ABL–T315I. (**A**) Treatment with the Hsp90 inhibitor IPI-504 prolonged the survival of CML mice. Mice with BCR–ABL–WT (*left panel*)- or BCR–ABL–T315I (*right panel*)-induced CML were treated with placebo ($n = 15$ for BCR–ABL–WT; $n = 13$ for BCR–ABL–T315I), imatinib (100 mg/kg, twice a day by gavage) ($n = 8$ for both BCR–ABL–WT and BCR–ABL–T315I), IPI-504 (50 mg/kg, once every 2 days by gavage) ($n = 20$ for both BCR–ABL–WT and BCR–ABL–T315I), IPI-504 (100 mg/kg, once every 2 days by gavage) ($n = 8$ for both BCR–ABL–WT; $n = 7$ for BCR–ABL–T315I), and imatinib+IPI-504 ($n = 12$ for both BCR–ABL–WT and BCR–ABL–T315I), respectively, beginning at day 8 post-transplantation. The IPI-504-treated mice with BCR–ABL–T315I-induced CML lived longer than those with BCR–ABL–WT-induced CML (comparing between *left* and *right panels*) (**B**) Photomicrographs of hematoxylin- and eosin-stained lung sections from drug-treated mice at day 14 post-transplantation. (**C**) Western blot analysis of spleen cell lysates for degradation of BCR–ABL in IPI-504-treated CML mice. IB, immunoblot. Adapted from [90]. (See color insert)

AML in NOD/SCID mice are exclusively $CD34^+CD38^-$ cells [95], which is characteristic of normal HSCs. The existence of similar biological characteristics between normal and leukemic stem cells is supported by the studies using *Bim-1*-deficient mice; *Bim-1* is required for maintenance of self-renewal of normal HSCs [96, 97] and stem cells for AML, as $Bim1^{-/-}$ bone marrow cells from AML mice are incapable of re-producing the disease in secondary recipients [96]. However, failure to repopulate malignant diseases to secondary recipients does not exclude the possibility that the transferred cancer stem cells with self-renewal capability did not engraft due to complex mechanisms related to the donor–recipient interactions, because the interaction between stem cells and their specific bone marrow microenvironment is critical for regulating the balance between self-renewal and differentiation of HSCs [98]. To better understand physiopathology of human hematologic malignancies, it is important to fully understand how leukemic stem cells communicate with bone marrow microenvironment.

Mouse CML stem cells have been recently identified and characterized using leukemia models (Fig. 7.3). C57BL/6 bone marrow cells transduced with BCR–ABL retrovirus were first sorted into Sca-1$^-$ or Sca-1$^+$ population, and only BCR–ABL-transduced Sca-1$^+$ cells transferred lethal CML to secondary B6 recipient mice [18], suggesting that early bone marrow progenitors contain CML stem cells. Because normal and leukemic stem cells share some common properties, HSCs (Lin$^-$c-kit$^+$Sca-1$^+$) are likely to be a candidate population. This idea is proven to be true, as BCR–ABL-expressing HSCs (GFP$^+$Lin$^-$c-Kit$^+$Sca-1$^+$) isolated from bone marrow cells of primary CML mice induce CML in recipient mice. Thus, BCR–ABL expressing HSCs function as CML stem cells. In the future, it is necessary to test whether other cell lineages serve as CML stem cells.

Because chronic phase CML can progress into lymphoid blast crisis and Ph$^+$ B-ALL can co-exist with CML [99], it is possible that Ph$^+$ B-ALL and CML develop from a common stem cell. This assumption is supported by the observation that an anti-serum that recognizes B-ALL cells also detects cells from CML patients [24]. Furthermore, lymphoid and myeloid leukemias induced by BCR–ABL originate from the same progenitor cells in mice [54]. However, P190-induced Ph$^+$ B-ALL is rarely present in CML [100], suggesting a possibility that early lymphoid progenitors serve as the stem cells for Ph$^+$ B-ALL. This hypothesis is supported by identification of B-ALL stem cells using mice with BCR–ABL-induced lymphoid leukemia. In this study, dasatinib remarkably prolonged survival of B-ALL mice, but a small percentage of leukemic cells ($<1\%$) remained in peripheral blood of these treated mice. These residual cells cause disease relapse after the treatment is stopped and are identified as B220$^+$/CD43$^+$ pro-B cells [18]. These progenitor leukemic cells have acquired self-renewal capacity and function as B-ALL stem cells.

Sensitivity of leukemic stem cells to kinase inhibitors. A critical question to ask is whether leukemic stem cells are sensitive to inhibition by kinase inhibitors, based on the fact that a complete and sustained molecular remission (undetectable levels of BCR–ABL transcripts) is difficult to attain in CML patients after a complete cytogenetic remission achieved through imatinib treatment [101–104]. These studies suggest that imatinib and probably other Abl kinase inhibitors can efficiently kill highly proliferating leukemic cells but are insufficient to eradicate leukemic stem cells. This idea is supported by the finding that neither imatinib nor dasatinib can completely eradicate leukemic stem cells in CML and B-ALL mice [18]. Consistent with the results from this study in mice,

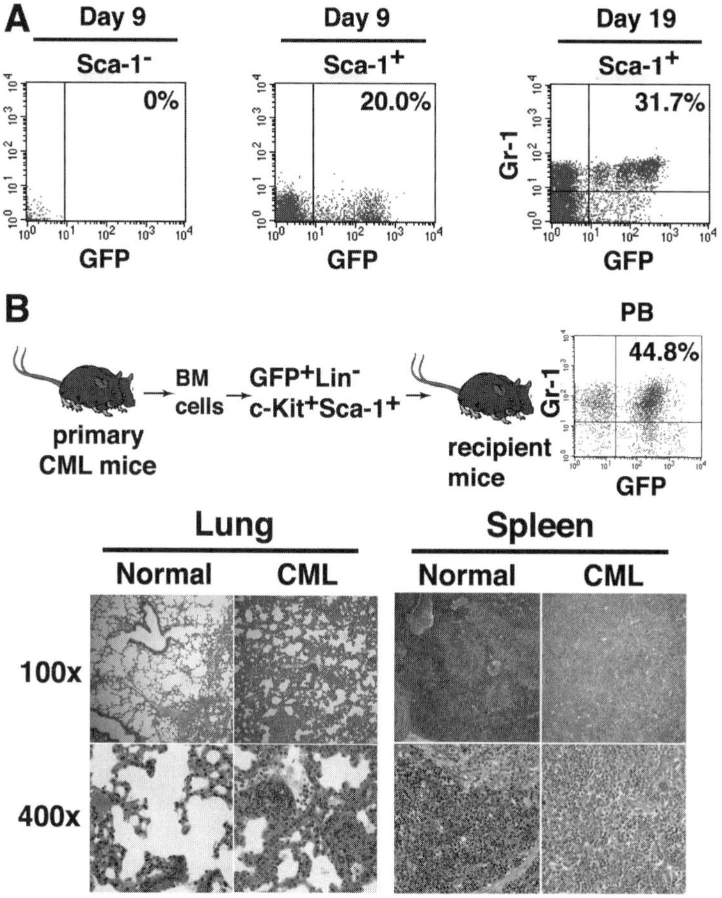

Fig. 7.3 Identification of bone marrow cell populations that function as CML stem cells. (**A**) BCR–ABL-transduced BM cells from B6 mice were sorted by Sca-1 MACS columns (Miltenyi Biotec), followed by transferring Sca-1$^-$ or Sca-1$^+$ population into B6 mice (1×10^5 cells/mouse; 4 mice per cell population group) to induce CML. GFP$^+$ myeloid cells (Gr-1$^+$) in peripheral blood (PB) of the mice were examined at days 9 and 19 after the induction of leukemia. All mice receiving Sca-1$^+$ population died of CML by day 42. (**B**) BCR–ABL-expressing HSCs function as CML stem cells. BM cells from CML mice in B6 background were sorted by FACS for BCR–ABL-expressing HSCs (GFP$^+$Lin$^-$c-kit$^+$Sca-1$^+$), followed by transferring into lethally irradiated B6 mice (2×10^4 cells/mouse). GFP$^+$ myeloid cells (Gr-1$^+$) were detected in peripheral blood. In contrast to the normal control mice, CML mice showed complete infiltration of the lungs with myeloid leukemic cells and complete disruption of follicular architecture of the spleen by infiltrating leukemic cells. Adapted from [18]. (See color insert)

the majority of B-ALL patients treated with imatinib have a marked but unsustained hematologic response [13, 14, 105, 106].

Src kinases as therapeutic targets for Ph$^+$B-ALL.Although allogeneic bone marrow transplantation (BMT) is the only established curative therapy for Ph$^+$ leukemia, this option is available to less than 15–20% of patients due to age restrictions and a lack of suitable donors. Imatinib was introduced to clinical trial for CML therapy more than a half decade ago [107, 108] and has been shown to induce a complete hematologic response in all interferon-resistant chronic phase CML patients [4]. Imatinib is, however, much less effective in treating patients with CML blast crisis and Ph$^+$ B-ALL [13, 14], and this type of insensitivity of leukemia to imatinib may not be associated with the development of imatinib-resistant BCR–ABL kinase domain mutations. To overcome this type of imatinib resistance, targeting BCR–ABL downstream signaling pathways that play an essential role in BCR–ABL leukemogenesis is likely a legitimate strategy. The success of this approach requires identification of key downstream signaling pathways utilized by BCR–ABL to induce leukemia. A good example that supports this idea is to identify Src kinases as key BCR–ABL downstream signaling molecules and to show that inhibition of Src kinases by the Src kinase inhibitor CGP76030 overcomes imatinib resistance to inhibit proliferation and induce apoptosis of pre-B-lymphoid cells that express BCR–ABL–T315I mutant [53]. These results are also supported by induction of apoptosis of leukemic cells from CML lymphoid blast crisis patients using anti-Lyn short interfering RNA [109].

7.6 Future Directions

Available mouse CML and B-ALL models have served as an excellent assay system in understanding the molecular basis of Ph$^+$ leukemia and in testing new therapeutic strategies. However, significant improvements are needed to allow answering some critical questions. First, Ph$^+$ leukemia is believed to be initiated from a stem cell that acquires Philadelphia chromosome. The mechanisms by which this stem cell accumulates other genetic mutations and subsequently develops into a fatal leukemia are largely unknown. The development of a model that allows studying the initial events of Ph$^+$ leukemia will be helpful. Second, most challenging issue in therapy of Ph$^+$ leukemia deals with leukemic stem cells. Although imatinib and dasatinib are effective in treating patients with Ph$^+$ leukemia and significantly prolong survival of leukemia mice, they are incapable of eliminating quiescent leukemic stem cells in patients [110] and in mice [18]. Study of biology of leukemic stem cells is key to developing anti-stem cell therapy for curing the disease and modeling Ph$^+$ leukemia using stem cells will provide a better model system for this area of research. Third, in human CML patients, the ineffectiveness of kinase inhibitors to completely eradicate leukemic cells can be caused by BCR–ABL mutations and could also be caused by the pre-existing BCR–ABL kinase domain mutations [111]. Investigation of developing mechanisms by which BCR–ABL mutations are initiated is critical to establishing curative therapy of Ph$^+$ leukemia. On the other hand, combination therapy using different kinase inhibitors to inhibit imatinib- or dasatinib-resistant leukemic cells is necessary [112–117]. It is also worth testing whether this strategy would help to inhibit leukemic stem cells. The development of a model system that focuses on elucidating imatinib-resistant mechanisms and developing novel therapies will be essential for curing Ph$^+$ leukemia.

References

1. Cobaleda C, Gutierrez-Cianca N, Perez-Losada J, Flores T, Garcia-Sanz R, Gonzalez M, Sanchez-Garcia I. A primitive hematopoietic cell is the target for the leukemic transformation in human philadelphia-positive acute lymphoblastic leukemia. *Blood.* 2000; 95: 1007–13.
2. van Rhee F, Hochhaus A, Lin F, Melo JV, Goldman JM, Cross NC. p190 BCR-ABL mRNA is expressed at low levels in p210-positive chronic myeloid and acute lymphoblastic leukemias. *Blood.* 1996; 87: 5213–7.
3. Roumier C, Daudignon A, Soenen V, Dupriez B, Wetterwald M, Lai JL, Cosson A, Fenaux P, Preudhomme C. p190 bcr-abl rearrangement: a secondary cytogenetic event in some chronic myeloid disorders? *Haematologica.* 1999; 84: 1075–80.
4. Druker BJ, Talpaz M, Resta DJ, Peng B, Buchdunger E, Ford JM, Lydon NB, Kantarjian H, Capdeville R, Ohno-Jones S, Sawyers CL. Efficacy and safety of a specific inhibitor of the BCR-ABL tyrosine kinase in chronic myeloid leukemia. *N Engl J Med.* 2001; 344: 1031–7.
5. Marley SB, Deininger MW, Davidson RJ, Goldman JM, Gordon MY. The tyrosine kinase inhibitor STI571, like interferon-alpha, preferentially reduces the capacity for amplification of granulocyte-macrophage progenitors from patients with chronic myeloid leukemia. *Exp Hematol.* 2000; 28: 551–7.
6. Gorre ME, Mohammed M, Ellwood K, Hsu N, Paquette R, Rao PN, Sawyers CL. Clinical resistance to STI-571 cancer therapy caused by BCR-ABL gene mutation or amplification. *Science.* 2001; 293: 876–80.
7. Weisberg E, Griffin JD. Mechanism of resistance to the ABL tyrosine kinase inhibitor STI571 in BCR/ABL-transformed hematopoietic cell lines. *Blood.* 2000; 95: 3498–505.
8. le Coutre P, Tassi E, Varella-Garcia M, Barni R, Mologni L, Cabrita G, Marchesi E, Supino R, Gambacorti-Passerini C. Induction of resistance to the Abelson inhibitor STI571 in human leukemic cells through gene amplification. *Blood.* 2000; 95: 1758–66.
9. Mahon FX, Deininger MW, Schultheis B, Chabrol J, Reiffers J, Goldman JM, Melo JV. Selection and characterization of *BCR-ABL* positive cell lines with differential sensitivity to the tyrosine kinase inhibitor STI571: diverse mechanisms of resistance. *Blood.* 2000; 96: 1070–9.
10. Shah NP, Nicoll JM, Nagar B, Gorre ME, Paquette RL, Kuriyan J, Sawyers CL. Multiple *BCR-ABL* kinase domain mutants confer polyclonal resistance to the tyrosine kinase inhibitor imatinib (STI571) in chronic phase and blast crise chronic myeloid leukemia. *Cancer Cell.* 2002; 2: 117–25.
11. Branford S, Rudzki Z, Walsh S, Grigg A, Arthur C, Taylor K, Herrmann R, Lynch KP, Hughes TP. High frequency of point mutations clustered within the adenosine triphosphate-binding region of BCR/ABL in patients with chronic myeloid leukemia or Ph-positive acute lymphoblastic leukemia who develop imatinib (STI571) resistance. *Blood.* 2002; 99: 3472–5.
12. von Bubnoff N, Schneller F, Peschel C, Duyster J. BCR-ABL gene mutations in relation to clinical resistance of Philadelphia-chromosome-positive leukaemia to STI571: a prospective study. *Lancet.* 2002; 359: 487–91.
13. Druker BJ, Sawyers CL, Kantarjian H, Resta DJ, Reese SF, Ford JM, Capdeville R, Talpaz M. Activity of a specific inhibitor of the BCR-ABL tyrosine kinase in the blast

crisis of chronic myeloid leukemia and acute lymphoblastic leukemia with the Philadelphia chromosome. *N Engl J Med.* 2001; 344: 1038–42.
14. Talpaz M, Sawyers CL, Kantarjain H, Resta D, Fernandes Rees S, Ford J, Bruker BJ. Activity of an ABL specific tyrosine kinase inhibitor in patients with BCR/ABL positive acute leukemias, including chronic myelogenous leukemia in blast crisis. *Oncologist.* 2000; 5: 282–3 (Abstr.).
15. Shah NP, Tran C, Lee FY, Chen P, Norris D, Sawyers CL. Overriding imatinib resistance with a novel ABL kinase inhibitor. *Science.* 2004; 305: 399–401.
16. O'Hare T, Pollock R, Stoffregen EP, Keats JA, Abdullah OM, Moseson EM, Rivera VM, Tang H, Metcalf CA, 3rd, Bohacek RS, Wang Y, Sundaramoorthi R, Shakespeare WC, Dalgarno D, Clackson T, Sawyer TK, Deininger MW, Druker BJ. Inhibition of wild-type and mutant Bcr-Abl by AP23464, a potent ATP-based oncogenic protein kinase inhibitor: implications for CML. *Blood.* 2004; 104: 2532–9.
17. Weisberg E, Manley PW, Breitenstein W, Bruggen J, Cowan-Jacob SW, Ray A, Huntly B, Fabbro D, Fendrich G, Hall-Meyers E, Kung AL, Mestan J, Daley GQ, Callahan L, Catley L, Cavazza C, Mohammed A, Neuberg D, Wright RD, Gilliland DG, Griffin JD. Characterization of AMN107, a selective inhibitor of native and mutant Bcr-Abl. *Cancer Cell.* 2005; 7: 129–41.
18. Hu Y, Swerdlow S, Duffy TM, Weinmann R, Lee FY, Li S. Targeting multiple kinase pathways in leukemic prognitors and stem cells is essential for improved treatment of Ph^+ leukemia in mice. *Proc Natl Acad Sci USA.* 2006; 103: 16870–75.
19. Advani AS, Pendergast AM. Bcr-Abl variants: biological and clinical aspects. *Leuk Res.* 2002; 26: 713–20.
20. Van Etten RA. Malignant transformation by abl and BCR/ABL. *Cancer Treat Res.* 1992; 63: 167–92.
21. Van Etten RA. The molecular pathogenesis of the Philadelphia-positive leukemias: implications for diagnosis and therapy. *Cancer Treat Res.* 1993; 64: 295–325.
22. Pane F, Frigeri F, Sindona M, Luciano L, Ferrara F, Cimino R, Meloni G, Saglio G, Salvatore F, Rotoli B. Neutrophilic-chronic myeloid leukemia: a distinct disease with a specific molecular marker (*BCR/ABL* with C3/A2 junction). *Blood.* 1996; 88: 2410–4.
23. Sawyers CL. Chronic myeloid leukemia. *N Engl J Med.* 1999; 340: 1330–40.
24. Janossy G, Roberts M, Greaves MF. Target cell in chronic myeloid leukaemia and its relationship to acute lymphoid leukaemia. *Lancet.* 1976; 2: 1058–61.
25. Towatari M, Adachi K, Kato H, Saito H. Absence of the human retinoblastoma gene product in the megakaryoblastic crisis of chronic myelogenous leukemia. *Blood.* 1991; 78: 2178–81.
26. Sill H, Goldman JM, Cross NC. Homozygous deletions of the p16 tumor-suppressor gene are associated with lymphoid transformation of chronic myeloid leukemia. *Blood.* 1995; 85: 2013–6.
27. Feinstein E, Cimino G, Gale RP, Alimena G, Berthier R, Kishi K, Goldman J, Zaccaria A, Berrebi A, Canaani E. p53 in chronic myelogenous leukemia in acute phase. *Proc Natl Acad Sci USA.* 1991; 88: 6293–7.
28. Deutsch E, Dugray A, AbdulKarim B, Marangoni E, Maggiorella L, Vaganay S, M'Kacher R, Rasy SD, Eschwege F, Vainchenker W, Turhan AG, Bourhis J. BCR-ABL down-regulates the DNA repair protein DNA-PKcs. *Blood.* 2001; 97: 2084–90.
29. Takeda N, Shibuya M, Maru Y. The BCR-ABL oncoprotein potentially interacts with the xeroderma pigmentosum group B protein. *Proc Natl Acad Sci USA.* 1999; 96: 203–7.
30. Canitrot Y, Lautier D, Laurent G, Frechet M, Ahmed A, Turhan AG, Salles B, Cazaux C, Hoffmann JS. Mutator phenotype of BCR-ABL transfected Ba/F3 cell lines and its association with enhanced expression of DNA polymerase beta. *Oncogene.* 1999; 18: 2676–80.
31. Slupianek A, Schmutte C, Tombline G, Nieborowska-Skorska M, Hoser G, Nowicki MO, Pierce AJ, Fishel R, Skorski T. BCR/ABL regulates mammalian RecA homologs, resulting in drug resistance. *Mol Cell.* 2001; 8: 795–806.

32. Dierov J, Dierova R, Carroll M. BCR/ABL translocates to the nucleus and disrupts an ATR-dependent intra-S phase checkpoint. *Cancer Cell.* 2004; 5: 275–85.
33. Huettner CS, Zhang P, Van Etten RA, Tenen DG. Reversibility of acute B-cell leukaemia induced by BCR-ABL1. *Nat Genet.* 2000; 24: 57–60.
34. Calabretta B, Perrotti D. The biology of CML blast crisis. *Blood.* 2004; 103: 4010–22.
35. Sawyers CL. Signal transduction pathways involved in BCR-ABL transformation. *Baillieres Clin Haematol.* 1997; 10: 223–31.
36. Anderson SM, Mladenovic J. The BCR-ABL oncogene requires both kinase activity and src-homology 2 domain to induce cytokine secretion. *Blood.* 1996; 87: 238–44.
37. Hariharan IK, Adams JM, Cory S. bcr-abl oncogene renders myeloid cell line factor independent: potential autocrine mechanism in chronic myeloid leukemia. *Oncogene Res.* 1988; 3: 387–99.
38. Skorski T, Nieborowska-Skorska M, Wlodarski P, Perrotti D, Martinez R, Wasik MA, Calabretta B. Blastic transformation of p53-deficient bone marrow cells by p210bcr/abl tyrosine kinase. *Proc Natl Acad Sci USA.* 1996; 93: 13137–42.
39. Honda H, Hirai H. Model mice for BCR/ABL-positive leukemias. *Blood Cells Mol Dis.* 2001; 27: 265–78.
40. Neshat MS, Raitano AB, Wang HG, Reed JC, Sawyers CL. The survival function of the Bcr-Abl oncogene is mediated by Bad-dependent and -independent pathways: roles for phosphatidylinositol 3-kinase and Raf. *Mol Cell Biol.* 2000; 20: 1179–86.
41. Majewski M, Nieborowska-Skorska M, Salomoni P, Slupianek A, Reiss K, Trotta R, Calabretta B, Skorski T. Activation of mitochondrial Raf-1 is involved in the antiapoptotic effects of Akt. *Cancer Res.* 1999; 59: 2815–9.
42. Sanchez-Garcia I, Martin-Zanca D. Regulation of Bcl-2 gene expression by BCR-ABL is mediated by Ras. *J Mol Biol.* 1997; 267: 225–8.
43. Dubrez L, Eymin B, Sordet O, Droin N, Turhan AG, Solary E. BCR-ABL delays apoptosis upstream of procaspase-3 activation. *Blood.* 1998; 91: 2415–22.
44. Amarante-Mendes GP, Naekyung Kim C, Liu L, Huang Y, Perkins CL, Green DR, Bhalla K. Bcr-Abl exerts its antiapoptotic effect against diverse apoptotic stimuli through blockage of mitochondrial release of cytochrome C and activation of caspase-3. *Blood.* 1998; 91: 1700–5.
45. McGahon AJ, Nishioka WK, Martin SJ, Mahboubi A, Cotter TG, Green DR. Regulation of the Fas apoptotic cell death pathway by Abl. *J Biol Chem.* 1995; 270: 22625–31.
46. Skorski T, Bellacosa A, Nieborowska-Skorska M, Majewski M, Martinez R, Choi JK, Trotta R, Wlodarski P, Perrotti D, Chan TO, Wasik MA, Tsichlis PN, Calabretta B. Transformation of hematopoietic cells by BCR/ABL requires activation of a PI-3 k/Akt-dependent pathway. *Embo J.* 1997; 16: 6151–61.
47. Jonuleit T, van der Kuip H, Miething C, Michels H, Hallek M, Duyster J, Aulitzky WE. Bcr-Abl kinase down-regulates cyclin-dependent kinase inhibitor p27 in human and murine cell lines. *Blood.* 2000; 96: 1933–9.
48. Parada Y, Banerji L, Glassford J, Lea NC, Collado M, Rivas C, Lewis JL, Gordon MY, Thomas NS, Lam EW. BCR-ABL and interleukin 3 promote haematopoietic cell proliferation and survival through modulation of cyclin D2 and p27Kip1 expression. *J Biol Chem.* 2001; 276: 23572–80.
49. Goetz AW, van der Kuip H, Maya R, Oren M, Aulitzky WE. Requirement for Mdm2 in the survival effects of Bcr-Abl and interleukin 3 in hematopoietic cells. *Cancer Res.* 2001; 61: 7635–41.
50. Danhauser-Riedl S, Warmuth M, Druker BJ, Emmerich B, Hallek M. Activation of Src kinases p53/56 lyn and p59hck by p210bcr/abl in myeloid cells. *Cancer Res.* 1996; 56: 3589–96.
51. Warmuth M, Bergmann M, Priess A, Hauslmann K, Emmerich B, Hallek M. The Src family kinase Hck interacts with Bcr-Abl by a kinase-independent mechanism and phosphorylates the Grb2-binding site of Bcr. *J Biol Chem.* 1997; 272: 33260–70.

52. Lionberger JM, Wilson MB, Smithgall TE. Transformation of myeloid leukemia cells to cytokine independence by Bcr-Abl is suppressed by kinase-defective Hck. *J Biol Chem.* 2000; 275: 18581–5.
53. Hu Y, Liu Y, Pelletier S, Buchdunger E, Warmuth M, Fabbro D, Hallek M, Van Etten RA, Li S. Requirement of Src kinases Lyn, Hck and Fgr for BCR-ABL1-induced B-lymphoblastic leukemia but not chronic myeloid leukemia. *Nat Genet.* 2004; 36: 453–61.
54. Li S, Ilaria RL, Jr., Million RP, Daley GQ, Van Etten RA. The P190, P210, and p230 forms of the *BCR/ABL* oncogene induce a similar chronic myeloid leukemia-like syndrome in mice but have different lymphoid leukemogenic activity. *J Exp Med.* 1999; 189: 1399–412.
55. Roumiantsev S, de Aos IE, Varticovski L, Ilaria RL, Van Etten RA. The src homology 2 domain of Bcr/Abl is required for efficient induction of chronic myeloid leukemia-like disease in mice but not for lymphoid leukemogenesis or activation of phosphatidylinositol 3-kinase. *Blood.* 2001; 97: 4–13.
56. Klejman A, Schreiner SJ, Nieborowska-Skorska M, Slupianek A, Wilson M, Smithgall TE, Skorski T. The Src family kinase Hck couples BCR/ABL to STAT5 activation in myeloid leukemia cells. *Embo J.* 2002; 21: 5766–74.
57. Warmuth M, Simon N, Mitina O, Mathes R, Fabbro D, Manley PW, Buchdunger E, Forster K, Moarefi I, Hallek M. Dual-specific Src and Abl kinase inhibitors, PP1 and CGP76030, inhibit growth and survival of cells expressing imatinib mesylate-resistant Bcr-Abl kinases. *Blood.* 2003; 101: 664–72.
58. Daigle I, Yousefi S, Colonna M, Green DR, Simon HU. Death receptors bind SHP-1 and block cytokine-induced anti-apoptotic signaling in neutrophils. *Nat Med.* 2002; 8: 61–7.
59. Yang W, McKenna SD, Jiao H, Tabrizi M, Lynes MA, Shultz LD, Yi T. SHP-1 deficiency in B-lineage cells is associated with heightened lyn protein expression and increased lyn kinase activity. *Exp Hematol.* 1998; 26: 1126–32.
60. Tauchi, Feng GS, Shen R, Song HY, Donner D, Pawson T, Broxmeyer HE. SH2-containing phosphotyrosine phosphatase Syp is a target of p210bcr-abl tyrosine kinase. *J Biol Chem.* 1994; 269: 15381–7.
61. Anderson SM, Jorgensen B. Activation of src-related tyrosine kinases by IL-3. *J Immunol.* 1995; 155: 1660–70.
62. Daley GQ, Baltimore D. Transformation of an interleukin 3-dependent hematopoietic cell line by the chronic myelogenous leukemia-specific P210bcr/abl protein. *Proc Natl Acad Sci USA.* 1988; 85: 9312–6.
63. Kabarowski JH, Allen PB, Wiedemann LM. A temperature sensitive p210 BCR-ABL mutant defines the primary consequences of BCR-ABL tyrosine kinase expression in growth factor dependent cells. *Embo J.* 1994; 13: 5887–95.
64. Bruecher-Encke B, Griffin JD, Neel BG, Lorenz U. Role of the tyrosine phosphatase SHP-1 in K562 cell differentiation. *Leukemia.* 2001; 15: 1424–32.
65. Gardai S, Whitlock BB, Helgason C, Ambruso D, Fadok V, Bratton D, Henson PM. Activation of SHIP by NADPH oxidase-stimulated Lyn leads to enhanced apoptosis in neutrophils. *J Biol Chem.* 2002; 277: 5236–46.
66. Park H, Wahl MI, Afar DE, Turck CW, Rawlings DJ, Tam C, Scharenberg AM, Kinet JP, Witte ON. Regulation of Btk function by a major autophosphorylation site within the SH3 domain. *Immunity.* 1996; 4: 515–25.
67. Rawlings DJ, Scharenberg AM, Park H, Wahl MI, Lin S, Kato RM, Fluckiger AC, Witte ON, Kinet JP. Activation of BTK by a phosphorylation mechanism initiated by SRC family kinases. *Science.* 1996; 271: 822–5.
68. Hariharan IK, Harris AW, Crawford M, Abud H, Webb E, Cory S, Adams JM. A bcr-v-abl oncogene induces lymphomas in transgenic mice. *Mol Cell Biol.* 1989; 9: 2798–805.
69. Heisterkamp N, Jenster G, ten Hoeve J, Zovich D, Pattengale PK, Groffen J. Acute leukaemia in bcr/abl transgenic mice. *Nature.* 1990; 344: 251–3.

70. Honda H, Fujii T, Takatoku M, Mano H, Witte ON, Yazaki Y, Hirai H. Expression of p210bcr/abl by metallothionein promoter induced T-cell leukemia in transgenic mice. *Blood*. 1995; 85: 2853–61.
71. Voncken JW, Kaartinen V, Pattengale PK, Germeraad WT, Groffen J, Heisterkamp N. BCR/ABL P210 and P190 cause distinct leukemia in transgenic mice. *Blood*. 1995; 86: 4603–11.
72. Castellanos A, Pintado B, Weruaga E, Arevalo R, Lopez A, Orfao A, Sanchez-Garcia I. A BCR-ABL(p190) fusion gene made by homologous recombination causes B-cell acute lymphoblastic leukemias in chimeric mice with independence of the endogenous bcr product. *Blood*. 1997; 90: 2168–74.
73. Heisterkamp N, Jenster G, Kioussis D, Pattengale PK, Groffen J. Human bcr-abl gene has a lethal effect on embryogenesis. *Transgenic Res*. 1991; 1: 45–53.
74. Honda H, Oda H, Suzuki T, Takahashi T, Witte ON, Ozawa K, Ishikawa T, Yazaki Y, Hirai H. Development of acute lymphoblastic leukemia and myeloproliferative disorder in transgenic mice expressing p210bcr/abl: a novel transgenic model for human Ph1-positive leukemias. *Blood*. 1998; 91: 2067–75.
75. Inokuchi K, Dan K, Takatori M, Takahuji H, Uchida N, Inami M, Miyake K, Honda H, Hirai H, Shimada T. Myeloproliferative disease in transgenic mice expressing P230 Bcr/Abl: longer disease latency, thrombocytosis, and mild leukocytosis. *Blood*. 2003; 102: 320–3.
76. Huettner CS, Koschmieder S, Iwasaki H, Iwasaki-Arai J, Radomska HS, Akashi K, Tenen DG. Inducible expression of BCR/ABL using human CD34 regulatory elements results in a megakaryocytic myeloproliferative syndrome. *Blood*. 2003; 102: 3363–70.
77. Koschmieder S, Gottgens B, Zhang P, Iwasaki-Arai J, Akashi K, Kutok JL, Dayaram T, Geary K, Green AR, Tenen DG, Huettner CS. Inducible chronic phase of myeloid leukemia with expansion of hematopoietic stem cells in a transgenic model of BCR-ABL leukemogenesis. *Blood*. 2005; 105: 324–34.
78. Sirard C, Lapidot T, Vormoor J, Cashman JD, Doedens M, Murdoch B, Jamal N, Messner H, Addey L, Minden M, Laraya P, Keating A, Eaves A, Lansdorp PM, Eaves CJ, Dick JE. Normal and leukemic SCID-repopulating cells (SRC) coexist in the bone marrow and peripheral blood from CML patients in chronic phase, whereas leukemic SRC are detected in blast crisis. *Blood*. 1996; 87: 1539–48.
79. Wang JC, Lapidot T, Cashman JD, Doedens M, Addy L, Sutherland DR, Nayar R, Laraya P, Minden M, Keating A, Eaves AC, Eaves CJ, Dick JE. High level engraftment of NOD/SCID mice by primitive normal and leukemic hematopoietic cells from patients with chronic myeloid leukemia in chronic phase. *Blood*. 1998; 91: 2406–14.
80. Shultz LD, Ishikawa F, Greiner DL. Humanized mice in translational biomedical research. *Nat Rev Immunol*. 2007; 7: 118–30.
81. Daley GQ, Van Etten RA, Baltimore D. Induction of chronic myelogenous leukemia in mice by the P210bcr/abl gene of the Philadelphia chromosome. *Science*. 1990; 247: 824–30.
82. Elefanty AG, Hariharan IK, Cory S. bcr-abl, the hallmark of chronic myeloid leukaemia in man, induces multiple haemopoietic neoplasms in mice. *Embo J*. 1990; 9: 1069–78.
83. Kelliher MA, McLaughlin J, Witte ON, Rosenberg N. Induction of a chronic myelogenous leukemia-like syndrome in mice with v-abl and BCR/ABL. *Proc Natl Acad Sci USA*. 1990; 87: 6649–53.
84. Pear WS, Miller JP, Xu L, Pui JC, Soffer B, Quackenbush RC, Pendergast AM, Bronson R, Aster JC, Scott ML, Baltimore D. Efficient and rapid induction of a chronic myelogenous leukemia-like myeloproliferative disease in mice receiving P210 bcr/abl-transduced bone marrow. *Blood*. 1998; 92: 3780–92.
85. Zhang X, Ren R. Bcr-Abl efficiently induces a myeloproliferative disease and production of excess interleukin-3 and granulocyte-macrophage colony-stimulating factor in mice: a novel model for chronic myelogenous leukemia. *Blood*. 1998; 92: 3829–40.

86. Ren R. Mechanisms of BCR-ABL in the pathogenesis of chronic myelogenous leukaemia. *Nat Rev Cancer*. 2005; 5: 172–83.
87. Li S, Gillessen S, Tomasson MH, Dranoff G, Gilliland DG, Van Etten RA. Interleukin 3 and granulocyte-macrophage colony-stimulating factor are not required for induction of chronic myeloid leukemia-like myeloproliferative disease in mice by *BCR/ABL*. *Blood*. 2001; 97: 1442–50.
88. Wolff NC, Ilaria RL, Jr. Establishment of a murine model for therapy-treated chronic myelogenous leukemia using the tyrosine kinase inhibitor STI571. *Blood*. 2001; 98: 2808–16.
89. Peng C, Brain J, Hu Y, Goodrich A, Kong L, Grayzel D, Park R, Read M, Li S. Inhibition of heat shock protein 90 prolongs survival of mice with BCR-ABL-T315I-induced leukemia and suppresses leukemic stem cells. *Blood*. 2007; 110: 678–85.
90. Reya T, Morrison SJ, Clarke MF, Weissman IL. Stem cells, cancer, and cancer stem cells. *Nature*. 2001; 414: 105–11.
91. Jamieson CH, Ailles LE, Dylla SJ, Muijtjens M, Jones C, Zehnder JL, Gotlib J, Li K, Manz MG, Keating A, Sawyers CL, Weissman IL. Granulocyte-macrophage progenitors as candidate leukemic stem cells in blast-crisis CML. *N Engl J Med*. 2004; 351: 657–67.
92. Reya T, Duncan AW, Ailles L, Domen J, Scherer DC, Willert K, Hintz L, Nusse R, Weissman IL. A role for Wnt signalling in self-renewal of haematopoietic stem cells. *Nature*. 2003; 423: 409–14.
93. Willert K, Brown JD, Danenberg E, Duncan AW, Weissman IL, Reya T, Yates JR, 3rd, Nusse R. Wnt proteins are lipid-modified and can act as stem cell growth factors. *Nature*. 2003; 423: 448–52.
94. Bonnet D, Dick JE. Human acute myeloid leukemia is organized as a hierarchy that originates from a primitive hematopoietic cell. *Nat Med*. 1997; 3: 730–7.
95. Lessard J, Sauvageau G. Bmi-1 determines the proliferative capacity of normal and leukaemic stem cells. *Nature*. 2003; 423: 255–60.
96. Park IK, Qian D, Kiel M, Becker MW, Pihalja M, Weissman IL, Morrison SJ, Clarke MF. Bmi-1 is required for maintenance of adult self-renewing haematopoietic stem cells. *Nature*. 2003; 423: 302–5.
97. Wilson A, Murphy MJ, Oskarsson T, Kaloulis K, Bettess MD, Oser GM, Pasche AC, Knabenhans C, Macdonald HR, Trumpp A. c-Myc controls the balance between hematopoietic stem cell self-renewal and differentiation. *Genes Dev*. 2004; 18: 2747–63.
98. Deininger M. Src kinases in Ph+ lymphoblastic leukemia. *Nat Genet*. 2004; 36: 440–1.
99. Deininger MW, Goldman JM, Melo JV. The molecular biology of chronic myeloid leukemia. *Blood*. 2000; 96: 3343–56.
100. Hughes TP, Kaeda J, Branford S, Rudzki Z, Hochhaus A, Hensley ML, Gathmann I, Bolton AE, van Hoomissen IC, Goldman JM, Radich JP. Frequency of major molecular responses to imatinib or interferon alfa plus cytarabine in newly diagnosed chronic myeloid leukemia. *N Engl J Med*. 2003; 349: 1423–32.
101. O'Brien SG, Guilhot F, Larson RA, Gathmann I, Baccarani M, Cervantes F, Cornelissen JJ, Fischer T, Hochhaus A, Hughes T, Lechner K, Nielsen JL, Rousselot P, Reiffers J, Saglio G, Shepherd J, Simonsson B, Gratwohl A, Goldman JM, Kantarjian H, Taylor K, Verhoef G, Bolton AE, Capdeville R, Druker BJ. Imatinib compared with interferon and low-dose cytarabine for newly diagnosed chronic-phase chronic myeloid leukemia. *N Engl J Med*. 2003; 348: 994–1004.
102. Lin F, Drummond M, O'Brien S, Cervantes F, Goldman J, Kaeda J. Molecular monitoring in chronic myeloid leukemia patients who achieve complete cytogenetic remission on imatinib. *Blood*. 2003; 102: 1143.
103. Drummond MW, Lush CJ, Vickers MA, Reid FM, Kaeda J, Holyoake TL. Imatinib mesylate-induced molecular remission of Philadelphia chromosome-positive myelodysplastic syndrome. *Leukemia*. 2003; 17: 463–5.

104. Sawyers CL, Hochhaus A, Feldman E, Goldman JM, Miller CB, Ottmann OG, Schiffer Ca, Talpaz M, Guilhot F, Deininger MW, Fischer T, O'Brien SG, Stone RM, Gambacorti-Passerini C, Russell NH, Reiffers JJ, Shea TC, Chapuis B, Coutre S, Tura S, Morra E, Larson RA, Saven A, Peschel C, Gratwohl A, Mandelli F, Ben-Am M, Gathmann I, Capdeville R, Paquette RL, Druker B. Imatinib induces hematologic and cytogeneic responses in patients with chronic myelogenous leukemia in myeloid blast crisis: results of a phase II study. *Blood.* 2002; 99: 3530–9.
105. Kantarjian HM, Cortes J, O'Brien S, Giles FJ, Albitar M, Rios MB, Shan J, Faderl S, Garcia-Manero G, Thomas DA, Resta D, Talpaz M. Imatinib mesylate (STI571) therapy for Philadelphia chromosome-positive chronic myelogenous leukemia in blast phase. *Blood.* 2002; 99: 3547–53.
106. Druker BJ, Lydon NB. Lessons learned from the development of an abl tyrosine kinase inhibitor for chronic myelogenous leukemia. *J Clin Invest.* 2000; 105: 3–7.
107. Lydon NB, Druker BJ. Lessons learned from the development of imatinib. *Leuk Res.* 2004; 28 Suppl 1: S29–S38.
108. Ptasznik A, Nakata Y, Kalota A, Emerson SG, Gewirtz AM. Short interfering RNA (siRNA) targeting the Lyn kinase induces apoptosis in primary, and drug-resistant, BCR-ABL1(+) leukemia cells. *Nat Med.* 2004; 10: 1187–9.
109. Elrick LJ, Jorgensen HG, Mountford JC, Holyoake TL. Punish the parent not the progeny. *Blood.* 2005; 105: 1862–6.
110. Pfeifer H, Wassmann B, Pavlova A, Wunderle L, Oldenburg J, Binckebanck A, Lange T, Hochhaus A, Wystub S, Bruck P, Hoelzer D, Ottmann OG. Kinase domain mutations of BCR-ABL frequently precede imatinib-based therapy and give rise to relapse in patients with de novo Philadelphia-positive acute lymphoblastic leukemia (Ph+ ALL). *Blood.* 2007; 110: 727–34.
111. Harrington EA, Bebbington D, Moore J, Rasmussen RK, Ajose-Adeogun AO, Nakayama T, Graham JA, Demur C, Hercend T, Diu-Hercend A, Su M, Golec JM, Miller KM. VX-680, a potent and selective small-molecule inhibitor of the Aurora kinases, suppresses tumor growth in vivo. *Nat Med.* 2004; 10: 262–7.
112. Doggrell SA. Dawn of Aurora kinase inhibitors as anticancer drugs. *Expert Opin Investig Drugs.* 2004; 13: 1199–201.
113. Carter TA, Wodicka LM, Shah NP, Velasco AM, Fabian MA, Treiber DK, Milanov ZV, Atteridge CE, Biggs WH, 3rd, Edeen PT, Floyd M, Ford JM, Grotzfeld RM, Herrgard S, Insko DE, Mehta SA, Patel HK, Pao W, Sawyers CL, Varmus H, Zarrinkar PP, Lockhart DJ. Inhibition of drug-resistant mutants of ABL, KIT, and EGF receptor kinases. *Proc Natl Acad Sci U S A.* 2005; 102: 11011–6.
114. Young MA, Shah NP, Chao LH, Seeliger M, Milanov ZV, Biggs WH, 3rd, Treiber DK, Patel HK, Zarrinkar PP, Lockhart DJ, Sawyers CL, Kuriyan J. Structure of the kinase domain of an imatinib-resistant Abl mutant in complex with the Aurora kinase inhibitor VX-680. *Cancer Res.* 2006; 66: 1007–14.
115. Giles FJ, Cortes J, Jones D, Bergstrom D, Kantarjian H, Freedman SJ. MK-0457, a novel kinase inhibitor, is active in patients with chronic myeloid leukemia or acute lymphocytic leukemia with the T315I BCR-ABL mutation. *Blood.* 2007; 109: 500–2.
116. Cheetham GM, Charlton PA, Golec JM, Pollard JR. Structural basis for potent inhibition of the Aurora kinases and a T315I multi-drug resistant mutant form of Abl kinase by VX-680. *Cancer Lett.* 2007; 251: 323–9.

Chapter 8
Mouse Models of Human Mature B-Cell and Plasma Cell Neoplasms

Siegfried Janz, Herbert C. Morse III, and Michael A. Teitell

Contents

S. Janz
Department of Pathology, Carver College of Medicine, University of Iowa,
500 Newton Road, 1046C ML, Iowa City, IA 52242, USA
Siegfried-janz@uiowa.edu

S. Li (ed.), *Mouse Models of Human Blood Cancers*,
DOI: 10.1007/978-0-387-69132-9_8, © Springer Science+Business Media, LLC 2008

8.1 Introduction

Developing mouse models that accurately reflect features of human B-cell lineage neoplasms has been a daunting but increasingly rewarding task. Studies of spontaneous tumors or those induced by chemicals, irradiation, or retroviruses performed before the 1980s provided remarkable insights into mechanisms and genetics of lymphomagenesis. With the advent of genetic engineering, it became possible to rapidly develop and explore new models and to enhance the value of established systems. Here, we will review past and present accomplishments in modeling mature human B-cell lymphomas and plasmas cell neoplasms (PCN) in mice, examine their strengths and limitations, and discuss obstacles that must be addressed in future work. These systems have accelerated our ability to understand the development of complex disease in vivo and to develop novel therapeutic approaches to diseases, many of which are almost uniformly lethal.

The cellular origins of human mature B cell and PCN defined by the consensus WHO classification (Jaffe, Harris et al. 2001a) are presented diagrammatically in Fig. 8.1. The lymphomas reflect various features of normal pregerminal center (pre-GC) and post-GC cells including anatomic location, expression patterns of differentiation markers, and mutational status of immunoglobulin gene variable region (IgV) sequences. Recently, further distinctions have been made based on the results of microarray gene expression profiling of normal B cells and lymphomas.

Most types of human B-cell lymphoma are derived from GC or post-GC B cells. A number of these are recognized as having close parallels among mouse B-lineage tumors classified according to the Bethesda proposals (Morse, Anver et al. 2002) including follicular B-cell lymphoma (FBL) and diffuse large B-cell lymphomas (DLBCL) as well as plasmacytomas (PCT) (Fig. 8.1). Human lymphomas of pre-GC origin, including a subset of chronic lymphocytic leukemia (CLL), termed small B-cell lymphoma (SBL) in mice and splenic marginal zone lymphoma (SMZL), also have parallels among spontaneous and induced tumors of mice. To date, there are no reports of mouse neoplasms with significant similarities to human Hodgkin, Burkitt, primary effusion or post-transplant lymphomas or to hairy cell or prolymphocytic leukemias. There are reports, however, of mouse models of marginal zone lymphomas (MZL) of

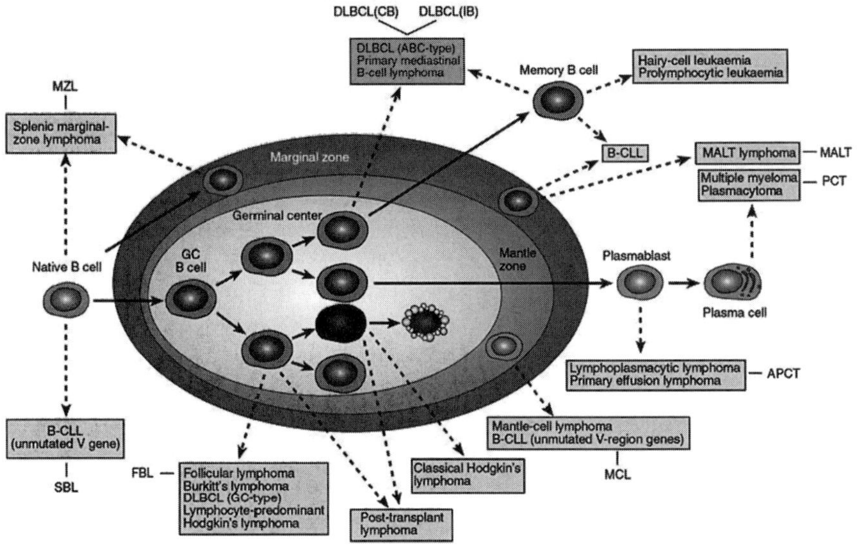

Fig. 8.1 Cellular origins of human and mouse mature B-cell lymphomas and plasma cell neoplasms. After undergoing early maturation in the bone marrow, naïve transitional B cells populate peripheral lymphoid tissues where they are recruited into the follicular and marginal zone B-cell subsets. Following interaction with antigen and helper T cells, follicular B cells establish germinal centers. There they undergo rapid clonal expansion and somatic hypermutation in the dark zone and move to the light zone where they undergo class switch recombination and positive selection on antigen-bearing follicular dendritic cells. Selected cells exit the germinal center to form memory B cells or to become plasma cells. Reciprocal chromosomal translocations involving *IgH* or *IgL* gene and a proto-oncogene, characteristic of most non-Hodgkin lymphomas (NHL), are thought to be generated as unfortunate by-products of the several mechanisms involved in *Ig* gene diversification that involves the generation of double-stranded DNA breaks. Some, such as IgH–BCL2 in follicular lymphoma, appear to occur as a consequence of aberrant V_HDJ_H recombination. Others, located adjacent to rearranged, somatically mutated V_HDJ_H genes, such as IgH–BCL6 in diffuse large B-cell lymphoma, most likely occur as a consequence of somatic hypermutation. A third group features breakpoint in IgH switch regions and appears to reflect aberrant class switch recombination, as in a subset of Burkitt lymphoma. The classes of human lymphomas and the mouse neoplasms most closely related when known are indicated. [Modified from Kuppers (2005).]

mucosa-associated lymphoid tissue (MALT) and mantle cell lymphomas (MCL) as well as lymphoplasmacytic lymphoma, termed anaplastic PCT (APCT) in mice. Systems that help define, explore, and extend these parallels are the subject of this chapter.

An ongoing challenge for developing accurate mouse models ofhuman NHL and PCN is the need to reproduce recurrent somatic mutations in the appropriate B-cell targets. Deciding which B cell to target—pre-GC, GC, or MZ B cell or extrafollicular plasmablast, for example—will be difficult as long as the precise nature and differentiation stage of the human tumor precursors remains unknown. Additional challenges for transgenic (TG) mouse models of NHL and PCN relate to the recapitulation of tumor progression pathways, mechanisms of stromal interactions, and responses to drugs used in human patients. Although mouse models of NHL and PCN might well be expected to phenocopy the human tumors, engineering the signaling pathways and responses is much more difficult than inducing rapid onset neoplasms such as those using retroviral transfer of classic oncogenes, which have remarkable value in their own right (Hu, Swerdlow et al. 2006).

A variety of TG techniques are now available to address the challenges mentioned above. It is possible to introduce into the mouse germ line gain-of-function mutations such as constitutively expressed oncogenes under control of B cell or plasma cell-specific enhancers and promoters. Conversely, normal mouse germ line genes can be replaced with loss-of-function alleles, which may take the form of classic null alleles ("knock-out" mice) or, of increasing importance, weak-efficiency alleles that retain some gene activity and thus more closely mimic alleles segregating in the human population. A more sophisticated method involves inducible transgenes, which provide for the temporal and spatial control of gene expression or gene attenuation, thereby circumventing potential developmental problems including embryonic toxicity and lethality that may be posed by constitutively expressed TG. Adenoviruses (Strair, Sheay et al. 2002) and retroviruses (Mikkers and Berns 2003) offer additional means for spatial and temporal gene regulation. A lesser known but very attractive example of the latter strategy takes advantage of cell type-specific retroviral binding to specific receptors of the subgroup A avian leucosis virus, affording introduction of several cancer genes into mouse target cells (Du, Podsypanina et al. 2006). Lentivirus-mediated transgenesis (Aronoff and Petersen 2006) represents yet another alternative to conventional technologies for generating the panel of TG mouse strains that may be required to accurately model human plasma cell tumors.

Mouse models of NHL and PCN should not only phenocopy their human counterparts at the histopathologic and molecular level but also exhibit desirable features including high tumor penetrance, short latencies, and predictable stages of tumor progression. Additional expectations, such as means for monitoring the tumor burden in live animals in a repeatable and reproducible manner, need also be considered.

Barriers to using TG mouse models of human mature B-cell lymphomas and PCN more widely are several and include the following:

1. *Problems related to establishment and maintenance of mouse colony*. Differences in genetic background of mice require costly and time-consuming backcrosses of individual TG from donor strains to desired recipient strains. In addition, differences in the microbial floras of mouse colonies frequently results in quarantine and monitoring of microbiological features and health status frequently resulting in rederivation of strains under specific pathogen-free (SPF) conditions in the recipient institution.
2. *Logistical problems*. There are limited financial and space resources for scaling up mouse breeding, husbandry, and genotyping to perform statistically robust

time course analyses of tumor development and drug testing. In addition, there are intellectual property issues that seriously affect time, cost, and mechanisms to negotiate and acquire mouse strains. The complexities of multiparty agreements and differing priorities of academic and commercial outfits lend an additional layer of difficulties. Finally, we are faced with problems related to data acquisition and analysis that include, as one example, a paucity of methods for high-throughput biomedical imaging and high-throughput microscopy.

8.2 Chronic Lymphocytic Leukemia/Small Lymphocytic Lymphoma

8.2.1 CLL/Small Lymphocytic Lymphoma in Humans

CLL and SLL are clonal, accumulative diseases of monomorphic, small, round, slowly proliferating $CD5^+$ B cells in peripheral blood, bone marrow, and lymph nodes admixed with smaller numbers of prolymphocytes and para-immunoblasts. Lymph nodes exhibit a pseudofollicular pattern. The term small lymphocytic lymphoma (SLL) is reserved for non-leukemic cases with similar tissue involvement and cellular phenotype. SLL is not considered to be the precursor to CLL. Rather, tissue involvement is thought to be almost always secondary to an established leukemia. Transformation to clonally related high-grade lymphoma, usually DLBCL, termed Richter syndrome, occurs in about 5% of cases (Jaffe, Harris et al. 2001). Interestingly, CLL may be preceded by a condition, tentatively designated benign monoclonal lymphocytosis (Victor Hoffbrand and Hamblin 2007), that may bear a similar relationship to CLL as monoclonal gammopathy of undetermined significance (MGUS) does to multiple myeloma (MM) (Kyle, Therneau et al. 2002).

Abnormal karyotypes are found by FISH in ~80% of cases with deletions of 13q14 (50%) and 12q trisomy (20%) being among the most common; translocation t(14q32) occurs in 5% of cases (Dohner, Stilgenbauer et al. 2000). The 13q14 deletion encompasses the micro-RNA genes, miR-15a, and miR-16-1 (miR15/16) (Calin, Sevignani et al. 2004). Familial aggregations of CLL are not uncommon. CLL/SLL is usually considered to be incurable with current therapy with an overall 5-year survival rate of around 50%. Molecular and phenotypic characterizations, however, have allowed the definition of subsets with clinically indolent and aggressive forms of the disease (Table 8.1). These are based on studies of IgV regions, cytogenetics, cell surface phenotype, and gene expression. Of particular interest is the observation that cases with mutated IgV genes and particular biases in V gene family utilization, such as V1-69, have a much more favorable course than cases with unmutated IgV genes and biased utilization of a separate set of V regions, such as V4-34 (Chiorazzi and Ferrarini 2003). This suggests that that the ability of BCRs to bind specific antigens might drive

Table 8.1 Features of indolent and aggressive chronic lymphocytic leukemia (CLL)

	Course of disease		
Variable	Indolent	Aggressive	Ref.
IgV regions	Mutated	Not mutated	Chiorazzi and Ferrarini (2003)
IgV preference	V1–69	V4–34	Chiorazzi and Ferrarini (2003)
Chr 11, Chr 17 aberrations	Less common	More common	Dohner, Stilgenbauer et al. (2000)
Chr 13q14 deletion	More common	Less common	Dohner, Stilgenbauer et al. (2000)
CD38 expression	Low	High	Damle, Wasil et al. (1999)
BCL2 expression	Low	High	Faderl, Keating et al. (2002)
ZAP70 expression	Low	High	Crespo, Bosch et al. (2003)
Serum thymidine kinase	Low	High	Hallek, Langenmayer et al. (1999)
Serum CD23	Low	High	Sarfati, Chevret et al. (1996)

expressing cells from a state of normality to the leukemic state. Studies of antigenic specificity have shown these BCRs to be poly- and autoreactive.

8.2.2 Mouse Models of CLL/SLL

8.2.2.1 Spontaneous Small B-Cell Lymphoma/Leukemia in Mice

Old mice of some strains spontaneously develop a clonal, mature B-cell disease termed SBL with many features reminiscent of CLL in humans (Fredrickson and Harris 2000; Hartley, Chattopadhyay et al. 2000). A predominant population of small lymphocytes with low mitotic activity associated with prolymphocytes and proliferation centers originates in the spleen. Advanced cases may exhibit involvement of lymph nodes, liver, and kidneys. A leukemic phase occurs in about 25% of cases and conversion to high-grade immunoblastic (IBL) lymphoma (Richter syndrome) is sometimes seen (Fredrickson and Harris 2000; Morse, Anver et al. 2002). The few cases that were phenotyped by flow cytometry were $CD5^{lo}$. There is no information on V_HDJ_H repertoire for these mice.

8.2.2.2 Models of CLL Based on Studies of New Zealand Mice

The first associations relating CD5 expression on B cells, neoplasia and NZB mice, were made in 1981with the finding that cultured B-lymphoma lines, including several from (BALB/c × NZB)F1 mice, expressed low levels of "Lyt-1" (Lanier, Warner et al. 1981). Later studies demonstrated that a subset of normal spleen cells expressed CD5 with spleens of NZB and (NZB × NZW)F1 mice having the highest frequencies (Manohar, Brown et al. 1982; Hayakawa, Hardy et al. 1983). $CD5^+$ B cells, now termed B1a cells, were later found to comprise a high proportion of peritoneal B cells and to share a distinctive $IgM^{hi}CD11b^+$

phenotype with another subset of functionally similar peritoneal B cells, now designated B1b B cells. B1b cells are not found in spleen, and splenic B1a cells do not express CD11b. Both subsets of peritoneal B1 cells derive from fetal/neonatal progenitors that are distinct from the B-cell progenitors in adult bone marrow that give rise to follicular and MZ B2 cells (Hardy 2006).

In spite of their differing origins, B1 cells share many features with MZ B cells including the ability to act as front-line responders to invading pathogens from the gut or circulating in the blood (Martin and Kearney 2000, 2001). The repertoires of both B1 and MZ B cells are also enriched for poly- or autoreactive antibody specificities. Importantly, the splenomegaly of aging NZB was shown in some cases to be the result of MZ enlargement, and NZB is the strain in which splenic MZL was first described (Yumoto 1980).

CLL cells were first shown to express CD5 in 1980 (Boumsell, Coppin et al. 1980). The fact that NZB mice were known to have high levels of normal splenic $CD5^+$ B cells prompted studies of the possible relationship of these cells to NZB lymphomas (East 1970). Soon, several laboratories reported the identification of clonal populations of $CD5^+$ B cells in aging NZB mice and showed that they were readily transplanted. In some mice, these lymphomas were associated with leukemic phases. This suggested that the $CD5^+$ lymphoma/leukemias of NZB mice might serve as a model for human CLL (Okada, Takiura et al. 1991; Phillips, Mehta et al. 1992; Stall, Farinas et al. 1988).

The clonal B-cell populations were found to develop in a characteristic fashion, first appearing in the peritoneal cavity in mice 2–3months of age; these peritoneal populations were usually oligoclonal. This was followed by successive spread to the spleen at 3–5months, peripheral blood at 5–7months, lymph nodes at 7–10 months, and bone marrow at 10–13 months (Stall, Farinas et al. 1988). The clones identified in spleens or lymph nodes were most often present among the several clones found in the peritoneum of the same animal. A similar pattern was seen in and NZW and (NZB × NZW)F1 mice (Stall, Farinas et al, 1988). Studies of congenic NZB and NZW and F1 mice showed that animals homozygous for $H\text{-}2^z$ had the highest frequencies of peritoneal $CD5^+$ B cells (Okada, Takiura et al. 1991). Other studies of NZB mice and progeny of crosses with DBA/2 demonstrated that the $CD5^+$ B cells accumulating in the spleens of aging mice were hyperdiploid and readily transplantable (Raveche, Lalor et al. 1988). Interestingly, this group did not identify hyperdiploid cells in the peritoneum of these mice.

Changes in expression of the cytokines IL-5 and IL-10were found to markedly affect the occurrence of $CD5^+$ lymphomas in NZB and (NZB × NZW)F1 mice. Studies of NZB mice homozygous for a null mutation of IL-10 showed that expansion of $CD5^+$ B cell outside the peritoneum and the development of clonal lymphomas was markedly reduced (Czarneski, Lin et al. 2004). In addition, (NZB × NZW)F1 mice overexpressing IL-5 from a transgene had greatly increased populations of $CD5^+$ B cells and were at increased risk for lymphoma development (Xiangshu Wen et al. 2004).

Two studies have examined the genetic basis for the lymphoma susceptibility of New Zealand mice. Analyses of backcross progeny from the crosses of (NZW × B10.NZW)F1 × B10.NZW indicted that the frequency of $CD5^+$ B cells in peripheral blood was governed by three susceptibility alleles (Hamano, Hirose et al. 1998). The first, *Bpal-1*, was closely linked to the MHC on Chr 17. This was consistent with earlier studies associating homozygosity for $H\text{-}2^z$ and $CD5^+$ B-cell frequency (Okada, Takiura et al. 1991). The second, *Bpal-2*, was located toward the centromeric end of Chr 13, and the third, *Bpal-3*, was close to the centromere on Chr 17 but not linked to the MHC (Hamano, Hirose et al. 1998). The development of leukemia in older mice was associated with elevated levels of $CD5^+$ B cells in blood at an early age. Each allele functioned independently and in an incompletely dominant fashion.

A second study examined mice from the cross (NZB × DBA/2)F1 × DBA/2, a low lymphoma strain (Raveche, Salerno et al. 2007). Lymphoproliferative disease occurred in 37% of the mice. Histologically, 94% of these cases were diagnosed as splenic MZL. Occurrence of disease was linked to three loci on chromosomes 14, 18, and 19. Sequence studies of Chr 14 identified a single base polymorphism 6 bp downstream of the pre-miR-16-1 sequence. This was associated with reduced expression of miR16 in NZB lymphoid cells and a NZB B-lymphoma cell line. Further studies suggested that miR-16-1normally functions in B cells to retard cell cycle progression and promote apoptosis. These results were very suggestive of an important tie between the lymphomas of NZB mice and human CLL as the miR15/16 locus is frequently deleted in the malignant B cells of CLL.

The IgH V region sequences of lymphomas occurring in New Zealand mice were examined for three cases (Mahboudi, Phillips et al. 1992). All lymphomas expressed unmutated V genes and DFL16.1, a D region gene frequently used by fetal B cells. No N additions were seen. This pattern resembles that of the normal fetal/neonatal B-cell repertoire (Feeney 1990).

Taken together, these studies indicate that the peritoneal and splenic $CD5^+$ B-cell populations of young New Zealand mice are considerably larger than those of most other strains. Over time, the peritoneal and splenic populations exhibit oligo- or monoclonal expansions of $CD5^+$ B cells that can spill into the blood as leukemia, seeding lymph nodes and other tissue but rarely affecting the bone marrow. For mice that have clonal populations in both spleen and peritoneum, the clones are sometimes common to the peritoneal and splenic B-cell populations, while in others they may be restricted to one site or the other (Stall, Farinas et al. 1988; Okada, Takiura et al. 1991). Numbers of $CD5^+$ B-cell numbers in young mice are tied to later development of lymphoma. $CD5^+$ B-cell numbers and lymphoma incidence are both under polygenic control but from genes that appear to differ between NZB and NZW. Little has been done to characterize Ig mutational state, but the few available sequences are very much like those of fetal/neonatal B cells.

Importantly, the lymphomas that develop in these mice have been diagnosed almost uniformly as splenic MZL. Pseudofollicles/proliferation centers, prolymphocytes, and para-immunoblasts are not features of the lymphomas of New Zealand mice, marking them as histologically quite distinct from human CLL.

8.2.2.3 The TCL1 TG Mouse Model of CLL

The *TCL1* oncogene was initially identified at Chr 14q32.1 as the gene commonly activated by translocations or inversions involving T-cell receptor loci (Fu, Virgilio et al. 1994). The development of T-cell lymphomas in mice with TCL1 expression driven by the *Lck* promoter in T cells established TCL1 as a true proto-oncogene (Virgilio, Lazzeri et al. 1998). TCL1 is also expressed in normal B-lineage cells from the pre-B to follicular B-cell stages and is then downregulated in GC B cells and extinguished in memory and plasma cells (Said, Hoyer et al. 2001; Virgilio, Narducci et al. 1994). High levels of expression have also been seen in a variety of immature and mature B-cell lymphomas (Teitell, Damore et al. 1999; Narducci, Pescarmona et al. 2000; Teitell 2005). The oncogenic effect of TCL1 is thought to be mediated, in part, by its interactions with AKT, enhancing its activation and stimulating downstream pathways that promote proliferation and survival (Teitell 2005).

In 2002, Bichi and her collaborators described features of mice bearing an Eμ–TCL1 TG (Bichi, Shinton et al. 2002) that included the development of late onset clonal $CD5^+$ lymphomas/leukemias. The general picture of this disease is remarkably similar to that described by Stall et al. for NZB mice (Stall, Farinas et al. 1988). Beginning around 2 months of age, the mice exhibited an expanded population of $CD5^+CD11b^+$ B cells in the peritoneum that became evident in the spleen at 4–5 months and then the bone marrow at 8 months. Analyses of Ig gene rearrangements in mice older than 7 months showed that the expanded populations were clonal and that clonal markers were sometimes shared between the peritoneum and spleen. All mice older than 13 months developed marked splenomegaly, hepatomegaly, lymphadenopathy, and leukemia with a mean WBC of 180×10^6/ml.

The B-cell expansion in mice younger than 7 months was polyclonal with a repertoire that was like that of normal $CD5^+$ B cells, including the recurrent use of specific V_HV_L combinations (Bichi, Shinton et al. 2002). The V_H11 sequences examined were essentially unmutated with only low levels of N-region additions, similar to V_H regions that characterize normal $CD5^+$ and fetal B cells to varying extents (Feeney 1990; Li, Hayakawa et al. 1993; Kantor, Merrill et al. 1997).

Histologic studies of mice 8 months of age and older showed a progressive enlargement of the splenic MZ by cells cytologically indistinsguishable from normal MZ B cells. The phenotype of the MZ B cells was atypical, however, as they were $CD21^{lo}CD5^{lo}$ rather than the $CD21^{hi}CD5^-$ phenotype of normal MZ B cells. In older mice, these cells extended into the red pulp in a manner similar to that seen with MZL in $NFS.V^+$ mice, but with no cytologic progression toward high-grade disease. Even cells from leukemic mice were unchanged.

More detailed studies of Ig utilization by the malignancies of older mice (Yan, Albesiano et al. 2006) revealed several important points: (1) sequences of the expressed V_H and V_L genes were identical to or differed minimally from germline; (2) utilization of V_H families 1, 11, and 12, D segment families, and the J_H segments, J_H1, diverged from that of the normal B-cell repertoire; (3) the HCDR3 and LCDR3 regions of the clones tended to be longer than for normal adult B cells and many contained two or more charged amino acids; (3) the cases exhibited stereotypic V_HDJ_H rearrangements that resembled sequences reported previously for certain autoantibodies and antibodies reactive with microbial antigens; and (4) cloned expressed sequences that were poly- and autoreactive and bound to a variety of polysaccharides. Almost all these features, except for reactivity with non-protein antigens, are similar to those of Ig genes from aggressive, unmutated CLL.

Other studies have forwarded the Eμ-TCL1 TG mouse as a tool for preclinical drug testing for human CLL (Johnson, Lucas et al. 2006). Leukemic mice responded initially to treatment with standard drug used in CLL, fludarabine, but then became resistant, similar to human CLL. Heightened expression of BCl2, MCL1, PDK1, and AKT1 in the transformed lymphocytes suggested that other potential drug targets were available. The importance of AKT signaling in this model was examined in studies of the effects of rapamycin, an mTOR inhibitor, on the survival of mice transplanted with expanded $CD5^+$ B-cell populations from the TG mice. Treated mice began to die significantly later than untreated animals although all animals in both groups were dead by ~200 days after transplantation (Zanesi, Aqeilan et al. 2006).

8.2.2.4 The BLC2/TRAF Model of CLL–the NFkB Connection

CLL and other NHL are characterized by overexpression of BCL2, which contributes to an apoptosis-resistant phenotype. TRAF1 is also overexpressed in a spectrum of NHL and in CLL is associated with aggressive disease (Zapata, Krajewska et al. 2000). TG mice overexpressing BCL2 or a dominant negative form of TRAF2 (TRAF2DN), which mimics the signaling features of TRAF1, develop expanded populations of B cells with occasional BCL2 TG mice developing long-latency, low-grade lymphomas (Strasser, Harris et al. 1993). Mice doubly TG for BCL2 and TRAF2DN were found to die between 6 and 18 months of age with marked splenomegaly, lymphadenopathy infiltration of non-lymphoid tissues, and in many cases, ascites and pleural effusions (Zapata, Krajewska et al. 2004). Leukemias WBC counts around 150×10^6/ml were common. The mice were diagnosed histologically as having SBL with a leukemic phase, and analyses of Ig gene organization showed the disease to be clonal. The tumor cells were $IgM^{hi}CD23^{-}CD21^{lo/-}CD5^{lo}$, consistent with an origin from B1a cells (Zapata, Krajewska et al. 2004). In addition, the cells were slowly proliferative and exhibited increased resistance to apoptosis due to effects of both BCL2 and TRAF2DN. These combined features were felt to be indicative of a CLL-like disease.

The use of double TG in preclinical drug studies was recently described (Kress, Martinez-Garcia et al. 2007). First, cells from double TG mice and humans with CLL were compared for their responses to treatment in vitro with synthetic triterpenoid derivatives. Both cell types were susceptible to induction of apoptosis. In addition, tests of the same drugs in double TG mice with leukemia resulted in marked decreases in WBC counts and reduced tissue burdens. These results were thought to support the testing of the drugs in patients with CLL.

A fascinating story that relates to that of the double TG mice comes from studies of mice bearing a mutant *NFkB2* gene (Zhang, Wang et al. 2007). Genomic alterations that result in truncation and constitutive activation of NFkB2 occur in a variety of human B- and T-cell malignancies (Zhang , Lombardi et al. 1994). TG mice developed marked splenomegaly, lymphadenopathy, and infiltration of non-lymphoid tissues and died with clonal B cell as well as some T-cell lymphomas between 5 and 18 months of age. The tumors were diagnosed histologically as SBL, but expression of CD5 was not evaluated and a leukemic phase was not described. The cells were non-proliferative and exhibited increased resistance to apoptosis. Interestingly, premalignant B cells and lymphoma exhibited significantly increased levels of TRAF1 and to a lesser extent TRAF2. TRAF1 was shown to be a direct transcriptional target of mutant NFkB2. Remarkably, TRAF1-deficient TG mice did not develop lymphoproliferation or lymphomas. These findings, together with the studies of the double TG mice, suggest a common pathway to development of SBL in mice.

8.2.2.5 APRIL and CLL?

APRIL (a proliferation inducing TNF ligand), also known as TNFSF13, is a secreted member of the TNF superfamily expressed by normal T cells, neutrophils, and dendritic cells as well as by a variety of cancers. APRIL binds to two receptors, BCMA and TACI, on the surface of B-lineage cells and is known to influence plasma cell survival, Ig switching, and the function of B1 B cells (Cancro 2004; Schneider 2005). Previous studies of human NHL showed that APRIL was expressed in association with high-grade DLBCL and Burkitt lymphoma but not with low-grade NHL including mantle cell and MZ lymphoma or CLL (Schwaller, Schneider et al. 2007). In contrast, Planelles, Carvalho-Pinto et al. (2004) found APRIL transcripts to be associated with nearly 50% of the CLL cases tested and demonstrated elevated levels of APRIL in serum from these patients. To investigate a role for APRIL in CLL, they generated TG mice with APRIL expressed from T cells.

Studies of APRIL TG mice older than 9 months revealed an expanded population of peritoneal B1a cells associated with enlargement of the mesenteric LN and Peyer's patches in about 40% of mice and splenomegaly and extralymphoid spread in fewer. The cells were non-proliferative but exhibited increased resistance to apoptosis. Comparisons with non-TG mice suggested that APRIL accelerates the expansion of peritoneal B1a cells seen in NZB and other strains.

Unfortunately, no studies were done to evaluate clonality, the mice were not identified as being leukemic, and none were said to have died of their disease.

8.2.2.6 Conclusions Regarding Mouse Models of CLL

As noted above, SBL, an uncommon spontaneous disease of old mice has many cytologic and histologic features in common with CLL. For mice suggested as models for CLL, some cases with histologic features of SBL are among those seen in BCL2/TRAF2DN mice (Zapata, Krajewska et al. 2004) but other lymphoma classes also develop in these mice, and the occurrence of ascites and pleural effusions is unusual. The description of the disease of mice carrying a mutant NFkB TG is like that of SBL, but the cells were not phenotyped or shown to be clonal. The diseases of NZB and TCL1 TG mice are histologically and cytologically quite distinct from SBL.

Many features of the malignant B-cell diseases of New Zealand mice and TCL1 TG mice are remarkably similar. They originate among oligoclonal populations of B1a cells in the peritoneum and progressively spread to spleen, peripheral blood, lymph nodes, and bone marrow. In the spleen, the histologic appearance is of MZL, but several features weigh against their origin from normal MZ B cells. First, the surface phenotype—$CD5^{lo}CD21^{lo/-}$—is not that of MZ B cells (Martin, Oliver et al. 2001; Bichi, Shinton et al. 2002). Second, the "MZL" often does not show the cytologic progression to high-grade disease seen in $NFS.V^{+}$ congenic mice. Instead, the cytology of cells in spleen, nodes, and even the blood of leukemic mice may differ little from those of mice with early expansion of the MZ. Third, MZL of $NFS.V^{+}$ almost never extend beyond the spleen. Finally, the V_HDJ_H sequences of the lymphomas are closer to those of normal B1a cells than to normal MZ B cells.

The process of peritoneal B1a B-cell transformation and subsequent spread may be accelerated by constitutive expression of TCL1, of the TRAF1 mimic, TRAF2DN, plus BCL2, and possibly of the mutant NFkB2 upstream of TRAF1 since CLL features heightened expression of TCL1, BCL2, and TRAF1. In this regard, it would be of interest to cross the TCL1 TG or mutant NFkB2 mice with NZB. The possible contributions of genetically determined changes in miR15/16 require confirmation but could relate the NZB disease to human CLL in yet another way. Caution is suggested by the understanding that NZW mice are like NZB in the development of clonal B1 populations but do not share the miR16 polymorphism with NZB.

The normal B-cell counterpart of the leukemic cell in CLL is not known but is clearly an issue of significant import. The candidates under consideration include resident or recirculating $CD5^{+}$ mantle zone B cells, MZ B cells, and lastly, the unidentified human equivalent of mouse B1a cells. Mantle cells seem unlikely as they exhibit little auto- or polyreactivity (Herve, Xu et al. 2005) while MZ and B1a cells of mice have this as a prominent feature (Martin, Oliver et al. 2001). A rationale for choosing between these cell subsets for one most like CLL is provided by extensive studies of V_HDJ_H sequences of purified peritoneal B1 and MZ B cells

(Kantor, Merrill et al. 1997; Schelonka, Tanner et al. 2007). Although the conclusions are based solely on analyses of the V_H7183 family, the CDR3s of MZ B cells were considerably shorter than for other B-cell subsets in spleen and bone marrow, D_H usage was biased toward DFL3, and J_H usage toward J_H2, N-region additions were fewer than for other B-cell subsets, and they had an increased proportion with charged amino acids. In contrast, B1a sequences revealed repertoires biased toward V_H1, V_H11 and V_H12, DSP D_H, and $J_H1$with fewer N-region additions than B1b or conventional B cells. In addition, CDR3 lengths were similar or slightly greater than those for B1b and B2 cells. These observations support a derivation of TCL1 lymphoma/leukemia from peritoneal B1a cells with the greatest discrepancy being the near-germline sequences of the clonal TCL1 TG populations. Human CLL might well derive from a parallel population of B1a cells. Efforts to develop an accelerated model of the NZB or TCL1 TG-based diseases would provide a superior preclinical model of CLL.

8.3 Marginal Zone Lymphomas

8.3.1 MZL in Humans

There are three general categories of MZL in humans: extranodal MZL of MALT lymphoma, nodal MZL, and splenic MZL (Jaffe, Harris et al. 2001). MALT and nodal MZL are characterized by accumulations of a heterogeneous population of small B cells infiltrating the marginal zones of reactive B-cell follicles. These centrocyte-like cells can be associated with occasional centroblasts and immunoblasts, and plasmacytoid differentiation is seen in some cases. In MALT lymphomas, the malignant cells characteristically infiltrate the epithelium-forming lymphoepithelial structures. Nodal MZL morphologically resembles lymph node infiltration by MALT but there is no evidence of extranodal involvement. Patients with MALT often have a history of autoimmune conditions, including Hashimoto's thyroiditis and Sjogren's syndrome, or inflammatory conditions, such as *Helicobacter pylori*-associated chronic gastritis or ocular infections with *Chlamydia psittaci*.

Splenic MZL is a rare disease in which small lymphocytes replace splenic white pulp GCs, infiltrate the surrounding marginal zones, and expand into the red pulp. Extension to splenic nodes and the bone marrow is common but involvement of peripheral nodes is not. These tumors may account for a high proportion of $CD5^-$ chronic lymphoid leukemias, sometimes featuring villous lymphocytes.

Two genes implicated in the development of MALT, *MALT1* and *BCL10*, were originally identified because of their involvement in recurring chromosomal translocations—t(11;18)(q21;q21) and t(14;18)(q32;q21) for MALT1 and t(1:14)(p22;q32) for BCL10—that occur specifically in MALT lymphomas. In normal B cells, MALT1 and BCL10 associate with CARMA1 downstream of the BCR to activate NFkB (Thome 2004).

8.3.2 Mouse Models of MZL

8.3.2.1 Spontaneous MZL in Mice

Splenic MZL is the only type of MZL that occurs spontaneously in mice (Fredrickson, Lennert et al. 1999). The disease, best characterized in NFS.V^+ mice more than a year of age (Hartley, Chattopadhyay et al. 2000), is a clonal disorder that initiates with expansion of the MZ by cells cytologically indistinguishable from normal MZ B cells and with almost no mitotic activity. Over time, these cells begin to finger into the red pulp and exhibit a more open chromatin pattern with more prominent nucleoli, and mitotic figures are more readily seen. This can progress to a high-grade lymphoma with a high mitotic index and cells cytologically indistinguishable from those of DLBCL of centroblastic (CBL) type. The lymphoma cells compress the white pulp and force out red pulp elements (Fredrickson, Lennert et al. 1999). The disease is almost always confined to the spleen but occasionally spreads to the splenic node and the liver. A leukemia phase is rare. FACS analyses have shown that the lymphomas cells are $CD5^{lo}IgM^{hi}B220^{lo}$ in the majority of cases.

Studies of NFS.V^+ MZL for somatically acquired proviral insertions of ecotropic MuLV identified a series of common integration sites (CIS) previously identified as candidate cancer genes (Shin, Fredrickson et al. 2004). Seven new CIS unique to MZL were also found including *Gfi1*, *Sox4*, and *Stat6* among others. Heightened expression of *Gfi1* distinguished MZL from other classes of B-cell lymphoma and was characteristic of MZL at all stages of progression suggesting a role in disease initiation.

8.3.2.2 Mouse Model of MALT

Mice infected with *Helicobacter felis* for 22 months or more developed a chronic gastritis associated with the development of lymphoid follicles, the appearance of lymphoepithelial lesions, and glandular destruction (Enno, O'Rourke et al. 1995). The later development of lymphoma was shown to be antigen-dependent since the incidence and severity of disease was significantly reduced in infected mice given anti-microbial therapy (Enno, O'Rourke et al. 1998). In addition, mice immunized against *H. felis* were protected from development of lymphoma (Sutton, O'Rourke et al. 2004). None of the lymphoid lesions were tested for clonality of the expanded B-cell populations, and upregulation of MALT or BCL10 was not described in reports of expression profiling (Mueller, O'Rourke et al. 2003).

8.3.2.3 Mouse Models of Splenic MZL

Aire-deficient mice replicate autoimmune features of patients with autoimmune polyendocrine syndrome type I, an inherited autosomal recessive disorder associated with progressive immune destruction of many tissues (Anderson,

Venanzi et al. 2002; Ramsey, Winqvist et al. 2002). More recent studies showed that mutant mice15–24 months of age exhibited expansion of the MZ (Hassler, Ramsey et al. 2006). Analyses of IgH D–J rearrangements revealed an oligoclonal pattern suggestive of early MZL. Interestingly, the cells populating the MZ were $CD21^{lo}$ and secreted autoantibodies on transfer, consistent with an activated phenotype. Unfortunately, expression of CD5 was not examined. These studies suggest a role for *Aire* as a tumor suppressor gene and stimulation with autoantigens as possibly contributory to development of MZL.

Interestingly, recent studies of mice with TG-induced expression of BCL10 in B cells were found to have significantly expanded populations of splenic MZ B cells, nuclear BCL10, and constitutive activation of the canonical NFkB signaling pathway (Stephen Morris, H. Morse, unpublished observations). Mice older than 18 months have started to develop lymphomas not seen in control littermates.

8.3.2.4 Conclusions Regarding Mouse Models of MZL

Spontaneous splenic MZL in mice has many similarities to splenic MZL in humans, but the latency for disease of greater than a year, the occurrence with other classes of B-cell lymphoma in $NFS.V^{+}$ mice, and the lack of demonstrable involvement of BCL10 or MALT1 make the model impractical for preclinical studies. The *Aire*-deficient mouse model of splenic MZL also suffers from long latency and low penitrance. *Helicobacter*-associated gastric lesions similar to those of gastric MALT never appears to evolve to clonal disease but appears to be useful for understanding the role of antigenic drive in early disease. The fact that there is no unequivocal evidence in mice for MZ B cells other than those in spleen may be responsible for the lack of models for nodal MZL. Mouse disorders with similarities to Sjogren's syndrome or Hashimoto's thyroiditis exhibit B-cell infiltrates of affected tissues but have never shown progression to clonal disease.

8.4 Mantle Cell Lymphoma

8.4.1 MCL in Humans

Human MCL is a mature B-cell neoplasm of small to medium-sized lymphocytes with irregular/cleaved nuclear contours that resemble centrocytes. Synonyms are morphologically descriptive and include intermediate or poorly differentiated lymphocytic lymphoma-diffuse or nodular type centrocytic (mantle cell) lymphoma, and malignant lymphoma diffuses small cleaved cell type. Human MCL typically involves lymph nodes and less frequently the spleen, bone marrow, and GI tract and is an intermediate to aggressive, usually incurable lesion with large cell blastoid variants of ominous prognosis

(Jaffe, Harris et al. 2001d). Until recently, there were no spontaneous or genetic mouse models of MCL, precluding development of a MMHCC classification although two MCL xenotransplant models have been reported (Bryant, Pham et al. 2000; M'Kacher, Farace et al. 2003). A t(11;14)(q13;32) between *IGH* and *CYCLIN D* loci is the hallmark aberration of human MCL, with dysregulated expression of the cyclin CCND1 protein (Williams, Westermann et al. 1990; Williams, Swerdlow et al. 1993). However, *Eμ–cyclin D1* TG mice have usual B-cell development and fail to develop tumors (Bodrug, Warner et al. 1994), indicating that cyclin D1 dysregulation may be necessary but not sufficient for developing a mouse model of MCL. By FACS or IHC, most human MCL are $IgM^{+}IgD^{+/-}CCND1^{+}BCL\text{-}2^{+}CD10^{-}BCL6^{-}CD23^{-}CD43^{+}FMC\text{-}7^{+}$ (Jaffe 2001). The cell(s) of origin are unknown although most cases show unmutated *IG* genes, suggesting a naïve or extrafollicular precursor B-cell type.

8.4.2 Mouse Models of MCL

8.4.2.1 MCL in Genetically Engineered Mice

Intraperitoneal injection of the tumor promoter pristane (2,6,10,14-tetramethyl-pentadecane) for 3 months into *Eμ–CCND1* TG mice >9 months of age resulted in a diffusely infiltrative, clonal, $IgM^{+}CD5^{+}CD20^{+}CD23^{-}$ B-cell lymphoma expressing the cyclin D1 transgene with intermediately sized, cleaved B cells reminiscent of MCL (Smith, Joshi et al. 2006) (Table 8.2). CD5 may represent an activation rather than differentiation marker in mouse B-cell tumors, and additional studies of tumor transplantability, aggression, and cell of origin are required to determine this model's resemblance to human MCL. Crossing *Eμ–IL-14α* with *Eμ–Myc* TG mice results in a disseminated, blastoid variant of MCL (MCL–BV) in almost 100% of mice by 3–4 months of age (Ford, Shen et al. 2007). Tumor cells are transplantable into SCID mice and show $sIgM^{+}CD5^{+}CD19^{+}CD21^{-}CD23^{-}$ by flow cytometry, with increased expression of endogenous CCND1, BCL2, ATM, RelA, and NF-κB2, and clonal Ig gene rearrangements, providing several molecular features that are observed in human MCL. However, the histology of these tumors is that of diffuse high-grade blastic B-cell lymphoma, frequently seen as a spontaneous disease in many strains of mice as well as in some genetically engineered strains (see below).

8.5 Follicular B-Cell Lymphoma

8.5.1 FBL in Humans

Follicular lymphoma in humans (FBL in mice) is mature B-cell lymphoma of GC origin comprised of a mixture of centrocytes and centroblasts with at least a partially follicular pattern (Jaffe, Harris et al. 2001). The cells are embedded in a

Table 8.2. Mouse models of human germinal center (GC) tumors[1]

Mode of tumor development	Tissue site of tumor development	GC B-cell tumor type	Mouse strain	Molecular alteration	Comments/other tumors	References
Transfer of human MCL	Peritoneal cavity	MCL	SCID	None	Xenotransplant of leukemic phase MCL cells	Bryant, Pham et al. (2000)
Transfer of human MCL	Lymphoid system	MCL [BV?]	NOD/SCID	None	Xenotransplant of peritoneal MCL cells	M'Kacher, Farace et al. (2003)
de novo	Peritoneal cavity, lymphoid system, metastases	MCL	C57BL/6	*Eμ–cyclin D1 TG*	Age dependent (>9-months), dependent on peritoneal inflammation (pristane)	Smith, Joshi et al. (2006)
de novo	Lymphoid system, metastases	MCL–BV	C57BL/6	*Eμ–IL–14α X, Eμ–Myc DTG*	Initial leukemia phase with blasts, lymphoma by 3–4 months in 100% DTG mice	Ford, Shen et al. (2007)
de novo	Lymphoid system, metastases	FBL, DLBCL	C57BL/6	*VavP–Bcl2* TG	Other tumors include PCT, LBL, HS	Egle, Harris et al. (2004)
de novo	Lymphoid system, metastases	FBL, DLBCL –CBL	C57BL/6	*Eμ–Pim1* TG	Other tumors include pre-T-LBL, HS	van Lohuizen, Verbeek et al. (1989) and Repacholi, Basten et al. (1997)
de novo	Lymphoid system, metastases	FBL, DLBCL	C57BL/6	*gMCL1* TG		Zhou, Levy et al. (2001)

Table 8.2. (continued)

Mode of tumor development	Tissue site of tumor development	GC B-cell tumor type	Mouse strain	Molecular alteration	Comments/other tumors	References
de novo	Lymphoid system, metastases	FBL, DLBCL, DBLL	C57BL/6 × C3H	*Eμ-B29–TCL1* TG	Other tumors include MZL, T-PLL	Hoyer, French et al. (2002); Shen, Ferguson et al. (2006); and Dawson, Hong et al. (2007)
de novo	Lymphoid system, metastases	FBL	C57BL/6 × FVB	*MLL–AF4* knock-in	Rare erythroid or myeloid leukemia	Chen, Li et al. (2006)
de novo	Lymphoid system metastases	FBL	C57BL/6	*Ing1* knock-out		Kichina, Zeremski et al. (2006)
de novo	Lymphoid system	DLBCL–CBL	C57BL/6 × 129 Sv	*Riz1* knock-out	Diverse non-lymphoid tumors	Steele-Perkins, Fang et al. (2001)
de novo	Lymphoid system	FBL, DLBCL –CBL	BALB/c	$H2\text{-}L^{d}\text{-}Il6$ TG	Occasional *IgH*/*Myc* gene rearrangements, co-existent PCT	Kovalchuk, Kim et al. (2002)
de novo	Lymphoid system, occasional metastases	DLBCL	C57BL/6 or 129/SvJ	*Bad* knock-out		Ranger, Zha et al. (2003)
de novo	Spleen, occasional lymph nodes	DLBCL, FBL	C57BL/6	*Bcl6* knock-in to *IgH* locus	Trisomy 13 and 15 common	Cattoretti, Pasqualucci et al. (2005)

Table 8.2. (continued)

Mode of tumor development	Tissue site of tumor development	GC B-cell tumor type	Mouse strain	Molecular alteration	Comments/other tumors	References
de novo	Lymphoid system	DLBCL, DBLL, FBL	C57BL/6	*Myc* knock-in 5' of $E\mu$ locus	Other tumors include LBL, PCT	Park, Kim et al. (2005) and Zhu, Qi et al. (2005)
de novo	Lymphoid system, variable metastases	DLBCL –CBL	C57BL/6	*AF4* invertor knock-in to *Mll* locus		Metzler, Forster et al. (2006)

[1]Mice are classified according to evolving criteria established initially by report of the Mouse Models of Human Cancer Consortium (MMHCC) study (Morse, Anver et al. 2002). Classifications in parentheses are not yet confirmed by MMHCC criteria or there are no MMHCC criteria yet developed for this entity. DBLL, diffuse high-grade blastic B cell lymphoma/leukemia; DLBCL, diffuse large B cell lymphoma; DTG, double transgenic; FBL, follicular B cell lymphoma; HS, histiocytic sarcoma; LBL, lymphoblastic lymphoma; MCL, mantle cell lymphoma; MCL-BV, mantle cell lymphoma-blastoid variant; MZL, marginal zone lymphoma; PCT, plasmacytoma; SCID, severe-combined immunodeficiency; TG, transgenic; T-PLL/CLL, T-prolymphocytic leukemia.

dense network of follicular dendritic cells. The disease appears to originate in lymph nodes, but spleen bone marrow and occasional blood involvement are not uncommon. The cells are usually $IgM^{+}CD5^{-}$ and, like normal GC B cells, express BCL6 and have mutated IgV region sequences. Almost all express BCL2, usually as the result of t(14;18)(q32;p21) translocations that bring the BCL2 gene under the control of IgL regulatory sequences (Tsujimoto, Finger et al. 1984; Hockenbery, Nunez et al. 1990). Morphologic transformation to aggressive DLBCL is common and is typically the cause of death. FBL makes up about 35% of adult NHL in the United States.

8.5.2 Mouse Models of FBL

8.5.2.1 Spontaneous FBL in Mice

FBL is a mature B-cell tumor characterized by a varying mixture of neoplastic centrocytes and centroblasts. Synonyms include follicular lymphoma, follicular center cell lymphoma mixed, CBL/centrocytic lymphoma, reticulum cell sarcoma type B, and lymphoma-pleomorphic. FBL is typically a low-grade lesion that resembles human follicular lymphoma and is the most frequent B-cell tumor of aging mice in many inbred strains, including $NFS.V^{+}$, CFW, and AKXD RI strains (Morse, McCarty et al. 2003). Distinct from human follicular lymphoma, spontaneous FBL is not associated with *Bcl2* gene rearrangements (Morse, Anver et al. 2002). Splenomegaly and variable enlargements of mesenteric lymph nodes and Peyer's patches are typically seen. Histologic examination reveals white pulp expansions that appear as white nodules and coalesce with advancing disease. Centroblasts and centrocytes are the main cell types present, with small follicular B cells pushed to the periphery and the T-cell zone reduced or eliminated. Blast cells should be less than 50% to distinguish FBL from diffuse high-grade blastic B-cell lymphoma/leukemia (DLBCL or DBLL). By FACS, most cases are $IgM^{+}IgD^{-}CD5^{dull}CD45R(B220)^{lo/+}$. By IHC, centroblasts and centrocytes are both $IgM^{+}CD45R(B220)^{+}CD19^{+}$. Tumor cells are mono- or oligoclonal for Ig gene rearrangements, with the presumed cells of origin being GC centrocytes and centroblasts.

8.5.2.2 FBL in Genetically Engineered Mice

Two independent lines of *Eμ-BCL2* TG mice develop follicular hyperplasia but rarely develop FBL and then with greatly prolonged latencies (McDonnell and Korsmeyer 1991; Strasser, Harris et al. 1993) (Table 8.2). In contrast, *VavP–Bcl2* TG mice that do not succumb to autoimmune disease develop follicular hyperplasia, followed by FBL at 10–18 months of age in up to 50% of mice. The disease is characterized by PCNA-positive, class-switched neoplastic B cells containing mutated IgV region genes (Egle, Harris et al. 2004). GC expansion and lymphomagenesis depended upon concurrent expansion of BCL2 transgene-expressing

$CD4^+$ T cells, suggesting that microenvironmental support was required for FBL development.

Eμ–Pim1 TG mice develop pre-T-lymphoblastic lymphoma (pre-T-LBL) at 7–10 months of age. Mice unaffected by pre-T-LBL demonstrating probable FBL and multiple subtypes of DLBCL at older ages using pre-Bethesda nomenclature criteria (van Lohuizen, Verbeek et al. 1989; Repacholi, Basten et al. 1997). A construct using the flanking regulatory elements of human *MCL1* caused lymphoma in 65% of TG mice by 24 months, with about 20% of cases diagnosed as FBL under pre-Bethesda criteria (Zhou, Levy et al. 2001).

Eμ-B29-TCL1 TG mice, encoding the AKT co-activator TCL1 oncoprotein, develop a spectrum of mature GC and non-GC B-cell lymphomas, with relatively rare FBL and more common DLBCL and DBLL generation (Hoyer, French et al. 2002; Shen, Ferguson et al. 2006). Similar to *VavP–Bcl2* TG mice, *Eμ-B29–TCL1* TG mice require concurrent *TCL1*-mediated $CD4^+$ T-cell expansion to transform GC B cells, because mice with only B-lineage *TCL1* transgene expression develop mainly a model of the aggressive form of B-CLL (Bichi, Shinton et al. 2002).

Knock-in of a human *MLL–AF4* fusion gene into the mouse *Mll* locus produces predominantly FBL with clonal $sIgM^+B220^+Pax5^+Bcl6^+CD19^+$ tumor cells arising from follicular centers following a mixed myeloid/lymphoid hyperplasia (Chen, Li et al. 2006). *MLL–AF4* tumor cells metastasized widely without a leukemic phase and are transplantable. Knock-out of the *Ing1* gene, which encodes a nuclear PHD finger-containing protein not yet associated with human lymphoid malignancies, results in 20% of mice developing lymphoma. Tumors originate in the spleen and contain a mixed population of $B220^+$ cells that histologically resemble centroblasts and centrocytes to suggest FBL (Kichina, Zeremski et al. 2006). However, additional marker studies, evaluation of *Ig* mutation status, and clonality and transplantation studies are required to confirm this diagnosis and to exclude a robust follicular hyperplasia instead of malignancy (Kichina, Zeremski et al. 2006).

8.5.2.3 Conclusions Regarding Mouse Models of FBL

Spontaneous FBL in mice and many of the disorders of TG mice models have a number of histologic and particularly cytologic features in common with the human disease. However, the true follicular pattern seen in humans is absent in all these cases including those with extensive lymph node involvement. None of the models exhibit chromosomal translocations affecting the *Bcl2* locus, and the *VavP–Bcl-2* TG is the only one with constitute Bcl2 expression. It may be important that the major breakpoint region (MBR) in the human *BCL2* locus bears is markedly different to the same general region in the mouse locus. These differences may preclude chromosomal rearrangements in the mouse. This possibility is being tested by knocking in 2 kb around the human MBR into the mouse *Bcl2* locus.

8.6 Diffuse Large B-Cell Lymphoma

8.6.1 DLBCL in Humans

DLBCL is characterized by a diffuse proliferation of large neoplastic B cells with nuclear size that exceeds that of normal histiocytes. A number of cytologic variants have been described including CBL, IBL, T-cell/histiocyte rich, plasmablastic, and anaplastic with CBL being the most common. Distinction among these variants suffers from poor interobserver reproducibility, and subsets have not been reliably tied to prognosis. Consequently, a designation simply as DLBCL is felt by pathologists to be most appropriate (Jaffe, Harris et al. 2001).The tumor cells express pan-B-cell markers and surface or cytoplasmic Ig, and about 10% are $CD5^+$. Nuclear BCL6 is expressed in almost all cases, and IgV region genes are mutated. Gene expression profiling by one group using microarrays delineated two major subsets that are related to cell of origin as activated B-cell-like and GC B-cell-like (Alizadeh, Eisen et al. 2000). The distinctions have prognostic significance as the prognosis for patients in the GC B-cell-like subset is considerably better than that of patients with the activated B-cell type. However, array-based studies of DLBCL by another group did not reproduce these associations, defining instead three discreet subgroups designated “oxidataive phosphorylation”, “B-cell receptor/proliferation,” and “host response” (Monti, Savage et al. 2005).

8.6.2 Mouse Models of DLBCL

8.6.2.1 Spontaneous DLBCL in Mice

DLBCL is an aggressive mature B-cell malignancy that demonstrates a diffuse proliferation of tumor cells with large nuclei and distinct cytologic features. Characteristic DLBCL variants occur spontaneously in aging mice and are classified as CBL, IBL, histiocyte-associated (HA), and primary mediastinal (PM, thymic) subtypes (Morse, Anver et al. 2002). CBL, IBL, and HA variants are common in $NFS.V^+$ mice and usually arise with splenomegaly or lymphadenopathy (Hartley, Chattopadhyay et al. 2000), whereas PM shows mainly thymic enlargement and has been seen only in mice infected with a unique replication-defective retrovirus (Morse, Anver et al. 2002).

8.6.2.2 Spontaneous Variants of DLBCL in Mice

DLBCL–CBL Variant

CBL synonyms include large cleaved follicular center cell lymphoma and CBL lymphoma. About 12% of spontaneous lymphomas in $NFS.V^+$ and 17% in CFW mice are CBL, whereas CBL was not detected in AKXD RI lymphomas and is not common in other inbred strains (Morse, McCarty et al. 2003). Histologically, the splenic white pulp is greatly expanded by tumor cells with round nuclei, often with one or two prominent nucleoli, basophilic cytoplasm, and numerous mitoses. These cells are admixed with varying amounts of smaller centrocytes. A diagnosis is made when >70% of the cells are blasts. When the proportion of centrocytes to blasts ranges from 40–70% and the ratio varies in different microscopic fields, a distinction between DLBCL and FBL is difficult although CBL may more completely destroy the usual GC architecture than FBL at advanced stages. CBL frequently infiltrates the lung, liver, and kidney and, less frequently, the bone marrow. By FACS, most cases are IgM^+ or IgG^+, $B220^+CD5^{low}CD19^+$. By IHC, they are usually $BCL6^+PAX5^+IRF8^+PU.1^+CD138^-$ $XBP1^-$ $Blimp1^-$. Tumors are clonal for *Ig* gene rearrangements, and oligonucleotide expression microarrays have shown no clear differences between follicular or diffuse CBL subtypes, suggesting that these subtypes may represent earlier and later stages of progression (Morse, unpublished results). By expression microarray analysis, CBL is readily distinguished from the CBL form of MZL and is similar to the CBL variant of human DLBCL.

DLBCL–IBL Variant

IBL lymphoma is the synonym ascribed to IBL. About 8% of spontaneous lymphomas in $NFS.V^+$ and 4% in CFW mice are IBL, whereas IBL was not detected in AKXD RI lymphomas (Morse, McCarty et al. 2003). Histologically, IBLs are highly aggressive and demonstrate large, round nuclei having dispersed chromatin and prominent nucleoli, abundant cytoplasm, and a high mitotic rate. A "starry sky" pattern may be seen with increased apoptotic cells. Tumor cells are clonal for Ig gene rearrangements and often admixed with centroblasts and centrocytes, which may reflect an origin from a FBL or post-GC immunoblast. By FACS, IBLs typically are $sIgM^{low}B220^{dull}$ and by IHC most cases are $BCL6^+PAX5^+IRF8^-PU.1^-XBP1^-IRF4^-Blimp1^-$.

DLBCL–HA variant

DLBCL–HA (histiocyte associated) is the acronym of HA variant. About 20% of spontaneous lymphomas in AKXD RI (and 1% in $NFS.V^+$) strain mice are HA, and HA is not common in other frequently used inbred strains (Fredrickson and Harris 2000; Morse, McCarty et al. 2003). Histologically, all mice show splenomegaly with a marked expansion of histiocytes (macrophages) that may obscure malignant B cells. Histiocytes may occupy the entire white pulp, obliterating the PALS and destroying the usual follicular architecture, thereby pushing B cells to the periphery. Malignant B cells usually have features of FBL or CBL although rare cases show tumor cells with features seen in MZL, SBL, or IBL. Lymphadenopathy is seen in half the cases, and HA may involve the liver early on. The pattern of tumor growth is mainly nodular rather than diffuse, and this lesion resembles human histiocyte/T-cell-rich DLBCL (Jaffe 2001). It may be difficult to distinguish DLBCL–HA from histiocytic sarcoma. By IHC, the histiocytes of HA are usually EMR1 (F4/80)$^+$LGALS (Mac-2)$^+$, whereas the malignant B cells express markers consistent with their origin and are typically Pax5$^+$. A clonal *Ig* gene rearrangement with PAX5$^+$ cells in a histologic picture dominated by histiocytes is diagnostic, with the main differential diagnosis being histiocytic sarcoma. The presumed cell of origin for the malignant B-cell component is usually a GC or post-GC B cell, whereas tissue macrophages comprise the non-malignant histiocytic component.

8.6.2.3 DLBCL in Genetically Engineered Mice

DLBCL may arise de novo or by aggressive transformation of FBL and possibly SMZL. Ionizing radiation causes an increased frequency of tumors with histologic features of pre-T-LBL, FBL, and DLBCL–CBL in *Eμ–Pim-1* TG mice (Repacholi, Basten et al. 1997). Targeted deletion of *Riz1*, encoding a Rb-binding zinc finger protein, results in 37% of null and 19% of heterozygous mice developing clonal, B220$^+$ B-cell lymphomas with histologic features of DLBCL–CBL by 18–22 months of age (Steele-Perkins, Fang et al. 2001) (Table 8.2). *H2-L*^{d}*-Il6* TG mice develop PCT between 6 and 19 months of age, frequently with co-existing FBL or DLBCL–CBL (Kovalchuk, Kim et al. 2002). By IHC, the lymphomas are IgM$^+$B220$^+$CD19$^+$ and several contained t(12;15) *IgH/Myc* gene rearrangements.

Eμ-B29–TCL1 TG mice develop clonal IgM$^+$B220$^+$CD5^{low}BCL6$^+$ DLBCL, most often HA and occasionally CBL or IBL subtypes with somatically mutated *Ig* genes and widespread dissemination (Hoyer, French et al. 2002). Equally frequent DBLL and rare FBL, SMZL, and T-PLL are also formed in this model (Hoyer, French et al. 2002; Dawson, Hong et al. 2007). B-cell lymphomas were eliminated by crossing the *TCL1* TG with an *OCA-B* null mouse that fare incapable of developing GC structures (Shen, Ferguson et al. 2006).

Knock-out of the proapoptotic BH3-only *Bad* gene results in 20% of mice developing clonal sIgM$^+$ or sIgG$^+$, B220$^+$CD19$^+$CD43$^-$BCL6$^+$ DLBCL of unclear subtype by 18–24 months of age (Ranger, Zha et al. 2003). Knock-in of the murine *Bcl6* gene into the *IgH* locus results in increased GC formation in spleens of non-immunized mice, followed successively by a benign lymphoproliferative disorder with expanded white pulp and then the development of DLBCL and FBL between 13 and 20 months of age (Cattoretti, Pasqualucci et al. 2005). Tumors were clonal and IgM$^+$IgD$^+$B220$^+$CD43$^-$CD138$^-$ with variable Mum1/IRF4 staining by IHC. They contained mutated *IgV* region genes and frequent trisomy of Chrs 13 and 15. More recent studies showed that mice bearing the *Bcl6* knock-in do not develop DLBCL when crossed onto an AID-deficient background (Pasqualucci and Dalla-Favera, unpublished observations)

Knock-in of the mouse *Myc* gene 5' of the *Eμ* intronic enhancer results in clonal IgM$^+$B220$^+$CD19$^+$Bcl6$^+$ DLBCL of unclear subtype developing between 6 and 21 months of age, along with FBL, DBLL, and PCT formation (Park, Kim et al. 2005; Zhu, Qi et al. 2005). Using an "invertor" conditional knock-in strategy to bypass embryonic lethality, a Cre-generated *Mll–AF4* fusion gene in the endogenous *Mll* locus results in IgM$^+$B220$^+$ CBL with clonal *Ig* gene rearrangements in 60% of cases (Metzler, Forster et al. 2006). Microarray profiling of tumor cells shows strong expression of *Pax5* and *Ebf* and variable expression of *Bcl2* and *Bcl6* differentiation markers (Metzler, Forster et al. 2006). The CBL tumor cells were transplantable into *Rag1*-deficient recipient mice.

8.6.2.4 Conclusions Regarding Mouse Models of DLBCL

The last several years have been marked by striking progress in the generation and validation of mouse DLBCL as shown by studies of *Eμ-B29–TCL1* TG and *Bcl6* knock-in mice. The lymphomas of these mice share histologic features with human DLBCL, carry mutated IgV regions, and are strikingly dependent on normally functioning GC for their development. They provide novel and important in vivo settings for furthering our understanding of the roles played by TCL1 and BCL6 in normal B-cell biology and lymphomagenesis.

8.7 Diffuse High-Grade Blastic B-cell Lymphoma/Leukemia (DBLL) in Mice

The human equivalent or parallel to this disorder is currently not known. DBLL is a highly aggressive lymphoma of medium-sized B cells that exhibit a high mitotic rate, extensive apoptosis, and sometimes a leukemic phase. Synonyms include lymphoblastic lymphoma, Burkitt and Burkitt-like lymphoma, and DLBCL of lymphoblastic lymphoma subtype [DLBCL(LL)]. About 20% of spontaneous lymphomas in NFS.V$^+$ and ~30% in AKXD RI strains and CFW mice are DBLL, but DBLL is not common in other frequently used inbred strains (Morse, McCarty et al. 2003). Cases present with lymphadenopathy, variable involvement of the spleen, and sometimes thymus, with frequent non-hematopoietic organ dissemination. Affected tissues show uniform-appearing lymphoblasts with little cytoplasm, dispersed chromatin, and indistinct nucleoli. Histologic sections show many mitotic figures typically with large numbers of tingible body macrophages ingesting apoptotic cells, leading to a "starry sky" appearance. Infiltration of the deep cortex in lymph nodes progresses to replacement of normal cells and growth outside the capsule into the fat. When involved, the spleen shows diffuse infiltration of both the red and the white pulp. Perivascular and peribronchial infiltrates of the lungs and periportal liver infiltrates are common. Histologically and cytologically, these mature B-cell neoplasms are indistinguishable from precursor T-cell lymphoblastic lymphomas that lack thymic involvement and precursor B-cell lymphoblastic lymphomas. Analyses of *Ig* and *TCR* gene organization and IHC studies provide definitive distinctions among these disorders.

There is a spectrum of IHC phenotypes for DBLL ranging from patterns similar to immature or transitional B cells (IgM$^+$IgD$^-$C1QR1(AA4.1)$^+$) to that of GC-experienced B cells that are *Ig* class-switched with *IgV* region mutations. DBLL are clonal for *Ig* gene rearrangements. Structural rearrangements of cellular genes, mostly due to proviral insertions, are seen from pooled studies of NFS.V$^+$ (Hartley, Chattopadhyay et al. 2000) and AKXD RI (Morse, Qi et al. 2001) lymphomas for *Zfp521* (*Evi3*) (11.9%), *Pim1* (5.6%), *Evi1* (4.8%), and *Myc* (0.8%). Lymphomas of *λ-MYC* were characterized by chromosomal instability and frequent biallelic deletions of *Cdkn2a* (p16) (Kovalchuk, Qi et al. 2000). Lymphomas of *Eμ–Myc* TG mice had frequent changes in the p19^{ARF}–MDM2–p53 tumor suppressor axis (Park, Kim et al. 2005). Immature or transitional B cells are the presumed cells of origin for *Eμ–Myc*, *IgH/c–myc YAC*, *EμIgH/c–myc YAC*, and *λ–MYC* TG mice. Probable GC or early post-GC B cells are the cells of origin for those with features similar to the DBLL of *Eμ-B29–TCL1* TG mice.

8.7.1 DBLL in Genetically Engineered Mice

An immature or transitional cell immunophenotype is characteristic of most lymphomas of *Eμ–Myc, IgH/c–Myc YAC*, *EμIgH/c–Myc YAC*, and *λ-MYC* TG mice. More mature immunophenotypes occur in spontaneous DBLL of NFS.V$^+$ mice and some lymphomas of *Eμ-B29–TCL1* TG and *Eμ–Myc* knock-in mice, along with many other genetically engineered mice. B-lineage lymphomas with lymphoblastic cytology but distinct from precursor B-lymphoblastic neoplasms are seen at low to high frequency in many strains of genetically engineered mice and a number of conventional inbred strains. The lymphomas of *λ-MYC* TG mice were originally designated Burkitt lymphoma (Morse, Anver et al. 2002), but *Ig* genes are not mutated and tumor cells have an immunophenotype of transitional or immature B cells indicating that they differ from human Burkitt cases. A change in nomenclature is clearly warranted. Mouse cases with similar histology and cytology occurring in mice other than the *λ-MYC* TGs were previously designated Burkitt-like (Morse, Anver et al. 2002). The findings that these tumors rarely have structural alterations in *Myc* and do not overexpress *Myc* distinguish them from human Burkitt-like lymphomas (Jaffe 2001).

8.8 Plasma Cell Neoplasms

8.8.1 Human PCN Including Multiple Myeloma

The evaluation of present mouse models of human PCN, and attempts to devise improved models, should be guided by insights into the natural history of PCN development in human beings (Mitsiades, Mitsiades et al. 2007) and the biologic and molecular genetic features of frank, untreated PCN at the time of clinical presentation (Carrasco, Tonon et al. 2006). In analogy to cancer development in general (Hanahan and Weinberg 2000), human PCN including MM are thought to be initiated by somatic mutations in oncogenes and/or tumor suppressor genes, followed by the stepwise accumulation of genetic and epigenetic alterations that comprise tumor progression events (Bergsagel and Kuehl 2005; Kuehl and Bergsagel 2005). The later changes alter the phenotype of the incipient tumor cell as well as its interactions with the local microenvironment until fully malignant transformation has occurred. As the acronym suggests, PCN comprise a spectrum of malignancies that share the rather uniform histopathology of the aberrant, neoplastic plasma cell. However, despite their morphologic similarities, PCN demonstrate a great deal of diversity at the molecular level associated with major differences in epidemiology, clinical behavior, and treatment options.

The classification of PCN in the World Health Organization (WHO) nomenclature includes the following:

1. *Plasma cell myeloma*. This is a bone marrow-based PCN, usually multifocal, thus commonly referred to as MM. MM is incurable with a survival rate of ~40% at 5 years after diagnosis. MM is defined by monoclonal Ig protein (M spike) in serum, bone destruction, hypercalcemia, and anemia. The standard of care includes low- and high-dose chemotherapy, bone marrow transplantation, and novel drugs. Tumor variants include non-secretory myeloma (no serum monoclonal Ig), indolent myeloma, smoldering myeloma, and plasma cell leukemia.
2. *PCT*. A solitary, localized, monoclonal PCN that grows either in bone (solitary bone PCT) or soft tissue (solitary extraosseous or extramedullary PCT). PCT is rare but curable with moderate-dose radiotherapy as the preferred treatment. The most common pattern of relapse is systemic, indicating progression to MM.
3. *Ig deposition diseases*. Primary amyloidosis and systemic IgL chain and IgH chain deposition diseases.
4. *Osteosclerotic myeloma (POEMS syndrome)*. POEMS, defined by *p*olyneuropathy, *o*rganomegaly, *e*ndocrinopathy, *m*onoclonal gammopathy, and *s*kin changes is very rare.
5. *Heavy chain diseases*. Distinguished according to the isotype (γ, μ, and α) of the monoclonal IgH chain produced by neoplastic plasma cells.

Among human PCN, MM is by far the most important and well-studied disease. MM is a neoplasm of mature post-GC, Ig-secreting, isotype-switched plasma cells (Zojer, Ludwig et al. 2003) that accumulate in the bone marrow and cause bone destruction (Roodman 2006). Recent molecular and cytogenetic studies have shown that MM is remarkably a heterogeneous disease that can be divided into a number of distinct categories based on global gene expression profiles, detection of reciprocal chromosomal translocations that recombine Ig loci with oncogenes, and ploidy status of tumor cells (Zhan, Hardin et al. 2002; Shaughnessy and Barlogie 2003). Depending on the criteria applied by different laboratories, it is possible to distinguish 5–8 subcategories of MM. Regardless of how these differences are resolved, the present molecular and cytogenetic subdivision of MM is already of clinical relevance because it predicts significant differences in the prognosis and response to therapy of MM patients, no matter whether treatment relies on standard, high-dose, or novel therapies (Mulligan, Mitsiades et al. 2007).

No definitive cause of MM has been identified. Genetic risk factors include gender (male > female), race (the incidence in African Americans in the United States is twice that of US whites), and age (median age at diagnosis is ~70 years). Familial clustering points to a hereditary predisposition consistent with an autosomal-dominant mode of inheritance, but tumor susceptibility alleles or "MM genes" have not been identified. Ionizing radiation is thought to be the strongest environmental risk factor for MM, but definitive studies have not been described. Although the evidence is not conclusive, there are reports of associations between MM and occupational exposure to various metals (nickel), chemical compounds (aromatic hydrocarbons, silicone, and petrochemical agents), pesticides and animal viruses (farming), protracted infections that can lead to sustained B-cell activation by microbial antigens (*H. pylori*, HHV8), acquired immunodeficiency syndromes, such as HIV/AIDS, that result in reduced immune surveillance by T cells, and autoimmune diseases, such as rheumatoid arthritis.

The neoplastic cell in MM appears to derive from an antigen-experienced isotype-switched post-GC B-lymphocyte that has undergone somatic hypermutation of the expressed *IgH* and *IgL* genes. Pathogenic factors implicated in MM include cytogenetic and molecular genetic alterations that result in the deregulated expression of oncogenes, such as *CCND1* (encoding cyclin D1), *FGFR3* (fibroblast growth factor receptor 3), and *WHSC1* (Wolf–Hirschhorn syndrome candidate 1; also known as *MMSET* or MM SET domain containing protein type III). The interaction of tumor cells with the bone marrow microenvironment is of crucial importance, as it leads to the production of cytokines including IL-6, IGF-1, VEGF, SDF-1α, TNF-α, and TGF-β.

The subgroups of MM are presently distinguished based on recurrent *IGH* translocations, ploidy status of tumor cells, and global gene expression patterns. Hyperdiploid tumors (40% of cases) contain 48–75 chromosomes and are characterized by multiple trisomies of Chr 3, 5, 7, 9, 11, 15, 19, and 21. Non-hyperdiploid tumors (nearly 50% of cases) carry one of seven recurrent chromosomal translocations that recombine *IGH* at 14q32 with seven different oncogenes. These translocations are thought to be very early if not the initiating oncogenic events and are caused by errors in Ig switch recombination or somatic hypermutation during the GC reaction. They fall into one of three groups.

1. D-type cyclins: *CCND1* (cyclin D1) at 11q13 in 15% of cases, *CCND2* (cyclin D2) at 12p13 in <15 of cases, and *CCND3* (cyclin D3) at 6p21 in 2% of cases.

2. MAF family genes: *MAF* (c-Maf) at 16q23 in 5% of cases, *MAFB* (Maf B) at 20q12 in 2% of cases, and *MAFA* (Maf A) at 8q24.3 in 1% of cases.
3. MMSET/FGFR3: *MMSET* (formally designated *WHSC1*) and *FGFR3* at 4p16 in 15% of cases.

Tumor progression events include chromosomal translocations that affect the *MYC* gene at 8q24 (15% of primary MM, 45% of advanced MM, and >90% of MM-derived cell lines) but do not involve aberrant isotype switching or somatic hypermutation and exhibit a similar prevalence in hyperdiploid and non-hyperdiploid tumors. They also include activating mutations of *NRAS*, *KRAS*, or *FGFR3*; amplifications of 1q; deletions of 13q and p53; constitutive activation of NFκB—e.g., via inactivation of TRAF3, constitutive overexpression of NIK (NFκB inducing kinase), or activation of NFKB2—perturbation of the RB pathway—e.g., via methylation of the $p16^{INK4a}$ promoter—and deletion of $p18^{INK4c}$.

MM is preceded in a sizable fraction of cases by a premalignant disorder that is characterized by the abnormal persistence, sometimes for decades, of a clone of Ig-producing plasma cells that are lodged in the bone marrow without causing osteoporosis or osteolytic lesions. This disorder is referred to as MGUS (Rajkumar, Lacy et al. 2007). MGUS is defined by a monoclonal serum Ig of <30 g/l, the presence of 10% or fewer plasma cells in the bone marrow, the absence of anemia and lytic bone lesions, and the absence of hypercalcemia and renal insufficiency related to the clonal plasma cell proliferation. The prevalence of MGUS in elderly patients is ~5%. The progression from MGUS to MM occurs at a slow but remarkably steady rate of 1% per year. The etiology of MGUS is not known, but epidemiologic evidence points to age, gender, and race as risk factors. The pathogenesis of MGUS is poorly understood. Approximately 50% of MGUS cell clones carry chromosomal translocations that rearrange *IGH* at 14q32 with oncogenes on one of five partner chromosomes also identified in MM: *CCND1*, *CCND3*, *FGFR3* and *MMSET*, *MAF*, and *MAFB*. These translocations are thought to play an important role in the initiation of MM. Approximately 40% of the plasma cell clones in MGUS smoldering MM and frank MM are hyperdiploid. This consistency suggests that hyperdiploid MM originates from hyperdiploid MGUS. Likewise, deletions of Chr 13q, which have an adverse prognostic association in MM, are found in similar frequencies in MGUS and MM, indicating a direct precursor–product relationship of $13q^-$ preneoplastic and neoplastic states. Empirical observations of this kind suggest that MGUS occurs as distinct molecular subtypes, which lead, in turn, to different forms of MM.

Evidence suggests that MGUS and MM develop along one of two distinct pathways that result in either non-hyperdiploid tumors that usually carry one of the seven recurrent *IGH* translocations or hyperdiploid tumors that usually are not associated with *IGH* translocations. Despite enormous progress in the past decade in our understanding of MM pathogenesis, many important questions remain. What are the molecular and microenvironmental mechanisms that drive the transition from MGUS to MM? How does hyperdiploidy contribute to plasma cell transformation? What genetic lesions underlie recurrent cytogenetic changes, such as gain of chromosome 1q or loss of chromosome 13q? Mouse models of human PCN may help to provide answers to these and other important questions.

8.8.2 Established and Newly Emerging Mouse Models of Human PCN

The presently available mouse models of human PCN can be divided into de novo and transplantation models. Although none of the genetically engineered strains recapitulate all features of a particular human PCN, several strains have emerged as useful platforms for mechanistic and therapeutic studies of alterations in signaling pathway found in human PCN (e.g., IL-6, Abl, and Myc). Furthermore, although the succession of oncogenic processes responsible for tumor development that occurs de novo does not completely match those in humans, the incipient tumor cells in mice interact with their microenvironment (immune cells, vascular and lymphatic networks, and extracellular matrix) in ways that mirror the interactions of neoplastic plasma cells in humans with their specific tissue microenvironment. Similarly, mouse models that have been developed to permit the outgrowth of fully transformed transplanted tumor cells in vivo are not suitable for studying mechanisms of tumor development. Nonetheless, they are highly valuable for many other purposes including preclinical drug testing. Table 8.3 shows mouse models of human PCN in chronological order of development, beginning with strains in which tumor development occurs de novo, followed by models that rely on tumor cell transfer.

The first mouse model of de novo PCN, peritoneal PCT in strain BALB/c, was discovered 50 years ago by Dr. Michael Potter of the National Cancer Institute and has been progressively developed and refined by him over the last half century Anderson and Potter (1969). Salient features of this model include dependency on chronic inflammation (usually induced by intraperitoneal application of pristane), genetic background (BALB/cAnPt is highly susceptible, NZB and BALB/cJ are weakly susceptible, and all other tested strains including DBA/2, C57BL/6, CBA/J, C3H, and 129 are solidly resistant), maintenance of mice in an antigen-rich conventional facility (SPF mice are refractory to tumor development), and the acquisition of *Myc*-deregulating chromosomal translocation in early tumor precursors. The penetrance of peritoneal PCT at 65% is incomplete and the average latency of 220 days is long. However, tumor development can be greatly accelerated by infection of mice with retrovirus expressing any of the series of oncogenes alone or in combination—Abelson-(v-*abl*), RIM (v-Ha-*Ras* and Eμ–c-*Myc*), J3V1 (v-*Raf1* and v-*myc*), and ABL–MYC (v-*abl* and human *MYC*).

Unfortunately, this model of PCN has been largely dismissed by the myeloma community as artificial and irrelevant for human MM, mainly due to

Table 8.3. Mouse models of human plasma cell neoplasms (PCN) including extraosseous plasmactyoma (PCT) and multiple myeloma (MM)

Mode of tumor development	Tissue site of tumor development	Tumor type	Mouse strain	Transgene	Comment	Reference
de novo	Peritoneal cavity	PCT	BALB/c	None	High impact on immunology and cancer research	Potter (2003)
					Dependent on peritoneal inflammation (pristane)	Potter and MacCardle (1964) and Anderson and Potter (1969)
					Dependent on *Myc* translocation	Potter and Wiener (1992) and Janz (2006)
					Accelerated by retroviruses, such as A-MuLV, RIM (c-myc + v-ras), J3V1 (v-myc + v-raf), and ABL–MYC	Potter, Sklar et al. (1973), Ohno, Migita et al. (1984), Clynes, Wax et al. (1988), Troppmair, Huleihel et al. (1988), Weissinger, Mischak et al. (1991)
de novo	Bone marrow	MM	C57BL/Ka	None	Spontaneous tumors Impractical due to long latency and low incidence Source of transplantable 5T tumors (see below) No *Myc* translocations	Radl, Croese et al. (1988), and Radl, Van Arkel et al. (1996)
de novo	Lymphoid system	PCT	BALB/c	Eμ–v-abl	Mice develop peritoneal tumors upon treatment with pristane	Rosenbaum, Harris et al. (1990)
de novo	Lymphoid system, GALT	PCT	BALB/c	H2-L^d-IL-6	Mice develop peritoneal tumors upon treatment with pristane	Kovalchuk, Kim et al. (2002)

Table 8.3. (continued)

Mode of tumor development	Tissue site of tumor development	Tumor type	Mouse strain	Transgene	Comment	Reference
de novo	Lymphoid system	PCT	BALB/c	Eμ–Bcl-2	Mice develop peritoneal tumors upon treatment with pristane	Silva, Kovalchuk et al. (2003)
de novo	Bone marrow, lymphoid system	MM > PCT	C57BL/6 and BALB/c	NPM–ALK	Transgene targeted to T lymphocytes	Chiarle, Gong et al. (2003)
de novo	Peritoneal cavity, lymphoid system, and bone marrow	PCT > MM	Mixed BALB/c	iMyc	Mice develop peritoneal tumors upon treatment with pristane	Park, Kim et al. (2005), Park, Shaffer et al. (2005), and Kim, Han et al. (2006)
de novo	Lymphoid system, bone marrow	PCT > MM	Mixed	iMyc + Bcl–X_L	3'KE–Bcl–X_L transgene	Cheung, Kim et al. (2004)
de novo	Lymphoid system, bone marrow	PCT > MM	FVB/N	Bcl–X_L	Accelerated tumorigenesis upon crossing in the Eμ/c-Myc transgene	Linden, Kirchhof et al. (2004) and Adams et al. (1985)
de novo	Bone marrow and lymphoid system	MM > PCT	C57BL/6	Bcl–X_L + virus		Linden, Kirchhof et al. (2005)
de novo	Bone marrow	MM > PCT	C57BL/6	Xbp1		Carrasco, Sukhdeo et al. (2007)
de novo	Not yet reported	Not yet reported	Not yet reported	TVA/TVB	Unpublished	F. Asimakopoulos and H.E. Varmus[1]
de novo	Bone marrow	MM	Not yet reported	Kappa*Myc	Unpublished	M. Chesi, A.K. Stewart, and P.L. Bergsagel et al.[1]

Table 8.3. (continued)

Mode of tumor development	Tissue site of tumor development	Tumor type	Mouse strain	Transgene	Comment	Reference
Transfer of mouse MM	Bone marrow	MM	C57BL/6	None	Relies on 5T tumor cells homing to mouse bone, extensively studied	Vanderkerken, Goes et al. (1996)
Transfer of human MM	Bone marrow	MM	SCID-hu	None	Human MM cells homing to human fetal bone implanted s.c. in mice, well established	Yaccoby, Barlogie et al. (1998)
Transfer of human MM	Bone marrow	MM	SCID-hu	None	Human MM bone cores implanted i.m. in mice	Campbell, Manyak et al. (2006)
Transfer of human MM	Bone marrow	MM	NOD/SCID-hu	None	Immunodeficiency more pronounced than SCID	Pilarski, Hipperson et al. (2000) and Huang, Tien et al. (2004)
Transfer of human MM	Bone marrow	MM	NOG = NOD/SCID/gammac(null)	None	Immunodeficiency more pronounced than NOD/SCID	Miyakawa, Ohnishi et al. (2004)
Transfer of human MM	Bone marrow	MM	SCID-rab	None	Human MM cells homing to rabbit fetal bone implanted s.c. in mice	Yata and Yaccoby (2004)

[1]Unpublished. Presented at the XI International Workshop on Multiple Myeloma, Kos Island, Greece, June 2007. NPM, nucleophosmin; PCT, plasmacytomas; SCID, severe-combined immunodeficiency.

the lack of bone marrow involvement. The dismissal may be premature, as certain properties of peritoneal PCT may be of great relevance for human MM. For example, peritoneal PCT formation is profoundly inhibited by anti-inflammatory agents, such as corticosteroids, which play an important role in the standard therapy of human MM. BALB/cAnPt mice deficient in IL-6 or treated with the cyclooxygenase inhibitors, indomethacin and sulindac, are also resistant to tumor induction. This suggests an intriguing parallel to the postulated tumor-promoting role of chronic inflammatory processes in the pathogenesis of human MM. Just as MM is preceded by MGUS, peritoneal PCT is preceded by a well defined and easily studied preneoplastic lesion, namely foci of aberrant plasma cells that reside in the inflammatory granulomas of the peritoneum where they can persist for months. Plasma cell foci of this sort may provide a good experimental opportunity to elucidate the enigmatic transition from preneoplastic to neoplastic plasma cell growth in a genetically defined and environmentally controlled study.

The 5T mouse myeloma of strain C57BL/KaLwRij was developed more than a quarter century ago by Dr. Jiri Radl (Radl 1981; Radl, Croese et al. 1988). In a survey of 2-year-old C57BL/Ka mice, he estimated that 0.5% of the mice developed aggressive PCN originating in the bone marrow. These tumors, designated as 5T myelomas, produced copious amounts of monoclonal Ig, were readily transplanted when injected intravenously into syngeneic mice, and, importantly, produced osteolytic lesions in recipient animals. Two serially transplanted neoplasms, called 5T2 and 5T33, are now in common use and are widely considered as the only mouse model that accurately recapitulates key properties of human MM [reviewed in Vanderkerken, Asosingh et al. (2003)]. 5T2 and 5T33 offer the unique advantage of testing new strategies for the treatment of MM in a neoplastic plasma cell that resides in the appropriate microenvironment of the bone marrow in an immunocompetent host. The 5T33 system has recently been adapted to tissue culture in presence of an adherent layer of stromal cells, further enhancing the suitability of this preclinical model system for drug testing. Another enhancement is provided by the continuous improvement of bioimaging methods that allow a more accurate evaluation of myeloma bone disease and tumor burden than was previously possible. Relevant methods include micro-CT of whole bone or bone explants and imaging techniques that detect 5T cells labeled with fluorochromes (GFP), luciferases (bioluminescence), or sodium iodide symporter (SPECT) with great sensitivity in vivo. Unlike BALB/c PCT, 5T myeloma does not harbor a chromosomal c-*Myc* translocation. This defines another intriguing parallel to human MM, in which *MYC* translocations, if they occur at all, appear as so-called secondary translocations involved in tumor progression.

The classic model of BALB/c PCT has been refined and accelerated by the development of a number of TGs that target oncogenes to the B-cell lineage. Among these are the H2-L^d-hu-IL-6, Eμ–Bcl-2, iMyc, and Eμ–v-abl transgenes. The Bcl2 and v-abl TG takes advantage of the intronic IgH enhancer, Eμ, to enforce the expression of the target genes in B-lineage cells. PCT incidence in

Eμ–v-abl mice approaches 100%, does not require treatment with inflammatory agents, is independent of genetic background, and has been reported to extensively involve the bone marrow. Some Eμ–v-abl mice were shown to present with only bone marrow PCT, developing hind limb paralysis as the result of tumor growth in vertebral marrow cavities. If further modification of this mouse were to succeed in reproducing this primary bone marrow manifestation of PCN growth more consistently, strain Eμ–v-abl may evolve into a true counterpart of human MM.

Among many attempts to express the plasma cell growth, differentiation and survival factor, IL-6, in the B cell and other cell lineages of TG mice, the H2-L^{d}-hu-IL-6 TG has emerged as the most promising for studying PCN. Deregulated expression of IL-6 in young TG mice causes progressive plasma cell hyperplasia in lymphoid tissues, hypergammaglobulinemia, kidney damage, and a histologic picture that resembles human multicentric Castleman's disease (Kovalchuk, Kishimoto et al. 2000). The transition from plasma cell hyperplasia to neoplasia occurs in older mice, usually in enlarged lymph nodes of the gut-associated lymphoid tissue, GALT (Kovalchuk, Kim et al. 2002). Bone marrow infiltration in mice bearing advanced tumors is often extensive. This mouse model may be useful for elucidating the molecular and cellular mechanisms of IL-6-driven plasma cell neoplasia and to test new treatments that target the IL-6 receptor (Yoshio-Hoshino, Adachi et al. 2007) or downstream elements of the IL-6 signaling pathway (Bhutani, Pathak et al. 2007; Hausherr, Tavares et al. 2007; Loffler, Brocke-Heidrich et al. 2007).

The EμSV–Bcl-2-22 TG contains a human *BCL2* cDNA driven by Eμ (Strasser, Whittingham et al. 1991). Transfer of the TG from PCT-resistant C57BL/6 mice onto the PCT-susceptible BALB/c genetic background resulted in a 24-fold increase in tumor incidence and a two-fold reduction in tumor latency. Similar to their IL-6 TG counterparts, *BCL2* TG PCT harbor *Myc*-deregulating T(12;15) translocations (Silva, Kovalchuk et al. 2003). Accelerated plasmacytomagenesis in strain Eμ-Bcl-2may facilitate the design and testing of BCL2 inhibition strategies of potential relevance to BCL2-overexpressing human PCN, such as Waldenström's macroglobulinemia and MM (Kline, Rajkumar et al. 2007).

TG mice, designated iMyc, contain a His$_6$-tagged mouse c-Myc cDNA, Myc$_{His}$, inserted head-to-head into different sites of the mouse *IgH* locus in ways that mimic the Myc-activating T(12;15) translocations of BALB/c PCT. A strain carrying the iMyc TG just 5′ of Eμ is the most thoroughly characterized to date (Park, Kim et al. 2005). In analogy to the experience with the IL-6 and Bcl-2 TG mentioned above, the transfer of the iMyc TG onto BALB/c rendered the mice hyper-susceptible to inflammation-induced peritoneal PCT (Park, Shaffer et al. 2005; Kim, Han et al. 2006). As expected, the PCT overexpressed Myc$_{His}$, produced monoclonal Ig, and exhibited a unique plasma cell signature upon gene expression profiling on mouse lymphochip.

A somewhat surprising observation was made in mice harboring a T-cell-targeted fusion gene joining nucleophosmin (NPM) and anaplastic lymphoma kinase (ALK). Predictably, these mice developed T-cell lymphomas; however, 20% developed PCN instead of T-cell lymphomas. The PCN arose in peripheral lymphoid tissues or the bone marrow. In the latter case, tumor growth resulted in peripheral neuropathy and hind leg paralysis. NPM–ALK TG mice are currently used primarily for studies on the T-cell neoplasm, anaplastic large cell lymphoma (Amin and Lai 2007). Further modification of this strain for modeling human MM has not been attempted.

With several newly developed TG models at their disposal, researchers began to generate double TG mice in efforts to develop robust models of human PCN. Other modifications, such as infecting TG mice with oncogenic virus or changing the genetic background, were also pursued to further accelerate tumor development and/or shift the tumor pattern from B-cell lymphoma to PCN. PCN formation is dramatically accelerated in double TG mice that carry the H2-L^d-hu–IL-6 TG and a Bcl-2 TG (Janz, unpublished finding), a Bcl-X_L TG (Fang, Mueller et al. 1996; Potter 2003) (Janz, unpublished finding) or iMyc TG (Janz, unpublished finding). The same findings were obtained in iMyc/Bcl-2 double TG mice (Janz, unpublished finding). An interesting alternative approach involved the infection of Bcl-X_L TG mice with ABL–MYC virus (Linden, Kirchhof et al. 2005). This resulted in a unique model of MM that recently was acknowledged by a panel of MM experts as holding promise for the validation of new therapeutics (Dalton and Anderson 2006). Additional research is warranted to better characterize double TG and virally accelerated mouse models of human PCN before recommendations can be made as to which model may be most suitable for elucidating specific aspects of the human disease.

Recent studies have shown that X-box-binding protein-1 (XBP1), a differentiation and unfolded protein/ergoplasmatic reticulum stress response factor essential for normal plasma cell development in mice, may also be implicated in human PCN. This prompted the development of a new model of human MM that relies on enforced expression of Xbp-1s ORF in the B-cell lineage under the control of the IgV_H promoter and Eμ enhancer. The mice are prone to a MGUS-like disorder followed by a type of PCN with many similarities to MM. Like all other TG strains susceptible to PCN, Eμ–Xbp1 TG also develop extraosseous PCN, either together with the MM-like tumors or on their own. Nonetheless, a number of features indicate that the Eμ–Xbp1 mice offer an attractive model of human MM. Among other applications, they may be useful to uncover the elusive genetic changes responsible for the transition of MGUS to MM.

A fresh, unorthodox approach to recapitulating the natural history of MM in a relevant cellular and physiologic milieu is a mouse model system that enables the delivery of stochastic, sequential, somatic mutations to precisely defined plasma cell precursors in vivo. Asimakopoulos and Varmus used BAC TG technology to express two distinct types of avian leukosis virus (ALV) receptors, TVA and TVB, in the expanding centroblasts of the GC dark zone and the committed plasmablasts of the light zone. Mouse cells are refractory to infection by retroviruses of the ALV family unless they ectopically express the cognate avian-derived receptors. To that end, TG mice were genetically developed that express TVA driven by regulatory elements of *Mybl1* (*A-Myb*), a transcription factor expressed in dividing blasts of the GC dark zone, and TVB under control of Blimp-1, a master regulator of plasma cell differentiation. As a result, the mice express TVA in dividing follicular B cells and TVB in cells of the GC light zone, extrafollicular plasma cells, and mature plasma cells in the bone marrow. Viral vectors have been engineered to carry dominant oncogenes or various inactivators of tumor suppressor genes, permitting the introduction of sequential oncogenic lesions in putative precursors of PCN.

Chesi, Bergsagel, and associates reported recently on a new mouse model of MM designated VK*MYC. This model is based on the VK*MYC TG that contains an inactive, non-coding human *c-MYC* gene under the transcriptional control of the Vκ promoter. TG MYC is activated sporadically in GC B cells undergoing somatic hypermutation. This approach has two potential benefits. First, in contrast to all previously generated MYC TG, expression of the VK*MYC TG occurs only at the GC stage of B-cell development. This circumvents the unwanted transformation of less mature B-lineage cells that occurs when Myc is expressed earlier in differentiation. Second, B cells in which MYC becomes activated are likely to participate in an ongoing T-cell-dependent immune response, because they were part of a GC reaction. This further restricts the pool of MYC target cells to those that define the postulated MM precursor pool in humans. Evidence indicates that virtually all Vk*MYC mice develop MGUS-like disease by 50 weeks of age. Plasma cells are fully differentiated ($CD19^-CD138^+$), have a very low proliferation index, and are found exclusively in the bone marrow. Vk*MYC mice also develop anemia, bone disease with low trabecular density as well as sporadic lytic bone lesions and hind limb paralysis. Similar to the Xbp1 TG mice, 30% of the Vk*MYC mice exhibit extramedullary disease. Importantly, VK*MYC mice responded to drugs known to be active against MM while demonstrating no response to drugs with little or no clinical activity. These features indicate that strain VK*MYC will be useful in the study of MM biology and the development of new pharmacological and immunological therapies.

8.8.3 Xenograft Models of Human Myeloma in Mice

In contrast to the models of de novo PCN formation in mice, xenograft models use MM cells or cell lines that are transplanted into SCID-Hu, NOD/SCID, or SCID-Rab mice. These systems offer the unique ability to test therapeutics in vivo against true MM (Tassone, Neri et al. 2005). The SCID-Hu mouse model that employs fetal bone permits studies on the interaction of MM cells with the microenvironment of human bone marrow. The NOD/SCID has been adapted to myeloma cells labeled with green fluorescent protein. Intravenous injection of these cells creates a model in which diffuse PCN dissemination can be visualized using whole-body, real-time fluorescence imaging to reproducibly quantify tumor burden. This allows serial, noninvasive monitoring of drug treatment. The SCID-Rab model avoids the ethical concerns about the use of human fetal bone in the SCID-Hu model by using rabbit bones. This model supports the growth of MM cells in a non-myelomatous, non-human, and non-fetal microenvironment. Although xenograft models are the current work-horses in preclinical testing of efficacy and mechanism of action of novel myeloma drugs, the xenograft implants have their own severe limitations, including the lack of an intact immune system, inability to model premalignant neoplastic stages, and imperfections in recapitulating the interactions between myeloma cells and surrounding stroma.

The SCID-hu mouse, which was originally developed for studies on human hematopoiesis in mice (Shultz, Ishikawa et al. 2007), has been adapted by Dr. J. Epstein, Y. Yaccoby, and their associates to investigate human MM cells in their native microenvironment of the human bone marrow (Yaccoby, Barlogie et al. 1998). In this system, myeloma growth is restricted to and dependent on human bone marrow and leads to osteolytic lesions in the transplanted human bone. The SCID-hu model contributed to our understanding of myeloma biology by demonstrating that myeloma alters the balanced expression of the osteoclast differentiation factor, RANKL/OPG, in the bone marrow (Pearse, Sordillo et al. 2001), depends on osteoclasts for growth and survival (Yaccoby, Pearse et al. 2002), relies, in part, on IL-6 to avoid programmed cell death (Yaccoby, Pearse et al. 2002), abolishes osteoblasts in the course of tumor progression (Yaccoby, Wezeman et al. 2006), and uses the serine phosphatase, fibroblast activation protein, to interact with stromal cells (Ge, Zhan et al. 2006). Importantly, the SCID-hu model was instrumental in showing that the anti-myeloma activity is dependent on its metabolism by liver microsomes (Yaccoby, Wezeman et al. 2006).

Progress in research on humanized mice (Shultz, Ishikawa et al. 2007) led to additional modifications of the SCID-hu model, such as NOD/SCID-hu (Huang, Tien et al. 2004), NOG (NOD/SCID/γ_c^{null}) (Miyakawa, Ohnishi et al. 2004), and SCID-rab (Yata and Yaccoby 2004), which permit the engraftment of human myeloma cells in endogenous human bone or implanted rabbit bone, respectively. The addition of the NOD genetic background to SCID mice enhances the immunodeficiency conferred by the SCID background, resulting in lack of B and T cells, lack of circulating complement, defective macrophage function, and low natural killer cell activity. The γ_c^{null} phenotype causes the complete loss of natural killer cells. Just like the original SCID-hu model, the newer models enhance our understanding of myeloma biology and are useful for evaluating novel drugs and drug candidates in a preclinical setting. The utility of the SCID-rab system to evaluate effects of antibody to DKK1, of bortezomib, and of bone anabolic agents on bone remodeling and myeloma growth illustrates this point (Yaccoby, Ling et al. 2007).

8.8.4 Conclusions Regarding Mouse Models of Human PCN

Recent progress in the design and development of genetically engineered mouse models of human PCN has resulted in two categories of experimental models systems. In the first or de novo category, PCN arise either spontaneously or are induced in inbred or TG mice. Tumor development occurs in predictable stages and is preceded by the expansion of premalignant plasma cells resembling benign monoclonal gammopathy (BMG), MGUS, Castleman's disease, or similar non-malignant human plasma cell disorders. The mouse models in this category are indispensable for mechanistic studies of plasma cell transformation and the design and testing of strategies for tumor prevention. The greatest weakness among these models is their failure to recapitulate the bone marrow manifestations of tumor growth that are typical of MM. Two recent models offer a glimmer of hope along this line (Cheung, Kim et al. 2004; Linden, Kirchhof et al. 2005; Boylan, Gosse et al. 2007; Carrasco, Sukhdeo et al. 2007). In the second or transplantation-based category, fully transformed plasma cells of mouse origin (5T) or human origin (primary MM cells and myeloma cell lines) are transferred into syngeneic, immunocompetent mice (5T) or immunodeficient SCID mice (xenotransplant system) that frequently harbor human or rabbit bone as a nesting ground for the incoming plasma cells. The mouse models in this category have made and continue to make important scientific contributions to the preclinical assessment of myeloma therapeutics and our understanding of myeloma bone disease. Nonetheless, technical and logistic barriers have prevented these models from having a significant economic effect on the process of anti-myeloma drug discovery. They are not extensively used in preclinical trials and have not gained wide acceptance in industry. In addition, transplantation models are not useful for studies on tumor development and prevention.

References

Alizadeh, A. A., M. B. Eisen, et al. (2000). "Distinct types of diffuse large B-cell lymphoma identified by gene expression profiling." *Nature* **403**: 503.

Amin, H. M. and R. Lai(2007). "Pathobiology of ALK+ anaplastic large-cell lymphoma." *Blood* **110**: 2259–2267

Anderson, P. N. and M. Potter (1969). "Induction of plasma cell tumours in BALB-c mice with 2,6,10,14-tetramethylpentadecane (pristane)." *Nature* **222**: 994–5.

Anderson, M. S., E. S. Venanzi, et al. (2002). "Projection of an Immunological Self Shadow Within the Thymus by the Aire Protein." *Science* **298**(5597): 1395–1401.

Aronoff, R. and C. C. Petersen (2006). "Controlled and localized genetic manipulation in the brain." *J Cell Mol Med* **10**(2): 333–52.

Bergsagel, P. L. and W. M. Kuehl (2005). "Molecular pathogenesis and a consequent classification of multiple myeloma." *J Clin Oncol* **23**(26): 6333–8.

Bhutani, M., A. K. Pathak, et al. (2007). "Capsaicin is a novel blocker of constitutive and interleukin-6-inducible STAT3 activation." *Clin Cancer Res* **13**(10): 3024–32.

Bichi, R., S. A. Shinton, et al. (2002). "Human chronic lymphocytic leukemia modeled in mouse by targeted TCL1 expression." *Proc Natl Acad Sci USA* **99**: 6955.

Bodrug, S. E., B. J. Warner, et al. (1994). "Cyclin D1 transgene impedes lymphocyte maturation and collaborates in lymphomagenesis with the myc gene." *EMBO J* **13**(9): 2124–30.
Boumsell, L., H. Coppin, et al. (1980). "An antigen shared by a human T cell subset and B cell chronic lymphocytic leukemic cells. Distribution on normal and malignant lymphoid cells." *J Exp Med* **152**(1): 229–34.
Boylan, K. L., M. A. Gosse, et al. (2007). "A transgenic mouse model of plasma cell malignancy shows phenotypic, cytogenetic, and gene expression heterogeneity similar to human multiple myeloma." *Cancer Res* **67**(9): 4069–78.
Bryant, J., L. Pham, et al. (2000). "Development of intermediate-grade (mantle cell) and low-grade (small lymphocytic and marginal zone) human non-Hodgkin's lymphomas xenotransplanted in severe combined immunodeficiency mouse models." *Lab Invest* **80**(4): 557–73.
Calin, G. A., C. Sevignani, et al. (2004). "Human microRNA genes are frequently located at fragile sites and genomic regions involved in cancers." *Proc Natl Acad Sci USA* **101**(9): 2999–3004.
Cancro, M. P. (2004). "The BLyS family of ligands and receptors: an archetype for niche-specific homeostatic regulation." *Immunol Rev* **202**(1): 237–49.
Carrasco, D. R., K. Sukhdeo, et al. (2007). "The differentiation and stress response factor XBP-1 drives multiple myeloma pathogenesis." *Cancer Cell* **11**(4): 349–60.
Carrasco, D. R., G. Tonon, et al. (2006). "High-resolution genomic profiles define distinct clinico-pathogenetic subgroups of multiple myeloma patients." *Cancer Cell* **9**(4): 313–25.
Cattoretti, G., L. Pasqualucci, et al. (2005). "Deregulated BCL6 expression recapitulates the pathogenesis of human diffuse large B cell lymphomas in mice." *Cancer Cell* **7**(5): 445–55.
Chen, W., Q. Li, et al. (2006). "A murine Mll-AF4 knock-in model results in lymphoid and myeloid deregulation and hematologic malignancy." *Blood* **108**(2): 669–77.
Cheung, W. C., J. S. Kim, et al. (2004). "Novel targeted deregulation of c-Myc cooperates with Bcl-X(L) to cause plasma cell neoplasms in mice." *J Clin Invest* **113**(12): 1763–73.
Chiarle, R., J. Z. Gong, et al. (2003). "NPM-ALK transgenic mice spontaneously develop T-cell lymphomas and plasma cell tumors." *Blood* **101**(5): 1919–27.
Chiorazzi, N. and M. Ferrarini (2003). "B cell chronic lymphocytic leukemia: Lessons learned from studies of the B cell antigen receptor." *Annu Rev Immunol* **21**: 841–94.
Clynes, R., J. Wax, et al. (1988). "Rapid induction of IgM-secreting murine plasmacytomas by pristane and an immunoglobulin heavy-chain promoter/enhancer-driven c-myc/v-Ha-ras retrovirus." *Proc Natl Acad Sci USA* **85**: 6067–71.
Crespo, M., Bosch, et al. (2003). "ZAP-70 expression as a surrogate for immunoglobulin-variable-region mutations in chronic lymphocytic leukemia." *N Engl J Med* **348**(18): 1764–1775.
Czarneski, J., Y. C. Lin, et al. (2004). "Studies in NZB IL-10 knockout mice of the requirement of IL-10 for progression of B-cell lymphoma." *Leukemia* **18**(3): 597–606.
Dalton, W. and K. C. Anderson (2006). "Synopsis of a roundtable on validating novel therapeutics for multiple myeloma." *Clin Cancer Res* **12**(22): 6603–10.
Damle, R. N., Wasil, et al. (1999). "Ig V gene mutation status and CD38 expression as novel prognostic factors in chronic lymphocytic leukemia." *Blood* **94**: 1837–1839.
Dawson, D. W., J. S. Hong, et al. (2007). "Global DNA methylation profiling reveals silencing of a secreted form of Epha7 in mouse and human germinal center B-cell lymphomas." *Oncogene* **26**(29): 4243–52.
Dohner, H., S. Stilgenbauer, et al. (2000). "Genomic aberrations and survival in chronic lymphocytic leukemia." *N Engl J Med* **343**(26): 1910–6.
Du, Z., K. Podsypanina, et al. (2006). "Introduction of oncogenes into mammary glands in vivo with an avian retroviral vector initiates and promotes carcinogenesis in mouse models." *Proc Natl Acad Sci USA* **103**(46): 17396–401.
East, J. (1970). "Immunopathology and neoplasms in New Zealand Black (NZB) and SJL/J mice." *Prog Exp Tumor Res* **13**: 84–134.

Egle, A., A. W. Harris, et al. (2004). "VavP-Bcl2 transgenic mice develop follicular lymphoma preceded by germinal center hyperplasia." *Blood* **103**(6): 2276–83.
Enno, A., J. L. O'Rourke, et al. (1995). "MALToma-like lesions in the murine gastric mucosa after long-term infection with Helicobacter felis. A mouse model of Helicobacter pylori-induced gastric lymphoma." *Am J Pathol* **147**(1): 217–22.
Enno, A., J. L. O'Rourke, et al. (1998). "Antigen-dependent progression of mucosa-associated lymphoid tissue (MALT)-type lymphoma in the stomach. Effects of antimicrobial therapy on gastric MALT lymphoma in mice." *Am J Pathol* **152**(6): 1625–32.
Faderl, S., Keating, et al. (2002). "Expression profile of 11 proteins and their prognostic significance in patients with chronic lymphocytic leukemia (CLL)." *Leukemia* **16**(6): 1045–1052.
Fang, W., D. L. Mueller, et al. (1996). "Frequent aberrant immunoglobulin gene rearrangements in pro-B cells revealed by a bcl-xL transgene." *Immunity* **4**(3): 291–9.
Feeney, A. J. (1990). "Lack of N regions in fetal and neonatal mouse immunoglobulin V-D-J junctional sequences." *J Exp Med* **172**(5): 1377–90.
Ford, R. J., L. Shen, et al. (2007). "Development of a murine model for blastoid variant mantle-cell lymphoma." *Blood* **109**(11): 4899–906.
Fredrickson, T. H., A. W. Harris (2000). *Atlas of Mouse Hematopathology*. Amsterdam, Harwood Academic Publishers.
Fredrickson, T. N., K. Lennert, et al. (1999). "Splenic marginal zone lymphomas of mice." *Am J Pathol* **154**(3): 805–12.
Fu, T. B., L. Virgilio, et al. (1994). "Characterization and localization of the TCL-1 oncogene product." *Cancer Res* **54**: 6297.
Ge, Y., F. Zhan, et al. (2006). "Fibroblast activation protein (FAP) is upregulated in myelomatous bone and supports myeloma cell survival." *Br J Haematol* **133**(1): 83–92.
Hallek, M., Langenmayer, et al. (1999). "Elevated serum thymidine kinase levels identify a subgroup at high risk of disease progression in early, nonsmoldering chronic lymphocytic leukemia." *Blood* **93**(5): 1732–1737.
Hamano, Y., S. Hirose, et al. (1998). "Susceptibility alleles for aberrant B-1 cell proliferation involved in spontaneously occurring B-cell chronic lymphocytic leukemia in a model of New Zealand white mice." *Blood* **92**(10): 3772–9.
Hanahan, D. and R. A. Weinberg (2000). "The hallmarks of cancer." *Cell* **100**(1): 57–70.
Hardy, R. R. (2006). "B-1 B cell development." *J Immunol* **177**(5): 2749–54.
Hartley, J. W., S. K. Chattopadhyay, et al. (2000). "Accelerated appearance of multiple B cell lymphoma types in NFS/N mice congenic for ecotropic murine leukemia viruses." *Lab Invest* **80**(2): 159–69.
Hassler, S., C. Ramsey, et al. (2006). "Aire-deficient mice develop hematopoetic irregularities and marginal zone B-cell lymphoma." *Blood* **108**(6): 1941–48.
Hausherr, A., R. Tavares, et al. (2007). "Inhibition of IL-6-dependent growth of myeloma cells by an acidic peptide repressing the gp130-mediated activation of Src family kinases." *Oncogene* **26**(34): 4987–98.
Hayakawa, K., R. R. Hardy, et al. (1983). "The -Ly-1 B— cell subpopulation in normal immunodefective, and autoimmune mice." *J Exp Med* **157**(1): 202–18.
Herve, M., K. Xu, et al. (2005). "Unmutated and mutated chronic lymphocytic leukemias derive from self-reactive B cell precursors despite expressing different antibody reactivity." *J Clin Invest* **115**(6): 1636–43.
Hockenbery, D., G. Nunez, et al. (1990). "Bcl-2 is an inner mitochondrial membrane protein that blocks programmed cell death." *Nature* **348**(6299): 334–6.
Hoyer, K. K., S. W. French, et al. (2002). "Dysregulated TCL1 promotes multiple classes of mature B cell lymphoma." *Proc Natl Acad Sci USA* **99**(22): 14392–7.
Hu, Y., S. Swerdlow, et al. (2006). "Targeting multiple kinase pathways in leukemic progenitors and stem cells is essential for improved treatment of Ph+ leukemia in mice." *Proc Natl Acad Sci USA* **103**(45): 16870–5.

Huang, S. Y., H. F. Tien, et al. (2004). "Nonirradiated NOD/SCID-human chimeric animal model for primary human multiple myeloma: a potential in vivo culture system." *Am J Pathol* **164**(2): 747–56.

Jaffe, E. S., N. L. Harris, et al. (2001a). *World Health Organization Classification of Tumours. Pathology and Genetics of Haematopoietic anbd Lymphoid Tissues*. Lyon, IARC Press.

Jaffe, E. S., N. L. Harris, et al. (2001b). "Burkitt lymphoma." *Pathology and Genetics of Tumours of Haematopoietic and Lymphoid Tissues*. P. a. S. Kleihues, L.H. Lyon, IARC Press: 181–4.

Jaffe, E. S., N. L. Harris, et al. (2001c). "Diffuse large B cell lymphoma." *Pathology and Genetics of Tumours of Haematopoietic and Lymphoid Tissues*. P. a. S. Kleihues, L.H. Lyon, IARC Press: 171–4.

Jaffe, E. S., N. L. Harris, et al. (2001d). "Mantle cell lymphoma." *Pathology and Genetics of Tumours of Haematopoietic and Lymphoid Tissues*. P. a. S. Kleihues, L.H. Lyon, IARC Press: 168–70.

Janz, S. (2006). "Myc translocations in B cell and plasma cell neoplasms." *DNA Repair (Amst.)* **5**(9–10): 1213–24.

Johnson, A. J., D. M. Lucas, et al. (2006). "Characterization of the TCL-1 transgenic mouse as a preclinical drug development tool for human chronic lymphocytic leukemia." *Blood* **108**(4): 1334–8.

Kantor, A. B., C. E. Merrill, et al. (1997). "An unbiased analysis of V(H)-D-J(H) sequences from B-1a, B-1b, and conventional B cells." *J Immunol* **158**(3): 1175–86.

Kichina, J. V., M. Zeremski, et al. (2006). "Targeted disruption of the mouse ingl locus results in reduced body size, hypersensitivity to radiation and elevated incidence of lymphomas." *Oncogene* **25**(6): 857–66.

Kim, J., S. Han, et al. (2006). "Plasma cell tumour progression in iMyc(Emicro) gene-insertion mice." *J Pathol* **209**(1): 44–55.

Kline, M. P., S. V. Rajkumar, et al. (2007). "ABT-737, an inhibitor of Bcl-2 family proteins, is a potent inducer of apoptosis in multiple myeloma cells." *Leukemia* **21**(7): 1549–60.

Kovalchuk, A. L., J. S. Kim, et al. (2002). "IL-6 transgenic mouse model for extraosseous plasmacytoma." *Proc Natl Acad Sci USA* **99**(3): 1509–14.

Kovalchuk, A. L., T. Kishimoto, et al. (2000). "Lymph nodes and Peyer's patches of IL-6 transgenic BALB/c mice harbor T(12;15) translocated plasma cells that contain illegitimate exchanges between the immunoglobulin heavy-chain mu locus and c-myc." *Leukemia* **14**: 1127–35.

Kovalchuk, A. L., C. F. Qi, et al. (2000). "Burkitt lymphoma in the mouse." *J Exp Med* **192**(8): 1183–90.

Kress, C. K., M; Martinez-Garcia, et al. (2007). "Tritrepenoids display single agent antitumor activity in a transgenic mouse model of chronic lymphocytic leukemia and small B cell lymphoma." *PLoS ONE* **2**: e559.

Kuehl, W. M. and P. L. Bergsagel (2005). "Early genetic events provide the basis for a clinical classification of multiple myeloma." *Hematology Am Soc Hematol Educ Program* : 346–52.

Kyle, R. A., T. M. Therneau, et al. (2002). "A Long-Term Study of Prognosis in Monoclonal Gammopathy of Undetermined Significance." *N Engl J Med* **346**(8): 564–9.

Lanier, L. L., N. L. Warner, et al. (1981). "Expression of Lyt-1 antigen on certain murine B cell lymphomas." *J Exp Med* **153**(4): 998–1003.

Li, Y. S., K. Hayakawa, et al. (1993). "The regulated expression of B lineage associated genes during B cell differentiation in bone marrow and fetal liver." *J Exp Med* **178**(3): 951–60.

Linden, M., N. Kirchhof, et al. (2004). "Targeted overexpression of Bcl-XL in B-lymphoid cells results in lymphoproliferative disease and plasma cell malignancies." *Blood* **103**(7): 2779–86.

Linden, M., N. Kirchhof, et al. (2005). "ABL-MYC retroviral infection elicits bone marrow plasma cell tumors in Bcl-X(L) transgenic mice." *Leuk Res* **29**(4): 435–44.

Loffler, D., K. Brocke-Heidrich, et al. (2007). "Interleukin-6-dependent survival of multiple myeloma cells involves the Stat3-mediated induction of microRNA-21 through a highly conserved enhancer." *Blood* **110**: 1330–1333

McDonnell, T. J. and S. J. Korsmeyer (1991). "Progression from lymphoid hyperplasia to high-grade malignant lymphoma in mice transgenic for the t(14; 18)." *Nature* **349**(6306): 254–6.

Mahboudi, F. P., J. A. Phillips, et al. (1992). "Immunoglobulin gene sequence analysis of B1 (CD5+B) cell clones in a murine model of chronic lymphocytic leukemia and Richter's syndrome." *Int J Oncol* **1**: 459–65.

Manohar, V., E. Brown, et al. (1982). "Expression of Lyt-1 by a subset of B lymphocytes." *J Immunol* **129**(2): 532–8.

Martin, F. and J. F. Kearney (2000). "B-cell subsets and the mature preimmune repertoire. Marginal zone and B1B cells as part of a "natural immune memory". *Immunol Rev* **175**: 70–79.

Martin, F. and J. F. Kearney (2001). "B1 cells: similarities and differences with other B cell subsets." *Cur Opin Immunol* **13**(2): 195–201.

Martin, F., A. M. Oliver, et al. (2001). "Marginal zone and B1B cells unite in the early response against T-independent blood-borne particulate antigens." *Immunity* **14**(5): 617–29.

Metzler, M., A. Forster, et al. (2006). "A conditional model of MLL-AF4 B-cell tumourigenesis using invertor technology." *Oncogene* **25**(22): 3093–103.

Mikkers, H. and A. Berns (2003). "Retroviral insertional mutagenesis: tagging cancer pathways." *Adv Cancer Res* **88**: 53–99.

Mitsiades, C. S., N. S. Mitsiades, et al. (2007). "Multiple myeloma: a prototypic disease model for the characterization and therapeutic targeting of interactions between tumor cells and their local microenvironment." *J Cell Biochem* **101**(4): 950–68.

Miyakawa, Y., Y. Ohnishi, et al. (2004). "Establishment of a new model of human multiple myeloma using NOD/SCID/gammac(null) (NOG) mice." *Biochem Biophys Res Commun* **313**(2): 258–62.

M'Kacher, R., F. Farace, et al. (2003). "Blastoid mantle cell lymphoma: evidence for nonrandom cytogenetic abnormalities additional to t(11;14) and generation of a mouse model." *Cancer Genet Cytogenet* **143**(1): 32–8.

Monti, S., K. J. Savage, et al. (2005). "Molecular profiling of diffuse large B-cell lymphoma identifies robust subtypes including one characterized by host inflammatory response." *Blood* **105**(5): 1851–61.

Morse, H. C., 3rd, M. R. Anver, et al. (2002). "Bethesda proposals for classification of lymphoid neoplasms in mice." *Blood* **100**(1): 246–58.

Morse, H. C., 3rd, T. McCarty, et al. (2003). "B lymphoid neoplasms of mice: characteristics of naturally occurring and engineered diseases and relationships to human disorders." *Adv Immunol* **81**: 97–121.

Morse, H. C., 3rd, C. F. Qi, et al. (2001). "Combined histologic and molecular features reveal previously unappreciated subsets of lymphoma in AKXD recombinant inbred mice." *Leuk Res* **25**(8): 719–33.

Mueller, A., J. O'Rourke, et al. (2003). "Distinct gene expression profiles characterize the histopathological stages of disease in Helicobacter-induced mucosa-associated lymphoid tissue lymphoma." *Proc Natl Acad Sci USA* **100**(3): 1292–7.

Mulligan, G., C. Mitsiades, et al. (2007). "Gene expression profiling and correlation with outcome in clinical trials of the proteasome inhibitor bortezomib." *Blood* **109**(8): 3177–88.

Narducci, M. G., E. Pescarmona, et al. (2000). "Regulation of TCL1 expression in B- and T-cell lymphomas and reactive lymphoid tissues." *Cancer Res* **60**: 2095.

Ohno, S., S. Migita, et al. (1984). "Chromosomal translocations activating myc sequences and transduction of v-abl are critical events in the rapid induction of plasmacytomas by pristane and abelson virus." *J Exp Med* **159**: 1762–77.

Okada, T. T., F; Tokushige, et al. (1991). "Major histocompatibility complex controls clonal proliferation of CD5+ B cells in H-2-congenic New Zealand mice: a model for B cell chronic lymphocytic leukemia and autoimmune disease." *Eur J Immunol* **21**: 2743–8.

Park, S. S., J. S. Kim, et al. (2005). "Insertion of c-Myc into Igh induces B-cell and plasma-cell neoplasms in mice." *Cancer Res* **65**(4): 1306–15.

Park, S. S., A. L. Shaffer, et al. (2005). "Insertion of Myc into Igh accelerates peritoneal plasmacytomas in mice." *Cancer Res* **65**(17): 7644–52.

Pearse, R. N., E. M. Sordillo, et al. (2001). "Multiple myeloma disrupts the TRANCE/osteoprotegerin cytokine axis to trigger bone destruction and promote tumor progression." *Proc Natl Acad Sci USA* **98**(20): 11581–6.

Phillips, J. A., K. Mehta, et al. (1992). "The NZB mouse as a model for chronic lymphocytic leukemia." *Cancer Res* **52**(2): 437–43.

Pilarski, L. M., G. Hipperson, et al. (2000). "Myeloma progenitors in the blood of patients with aggressive or minimal disease: engraftment and self-renewal of primary human myeloma in the bone marrow of NOD SCID mice." *Blood* **95**(3): 1056–65.

Planelles, L., C. E. Carvalho-Pinto, et al. (2004). "APRIL promotes B-1 cell-associated neoplasm." *Cancer Cell* **6**(4): 399–408.

Potter, M. (2003). "Neoplastic development in plasma cells." *Immunol Rev* **194**: 177–95.

Potter, M. and R. C. MacCardle (1964). "Histology of developing plasma cell neoplasia induced by mineral oil in BALB/c mice." *J Natl Cancer Inst* **33**: 497.

Potter, M., M. D. Sklar, et al. (1973). "Rapid viral induction of plasmacytomas in pristane-primed BALB-c mice." *Science* **182**: 592–4.

Potter, M. and F. Wiener (1992). "Plasmacytomagenesis in mice: model of neoplastic development dependent upon chromosomal translocations." *Carcinogenesis* **13**: 1681–97.

Radl, J. (1981). "Animal model of human disease. Benign monoclonal gammopathy (idiopathic paraproteinemia)." *Am J Pathol* **105**(1): 91–3.

Radl, J., J. W. Croese, et al. (1988). "Animal model of human disease. Multiple myeloma." *Am J Pathol* **132**(3): 593–7.

Radl, J., C. Van Arkel, et al. (1996). "Tenfold increased incidence of spontaneous multiple myeloma in long-term immunosuppressed aging C57BL/KaLwRij mice." *Clin.Immunol. Immunopathol* **79**: 155–62.

Rajkumar, S. V., M. Q. Lacy, et al. (2007). "Monoclonal gammopathy of undetermined significance and smoldering multiple myeloma." *Blood Rev* **21**: 255–265

Ramsey, C., O. Winqvist, et al. (2002). "Aire deficient mice develop multiple features of APECED phenotype and show altered immune response." *Hum Mol Genet* **11**(4): 397–409.

Ranger, A. M., J. Zha, et al. (2003). "Bad-deficient mice develop diffuse large B cell lymphoma." *Proc Natl Acad Sci USA* **100**(16): 9324–9.

Raveche, E. S., P. Lalor, et al. (1988). "In vivo effects of hyperdiploid Ly-1+ B cells of NZB origin." *J Immunol* **141**(12): 4133–9.

Raveche, E. S., E. Salerno, et al. (2007). "Abnormal microRNA-16locus with synteny to human 13q14 linked to CLL in NZB mice." *Blood* **109**(12): 5079–86.

Repacholi, M. H., A. Basten, et al. (1997). "Lymphomas in E mu-Pim1 transgenic mice exposed to pulsed 900 MHZ electromagnetic fields." *Radiat Res* **147**(5): 631–40.

Roodman, G. D. (2006). "New potential targets for treating myeloma bone disease." *Clin Cancer Res* **12**(20 Pt 2): 6270s–6273s.

Rosenbaum, H., A. W. Harris, et al. (1990). "An E mu-v-abl transgene elicits plasmacytomas in concert with an activated myc gene." *EMBO J* **9**: 897–905.

Said, J. W., K. K. Hoyer, et al. (2001). "TCL1 oncogene expression in B cell subsets from lymphoid hyperplasia and distinct classes of B cell lymphoma." *Lab Invest* **81**(4): 555–64.

Sarfati, M., Chevret, et al. (1996). "Prognostic importance of serum soluble CD23 level in chronic lymphocytic leukemia." *Blood* **88**(11): 4259–4264.

Schelonka, R. L., J. Tanner, et al. (2007). "Categorical selection of the antibody repertoire in splenic B cells." *Eur J Immunol* **37**(4): 1010–21.

Schneider, P. (2005). "The role of APRIL and BAFF in lymphocyte activation." *Cur Opin Immunol* **17**(3): 282–9.

Schwaller, J., P. Schneider, et al. (2007). "Neutrophil-derived APRIL concentrated in tumor lesions by proteoglycans correlates with human B-cell lymphoma aggressiveness." *Blood* **109**(1): 331–8.

Shaughnessy, J. D. and B. Barlogie (2003). "Interpreting the molecular biology and clinical behavior of multiple myeloma in the context of global gene expression profiling." *Immunol Rev* **194**: 140–63.

Shen, R. R., D. O. Ferguson, et al. (2006). "Dysregulated TCL1 requires the germinal center and genome instability for mature B-cell transformation." *Blood* **108**(6): 1991–8.

Shin, M. S., T. N. Fredrickson, et al. (2004). "High-throughput retroviral tagging for identification of genes involved in initiation and progression of mouse splenic marginal zone lymphomas." *Cancer Res* **64**(13): 4419–27.

Shultz, L. D., F. Ishikawa, et al. (2007). "Humanized mice in translational biomedical research." *Nat Rev Immunol* **7**(2): 118–30.

Silva, S., A. L. Kovalchuk, et al. (2003). "BCL2 accelerates inflammation-induced BALB/c plasmacytomas and promotes novel tumors with coexisting T(12;15) and T(6;15) translocations." *Cancer Res* **63**(24): 8656–63.

Smith, M. R., I. Joshi, et al. (2006). "Murine model for mantle cell lymphoma." *Leukemia* **20**(5): 891–3.

Stall, A. M., M. C. Farinas, et al. (1988). "Ly-1 B-cell clones similar to human chronic lymphocytic leukemias routinely develop in older normal mice and young autoimmune (New Zealand Black-related) animals." *Proc Natl Acad Sci USA* **85**: 7312.

Steele-Perkins, G., W. Fang, et al. (2001). "Tumor formation and inactivation of RIZ1, an Rb-binding member of a nuclear protein-methyltransferase superfamily." *Genes Dev* **15**(17): 2250–62.

Strair, R. K., W. Sheay, et al. (2002). "Adenovirus infection of primary malignant lymphoid cells." *Leuk Lymphoma* **43**(1): 37–49.

Strasser, A., A. W. Harris, et al. (1993). "E mu-bcl-2 transgene facilitates spontaneous transformation of early pre-B and immunoglobulin-secreting cells but not T cells." *Oncogene* **8**(1): 1–9.

Strasser, A., S. Whittingham, et al. (1991). "Enforced BCL2 expression in B-lymphoid cells prolongs antibody responses and elicits autoimmune disease." *Proc Natl Acad Sci USA* **88**: 8661–5.

Sutton, P., J. O'Rourke, et al. (2004). "Immunisation against Helicobacter felis infection protects against the development of gastric MALT Lymphoma." *Vaccine* **22**(20): 2541–6.

Tassone, P., P. Neri, et al. (2005). "Combination therapy with interleukin-6 receptor superantagonist Sant7 and dexamethasone induces antitumor effects in a novel SCID-hu In vivo model of human multiple myeloma." *Clin Cancer Res* **11**(11): 4251–8.

Teitell, M. A. (2005). "The TCL1 family of oncoproteins: co-activators of transformation." *Nat Rev Cancer* **5**(8): 640–8.

Teitell, M., M. A. Damore, et al. (1999). "TCL1 oncogene expression in AIDS-related lymphomas and lymphoid tissues." *Proc Natl Acad Sci USA* **96**(17): 9809–14.

Thome, M. (2004). "CARMA1, BCL-10 and MALT1 in lymphocyte development and activation." *Nat Rev Immunol* **4**(5): 348–59.

Troppmair, J., M. Huleihel, et al. (1988). "Plasmacytoma induction by J series of v-myc recombinant retroviruses: evidence for the requirement of two (raf and myc) oncogenes for transformation." *Curr Top Microbiol Immunol* **141**: 110–4.

Tsujimoto, Y., L. R. Finger, et al. (1984). "Cloning of the chromosome breakpoint of neoplastic B cells with the t(14;18) chromosome translocation." *Science* **226**(4678): 1097–9.

van Lohuizen, M., S. Verbeek, et al. (1989). "Predisposition to lymphomagenesis in pim-1 transgenic mice: cooperation with c-myc and N-myc in murine leukemia virus-induced tumors." *Cell* **56**(4): 673–82.

Vanderkerken, K., K. Asosingh, et al. (2003). "Multiple myeloma biology: lessons from the 5TMM models." *Immunol Rev* **194**: 196–206.

Vanderkerken, K., E. Goes, et al. (1996). "Follow-up of bone lesions in an experimental multiple myeloma mouse model: description of an in vivo technique using radiography dedicated for mammography." *Br J Cancer* **73**: 1463–5.

Victor Hoffbrand, A. and T. J. Hamblin (2007). "Is "leukemia" an appropriate label for all patients who meet the diagnostic criteria of chronic lymphocytic leukemia?" *Leukemia Res* **31**(3): 273–5.

Virgilio, L., C. Lazzeri, et al. (1998). "Deregulated expression of TCL1 causes T cell leukemia in mice." *Proc Natl Acad Sci USA* **95**(7): 3885–9.

Virgilio, L., M. G. Narducci, et al. (1994). "Identification of the TCL1 gene involved in T-cell malignancies." *Proc Natl Acad Sci USA* **91**(26): 12530–4.

Weissinger, E. M., H. Mischak, et al. (1991). "Induction of plasmacytomas secreting antigen-specific monoclonal antibodies with a retrovirus expressing v-abl and c-myc." *Proc Natl Acad Sci USA* **88**: 8735–9.

Williams, M. E., S. H. Swerdlow, et al. (1993). "Chromosome 11 translocation breakpoints at the PRAD1/cyclin D1 gene locus in centrocytic lymphoma." *Leukemia* **7**(2): 241–5.

Williams, M. E., C. D. Westermann, et al. (1990). "Genotypic characterization of centrocytic lymphoma: frequent rearrangement of the chromosome 11 bcl-1locus." *Blood* **76**(7): 1387–91.

Xiangshu Wen, D. Z., Yuji Kikuchi, et al. (2004). "Transgene-mediated hyper-expression of IL-5 inhibits autoimmune disease but increases the risk of B cell chronic lymphocytic leukemia in a model of murine lupus." *Eur J Immunol* **34**(10): 2740–9.

Yaccoby, S., B. Barlogie, et al. (1998). "Primary myeloma cells growing in SCID-hu mice: a model for studying the biology and treatment of myeloma and its manifestations." *Blood* **92**(8): 2908–13.

Yaccoby, S., W. Ling, et al. (2007). "Antibody-based inhibition of DKK1 suppresses tumor-induced bone resorption and multiple myeloma growth in vivo." *Blood* **109**(5): 2106–11.

Yaccoby, S., R. N. Pearse, et al. (2002). "Myeloma interacts with the bone marrow micro-environment to induce osteoclastogenesis and is dependent on osteoclast activity." *Br J Haematol* **116**(2): 278–90.

Yaccoby, S., M. J. Wezeman, et al. (2006). "Inhibitory effects of osteoblasts and increased bone formation on myeloma in novel culture systems and a myelomatous mouse model." *Haematologica* **91**(2): 192–9.

Yan, X.-j., E. Albesiano, et al. (2006). "B cell receptors in TCL1 transgenic mice resemble those of aggressive, treatment-resistant human chronic lymphocytic leukemia." *Proc Natl Acad Sci USA* **103**(31): 11713–8.

Yata, K. and S. Yaccoby (2004). "The SCID-rab model: a novel in vivo system for primary human myeloma demonstrating growth of CD138-expressing malignant cells." *Leukemia* **18**(11): 1891–7.

Yoshio-Hoshino, N., Y. Adachi, et al. (2007). "Establishment of a new interleukin-6 (IL-6) receptor inhibitor applicable to the gene therapy for IL-6-dependent tumor." *Cancer Res* **67**(3): 871–5.

Yumoto, T. Y., Y. Yoshida, et al.(1980). "Prelymphomatous and lymphomatous changes in splenomegaly of New Zealand Black mice." *Acta Pathol Japan* **30**(2): 171–6.

Zanesi, N., R. Aqeilan, et al. (2006). "Effect of rapamycin on mouse chronic lymphocytic leukemia and the development of nonhematopoietic malignancies in E{micro}-TCL1 transgenic mice." *Cancer Res* **66**(2): 915–20.

Zapata, J. M., M. Krajewska, et al. (2000). "TNFR-associated factor family protein expression in normal tissues and lymphoid malignancies." *J Immunol* **165**(9): 5084–96.

Zapata, J. M., M. Krajewska, et al. (2004). "TNF receptor-associated factor (TRAF) domain and Bcl-2 cooperate to induce small B cell lymphoma/chronic lymphocytic leukemia in transgenic mice." *Proc Nat Acad Sci USA* **101**(47): 16600–5.

Zhan, F., J. Hardin, et al. (2002). "Global gene expression profiling of multiple myeloma, monoclonal gammopathy of undetermined significance, and normal bone marrow plasma cells." *Blood* **99**(5): 1745–57.

Zhang, B., Z. Wang, et al. (2007). "NF-{kappa}B2 mutation targets TRAF1 to induce lymphomagenesis." *Blood* **110**(2): 743–51.

Zhang, J. C., CC; Lombardi, et al. (1994). "Rearranged NFKB2 gene in the HUT78 T-lymphoma cell line codes for a constitutive nuclear factor lacking transcriptional repressor functions." *Oncogene* **9**(7): 1931–7.

Zhou, P., N. B. Levy, et al. (2001). "MCL1 transgenic mice exhibit a high incidence of B-cell lymphoma manifested as a spectrum of histologic subtypes." *Blood* **97**(12): 3902–9.

Zhu, D., C. F. Qi, et al. (2005). "Deregulated expression of the Myc cellular oncogene drives development of mouse "Burkitt-like" lymphomas from naive B cells." *Blood* **105**(5): 2135–7.

Zojer, N., H. Ludwig, et al. (2003). "Patterns of somatic mutations in VH genes reveal pathways of clonal transformation from MGUS to multiple myeloma." *Blood* **101**(10): 4137–9.

Chapter 9
Genetic and Virological Predisposition to Pre-B Lymphomagenesis in SL/Kh

Hiroshi Hiai

Contents

List of Abbreviations

BM	bone marrow
Bomb-1	*bone marrow pre-B-1*
Esl-1	*early lymphoma in SL/Kh-1*
Foc-1	*follicular center lymphoma-1*
Ig	immunoglobulin
Lla	*lymphoma latency acceleration*
MCF	mink cell focus

H. Hiai
Shiga Medical Center Research Institute, 5-4-30 Moriyama, City of Moriyama, Shiga 524-8524, Japan
hiai6029@shigamed.jp

S. Li (ed.), *Mouse Models of Human Blood Cancers*,
DOI: 10.1007/978-0-387-69132-9_9, © Springer Science+Business Media, LLC 2008

MHC	major histocompatibility complex
MMMTV	mouse mammary tumor virus
MRF	maternal resistance factor
MuLV	murine leukemia virus
PMA	phorbol myristic acetate
RI	recombinant inbred
QTL	quantitative trait locus
Svi-1	*SL/Kh virus integration-1*
Tlsm-1	*thymic lymphoma susceptible mouse-1*

9.1 Introduction

Spontaneous pre-B lymphoma is a relatively infrequent hematopoietic malignancy in mice. Pre-B lymphomas are occasionally observed in some mouse models such as AKXD recombinant inbred (RI) strains, Eμ–myc transgenic mice, and Abelson virus-injected mice. In an inbred strain SL/Kh, pre-B lymphomas develop at an unusually high incidence (>90%) by 6 months of age [10]. Reintegration of the endogenous ecotropic murine leukemia virus (MuLV) provirus to host DNA is a pathogenetic mechanism [16, 36], but lymphoma development is largely dependent on a number of host loci as well as on epigenetic factors [8, 13]. Therefore, SL/Kh pre-B lymphoma is an excellent multifactorial disease model. In this article, we will review the origin of SL/Kh mice, the biological features of lymphomas in this strain, the virology and genetics of lymphomagenesis, the unusual transient expansion of pre-B cells in pre-cancerous bone marrow (BM), and provirus integration in lymphoma DNA leading to the activation of cancer-related genes. Contained in this report are historical descriptions of our previous research; however, many important questions remain to be answered as technology and genome informatics advance.

9.2 Origin of SL/Kh and Related Strains of Mice

The SL has been established in Japan as a mouse strain prone to spontaneous leukemia. Their origin, history of establishment, and genetic interrelationship have been extensively studied [1]. The ancestors of the SL family were outbred Swiss mice and probably A2G mice, which were imported to Japan from an anonymous US source in approximately 1941 and have been maintained at several institutions. To date, four substrains with distinctive biological properties have been reported, that is, SL/Am, SL/Ni, SL/Kh, and SL/QDg. Some parameters relevant to lymphomagenesis are listed in Table 9.1. At present, the SL/Kh and SL/Ni strains are deposited at the RIKEN Bioresource Center at Tsukuba, but SL/Am and SL/QDg have been terminated.

Table 9.1 Parameters for lymphomagenesis in AKR and SL family mice

	AKR/Ms	SL/Kh	SL/Ni	SL/Am	SL/QDj
Lymphoma type, incidence	T, 85%	Pre-B, >95%	Mature B, <10%	Mature B and myelogenous, 56.4%	None
Ecotropic MuLV genome (kb size of EcoRI fragments)	27, 14.5, 10.5	27, 21, 19, 14.5, 13,[a] 10.5	21, 19	21, 19	21, 14.5, 8.8
ecotropic virus expression	High	High	High or None	High	None
xenotropic virus expression	High	High	None	High	None
MHC	k	q	q	q	Q
Thy1	Thy1.1	Thy1.1	Thy1.2	Thy1.2	Thy1.2
Mx	Type-2	Type-2	Type-1	Type-1	Type-2

[a]A duplet in Southern blot (37)

The SL/Kh strain originated from a pair of SL mice introduced to the Aichi Cancer Center Research Institute (Nagoya, Japan) from Kyushu University (Fukuoka, Japan) by Nishizuka in the 1970s. SL/Kh mice share alleles at 59% microsatellite loci with SL/Am and SL/Ni, showing a closer relation than any other unrelated inbred strains [1]. However, the genetic profiles of the endogenous MuLV, the mammary tumor virus (MMTV), and the Mx gene allele are different from those of other SL family members. Moreover, many distinct microsatellite alleles are shared with AKR mice. For instance, Thy1, a marker antigen for T-cells, is Thy1.1 in SL/Kh, a rare genotype carried by AKR. When EcoRI-digested genomic DNA is Southern blotted with an Akv1 *env* probe, SL/Kh shows seven copies of ecotropic virus fragments, of which the 27-kb band is shared with the AKR endogenous ecotropic virus Emv11. SL/Ni and SL/Am do not have this band. These observations suggest that the SL/Kh strain is a RI strain derived from an intercross of proto-SL mice and AKR at an earlier stage of maintenance. The provirus yielding the 27-kb band is presumably acquired genetically from the AKR ancestor. We have shown that a high level of the infectious ecotropic virus is produced from two provirus loci in crosses with NFS mice without an endogenous ecotropic provirus and that one of the viruses producing the loci is at the proximal end of chromosome 7, where Emv11 is located [37].

9.3 Immunopathology of SL/Kh Pre-B Lymphomas

The most prevalent form of hematopoietic neoplasm in the mouse is the T lymphoma, which develops spontaneously or is induced by a virus, a chemical, radiation, or gene manipulation. SL/Kh mice are unique, as they develop

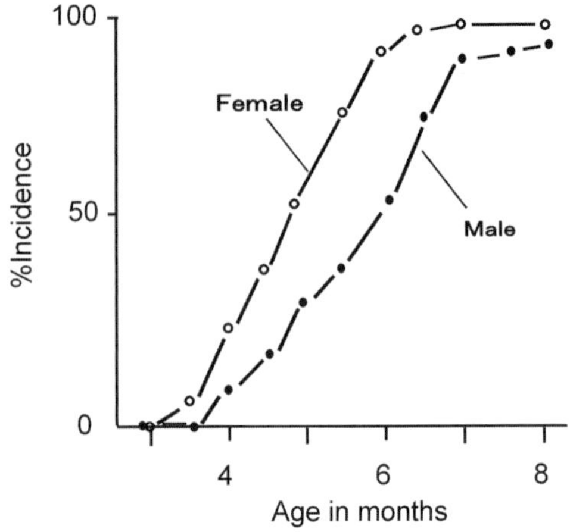

Fig. 9.1 Cumulative percent incidence of spontaneous pre-B lymphomas in SL/Kh mice [10]

exclusively pre-B lymphomas early in life at a high incidence (Fig. 9.1) [10]. There are two clinically distinct types among them. In the major type (83.7%), lymph node swelling and hepatosplenomegaly are the main features, while, in the minor type (16.3%), no macroscopically overt lymphoid organ involvement was evident although spinal paraplegia and incontinence were remarkable. BM is the main site of lymphoma cell proliferation in both types. In the minor type, the growth of lymphoma cells is limited in BM, and it compresses the spinal cord to cause spinal paralysis. Both types of lymphomas are readily transplantable in syngenic adult mice and kill recipients in as little as 2 weeks. The macroscopic types of lymphoma remain the same as primary lymphomas for at least three generations of in vivo passage. Both types of lymphomas are diffuse lymphoblastic lymphomas (Fig. 9.2a) but indistinguishable from each other except for tissues of infiltration.

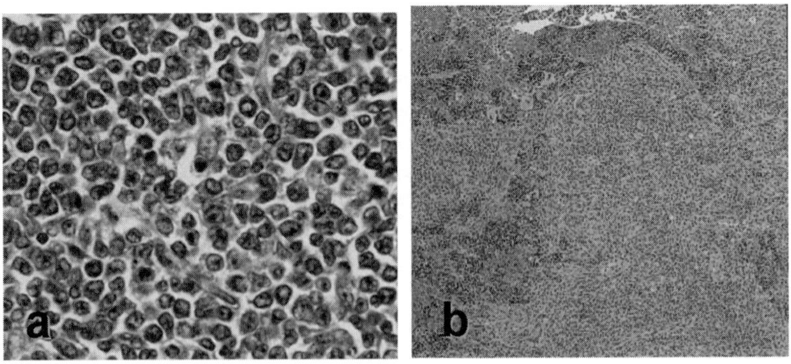

Fig. 9.2 (**a**) Histopathology of a major type pre-B lymphoma in a SL/Kh mouse. ×400, H.E. (**b**) Follicular center cell lymphoma in a (SL/Kh × NFS)F1 × NFS mouse [8]. ×100, H.E. (See color insert)

Both types of lymphomas show typical pre-B-cell phenotypes, that is, positive for B220, a pan-B cell antigen, and BP1, a pre-B cell antigen, and negative for surface immunoglobulin (Ig) [32]. The Ig heavy-chain gene is rearranged either mono- or oligoclonally, but the light-chain gene remains in a germ-line configuration. Products of the *lambda 5* and $V_{\text{pre-B}}$ gene form a receptor-like complex on the cell surface by which pre-B lymphocytes transmit a signal for proliferation. *RAG-1* and *RAG-2* genes code for key enzymes inducing the Ig gene recombination. SL/Kh lymphomas express *Lambda 5*, $V_{\text{pre-B}}$, *RAG-1*, and *RAG-2* genes. Unlike normal pre-B cells, SL/Kh neoplastic pre-B cells express adhesion molecules LECAM-1 and LFA-1, but their expression is also shared by both types of lymphomas [24]. To date, no parameter has been found to explain the distinctive in vivo behavior of these two types of pre-B lymphomas.

9.4 Host Genetic Factors Affecting Types of Lymphomas

9.4.1 Pre-B Lymphoma vs. Follicular Center Cell Lymphoma

It is well known that lymphoma development is significantly affected by host genes. Among particularly important genes, *Fv1* determines the tropism of MuLV and *H-2*, the major histocompatibilty complex gene, affects the immune responsiveness to MuLV and lymphoma cells. Investigations to find loci affecting lymphomagenesis have been extensive in chemical- and radiation-induced lymphomagenesis.

In order to analyze host genetic predisposition to pre-B lymphomas in SL/Kh, we studied lymphomagenesis in F1 and a backcross to NFS, a mouse strain without the endogenous ecotropic MuLV genome and without spontaneous lymphoma by 12 months of age [37]. In (SL/Kh × NFS)F1, all lymphomas were of the pre-B type, but their incidence was lower (53.8%). Furthermore, the latent period was longer (8.4 months). In 83 backcross mice, 22 (26.5%) developed hematopoietic malignancies, including 8 pre-B lymphomas, 2 myeloid leukemias, and 12 follicular center cell lymphomas (Fig. 9.2b). All individuals developing lymphomas expressed a high level of ecotropic MuLV. Genome-wide screening with microsatellite and biochemical genetic markers revealed that all the backcross mice developing any tumor had an SL/Kh-derived allele at *Gpi1* at the proximal end of chromosome 7. It is known that *Gpi1* is closely linked with *Akv1* (*Emv11*), which is an endogenous ecotropic MuLV in AKR mice. As previously stated, one of the seven ecotropic provirus in SL/Kh is genetically acquired from an AKR ancestor. Further genetic analysis showed that, without exception, the backcross mice developing pre-B lymphomas had a dominant SL/Kh-derived allele on the chromosome 17 segment bearing the MHC locus. This locus is called *Esl-1* (*early lymphoma in SL/Kh-1*). We concluded that the presence of an *Akv1*-like provirus and the SL/Kh-derived allele at *Esl-1* is required for pre-B lymphomas to develop. On the other hand, the

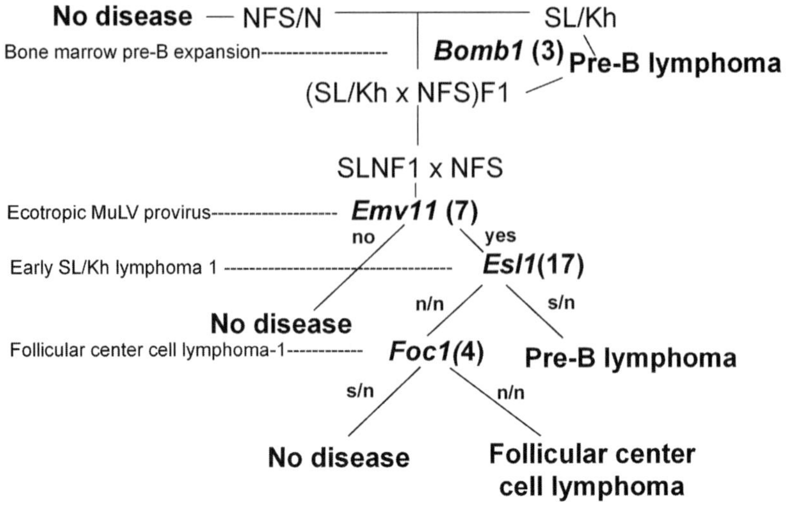

Fig. 9.3 Genetic determination of lymphomagenesis in a cross of SL/Kh × NFS [13]. Chromosome numbers for relevant loci are shown in parentheses

backcross mice developing follicular center lymphomas have a recessive NFS-derived allele at *foc-1* (*follicular center lymphoma-1*) on the proximal segment of chromosome 4. Therefore, the requirements for follicular center cell lymphomas are the presence of the *Akv1*-like provirus and the homozygosity of the NFS-derived allele at foc-1. The majority of hematopoietic neoplasms developing in NFS mice into which *Akv1* was introgressed by extensive backcrossing are mature B-cell type [3, 6]. The observations of the two groups of researchers indicated above are consistent with our findings. Two myeloid leukemias have genotypes $Esl\text{-}1^{SL/Kh/NFS}$ and $foc\text{-}1^{NFS/NFS}$. Thus, the forms of lymphomas are determined by combinations of the host loci genotype as summarized in Fig. 9.3. Unfortunately, the genes corresponding to these loci have not been identified; therefore, the mechanism of the disease type determination remains hypothetical.

9.4.2 T Lymphoma vs. B Lymphoma

Subsequently, we investigated lymphomagenesis in the cross between SL/Kh and AKR mice to analyze the possible genetic mechanism determining the type of lymphomas to the B- or T-cell type. Before discussion of the primary topic, a brief review of the role of the thymus in T-lymphomagenesis will be presented.

The lymphomas developing spontaneously in AKR mice are T lymphomas arising in the thymus and secondarily infiltrating into other lymphoid organs. These lymphoma cells show an immunocytological profile of primitive thymic cortical lymphocytes. Gross first found that cell-free extracts of AKR lymphoma induced T lymphomas when injected into newborn C3H mice as reviewed in 1958 [5]. A pathogenetic virus is derived from endogenous ecotropic MuLVs; however, it was later shown that, ultimately, a leukemogenic virus is generated in the pre-leukemic thymus through complicated recombination events among endogenous MuLVs [7, 21, 34]. This virus is called a mink cell focus (MCF)-forming virus, as it induces morphological changes in infected mink lung cells. The MCF virus is thymotropic, has a dualtropic host range, and induces T lymphomas by injection to appropriate recipients. Similar viruses have been detected in high leukemia strains, such as C58 and HRS/J.

The thymus is essential for T lymphomagenesis in the mouse. Thymectomy remarkably suppresses lymphoma development, and a thymus graft from an appropriate donor restores lymphomagenesis. There are three explanations for the essential role of the thymus. First, the thymus provides the target cells for lymphomagenesis, since lymphoma cells have the properties of primitive thymic cortical lymphocytes. However, whether or not a thymic lymphocyte per se is the direct target of a carcinogen is controversial. It is possible that the initial transformation may occur at the level of pre-T or lymphoid precursors residing in BM and that the cells later colonize and grow in the thymic microenvironments. Second, recombination events among endogenous MuLVs and their infection to target cells take place in the thymus. The thymus is also required for T lymphomagenesis induced by radiation or chemical carcinogens, in which direct involvement of recombinant viruses is not likely. Third, the thymus physiologically provides tissue microenvironments to support the growth and differentiation of thymic lymphocytes. This function is applicable to transformed thymic lymphocytes. From AKR primary lymphoma thymuses, we could consistently isolate cellular complexes of neoplastic thymocytes and thymic stromal cells [11] and maintain them in tissue culture for a long term. Neoplastic lymphocytes survive and grow in close contact with stromal cells in the form of pseudo-emperipolesis (Fig. 9.4) for a few weeks in culture. When

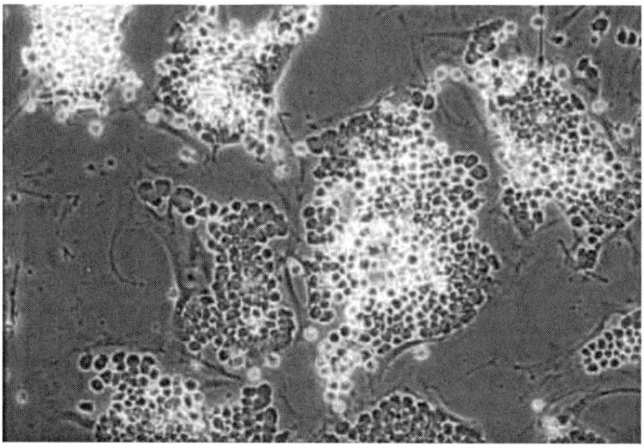

Fig. 9.4 Symbiotic complexes isolated from a primary lymphoma thymus of an AKR mouse. Note most T-lymphoma cells are crawling under cytoplasm of thymic stromal cells (pseudo-emperipolesis). Phase contrast,. ×200

they are separated from the stromal cells, they quickly become apoptotic. However, they can survive and grow when phorbol myristic acetate (PMA) or a related tumor promoter is supplemented to the culture [12, 18]. It is possible to maintain microenvironment-dependent lymphoma cells in a PMA-containing medium for more than a year [19]. Lymphoma cells complexed with stromal cells gradually acquire the capability of autonomic growth. The cellular complex of neoplastic lymphocytes and stromal cells is called symbiotic complex. Stromal cells are one of the subsets of thymic epithelial cells residing in the thymic subcapsular zone and medulla [11, 20]. Based on these observations, we postulate that developing T lymphomas requires some support of thymic microenvironments. In their natural history, they form a symbiotic complex with thymic stromal cells. Under close cell-to-cell interaction in the complex, lymphoma cells survive, grow, and are selected for autonomic growth. These three functions of thymus may not be mutually exclusive, but they contribute to thymic lymphomagenesis by a variety of etiologies.

The lymphomas in AKR and SL/Kh are distinct in immunocytology; therefore, they provide an excellent tool to study the genetic factor determining types of lymphomas [38]. Of 84 lymphomas developing in 91 (AKR × SL/Kh)F_1 mice, 75 were T lymphomas. In 75 (AKR × SL/Kh)F_1 × SL/Kh backcross mice, 74 developed lymphomas, including 35 T (47.3%), 34 B (45.9%), and 5 mixed T and B lymphomas (6.8%). Of 144 lymphomas in the (AKR × SL/Kh)F_2 intercross, 96 (66.7%) were T lymphomas, 38 (26.4%) B lymphomas, and 10 (6.8%) mixed T and B lymphomas. The segregation data are best explained by assuming a single dominant *AKR* gene determining the type of lymphoma to the T-cell type. We call this gene *Tlsm-1* (*thymic lymphoma susceptible mouse-1*) (Fig. 9.5). By genome-wide screening with microsatellite genetic markers, *Tlsm-1* is mapped on a 7 cM segment between *D7Mit8* and *D7Mit13* on chromosome 7.

The AKXD strains are a set of RI strains between AKR/J and DBA/2 J. AKXD RI mice develop spontaneous lymphomas of various pathological forms [4]. We tried to determine whether the above locus is involved in the determination of the type of lymphoma by examining the allele type of microsatellite loci in the *Tlsm-1* segment on chromosome 7. Out of 20 AKXD RI

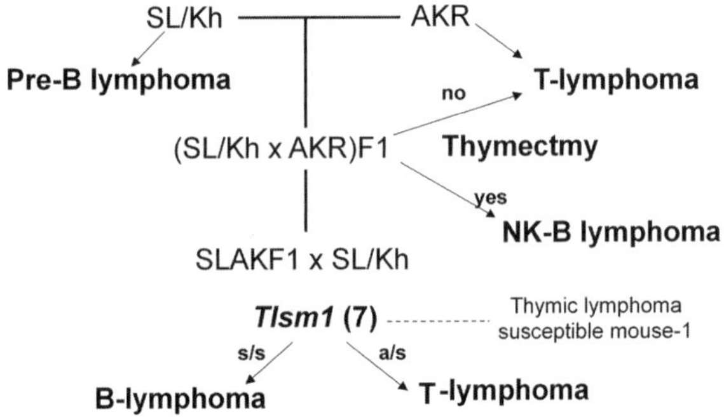

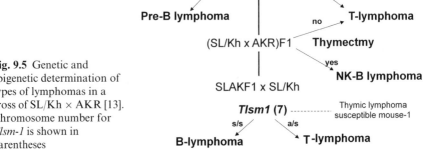

Fig. 9.5 Genetic and epigenetic determination of types of lymphomas in a cross of SL/Kh × AKR [13]. Chromosome number for *Tlsm-1* is shown in parentheses

strains, 9 strains with high T-lymphoma incidence had an AKR-derived allele between *D7Mit71* and *D7Mit13*, where *Tlsm-1* is located [38]. It is highly likely that AKR mice have a dominant locus for susceptibility to T lymphomas rather than B lymphomas not only in crosses to SL/Kh but also in those to DBA/2 J.

The length of the latent period is determined by *MHC* rather than by *Tlsm-1* [38]. By quantitative trait locus (QTL) analysis of the latent period of lymphomas in the F2 intercross, a locus on chromosome 17 was mapped with an LOD score of 7 and called *Lla (lymphoma latency acceleration)* [17]. The QTL peak for *Lla* is located in the MHC class II. Homozygosity of the SL/Kh recessive allele of *Lla* is associated with significant shortening of lymphoma latency. The MHC haplotype of SL/Kh is q, which has a defect in I-E. SL/Kh mice responded well to the I-A-dependent antigen but not to the I-E-dependent antigen (Shimada, unpublished observation). The MHC class II molecule is involved in an immune response to a retrovirus-enveloping antigen. A defect in I-E may reduce the immune response to an infectious virus.

9.4.3 Unusual Mixed-Type Lymphoma in Thymectomized (SL/Kh × AKR)F1 Mice

To study the role of the thymus in T lymphomagenesis in (SL/Kh × AKR)F1 mice, we compared the lymphomas in F1 mice intact or thymectomized at 3–5 days of age [23]. In AKR, thymectomy remarkably reduces the incidence of lymphomas except for the low incidence of B1 lymphomas after a long latent period [31]. In contrast, thymectomy does not reduce lymphoma development in (SL/Kh × AKR)F1. Of 39 intact F1 mice, 36 developed lymphomas (92.3%), of which 30 were T lymphomas. In contrast, 39 of 41 thymectomized mice (95.1%) developed lymphomas with an unusual phenotype, $NK1.1^+Mac1^+ CD16^+$. Resembling large granular lymphocytes (Fig. 9.6), these lymphoma cells had large lysosomal granules and expressed IL4, perforin, and interferon-γ. To our knowledge, unusual $NK1^+$ B1 lymphomas have not been reported.

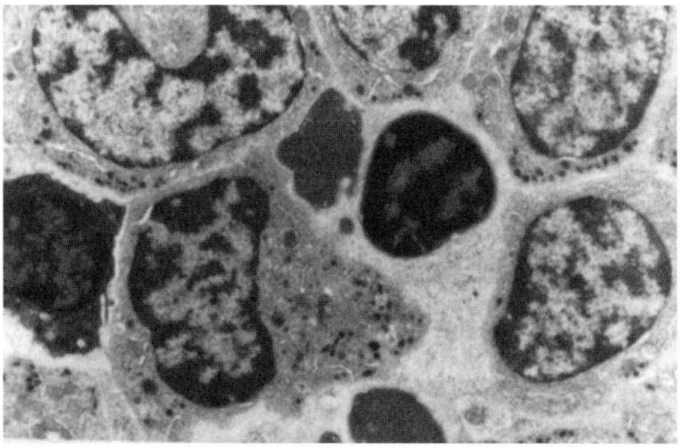

Fig. 9.6 Large granular-cell lymphomas with unusual NK-B phenotype in thymectomized (SL/Kh × AKR)F1 mice [23]. Electron microscopy, ×5000

An increase of NK or NK-T cells is known in thymectomized mice, suggesting that the thymus may well play a role in negative regulation to NK-related cells. However, grafting of a newborn thymus from AKR or SL/Kh to thymectomized F1 mice at 4 weeks of age did not prevent $NK1^+$ B1 lymphomas from developing (Lu, unpublished data). Further study is thus indicated to understand the role of the thymus in modulating the type of lymphomas.

9.4.4 Other Host Loci Affecting Lymphomagenesis

Subsequently, we explored other host loci affecting lymphomagenesis in crosses to a variety of inbred laboratory mice [2]. F1 mice between SL/Kh and low-lymphoma strains, such as BALB/c, B10, NZB, A/J, C3H, CBA, SJL, DBA/2, and MSM/Ms, expressed endogenous ecotropic MuLV depending on the allelotype of *Fv1*. F1 mice with BALB/c ($Fv1^b$), B10 ($Fv1^b$), or NZB ($Fv1^{nr}$) did not show virus expression, whereas those with C3H, CBA, SJL, DBA/2, or MSM/Ms ($Fv1^n$) did. In these F1 mice, lymphoma incidence was very low or null. For lymphoma development, the *Fv1* allelotype and ecotropic MuLV expression are not sufficient, but there should be dominant resistance to lymphomagenesis in low-lymphoma strains.

9.4.4.1 Two Dominant Resistance Loci in MSM/Ms Mice

The MSM/Ms is an inbred mouse strain established from Japanese wild mice, *Mus. Molossinus*. This strain is the most remote from laboratory mice from a genetic standpoint [1]. During 2 years of observation, no spontaneous tumor was observed. As stated above, (SL/Kh × MSM)F1 expressed ecotropic virus expression, but lymphoma development was tightly suppressed [2]. A genome-wide screening for the resistant loci was carried out in 60 SL/Kh × (SL/Kh × MSM)F1, and we mapped two loci *Msmr1* and *Msmr2* on chromosomes 17 and 18, respectively. Of 14 backcross mice developing pre-B lymphomas, 13 were homozygous for the SL/Kh allele at both loci. The map location of *Msmr1* showed overlapping with those of *MHC*, *Esl-1*, and *Lla*. In *Esl-1* and *Lla*, the SL/Kh allele was associated with dominant susceptibility. Judging from the mode of inheritance, *Msmr1* is distinct from *Esl-1* and *Lla*. This, however, does not exclude the possibility that *Msmr1* is a part of *MHC*. Candidate genes for *Msmr2*, *li*, and *CD14* are being considered, but so far, no direct evidence has been obtained.

9.4.4.2 Lymphoma Resistance of the SL/Ni Strain

The SL/Ni strain is a member of the SL family and is closely related to the SL/Am strain. They have been carefully maintained as an inbred strain, but from 1970 to 1990, a variety of changes in the virus–host relationship were observed. When

SL/Ni mice [28] were obtained from Nishizuka at the Aichi Cancer Center Research Institute (Nagoya, Japan), some SL/Ni mice expressed a high level of endogenous ecotropic virus, but others did not [9]. We found that the virus-negative individuals had a maternal resistance factor (MRF), namely, a natural antibody to ecotropic virus Gp70. A similar factor has been described regarding the RF strain [26, 27]. This factor is transmitted from mother to pups via maternal milk. Therefore, newborn mice from a highly viremic mother became virus-free when they were nursed by a virus-negative foster mother or injected with the serum of virus-free SL/Ni mice immediately after birth. When SL/Kh newborn mice were injected with an MRF-containing serum, ecotropic virus expression was intensely inhibited, but xenotropic virus expression was not affected. Pre-B-lymphoma development was remarkably delayed [9]. This is another clue providing evidence that the expression of an ecotropic virus is essential for SL/Kh pre-B lymphomas.

SL/Ni mice without MRF express an ecotropic virus as highly as SL/Kh mice, but they develop follicular center cell lymphomas or myeloid leukemias at a very low incidence ($<10\%$ at 18 months of age). Genetic analysis of (SL/Kh $\times$ SL/Ni)F1 $\times$ SL/Ni backcross mice revealed that lymphoma resistance of SL/Ni is associated with the homozygosity of recessive SL/Ni allele at locus *nir1* on chromosome 4 weakly but significantly [33]. The map position of *nir1* shows overlapping with that of *foc-1* described previously [37], but it remains obscure whether or not these are identical.

9.5 Bone Marrow Pre-B-Cell Expansion

9.5.1 Genetically Determined Pre-B-cell Expansion

Studying the characteristics of a hemo-lymphopoietic system of SL/Kh, we noted that young SL/Kh mice have an unusually high proportion of pre-B cells among BM lymphocytes [30]. In most laboratory strain mice, $BP1^{+}B220^{+}$ pre-B cells in BM are 2–5%, whereas the percentage in SL/Kh is nearly 30% (Fig. 9.7). The percentage of pre-B cells changes by age, with a peak at 4–6 weeks. Thereafter, it somehow declines, but after 12 weeks of age, it increases,

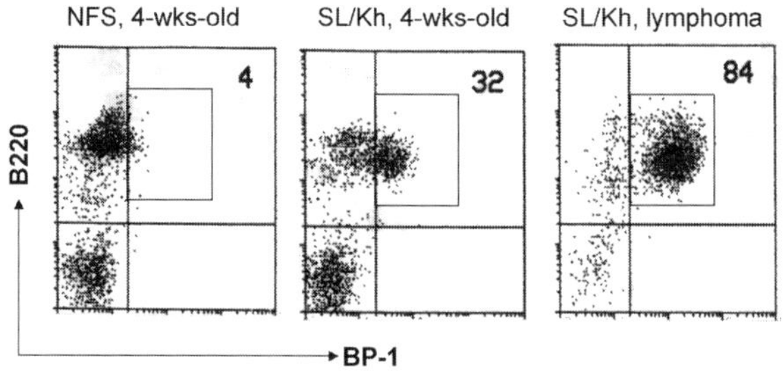

Fig. 9.7 Bone marrow pre-B cells in NFS (4-week-old), SL/Kh (4-week-old), and a SL/Kh lymphoma [8]. Percentage of $BP1^{+}B220^{+}$ cells is shown in right upper quadrant

and pre-B lymphomas ultimately develop. These observations suggest that pre-B expansion in BM may be a precursor lesion of lymphoma or abnormal differentiation of early B cells predisposing to lymphomagenesis, as suggested in Abelson virus-injected mice [35] and Eμ–*myc* transgenic mice [22]. When either of these hypotheses is correct, pre-B lymphomagenesis in SL/Kh mice should occur in two steps.

We next set out to determine whether pre-B expansion is induced by ecotropic MuLV essentially required for lymphomagenesis. To examine this hypothesis, we prepared F1 hybrids of SL/Kh and C4W, a BALB/c congenic for *Fv4*, and used (SL/Kh × BALB/c)F1 as a control. *Fv4* is a fragment of the Gp70 gene derived from wild-mice MuLV and is inherited as a dominant host gene [29]. The product of *Fv4* binds a cellular receptor for an ecotropic virus and thus, intensely inhibits infection by an ecotropic virus [15]. The level of an endogenous ecotropic virus is also suppressed as horizontal infection is inhibited. In (SL/Kh × C4W)F1, an ecotropic virus was not detectable, but the expansion of pre-B cells was as strong as that in (SL/Kh × BALB/c)F1 mice. Furthermore, pre-B cells in SL/Kh BM were not reduced when the expression of ecotropic MuLV was inhibited by neonatal injection of the MRF. These observations exclude the hypothesis that pre-B cell expansion is induced by ecotropic MuLV.

To determine whether the pre-B cell expansion is a geneticproperty of BM stem cells or is induced by BM microenvironments, we produced reciprocal radiation chimeras between SL/Kh and BALB/c mice by transferring BM cells and one month later, evaluating the percentage of pre-B cells. The lethally irradiated and BALB/c and SL/Kh mice receiving SL/Kh BM cells showed a high level of pre-B cells, whereas those receiving BALB/c BM cells did not. Therefore, the genetic property of BM stem cells is essential for pre-B-cell expansion [30].

The levels of pre-B cells in BM of 4-week-old (SL/Kh × NFS)F1 and (NFS × SL/Kh)F1 mice are comparable and an intermediate between those of SL/Kh and NFS, suggesting that the mode of inheritance is semidominant or polygenic. We measured the percentage of $BP1^{+}B220^{+}$ cells in BM of 4-week-old (SL/Kh × NFS)F2 and SL/Kh × (SL//Kh × NFS)F1 mice. A genome-wide screening for QTL responsible for increased pre-B cells revealed a QTL peak on chromosome 3 with an LOD score 22.0. It was named as *Bomb-1* (*bone marrow pre-B-1*) [25].

9.5.2 *Pre-B-Cell Expansion is Not Sufficient for Lymphomagenesis*

Determining the significance of pre-B-cell expansion in SL/Kh pre-B lymphomagenesis is important. The fact that expanded pre-B cells show a similar phenotype to lymphoma cells suggests the hypothesis that they represent an early lymphoma and start to grow with an appropriate second hit, for instance, the insertion of a retrovirus genome, but are destined to die without this second hit. The second hypothesis is that the transient pre-B-cell expansion is due to a genetic abnormality that expands the target cells for virus insertion. To examine these possibilities, we generated NFS mice into which a chromosomal segment carrying SL/Kh *Bomb-1* was introgressed using a speed congenic procedure [14]. The NFS.SL/Kh-*Bomb-1* mice showed BM pre-B expansion at an equivalent level to that of SL/Kh mice. However, none of the NFS.SL/Kh-*Bomb-1* mice developed lymphomas within 1 year of observation. Injection of infectious ecotropic MuLV from an SL/Kh lymphoma to neonates induced viremia but not lymphoma.

To determine whether or not BM pre-B cells in the prelymphoma stage are clonal, $BP1^{+}B220^{+}$ cells were collected from BM of SL/Kh and NFS.SL/Kh-*Bomb-1* at 4, 10, and 15 weeks of age using a cell sorter, and the *Ig* heavy-chain gene was examined for recombination by PCR Southern blot. The pre-B cells in NFS.SL/Kh-*Bomb-1* remained polyclonal at all ages, whereas in SL/Kh, a monoclonal population appeared in SL/Kh at 10 weeks of age and thereafter, gradually prevailed. Therefore, the pre-B expansion induced by *Bomb-1* is polyclonal in nature and not sufficient in itself for lymphoma development [14]. As previously reported, in the cross between SL/Kh and NFS, a dominant SL/Kh allele at *Esl-1* [37] is required for a pre-B lymphoma to occur. This may explain why NFS.SL/Kh-*Bomb-1* mice failed to develop lymphomas.

Although the gene for the *Bomb-1* locus has not been identified, it is a useful target for the investigation of the growth requirement of the normal early B lymphocytes as well as their lymphomagenesis.

9.6 Molecular Pathogenesis: Retrovirus Integrations in Lymphoma

The etiologic role of endogenous ecotropic MuLV in SL/Kh lymphomagenesis has been recognized since earlier genetic analysis [37], as has the inhibition of lymphomagenesis by MRF [9]. However, its molecular mechanism remained obscure until the start of systemic study on viral genome integration at strategic sites in the DNA of target cells. After the introduction of inverse PCR technology, we amplified the virus–host junctions and characterized the host flanking sequence very effectively. In this way, a number of cancer-related genes, including *Stat5a*, *Evi3*, *c-myc*, *N-myc*, and *Stat5b*, were identified as genes activated by provirus integration. The plethora of genes activated by retrovirus in SL/Kh pre-B lymphomas was beyond our expectations to some extent.

In SL/Kh pre-B lymphomas, *Stat5a* is the first gene found to be activated by provirus integration [36]. *Stat5a* is translated from the third exon, and the integrations are concentrated in the second intron of *Sta5a*; therefore, it is called *Svi-1* (*SL/Kh virus integration-1*). In *Svi-1* lymphomas, *Stat5a* mRNA and the STAT5a protein are expressed at a high level. The intensely phosphorylated STAT5a protein is translocated to the nucleus, where it binds to an interferon-γ–activated sequence (GAS) element on host genomic DNA, as

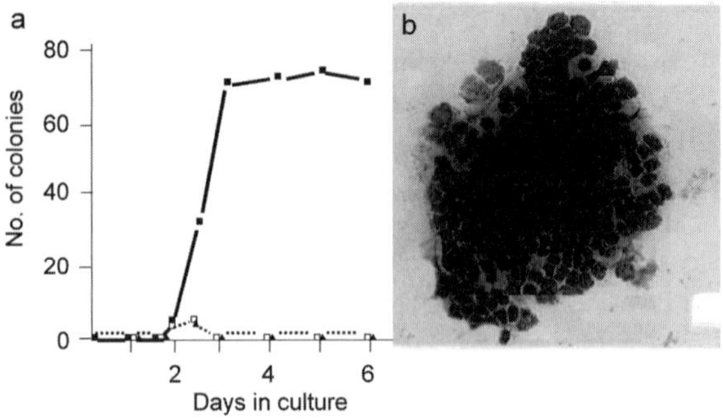

Fig. 9.8 (**a**) Kinetics of colony formation by pre-B cells after transfection of SL/Kh BM cells with constitutively activated mutant Stat5a cDNA [36]. Closed square, transfected with mutant Stat5a cDNA; open square, with wild type Stat5a cDNA; closed triangle, mock transfection. (**b**) A colony of pre-B cells in semisold medium [36]. (See color insert)

shown by a gel-shift assay. Genes with a GAS element, such as *c-myc*, *pim1*, and Bcl_{XL}, increase their expression. Such genes are known to have anti-apoptotic activity.

The *Svi-1* lymphomas express B220, BP1, CD19, CD24, CD43, Igα, and IL7R and thus share the characteristics of pre-B lymphocytes. On the other hand, many non-*Svi-1* lymphomas are $CD43^{-}IL7R^{-}$; thus, they seem to be pre-B lymphocytes in a later stage of maturation. The activation of STAT5a in *Svi-1* lymphoma occurs via the IL7-signaling pathway because the addition of IL7 to cultured *Svi-1* lymphoma cells intensifies the phosphorylation of STAT5a.

Evidence for the direct contribution of activated STAT5a to lymphomagenesis is given by the fact that transfection of constitutively activated mutant *Stat5a* cDNA to normal SL/Kh BM cells induces selective colonial growth of pre-B cells in a semisolid medium (Fig. 9.8a, 9.8b) [36]. By transfection of wild-type *Stat5a* cDNA or mock transfection, pre-B cells die and colonial growth fails to occur. The presence of IL7 is essential for the early stage of in vitro growth of the transfectant. On transfer to an IL7-free medium, within the first 48 hours in the culture, the transfected BM cells quickly become apoptotic, but after 96 hours, they lose dependence on IL7.

The transfectants growing in colonies express STAT5a intensely and also B220, BP1, CD19, CD24, CD43, and IL7R. The phenotype is common to *Svi-1* lymphoma cells and early pre-B cells in normal BM. Colonial growth of pre-B cells by constitutively activated mutant Stat5a cDNA occurs exclusively in SL/Kh BM, but not in NFS, C57BL/6, C3H, or AKR BM. This indicates that some host factor proper to SL/Kh is essential for this phenomenon, but its nature has not been clarified.

9.7 Discussion

We have shown that pre-B lymphomagenesis in SL/Kh strain mice is an excellent model of multifactorial diseases. Reintegration of endogenous ecotropic MuLV to several strategic sites for pre-B cell growth, including *Stat5a*,

Evi3, *c-myc*, *N-myc*, and *Stat5b*, is pathogenetic. From the viewpoint of a pathobiologist, the attention here has been focused on host genetic and epigenetic factors affecting pre-B lymphomagenesis. As reviewed in this article, virus expression, immunity to virus and their spread, types of lymphomas, and growth regulation of the BM pre-B cells, which are possible target cells of lymphomagenesis, are under host control. In SL/Kh, all these steps are destined to favor the development of pre-B lymphomas. Most of this study was conducted in the 1990s, before the author's retirement from Kyoto University. Regretfully, none of these host loci have been cloned; therefore, their functions have not been clarified at the molecular level. It is obvious that future study should be directed to the molecular cloning of these genes. Research involving *Esl-1*, *foc-1*, *Tlsm-1*, and *Bomb-1* would be particularly rewarding. SL/Kh, SL/Ni, SL/Kh.AKR-*Tlsm-1*, NFS.SL/Kh-*foc-1*, and NFS.SL/Kh-*Bomb-1* mice are maintained either as live stocks or frozen embryos at the National Bioresource Center in RIKEN Tsukuba Institute (http://www.brc.riken.go.jp/lab/animal/) and are available on request.

Acknowledgments I am very grateful to all of my colleagues who have contributed to the understanding of pre-B lymphomagenesis in SL/Kh mice. This study was supported by grants-in-aid for Scientific Research by the Ministry of Education, Culture, Sports, and Science and Grants for Cancer Research by the Ministry of Health, Labor, and Welfare, Japan.

References

1. Abujiang P, Yamada Y, Haller O, Kobayashi K, Kamoto T, Lu L-M, Ogawa M, Ishimoto A, Katoh H, Kanehira K, Ikegami S, Fukumoto M, Hiai H (1996a) The origin of the SL family mice. Lab Anim Sci 46: 410–417
2. Abujiang P, Kamoto T, Lu L-M, Yamada Y, Hiai H (1996b) Two dominant resistance genes to pre-B lymphoma in a wild-derived inbred mouse strain MSM/Ms. Cancer Res 56: 3716–3720
3. Fredrickson TN, Morse HC 3rd, Yetter RA, Rowe WP, Hartley JW, Pattengale PK (1985) Multiparameter analyses of spontaneous nonthymic lymphomas occurring in NFS/N mice congenic for ecotropic murine leukemia viruses. Am J Pathol 121:349–360.
4. Gilbert DJ, Neumann PE, Taylor BA, Jenkins NA, Copeland NG (1993) Susceptibility of AKXD recombinant inbred mouse strains to lymphoma. J Virol 67: 2083–2090.
5. Gross L (1958) Viral etiology of spontaneous leukemia: a review. Cancer Res 18: 371–381.
6. Hartley JW, Chattopadhyay SK, Lander MR, Taddesse-Heath L, Naghashfar Z, Morse HC 3rd, Fredrickson TN (2000) Accelerated appearance of multiple B cell lymphoma types in NFS/N mice congenic for ecotropic murine leukemia viruses. Lab Invest 80:159–169
7. Hartley JW, Wolford NK, Old LJ, Rowe WP (1977) A new class of murine leukemia virus associated with development of spontaneous lymphomas. Proc Natl Acad Sci USA 74: 789–792.
8. Hiai H (1996) Genetic predisposition to lymphomas in mice. Pathol Intern 46: 707–718
9. Hiai H, Buma YO, Ikeda H, Moriwaki K, Nishizuka Y (1987) Epigenetic control of endogenous ecotropic virus expression in SL/Ni strain mice. J Natl Cancer Inst 79: 781–787.

10. Hiai H, Kaneshima H, Nakamura H, Oguro BY, Moriwaki K, Nishizuka Y (1982) Unusually early and high rate of spontaneous occurrence of non-thymic leukemias in SL/Kh mice, a subline of SL strain. Jpn J Cancer Res 73: 603–613.
11. Hiai H, Nishi Y, Miyazawa T, Matsudaira Y, Nishizuka Y (1981) Mouse lymphoid leukemias: Symbiotic complexes of neoplastic lymphocytes and their microenvironments. J Natl Cancer Inst 66: 703–722.
12. Hiai H, Nishizuka Y (1981) Growth stimulation of microenvironment-dependent mouse leukemias by tumor-promoting phorbol esters. J Natl Cancer Inst 67: 1333–1340.
13. Hiai H, Tsuruyama T, Yamada Y (2003) Pre-B lymphomas in SL/Kh mice: A multifactorial disease model. Cancer Sci 94: 847–850
14. Hiratsuka T, Tsuruyama T, Kaszynski R, Kometani K, Minato N, Nakamura T, Tamaki K, Hiai H (2008) Bone marrow pre-B expansion by SL/Kh Bomb1 locus: Not sufficient for lymphomagenesis. Leuk Res 32: 309-14
15. Ikeda H, Odaka T (1983) Cellular expression of murine leukemia virus gp70-related antigen on thymocytes of uninfected mice correlates with *Fv4* gene-controlled resistance to Friend leukemia virus infection. Virology 128: 127–139
16. Jin G, Tsuruyama T, Yamada Y, Hiai H (2003) *Svi3*: a provirus common integration site in c-myc of SL/Kh pre-B lymphomas. Cancer Sci 94: 791–795
17. Kamoto T, Shisa H, Abujiang P, Lu L-M, Yoshida O, Yamada Y, Hiai H (1996) A quantitative trait locus in major histocompatibility complex determining latent period of mouse lymphomas. Jpn J Cancer Res 87: 401–404
18. Kaneshima H, Hiai H, Fujiki H, Iijima S, Sugimura T, Nishizuka Y (1983) Teleocidine-induced modulation of growth and cell interaction in microenvironment-dependent mouse leukemias. Leuk Res 7: 287–293.
19. Kaneshima H, Hiai H, Fujiki H, Oguro BY, Iijima S, Sugimura T, Nishizuka Y (1983) Tumor-promoter dependent mouse leukemia cell line. Cancer Res 43: 4676–4680
20. Kaneshima H, Ito M, Asai J, Taguchi O, Hiai H (1987) Thymic epithelial reticular cell sub-populations in mice defined by monoclonal antibodies. Lab Invest 56: 372–380
21. Kawashima K, Ikeda H, Hartley JW, Stockert E, Rowe WP, Old LJ (1976) Changes in expression of murine leukemia virus antigens and production of xenotropic virus in the late preleukemic period in AKR mice. Proc Natl Acad Sci USA. 73: 4680–4684
22. Langdon WY, Harris AW, Cory S, Adams JM (1986) The *c-myc* oncogene perturb B lymphocyte development in Eμ-*myc* transgenic mice. Cell 47: 11–18
23. Lu L-M, Hiai H (1999). Mixed phenotype lymphomas in thymectomized (AKR x SL/Kh) F1 mice. Jpn J Cancer Res 90: 1218–1223
24. Lu L-M, Ogawa M, Kamoto T, Yamada Y, Abujiang P, Hiai H (1997) Expression of LECAM-1 and LFA-1 on pre-B lymphoma cells but not on preneoplastic pre-B cells in SL/Kh mice. Leuk Res 21: 337–342
25. Lu L-M, Shimada M, Higashi S, Zeng Z-Z, Hiai H (1999) Bone marrow pre-B-1 (Bomb1): a quantitative trait locus inducing bone marrow pre-B cell expansion in lymphoma-prone SL/Kh mice. Cancer Res 59: 2593–2595
26. Mayer A, Struuck FD, Duran-Reynals ML, Lilly F (1980) Maternally transmitted resistance to lymphoma development in mice of reciprocal crosses of the RF/J and AKR/J strains. Cell 19: 431–436.
27. Melamedoff M, Lilly F, Duran-Reynals ML (1983) Suppression of endogenous murine leukemia virus by maternal resistance factor. J Exp Med. 1983 158; 506–14
28. Nishizuka Y (1979) Origin and use of SL strain mice: an animal model of disease. Exp Anim 28: 185–191 (In Japanese)
29. Odaka T, Ikeda H, Yoshikura H, Moriwaki K, Suzuki S (1981) Fv-4: Gene controlling resistance to NB-tropic Friend leukemia virus. Distribution in wild mice, introduction into genetic background of BALB/c mice and mapping of chromosome. J Natl Cancer Inst 67: 1123–1127

30. Okamoto K, Yamada Y, Shimada MO, Nakakuki Y, Nomura H, Hiai H (1994) Abnormal bone marrow B-cell differentiation in pre-B lymphoma- prone SL/Kh mice. Cancer Res 54:399–402
31. Peled A, Haran-Ghera N (1985) High incidence of B cell lymphomas derived from thymectomized AKR mice expressing TL.4 antigen. J Exp Med 162:1081–1086.
32. Shimada MO, Yamada Y, Nakakuki Y, Okamoto K, Fukumoto M, Honjo T, Hiai H. (1993) SL/Kh strain mice: A novel animal model of pre B lymphomas. Leuk Res 17: 573–578
33. Shisa H, Yamada Y, Kawarai A, Terada N, Kawai M, Matsushiro H, Hiai H (1996) Genetic and epigenetic resistance of SL/Ni mice to lymphomas. Jpn J Cancer Res 87: 258–262
34. Stoye JP, Moroni C, Coffin JM (1991) Virological events leading to spontaneous AKR thymomas. J Virol 65: 1273–1285.
35. Tidmarsh G, Dailey MO, Whitlock CA, Pilemer E, Weissman IL (1985) Transformed lymphocytes from Abelson-diseased mice express levels of a lineage transformation associated antigen elevated from that found on normal lymphocytes. J Exp Med 162: 1421–1343
36. Tsuruyama T, Nakamura T, Jin G, Ozeki M, Yamada Y, Hiai H (2002) Constitutive activation of Stat5a by retrovirus integration in early pre-B lymphomas of SL/Kh strain mice. Proc. Natl. Acd. Sci. USA 99: 8253–8258
37. Yamada Y, Shimada MO, Toyokuni S, Okamoto K, Fukumoto M, Hiai H (1994) Genetic predisposition to pre-B lymphoma in SL/Kh strain mice. Cancer Res 54:403–407
38. Yamada Y, Shisa H, Matsushiro H, Kamoto T, Kobayashi Y, Kawarai A, Hiai H (1994) T-lymphomagenesis is determined by a dominant host gene Thymic Lymphoma Susceptible Mouse-1 (Tlsm-1) in murine models. J Exp Med 180: 2155–2162

Chapter 10
Animal Cancer Models in Anticancer Drug Discovery and Development

Francis Lee and Roberto Weinmann

Contents

10.1 Introduction

The prevention and treatment of cancer continues to pose great challenges to modern medical science. Long dreaded, cancer remains one of most lethal diseases in the United States and is poised to overtake heart diseases as the most common cause of death in the very near future [1]. Despite great advances over the last 50 years in our understanding of the cause (the genetics of cancer) and pathological progression (the physiology of cancer), efforts in the clinic to effectively control the disease have met with uneven successes in prolonging patients survival, ranging from the highly effective (in the treatment of even advanced stages of choriocarcinoma, testicular cancers, and some lymphomas), to the partially effective (when used as an adjuvant to surgery in the early stages of some common carcinomas of adults), to the modest at best (in the treatment

F. Lee
Bristol-Myers Squibb Research and Development, Oncology Discovery, Princeton, NJ 08543, USA
francis.lee@bms.com

S. Li (ed.), *Mouse Models of Human Blood Cancers*,
DOI: 10.1007/978-0-387-69132-9_10, © Springer Science+Business Media, LLC 2008

of the most common advanced stages adult solid malignancies). In recent years, through unprecedented collaborative efforts between academic- or government-funded laboratories and the pharmaceutical industries, the discovery and development of anticancer drugs has undergone a drastic change. The commonly held perception regarding the slow pace of therapeutic advances is rapidly changing with the recent successful drugs such as Herceptin (trastuzumab), Gleevec (imatinib), Erbitux (cetuximab), Avastin (bevacizumab), and Sprycel (dasatinib). Nonetheless, the overall success with oncology drug discovery and development in recent years has been mixed. Indeed, the failure rates for oncology drugs in the clinic are among the worst overall in comparison with other disease areas, with only 5% of drugs that enter the clinic make it to marketing approval [2] compared with the pharmaceutical industry overall success rate of 11%. Although this book focuses on blood cancers, it is necessary to use some examples for solid tumors to help express our points.

10.2 Identifying the Main Causes of Failure of Anticancer Drug Candidates

Why do drug development candidates fail? Some of the main reasons for failure have been identified and it is informative to review this (Fig. 10.1). Patents and intellectual property issues are responsible for 5% of the total causes of attrition.

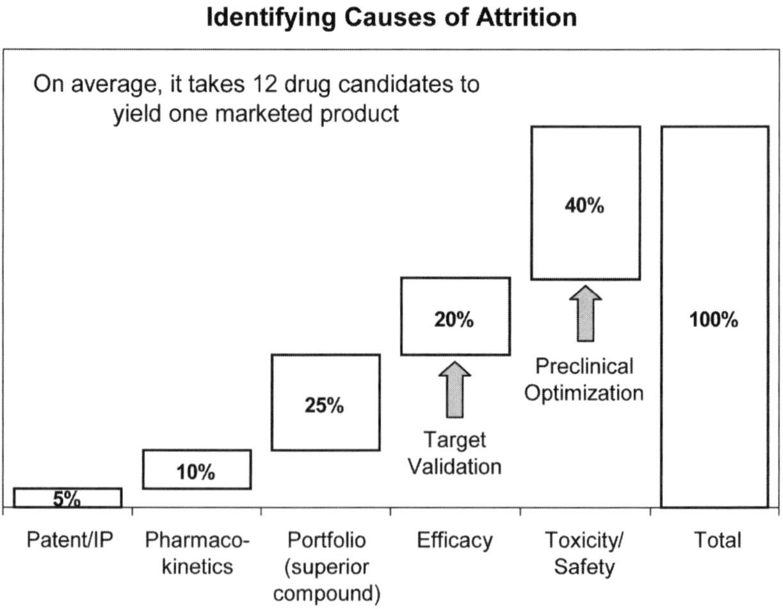

Fig. 10.1 Rates and causes for attrition of clinical candidates during discovery and development in oncology

In addition, approximately 25% of compounds are terminated for portfolio reasons. Some of this attrition represents changes in internal strategy, while other terminations are due to changes in the commercial environment. Before the 1990s, drug candidates frequently failed (at a rate of 25%) due to poor pharmacokinetic behavior, that is, the inability to deliver the required amount of drug to the target site for the required amount of time. This may be due to insufficient oral bioavailability or to differences in pharmacokinetics or metabolism between test animals and human subjects. With the availability of sophisticated technology of monitoring drug fate in biologic samples (e.g., HPLC-MS) and powerful PK modeling tool [3], this deficiency in drug development had been greatly improved and accounts for approximately only 10% of attrition for the last 10 years compared to over 25% 15 years ago. The last two causes of attrition, namely lack of efficacy and/or toxicity and safety concerns, represent approximately 60 percent of attrition. Moreover, lack of efficacy in the target disease at maximum-tolerated dose (MTD), which usually only becomes evident late in development and is therefore costly, is a failure of on-target hypotheses and should be addressable by rigorous target identification and validation during the drug discovery process. The inability to gain signal during early development about the efficacy of a candidate compound, clearly points to a deficiency of the animal models utilized to evaluate its developmental potential. Thus, a last portion of the risks can be reduced by identifying better predictive cancer models.

10.3 The Modern Paradigm for Anticancer Drug Discovery

To gain a better understanding of how more predictive animal models may help to reduce risk, it is instructive to gain an understanding of the sea of change that has taken place in the pharmaceutical industry with regard to drug discovery approach. The modern paradigm for anticancer drug discovery comprises a series of carefully constructed steps that are designed to rapidly and efficiently allow the demonstration of the so-called proof of principle of a particular target, through the evaluation of large number of pharmaceutically tractable molecules, culminating in phases I and II clinical trials of the final drug candidate (Fig. 10.2). This cascade of steps, called a decision network, can be envisioned as molecules feeding into a series of iterative stop/go tests of increasing biological complexity. The concept of "therapeutic index," that is the demonstration of antitumour efficacy at doses well below those causing severe toxicities, is also a long-established paradigm in preclinical drug discovery [4]. A key part of the preclinical stage of the process, and often representing a significant bottleneck, is the demonstration of antitumour efficacy in a "relevant" tumour model in vivo.

Mouse cancer models are critical tools for elucidating mechanisms of cancer development, as well as for assessment of putative cancer therapies. However, validation studies of these model systems for their ability to adequately predict therapeutic responses in patients have been rare [5]. Consequently, design and interpretation of preclinical studies for tumor modeling must be undertaken

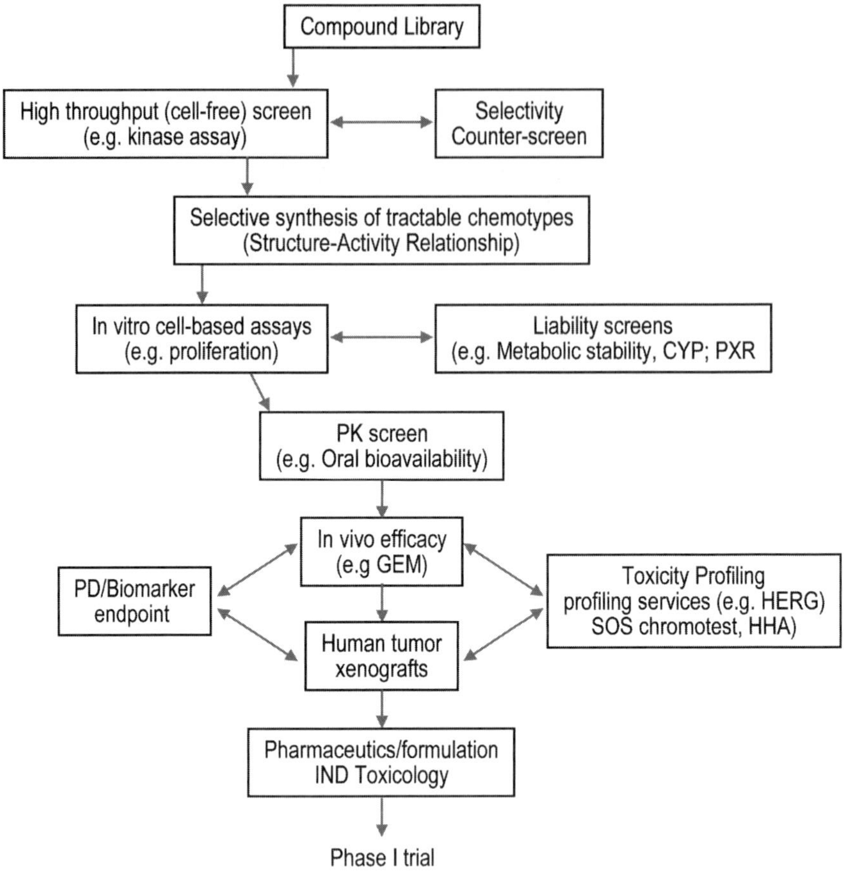

Fig. 10.2 Example of the flow of compounds in a decision network for drug discovery in oncology

carefully. This chapter briefly reviews the most commonly used transplanted tumor models (the human tumor xenografts). It also reviews commonly utilized in vivo study endpoints. Even small improvements in predictive value achieved through careful selection of models and endpoints have the potential to have large impacts on productivity and overall drug development costs.

10.4 Typical Protocol for Drug Evaluation Utilizing Tumor Xenografts-Commonality and Variables

10.4.1 Site of Implant

Most transplantable human tumor xenografts are placed heterotopically (ectopically) in host systems. Tumor lines in use have been specifically selected for mutations that allow heterotopic growth in mice. Although these tumors will grow and respond to therapeutics, the selection of the transplantation site may modulate tumor growth [6] and success of therapeutic intervention [7]. The subcutaneous (SC) site is by far the most commonly utililized for primary tumors for reasons of accessibility, lack of distress and interference with mobility in mice, and visibility for monitoring. Generally, SC refers to placement by injection or surgical implantation in the flank, a region referring to the posterior lateral abdominal quadrant. Placement is generally done in fat and mammary gland tissues near popliteal, inguinal, or accessory axillary lymph nodes.

10.4.2 Origin of the Model

From the early days, human tumour xenografts were established either by direct implantation of patient biopsy material or via inoculation of continuous human tumour cell lines. A particularly important large panel of xenografts, derived directly from biopsies, has been established by HH Fiebig and colleagues at the University of Freiburg in Germany [8]. More than 1600 tumors have been transplanted SC into nude mice and more than 300 xenografts established, representative of all of the major tumour types [8].

A comparison of drug response in the xenograft compared with that in the patient was made in 80 cases in 55 xenografts using either an in vivo assay (a comparison of treated versus control tumour volumes) or ex vivo using a soft agar clonogenic assay from disaggregated tumors. In accordance with the earlier studies of Steel and colleagues alluded to above, the xenografts predicted correctly for clinical response in 19/21 (90%) of occasions when using the in vivo assay (this was reduced a little to 60% using the clonogenic assay) and predicted for resistance in 57/59 (97%) of occasions when using the in vivo assay (92% for the clonogenic assay) [8].

In addition, the response pattern of more recently discovered clinically active drugs, paclitaxel, gemcitabine, docetaxel, vindesine and topotecan, was determined in 187 xenografts. Overall, the five drugs induced remissions in 24% (45/187) of the xenografts studied, whereas minor regressions or no change occurred in 13% of cases while 63% (117/187) of xenografts progressed on treatment. These findings are similar to the overall response rates recorded for monotherapy clinical trials with these agents. In addition, more responses (37%) were seen in a subgroup of tumors classified by the authors as clinically sensitive (small cell and non-small cell lung, breast, head and neck, leukaemia, melanoma, non-Hodgkin's lymphoma, gastric, testis) in comparison with those designated as resistant [4%; bladder, colon, cervix, central nervous system (CNS), hepatoma, mesothelioma, ovary, pancreas, prostate, renal soft tissue sarcoma].

10.4.3 Study Endpoints

The ultimate goal of cancer chemotherapy is to reduce the tumor burden to the lowest possible level without intolerable toxicity, improve survival, and quality of life. More stringent criteria than curability of experimental tumors in mice need to be assessed to determine therapeutic efficacy. Measurement of tumor burden is the easiest and most frequently used outcomes of efficacy in preclinical studies. In reality, endpoints need to be matched to type of tumor (solid, leukemia, or metastatic), context of the study, accessibility of the implantation site, type of implantation, and therapeutic class. Simplistic criteria used in mouse models do not match criteria of partial and complete responses used in clinical oncology, and they contribute to the conflicting opinions about the relevance and predictability of mouse models. Therefore, use of other metrics and evaluations of angiogenesis, immunomodulation, metastases, and detailed histopathology need to be incorporated into most study designs for preclinical testing. Despite the technical difficulty, labor-intensive nature, and expense commonly cited as limitations for detailed examinations, the utility of mouse models is improved by multiple and appropriate endpoints.

Tumor growth inhibition studies where treatment is prophylactically administered before or on the day of tumor induction are not realistic for preclinical evaluation of clinical responses. Typically, preclinical efficacy studies use tumor growth delay in which tumors are initiated by injection or surgical implantation of cells or tissue fragments and allowed to establish for a number of days prior to initiation of treatment. Solid tumors in accessible sites are amenable to a variety of metrics that are not applicable to primary and metastatic tumors of internal organs and hematologic neoplasms. Spontaneous regressions and failure of tumors to become established may account for a small percentage of false cures. For this reason, tumor onset and progression should be monitored frequently to ensure adequate and similar tumor masses prior to treatment and monitor onset of regression in each group of a sufficient number of animals. In models with log-phase tumor growth, animals can be randomized into treatment groups after a predictable period of development, usually 4–45 days. Conversely, less well-developed tumor models may require enrollment of individual animals into the study when the tumor burden reaches a minimum size. Such enrollment studies are more difficult to evaluate. Allowing extra days for tumor growth may be as misleading as starting treatment on small tumor masses that have not yet established and show enhanced regression after onset of treatment. In vivo progression of tumor burden should be evaluated on a frequent basis. Tumor size estimates (e.g., length $\times$ width^2/2) is performed with a caliper at least twice a week. Tumor response endpoint is expressed in terms of tumor growth delay (T–C value), defined as the difference in time (days) required for the treated tumors (T) to reach a predetermined target size, usually 0.5–1.0 cm^3 (Fig. 10.3), compared to those of the control group (C). This value has been suggested to mimic clinical endpoints and disease progression. Tumor cell kill

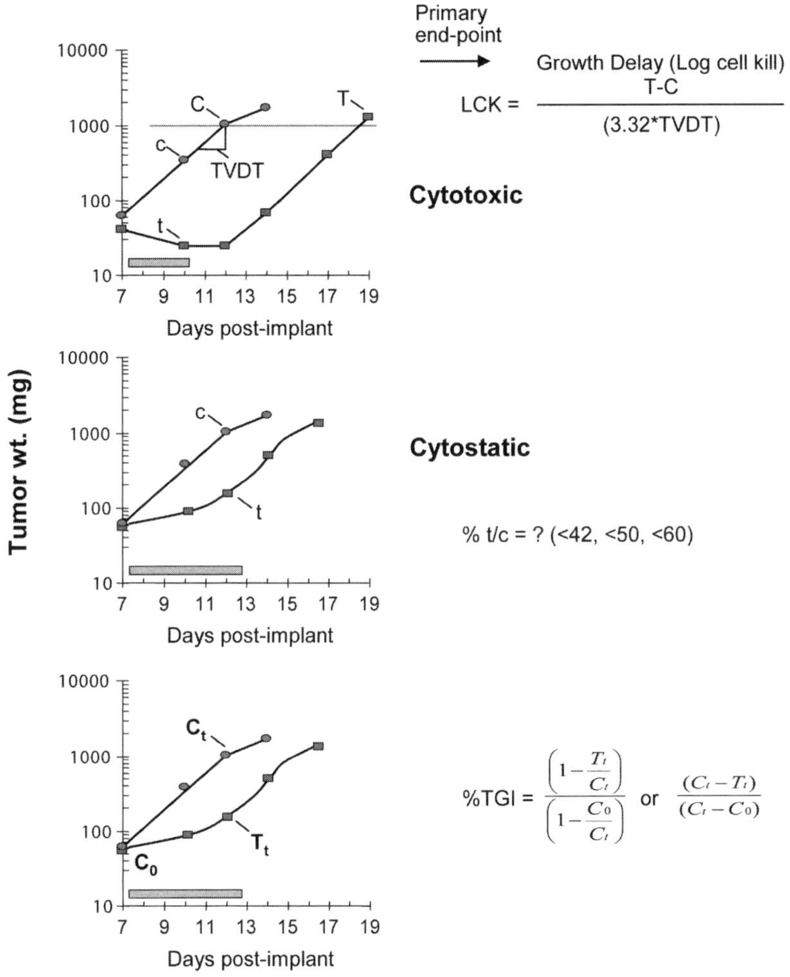

Fig. 10.3 Examples of xenograft tumor response to a cytotoxic drug (*upper panel*) and the calculations required to determine log cell kill (LCK). In the case of cytostatic drugs (*two lower panels*), the relative difference between treated and controls is smaller and a therapeutic growth index (TGI) can be calculated

(net and total) can also be estimated based on assumed exponential tumor growth kinetics as follows:

And,

$$\text{Log cell kill (LCK)} = \text{T} - \text{C} \div (3.32 \times \text{tumor volume doubling time})$$

Today, in contemporary oncological therapy, there is a far less emphasis on the development of cytotoxic agent. Instead, modern chemotherapy includes diverse approaches, with particular focus on attacking specific molecular targets where often cytostatic rather than cytotoxic effects may be predicted. Thus, a slowing of tumour growth rather than shrinkage may occur. This may require a re-evaluation of the in vivo models developed and validated using cytotoxic drugs when testing such agents. Targeted compounds are not potent to produce tumor regressions by themselves, as the tumor may be driven by multiple changes in its genetic makeup and only result in stasis or delay in tumor growth. Moreover, changes in response to the agent may only occur in a subset of models in which the target(s) of the agent is the driving force for tumor growth.

For targeted agents that induce cytostasis, tumor response is more appropriately measured in terms of relative growth inhibition and may be expressed as % t/c or more rigorously as percent tumor growth inhibition (%*TGI*) and calculated as follows:

$$\%TGI = \frac{\left(1 - \frac{Tt}{Ct}\right)}{\left(1 - \frac{C0}{Ct}\right)} \text{ or } \frac{(Ct - Tt)}{(Ct - C0)}$$

where, C_t is the median control tumor size at end of treatment, C_0, median control tumor size at treatment initiation, T_t, median tumor size of treated group at end of treatment, and T_0, median tumor size of treated group at treatment initiation.

10.5 The Value of the Xenograft Models in Contemporary Cancer Drug Discovery

In the post-genomic era, there has been a considerable move away from the "black-box" approach to phase I clinical trials where many agents of unknown mechanisms of action and poorly defined preclinical pharmacokinetics were introduced into the clinic. Does this necessarily mean that the xenograft model is of no further value in contemporary mechanism-directed cancer drug development? This may not be the case as long as care is taken to ensure the xenografts used are a faithful representation of the pathophysiology of the tumor of origin. In careful mechanism-based studies, combined with sound pharmacological principles (as described above), xenograft model remains of great value, both for assisting in the selection of leads for clinical evaluation and for guiding clinical studies (e.g., scheduling and combination strategies). Some of the other advantages are the speed of tumor development and response, as well as the easier timing of large cohorts of experimental animals for testing purposes.

Here, two examples will be given of where xenograft studies have proven invaluable in selecting candidate agents that ultimately received FDA approval in the last 2 years and, moreover, potentially guiding their clinical utility. It should be pointed out here that the number of new cancer drugs entering clinical development more than doubled between the early 1990s and the mid-2000s, from 33/year to 73/year, respectively. At the same time, patients with diseases such as breast cancer where in the past effective therapy was lacking now have multiple options and will likely receive multiple lines of therapy. Thus, the hurdle for developing a successful agent that can gain regulatory approval has been raised considerably and the competition for eligible patients for clinical trials has dramatically increased. This has adversely affected approval rate in recent years and lengthened the time taken to complete the clinical development and approval process [9]. It is thus highly advantageous, if at all possible, to define the medical need (i.e., the patient population) at the outset of a drug development program. Moreover, with the increasing move of clinical oncology practice and the regulatory process toward evidence-based approach to treatment, the ability to identify the patient population that is likely to benefit and then to develop tumor models that faithfully reflect that population is likely to be attractive to investigators and regulatory agencies. Such approaches remove much of the uncertainties regarding the predictability of the models being used to predict outcome and increase the confidence that the agent under investigation may recapitulate similar degree of activity in clinical trials.

10.6 Taxane Resistance in Breast Cancer

The first example concerns the development of ixabepilone (Ixempra) for the treatment of metastatic breast cancer in patients who have failed prior therapy, primarily taxanes. Since the antitumor activity of the taxanes was discovered in the 1990s, the rationale for using microtubule-stabilizing agents in the treatment of cancer is undisputed. Taxanes are clinically active against a wide range of tumor types and play a key role in the treatment of both primary and metastatic breast cancer. However, resistance to cytotoxic drugs (including taxanes) is common and results in reduced response rates and ultimately disease progression in up to 90% of patients with metastatic cancer. While some tumors display intrinsic resistance to chemotherapeutic drugs, and thus show no response, others are initially responsive to chemotherapy, but subsequently develop acquired resistance. Both intrinsic and acquired resistance lead to a requirement for alternative treatment options [10].

In the laboratory, a major mechanism by which tumors display resistance to commonly used agents such as taxanes and anthracyclines is through overexpression of multidrug resistance (MDR) proteins including *P*-glycoprotein (P-gp) and multidrug resistance-associated protein (MRP)-1 [11]. Overexpression of these efflux pump proteins causes retention of subtherapeutic concentrations of drug in tumor cells, which results in a lack of efficacy. In some tumors that are intrinsically resistant to chemotherapy, expression of MDR proteins reflects the constitutive expression of these proteins by the tissues from which the tumors are derived (e.g., liver and kidney). However, in tumors derived from tissue types that do not express MDR proteins physiologically, treatment with chemotherapy can induce expression of these proteins. This results in acquired resistance to the chemotherapy agent used, in addition to drugs of the same class and, on occasion, of different classes. In addition, at least two additional mechanisms of drug resistance are known to exist for taxanes, both of which are related to tubulin, the therapeutic target for the taxanes. Firstly, mutations in beta-tubulin can prevent taxanes from binding to their target. Secondly, overexpression of the beta-III tubulin isoform in preference to the beta-II isoform reduces the efficacy of taxanes, as these drugs specifically target the beta-II isoform [12]. Thus, as described above, multiple mechanisms can lead to taxane resistance in preclinical laboratory models; however, it is not at all clear which of the potential mechanisms play key roles in clinical resistance found in patients.

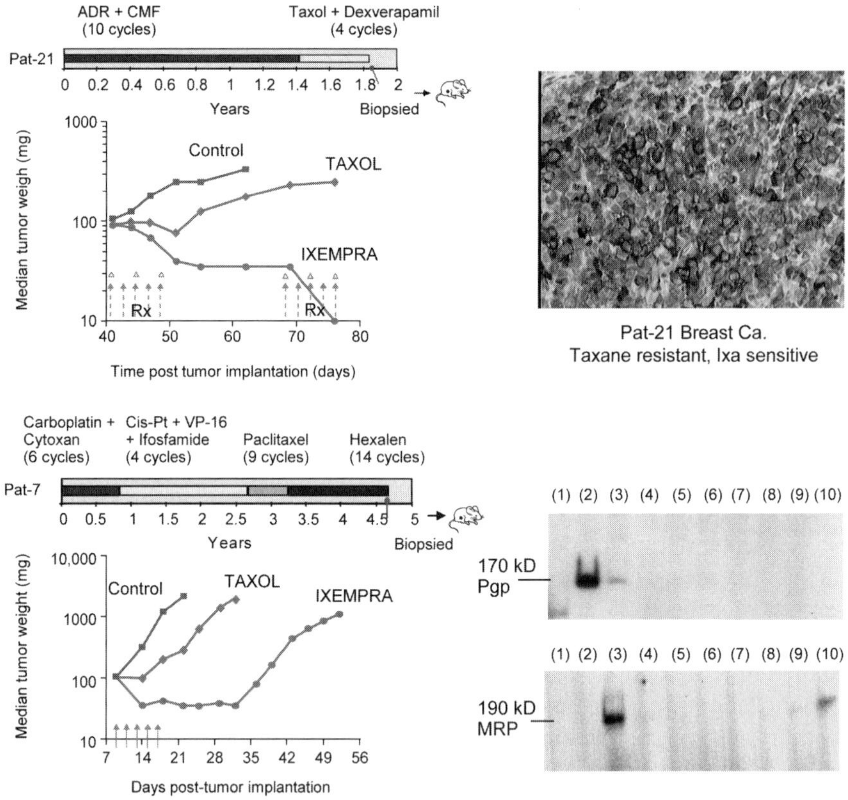

Fig. 10.4 Examples of xenografts used for development of Ixempra. The history of treatment for the tumor of Pat-21 (patient-21) and Pat-7 (patient-7) followed by biopsy and transplant to mice is shown in the bar graph. The *upper graph* shows the response in xenografts to paclitaxel or Ixempra® of Pat-21 tumors, the *lower graph* indicates the response of Pat-7 tumors. On the *right* is a stained section of the Pat-21 xenograft grown in mice (*upper panel*) and the *lower two panels* show a western blot reacted with anti-pGp (*upper*) and anti-MRP (*lower*). Lane 2 contains proteins from Pat-21 and lane 3 from Pat-7

In the early 1990s, natural epothilones, produced by the myxobacterium *Sorangium cellulosum* and their analogs, were identified and were found to have antineoplastic activities [13]. Like the taxanes, epothilones promote tumor cell death by stabilizing microtubules and inducing apoptosis. However, as macrolide antibiotics, the epothilones are structurally unrelated to taxanes and were shown to have activity against several laboratory cell models of taxane resistance. At BMS, we initiated an epothilone analog program in order to optimize the in vivo antitumor efficacy and therapeutic index of this chemical class. Over 300 semisynthetic analogs were made and tested in various in vitro and in vivo systems. From these efforts, BMS-247550 (ixabepilone), a lactam analog of epothilone B, emerged as the most efficacious epothilone in a battery of in vivo preclinical chemotherapy studies, outperforming paclitaxel in each of the paclitaxel-resistant tumor models tested. The discovery of ixabepilone with the accompanying confidence that it has good potential to overcome clinically relevant taxane resistance was tremendously helped by the availability of two early passage human xenografts obtained from a breast and ovarian cancer patient, respectively, who either was intrinsically resistant (Pat-21) or had acquired resistance to TAXOL (Fig. 10.4). These two models recapitulate the taxol resistance observed in the patients of origin, demonstrating two differing mechanisms of taxane resistance—overexpression of beta-III tubulin in Pat-21 and Pgp in Pat-7 (Fig. 10.4). These results obtained preclinically predicted the clinical activity of ixabepilone which showed, in a pivotal phase II study of ixabepilone in patients with metastatic breast cancer refractory to an anthracycline, a taxane, and capecitabine, that it possessed significant antitumor activity as a single agent in this highly drug refractory population. These data became part of the basis for which ixabepilone was approved.

10.7 Imatinib Resistance in Chronic Myeloid Leukemia

BCR–ABL, a fusion oncogene generated by a reciprocal translocation between chromosomes 9 and 12, encodes the BCR–ABL fusion protein, a constitutively active cytoplasmic tyrosine kinase present in >90% of all patients with chronic myelogenous leukemia (CML) and in 15–30% of adult patients with acute lymphoblastic leukemia (ALL). Numerous studies have demonstrated that the underlying pathophysiology of CML is the kinase activity of BCR–ABL. The clinical success of the BCR–ABL kinase inhibitor imatinib (Gleevec®) has validated its use in the management of CML. Imatinib is particularly effective in the early (chronic) phase of the disease, where the complete hematologic response (CHR) rate can be in excess of 90%. However, patients with advanced disease (accelerated phase and blast crisis) and Philadelphia chromosome-positive ALL (Ph+ ALL) have been less sensitive to imatinib. Furthermore, responses are transient, generally lasting less than 6 months and, clinical resistance to imatinib both innate and acquired, has been observed in all phases of disease, which may limit treatment benefits of imatinib in the long term. In light of these limitations of imatinib therapy in CML, and the lack of therapeutic options for patients who are refractory to, or intolerant of, imatinib treatment, a clear medical need exists for more effective therapeutic options, particularly in advanced disease and Ph+ ALL. In particular, use of agents that inhibit both BCR–ABL-dependent and BCR–ABL-independent mechanisms of imatinib resistance would be a favorable approach. The use of combinations of BCR–ABL and SRC inhibitors, or multi-targeted inhibitors of both kinases, to address these problems has been suggested in some cases assessed preclinically. However, it is necessary to gain proof-of-confidence that such an approach would result in a clinically useful agent. Here, the availability of a human CML xenograft,

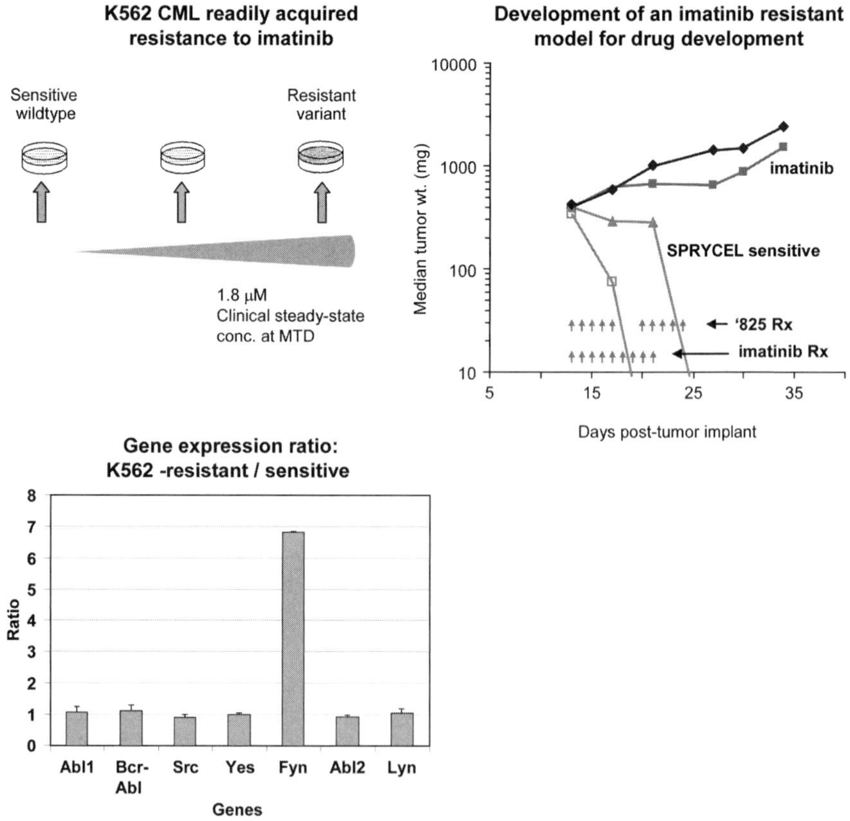

Fig. 10.5 Development of an imatinib-resistant CML cell line. By growing K562 cells in increasing imatinib concentrations (up to 1.8 μM], an imatinib-resistant cell line was generated (*upper left*). When this was grown as a xenograft and treated (*upper right*) with imatinib (*green line*), the tumors were also imatinib resistant and SPRYCEL sensitive [*orange lines*]. Quantitative PCR of Abl and Src family kinases of the resistant versus the sensitive k562 line showed (*lower left*) overexpression of Fyn

K562/IM/R, derived from the originally sensitive CML line K562, with acquired resistance to imatinib through activation of FYN, a SRC family kinase, proved high valuable. SRC family kinase activation is known to be a frequent finding in patients in the blast phase of CML that does not respond well to imatinib. Thus, the demonstration that dasatinib (Sprycel®) is completely effective in inhibiting the growth of the resistant human tumor xenografts in mice, causing cures in some instances (Fig. 10.5), provided high confidence of its clinical utility and set the stage for its candidacy for clinical development.

10.8 Summary

In cancer drug discovery, perhaps more than in any other therapeutic areas, the transition from in vitro to animal models and then to clinical evaluation of a candidate anticancer agent is thwart with difficulties. Often the unavailability of animal cancer models that is predictive of the tumor types that the agent is intended to treat results in disappointing clinical outcome in human trial and a low rate of success for marketing approval. In this chapter, we argued and provided examples that human tumor xenografts in its various guises should remain the cornerstone of any in vivo drug evaluation program, so long as careful attention is paid to select the "right" xenograft for the drug target that the experimental agent is proposed to treat. Human tumor xenograft is particularly invaluable in settings where it is necessary to obtain in vivo "proof of principle" for a particular target as well as in optimizing the in vivo activity of pharmaceutically tractable chemotypes. Lastly, human tumor xenograft that faithfully represents the pathophysiology of its origin, when available, can provide invaluable information regarding the PK–PD relationship of the drug-target effects and therefore will assist greatly the logistics and speed of the clinical development of a candidate anticancer agent.

References

1. http://www.cancer.org/docroot/PRO/content/PRO_1_1_Cancer_Statistics_2006_Presentation.asp.
2. Kola, I. and J. Landis (2004). "Can the pharmaceutical industry reduce attrition rates?" *Nature Reviews. Drug Discovery* **3**(8): 711–716.
3. Bourne, D. and L. Dittert (1995). Pharmacokinetics. *Modern Pharmaceutics*. G. Banker and C. Rhodes. New York, NY, Marcel Dekker.
4. Double, J. A. and M. C. Bibby (1989). "Therapeutic index: A vital component in selection of anticancer agents for clinical trial." *Journal of the National Cancer Institute* **81**(13): 988–994.
5. Hann, B. and A. Balmain (2001). "Building 'validated' mouse models of human cancer." *Current Opinion in Cell Biology* **13**(6): 778–784.
6. Corbett, T. H., L. Polin, et al. (2002). Transplantable syngeneic rodent tumors: solid tumors in mice. *Tumor Models in Cancer Research*,. T. B. A. Totowa, NJ., Humana Press.

7. Averbook, B. J., J. L. Schuh, et al. (2002). "Antitumor Effects of Flt3 Ligand in Transplanted Murine Tumor Models." *Journal of Immunotherapy* **25**: 27–35.
8. Fiebig, H. and A. Burger (2002). Human tumor xenografts and explants. *Tumor Models in Cancer Research*. B. A. Teicher. Totowa, NY, Humana Press Inc: 113–137.
9. Kaitin, K. (Ed.) (2007). "Despite more cancer drugs in R&D, overall U.S. approval rate is 8%." *Tufts Center for the Study of Drug Development Impact Report* **9**(5).
10. Longley, D. and P. Johnston (2005). "Molecular mechanisms of drug resistance." *Journal of Pathology* **205**: 275–92.
11. Leonessa, F. and R. Clarke (2003). "ATP binding cassette transporters and drug resistance in breast cancer." *Endocrine-Related Cancer* **10**(1): 43–73.
12. Jordan, M., H. Miller, et al. (2006). "The Pat-21 breast cancer model derived from a patient with primary Taxol® resistance recapitulates the phenotype of its origin, has altered beta-tubulin expression and is sensitive to ixabepilone." *Proceedings of the American Association for Cancer Research* 97th Annual Meeting: LB-280.
13. Höfle, G., N. Bedorf, et al. (1996). "Epothilone A and B – novel 16-membered macrolides and cytotoxic activity: Isolation, crystal structure, and conformation in solution." *Angewandte Chemie* (*International ed. in English*) **35**: 1567–1569.
14. Sawyers, C. L. (1999). "Chronic myeloid leukemia." *N Engl J Med* **340**: 1330–1340.

Chapter 11
DGL Global Strategies in DNA Microarray Gene Expression Analysis and Data Mining for Human Blood Cancers

Dongguang Li

Contents

11.1 Introduction

Computation is required to extract meaningful information from the large amount of data generated by gene expression profiling [1, 2, 3]. Most of the algorithms commonly applied to microarray data analysis have been correlation-based approaches named cluster analysis [4]. For example, an efficient two-way clustering algorithm was applied to a colon cancer data set consisting of the expression patterns of different cell types. Gene expression in 40 tumour and 22 normal colon tissue samples was analysed across 2000 genes [4]. Cluster

D. Li
School of Computer and Information Science, Faculty of Computing, Health and Science, Edith Cowan University, Mount Lawley, WA 6050, Australia
d.li@ecu.edu.au

S. Li (ed.), *Mouse Models of Human Blood Cancers*,
DOI: 10.1007/978-0-387-69132-9_11, © Springer Science+Business Media, LLC 2008

analysis groups the genes involved in microarray data. Those clustered genes are likely to be functionally linked and need to be looked into closely. Although cluster analysis has widely been accepted in analysing the patterns of gene expression, the methods developed may not be able to fully extract the information from the microarray data corrupted by high-dimensional noise. If the noise from the genes that are irrelevant is not sufficiently reduced, incorrect classification for samples or misleading information on selecting informative genes may result. For selecting informative genes for sample classification, a neighbourhood analysis method was developed to obtain a subset of genes that discriminate between the acute lymphoblastic leukaemia (ALL) and the acute myeloid leukaemia (AML) successfully [5]. In the microarray data set containing 7129 genes, those genes whose expression levels differ significantly in ALL and AML were identified and then they were subsequently used to predict the class membership (either ALL or AML) of new leukaemia cases. Both approaches described above [4, 5] were focused on comparing samples in each single gene dimension and assumed that the relevant genes were similarly and uniformly expressed among samples of each type. To overcome these defects, a multi-variate approach that compares samples in a multi-gene dimension using the genetic algorithms (GAs) was proposed [6]. Samples were classified based on the class membership of their k-nearest neighbours (KNN) in the gene space. The dimensionality (length) of the gene subset was arbitrarily set to 50. GA was used to select hundreds and thousands of subsets of 50 genes that could potentially discriminate between two classes of samples (tumour and normal tissues). The frequency with which genes were selected was statistically analysed in the large number of 50-dimension gene subsets. The most frequently selected 50 genes were used to predict 34 new samples. Although the performance of GA predictor with 50 genes was remarkable, only 29 of 34 test samples were correctly predicted with high confidence [7]. To improve the successful rate of classification, more reliable and accurate algorithms are needed.

During the past five decades, the field of the global optimisation has been growing at a rapid pace and many new theoretical, algorithmic, and computational contributions have resulted [8]. Global optimisation is concerned with the computation and characterisation of global minima (or maxima) of nonlinear functions. Global optimisation problems are widespread in the mathematical modelling of real world systems for a very broad range of applications. The majority of problems can be described as some form of global optimisation procedures. In the gene selection problem, one would need to find how to form gene subsets to obtain the optimum classification response – changing one gene element in a given subset may improve the classification performance of the subset at one testing sample, but worsen it at another.

An objective function is necessary to evaluate how close each gene subset gets to the target requirement. The gene selecting process involves finding the gene subset that corresponds to the minimum (or maximum) of the objective function. Plotting the objective function against the gene search space of each element gene in the gene subset, one axis per element gene would be needed, plus the orthogonal axis for the objective function. The objective function plot would appear as a multi-peak, multi-variable plot. Because there are an enormous number of inter-related possible gene combinations, the best gene subset cannot be found by any simple process. It is not obvious how to select the genes analytically to find the best solution. The methods currently used in gene selection, such as the clustering, neighbourhoods analysis, and GAs, almost all depend on a starting condition either selected by the user or generated internally by the program that is sometimes not obvious. Changing the initial conditions will give a different result, and one has no way of knowing how much improvement could be effected.

Currently available multi-variable optimisation algorithms for selecting the gene subset may not give optimum solutions. Usually, those algorithms obtain their final solutions either from optimising a starting guess or by techniques, which may or may not involve a pseudo-random process that gives different answers every time, depending upon the initial conditions. A true global optimisation algorithm should always find the very best solution possible within the boundary conditions stipulated. The possibility of creating a true global optimisation algorithm for a large number of inter-dependent variables has been preposed in this study. Although many optimisation algorithms may be appropriate for the gene classification problem, DGL (DGL is the abbreviation for Dongguang Li) global optimisation was proposed and applied to the cancer classification in this study for its superb performance in theory and applications.

Some of strategies of DGL global optimisation were firstly successfully applied to the optical thin film design problem [9]. It was also a candidate for the real function test bed of the First International Contest on Evolutionary Optimisation in order to solve 10 hard mathematical multi-variable optimisation problems [10]. It is of great interest to develop techniques for extracting useful information from the microarray data sets. In this chapter, I report the application of the DGL global optimisation approach for classifying and validating two well-known data sets [4, 5] consisting of the expression patterns of different cell types.

In previous years, many clinicians have been unable to provide a clear cut classification of cancerous patients, based upon the biopsy. However, with the system proposed here, the surveying of the expression of thousands of genes is made practical.

This chapter is concerned with the challenge of mining knowledge from DNA microarray expression data. With the objective to discover unknown patterns from microarray data, methodologies are derived from machine learning, artificial intelligence, and statistics. Nowadays, microarray expression data accumulate at an alarming speed in various storage devices, and so does valuable information. However, it is difficult to understand information hidden in data without the aid of data analysis techniques. Both the machine learning and the data mining have been applied to the field in order to better understand the microarray expression data sets. A data mining system usually enables one to collect, store, access, process, and ultimately describe and visualise data sets.

The discussion of data collection and storage is not included here though it is important for mining microarray expression data. In particularly, data mining has successfully provided solutions for finding information from data in many medical research fields such as bioinformatics and pharmaceuticals. Many important problems have been addressed by data mining methods, such as neural networks, fuzzy logic, decision trees, GAs, and statistical methods. Data mining tasks can be descriptive and predictive. In other words, it is an inter-disciplinary field with a general goal of predicting outcomes and uncovering relationships in data [11, 12, 13, 14].

Microarray data analysis is one of the most attractive fields of data mining. With the help of gene expressions obtained from microarray technology, heterogeneous cancers can be classified into appropriate subtypes [15]. Many different kinds of machine learning and statistical methods have recently been applied to analyse gene expression data [16, 17, 18, 19]. Data mining tasks normally include data pre-processing, data modelling, and knowledge description. One more example application to classify the publicly available data on leukaemia has also been described in detail to take the advantages of data mining.

11.2 Microarray Gene Expression and Experimental Design

DNA microarrays, also called gene arrays or gene chips, usually consist of thin glass or nylon substrates containing specific DNA gene samples spotted in an array by a robotic printing device [20]. Researchers spread fluorescently labelled m-RNA from an experimental condition onto the DNA gene samples in the array. This m-RNA bins strongly with some DNA gene samples and weakly with others, depending on the inherent double helical characteristics. A laser scans the array and sensors detect the fluorescence levels (using red and green dyes), indicating the strength with which the sample expresses each gene. The logarithmic ratio between the two intensities of each dye is used as the gene expression data. The relative abundance of the spotted DNA sequences in a pair of DNA or RNA samples is assessed by evaluating the differential hybridisation of the two samples to the sequences on the array. Gene expression levels can be determined for samples taken at multiple time instants of a biological process or under various conditions. Each gene corresponds to a high-dimensional row vector of its expression profile [21]. The fundamental goal of microarray experiments is to identify genes that are differentially expressed in the conditions being studied [22].

11.2.1 Fold Change Analysis

Fold change is defined as follows:

Take log2 transformed normalised intensities from robust multi-chip averaging (RMA) for two samples;

Let a = log2 (intensity sample 1)
b = log2 (intensity sample 2)
If $a > b$: fold change = 2 (| a–b |)
If $a <$ b: fold change = –2 (| a–b |)
If $a = b$: fold change = 0

The pre-processing of gene expression profile is often necessary to reach the goal of converting from raw data to biological significance. The following steps are common:

- normalising the hybridisation intensities within a single array experiment;
- transforming the data using a nonlinear function, like the logarithm in case of expression ratios;
- estimating and replacing missing values in expressions or adapting existing algorithms to handle missing values;
- filtering gene expression profile to eliminate those that do not satisfy some simple criteria;
- standardising or rescaling the profiles to generate vectors of length one.

Mouse 430 v2 Affymetrix GeneChip® arrays are used for all experiments. Probe intensity data as CEL files are imported into the R software environment (http://www.R-project.org). Probe level data quality is assessed using image reconstruction, histograms of raw signal intensities, and MA plots. Normalisation is performed for each batch separately using the robust multi-chip average (affy/RMA, http://www.bioconductor.org) method using all probe intensity data sets together to form one expression measure per probe set per array. Fold change analysis is conducted for each pair of comparisons as listed above.

11.2.2 Classification and Clustering – Molecular Classification of Leukaemia

Since the fold change does not address the reproducibility of the observed difference and cannot be used to determine the statistical significance, raw data are rarely of direct benefit. Its true value is predicated on the ability to extract information useful for decision support or exploration and understanding the phenomenon governing the data source. In the microarray domain, data analysis was traditionally a manual process. One or more analyst(s) would become intimately familiar with the data and, with the help of statistical techniques, provide summaries and generate reports. However, such an approach rapidly broke down as the size of data grew and the number of dimensions increased. When the scale of data manipulation and exploration goes beyond human capacities, people need the aid of computing technologies for automating the process. All these have prompted the need for intelligent data analysis methodologies, which could discover useful knowledge from data.

Classification is also described as supervised learning [23]. Classification and clustering are two data mining tasks with close relationships. A class is a set of data samples with some similarity or relationship, and all samples in this class are assigned the same class label to distinguish them from samples in other classes. A cluster is a collection of objects that are similar locally. Clusters are usually generated in order to further classify objects into relatively larger and meaningful categories. Clustering is also called unsupervised classification, where no predefined classes are assigned [23]. According to a data set with class labels, data analysis builds classifiers as predictors for future unknown objects. A classification model is formed first based on available data. Future trends are predicted using the learned model. In the following case, the data sets used are from a public microarray database and the samples are collected to build a model that can be used to classify new samples into categories of ALL or AML for leukaemia.

Classification of acute leukaemia, having highly similar appearance in gene expression data, has been made by combining a pair of classifiers trained with mutually exclusive features [24]. Gene expression profiles were constructed from 71 patients having ALL or AML, each constituting one sample of the DNA microarray. Each pattern consists of 7129 gene expressions. Feature selection was employed to generate 25 top-ranked genes for the experiment. In the following sections, a case study from theory to practice is presented in detail.

11.3 Genetic Algorithms

GAs is motivated by the natural evolutionary process. Most of classification with artificial intelligence uses GAs as core algorithms. Solutions of the problem at hand are encoded in chromosomes or individuals. An initial population of individuals is generated at random or heuristically. The operators in GAs include selection, crossover, and mutation. To generate a new generation, chromosomes are selected according to their fitness score. The selection operator gives preference to better individuals as parents for the next generation. The crossover operator and the mutation operator are used to generate offspring from the parents. A crossover site is randomly chosen in the parents. The mutation operator is used to prevent premature convergence to local optima [25]. The basic concept in GAs is to introduce effective parallel searching in the high-dimensional problem space.

To solve the problem of mining microarray expression data, GAs are especially useful for the following reasons:

- the problem space is large and complex;
- prior knowledge is scarce;
- it is difficult to determine a machine learning model to solve the problem due to complexities in constraints and objectives;
- traditional search methods, such as stochastic, combinatorial, and classical so-called hard optimisation-based techniques, perform badly.

11.4 DGL Global Optimisation Algorithms

Although GAs is popular and useful, many problems at hand cannot be resolved easily and accurately. This section combines a powerful algorithm, called DGL global optimisation [26], with the methods of cancer diagnosis through gene selection and microarray analysis. A generic approach to cancer classification based on gene expression monitoring by DNA microarrays is proposed and applied to a test leukaemia case.

By using the orthogonal arrays (OAs) for sampling and a search space reduction process, a computer program has been written that can operate on a personal laptop computer. The leukaemia microarray data can be classified 100% correctly without previous knowledge of their classes.

11.4.1 Leukeamia Data

The original data were downloaded from the web (http://www.broad.mit.edu/cgi-bin/cancer/datasets.cgi). The data contain the expression levels of 7129 genes across the 72 samples, of which 47 are the ALL samples and 25 the AML samples. These data sets contain measurements corresponding to ALL and AML samples from bone marrow and peripheral blood that is divided into a training set (38 samples) and a test set (34 samples).

11.4.2 Overall Methodology

The proposed DGL global optimisation method in this study includes following major steps:

- sampling within search spaces by using a suitable OA instead of conducting a random search
- constructing objective function for optimisation algorithms;
- searching spaces reduction strategies;
- searching for global optimal solutions;
- building up a multi-subsets pyramidal hierarchy class predictor for classification;
- predicting through a voting mechanism.

11.4.3 Orthogonal Arrays and Sampling Procedure

The OA used in this research is L242(1123) that is too large to be shown here. The OA L242(1123) has 242 rows (observations or tests), 23 columns (factors or variables), and 11 levels for each factor. The complete L242(1123) is available on the website http://www.scis.ecu.edu.au/dli/. The L242(1123) was initially used in selecting a gene subset with 23 gene elements. The search space of 2000 genes in the colon data was divided into 11levels equally. If all the genes are assigned a unique ID number from 1 to 2000 and the initial search space ranges from 1 to 2000, then the selected gene IDs are 1, 200, 400, 600, 800, 1000, 1200, 1400, 1600, 1800, and 2000. As the first row of L242(1123) reads (1, 10, 2, 3, 8, 8, 2, 4, 8, 9, 5, 4, 10, 5, 7, 1, 5, 5, 8, 1, 10, 11, 2), the constructed gene subset will read (1, 1800, 200, 400, 1400, 1400, 200, 600, 1400, 1600, 800, 600, 1800, 800, 1200, 1, 800, 800, 1400, 1, 1800, 2000, 200). Since the duplicated gene IDs are not allowed in a gene subset, those repeated gene IDs are shifted forwards or backwards a little. The modified 23-gene subset now reads (1, 1800, 200, 400, 1400, 1399, 199, 600, 1401, 1600, 800, 599, 1799, 799, 1199, 2, 801, 798, 1401, 3, 1798, 2000, 201). According to the L242(1123), 242 different 23-gene subsets were created and evaluated with the defined objective function. All the 242 subsets were ranked based on their values of objective function. Ten percent of top performers in classifying the training set were kept, and those gene IDs included in the top 10% gene subsets were ranked in order to work out the minimum ID and the maximum ID. The new and reduced search space ranged from the minimum ID to the maximum ID. The above process was repeated until the search space was small enough (e.g. less than 11 genes left) or the objective function could not be improved any further. The rank no.1gene subset in the last round of optimisation was chosen as the optimal solution for the 23-gene subsets. The optimisation was run 23 times with different lengths (23, 22, ..., 2, 1) of gene subsets at each run. Total of 23 optimal solutions were obtained. All the 23 optimal solutions constructed a multi-subset cancer class predictor and then were used to classify the samples in the test data set. All the 23 gene subsets were arranged to form a pyramidal layer-by-layer hierarchy with the shortest subset (1gene) on the top and the longest subset (23 genes) in the bottom (see Table 11.2 for details).

11.4.4 Objective Function

An objective function is also called a fitness or merit function, which is a measure of the ability for a selected gene subset to classify the training set samples according to the DGL optimisation procedure. There are several ways, such as neighbourhood analysis [5], support vector machines [27, 28], and KNN [6], to construct an objective function for the optimisation and gene selection algorithms. Among them, KNN is used for the proposed DGL global optimisation because it is easy to compute. The Euclidean distance between a single sample (represented by its pattern vector *Vm*) and each of the pattern vectors of the training set containing *M* samples is calculated: $Vm = (g1, g2, \ldots, gn)$, where *n* is the number of genes in the vector that can be set to from 1 to 23 in order to form the gene vectors (or subsets) with different lengths, *gn* is the expression level of the *n*th gene in the *m*th sample, $m = 1, 2, \ldots, M$. For

Table 11.1 k-nearest neighbour (KNN) rules (k = 5)

Among the ranked 5 nearest neighbours	Classification	Class code
All 5 are ALL samples	ALL	1
All 5 are AML samples	AML	–1
4 are ALL and 1 is AML	ALL	1
4 are AML and 1 is ALL	AML	–1
3 are ALL and 2 are AML	Unknown	0

the leukaemia data set $M = 40$, each sample is classified according to the class membership of its KNNs as determined by the Euclidean distance in n-dimensional space. If all or majority of the KNNs of a sample belongs to the same class, the sample is classified as that class. Otherwise, the sample is considered unclassifiable. The k was arbitrarily set to 5 in this study. The detailed rules are shown in Table 11.1.

If the class membership of a training set sample and its five nearest neighbours in the particular n-dimensional space defined by a gene subset agree or four out of five nearest neighbours agree, the sample is classified and a score of 1 is assigned to that sample. These agreement scores are summed across the training set. For convenience, this sum is divided by the number of training samples as the value of the objective function for the selected gene subset. The bigger the value is, the better the selected gene subset performs in classification. A maximal objective function value is 1, which means all the samples in the training set is classified correctly by the gene subset under testing. The goal of the optimisation procedure is to discover the optimal gene subset (optimal solution) with the maximal value of the objective function. As in other methods, an objective function is calculated for each subset of genes by the sum over all classifying scores of the samples in the training data set. The optimisation process then conducts the searching for the gene subset that has the best objective function value (minima or maxima). Therefore, by finding the lowest or highest value of the objective function, one will have the best performing gene subset discovered. This procedure can be made more sophisticated by introducing weighting factors to increase the importance of user-specified samples in training sets, as well as using other forms of the distance formula between one subset and another.

11.4.5 Search Spaces Reduction for Global Search

With local optimisation (a fast method for a large number of genes), the program finds the nearest minimum and stops. For some so-called global optimisation procedures, the algorithm not only finds a local minimum but can also find some neighbouring minima. The processes, however, is a hit and miss situation, because starting at a different place can result in different solutions. The global algorithm in DGL repeatedly narrows the region where the global minimum is known to lie by using a special OA's sampling that operates simultaneously in all orthogonal dimensions, one for each gene in the gene subset to find the optimum solution. As the process runs, one can observe the range of genes for each gene variable in an n-dimensional subset being reduced.

11.4.6 Mathematical Form of DGL Optimisation

Consider a multi-dimensional continuous function $f(x)$ with multiple global minima and local minima on subset G of Rn

(i) A local minima is defined as follows

For a given point $x^* \in G$, if there exists a δ-neighbourhood of x^*, $O(x^*, \delta)$, such that for
$x \in O(x^*, \delta)$,

and $f(x^*) \leq f(x)$ (1)

then x^* is called a local minimal point of $f(x)$.

(ii) Definition of global minima:

If for every $x \in$ G the inequality (1) is correct, then x^* is called a global minimum of $f(x)$ on G, and the global minima of $f(x)$ on G form a global minimum set.

(iii) How to find the global minima:

Now for a given constant $C0$ such that the level set

$H0 = \{x|f(x) < C0, x \in G\}$ is nonempty,

if $\mu(H0) = 0$, where μ is the Lebesque measure of $H0$, then $C0$ is the minimum of $f(x)$ and $H0$ is the global minimum set.
Otherwise, assume that $\mu(H0) > 0$ and $C1$ is the mean value of $f(x)$ on $H0$.

$$\text{Then } C1 = 1/\mu(H0) \int_{Ho} f(x)d\mu \qquad (2)$$

and

$$C0 \geq C1 \geq f(x^*) \qquad (3)$$

One then gradually constructs the level set Hk and mean value $Ck+1$ of $f(x)$ on Hk as follows:

$$Hk = \{x|f(x) < Ck, x \in G\} \qquad (4)$$

and

$$Ck+1 = 1/\mu(Hk) \int_{Hk} f(x)d\mu \qquad (5)$$

With the assistance of OA's sampling, a decreasing sequence of mean values $\{Ck\}$ and a sequence of level sets $\{Hk\}$ are obtained.

Let $$\lim_{k\to\infty} Ck = C^* \tag{6}$$
and
$$\lim_{k\to\infty} Hk = H^* \tag{7}$$

It can be proved that C^* is the minimum of $f(x)$ on G, and H^* is the global minimum set. There are several strategies to avoid missing the global optimum when seeking the minimum solution. Among these, the most important step is to select or design a suitable OA with which the function within domains can be repeatedly sampled. The algorithm is automatically constrained to stay within the function domain and will not request function evaluations outside this domain.

There are two stopping criteria possible, either when the target objective function value is reached or when the maximum domain length is smaller than the user selected value. In this research, one uses the latter stop criteria, corresponding to the variation possible for each gene element in the subset – which can be as little as one gene. This means that the global minimum has been found for a particular gene selection range of each gene element, with a variation of less than one gene for each gene element. Strictly speaking then, the global optimum is not defined at a point but as lying within a region.

11.4.7 Multi-Subsets Class Predictor

Although DGL optimisation will result in an optimal gene subset with a given length, the classification performance varies. It seems that for both the colon and the leukaemia data sets, there is no guarantee to name a single gene subset that is capable of classifying all the samples in the testing set correctly. It is observed that the gene subsets with different lengths tend to misclassify or un-classify the different samples in the testing data sets. In another words, the gene subsets with the same length will always misclassify a few same samples in the testing data sets although those are all the optimal subsets identified by optimisation procedures. This fact indicates that the key factor to improve the signal to noise ratio in classifying the very noisy data, such as the microarray gene expressions, is the length of the gene subset. Based on the above observation, a multi-subsets class predictor was constructed for classification by using all the 23 optimal gene subsets with the lengths from 1 to 23 genes. The maximal number of genes involved in the predictor is 276 in total. As some of genes may appear more than one time, the actual number of the unique gene IDs is a bit less and varies from case to case.

11.4.8 Validation (Predicting Through a Voting Mechanism)

The established multi-subsets class predictor is validated with the testing data sets for both the colon and the leukaemia data. Each gene subset in the predictor predicts the class of every sample in the testing data sets independently according to the same KNN rules ($k = 5$) used in the training stage. The predicted class code (in leukaemia data: 1 for ALL, –1 for AML, and 0 for unknown) is assigned to the particular sample accordingly. Each single class code is treated as a single vote. For each sample in the testing data sets, up to 23 votes contributed by 23 gene subsets in the predictor can be obtained. The final class predicted by the predictor depends on the sign of the sum of the 23 votes of the sample under test. A positive sign indicates that there are more gene subsets in the predictor vote for class 1, and the sample is finally classified as 1 by the multi-subsets predictor. A negative sign indicates that there are more gene subsets in the predictor vote for class –1, and the sample is finally classified as –1 by the multi-subsets predictor. When the sum is zero, there are equal numbers of gene subsets among the 23 gene subsets for the class 1 and the class –1. In this case, the corresponding sample should be classified as 0 (unknown or unclassified). It is not difficult to interpret the actual values of the classification results. The absolute value of the sum of the 23 votes should indicate the predicting strength. The larger the value is, the more confident the prediction is.

11.4.9 Experimental Results

A Microsoft Windows based computer program with a user-friendly graphic interface has been written. The entire experimental computation was carried out on a personal laptop computer (1.7 GHz Intel Pentium Pro/II/III). The software can be downloaded from the supporting website of this chapter [29] and is available free to researchers. Both the colon cancer and the leukaemia samples were classified 100% correctly. The classification processes are automated after the gene expression data being inputted. It can find the global optimum solutions and construct a multi-subsets class predictor containing up to 23 gene subsets based on a given microarray gene expression data collection, such as the colon or leukaemia data, within a period of several hours.

For the convenience of computation, every gene was assigned a unique integer ID number, from 1 to 7129, according to the order in their original data sets. The aim was to study how changes in the choices of various gene element variables for a gene subset with a given length affect a response variable (success rate in classifying training samples). For each of the gene elements that are used to form a gene subset, 11 choices (levels) were selected for inclusion in the OA's sampling based on L242(1123). Those eleven choices of gene IDs were generated by the formula (the length of the current search space divided by 10) at an equal distance. Some shifting on the selected gene IDs was necessary to

Table 11.2 Optimal gene subsets and selected genes for the leukaemia data class predictor

Gene subsets	Gene IDs																						
1-gene-subset	5501																						
2-gene-subset	3320	1068																					
3-gene-subset	2020	4782	2348																				
4-gene-subset	4270	2039	4050	2642																			
5-gene-subset	2642	1837	4050	1488	5605																		
6-gene-subset	3137	2642	3336	2368	2852	4050																	
7-gene-subset	2020	1725	2531	2096	4991	2348	2120																
8-gene-subset	2642	4492	307	6368	3753	4708	5655	4050															
9-gene-subset	1481	4991	2224	2642	109	4050	5094	3565	6441														
10-gene-subset	2619	3119	3056	2971	4339	5297	2861	2020	5247	2001													
11-gene-subset	1584	4023	2020	1506	2852	4459	1060	6467	2295	2348	2483												
12-gene-subset	6910	4669	2642	6939	1891	4050	2020	4916	6487	1442	4950	2128											
13-gene-subset	1934	3906	3010	3392	5906	7129	4453	4724	4961	2280	2642	1	4050										
14-gene-subset	1362	2642	6771	4050	2090	6681	2811	988	4574	4727	5673	3191	1427	3565									
15-gene-subset	2020	1853	501	1387	4414	3565	3056	1630	6243	1143	2342	5251	4139	4720	1834								
16-gene-subset	4751	6438	3414	4224	5949	4889	1056	6559	2642	2648	5210	5166	1	4050	3888	5134							
17-gene-subset	7129	1834	4640	3189	6872	3118	2433	4050	1740	5326	4768	2469	6042	1	4444	2642	4252						
18-gene-subset	5828	442	3299	6548	2400	2378	3525	5452	4127	2642	5770	5342	6319	1945	4050	2780	6136	4464					
19-gene-subset	714	1714	5912	4711	3839	3215	2506	2642	3804	1900	5299	5609	4050	1	6655	6372	2791	1211	3068				
20-gene-subset	3515	7129	3854	6762	5826	4050	1250	2416	1021	3322	5451	5508	4410	2642	2327	4037	6639	4278	4334	5745			
21-gene-subset	92	6833	2642	1385	1801	3102	4251	4050	6832	5651	2449	4189	1925	5826	301	1126	3034	6940	1594	3342	5384		
22-gene-subset	5064	5692	6034	4050	6435	2642	628	501	4960	4908	5882	2227	3565	3998	2004	4723	7021	1	2829	1513	3423	3642	
23-gene-subset	7129	5477	714	4534	4572	643	3066	4991	2327	1229	4050	1425	1	4634	3565	6416	4452	3149	1250	4063	3026	2642	3780

Table 11.3 Validation of the leukaemia data with the multi-subset class predictor

	Prediction of 34 test samples (no. 39–72)																																		Results of Classification			
Gene subsets	39	40	41	42	43	44	45	46	47	48	49	50	51	52	53	54	55	56	57	58	59	60	61	62	63	64	65	66	67	68	69	70	71	72	Correct	Incorrect	Unknown	Success rate %
1-gene subset	+1	0	+1	0	+1	+1	+1	+1	+1	+1	+1	0	0	−1	0	0	0	+1	0	−1	+1	0	0	0	0	+1	−1	0	+1	+1	+1	0	0	+1	18	2	14	52.9
2-gene subset	+1	+1	+1	+1	+1	+1	+1	+1	+1	+1	+1	−1	−1	+1	−1	0	+1	+1	0	−1	+1	+1	+1	+1	−1	−1	−1	+1	+1	+1	+1	+1	+1	+1	27	5	2	79.4
3-gene subset	+1	+1	+1	−1	+1	+1	+1	+1	+1	+1	+1	−1	−1	+1	−1	−1	+1	+1	0	−1	+1	+1	0	0	0	−1	+1	+1	+1	+1	+1	+1	+1	+1	25	5	4	73.5
4-gene subset	+1	0	+1	+1	+1	+1	+1	+1	+1	+1	+1	−1	−1	−1	−1	−1	0	+1	−1	−1	+1	−1	−1	0	−1	−1	−1	−1	+1	+1	+1	+1	+1	+1	31	0	3	91.2
5-gene subset	+1	0	+1	+1	+1	+1	+1	+1	+1	+1	+1	−1	−1	−1	−1	−1	0	+1	−1	−1	+1	−1	−1	0	−1	−1	−1	−1	+1	+1	+1	+1	+1	+1	31	0	3	91.2
6-gene subset	+1	−1	+1	+1	+1	+1	+1	+1	+1	+1	+1	−1	−1	−1	−1	−1	0	+1	−1	−1	0	−1	−1	−1	−1	−1	−1	−1	0	+1	+1	+1	+1	+1	30	1	3	88.2
7-gene subset	+1	+1	+1	0	+1	+1	+1	+1	+1	+1	+1	−1	−1	+1	−1	−1	+1	+1	−1	−1	+1	+1	0	0	−1	−1	+1	+1	+1	+1	+1	+1	+1	+1	27	4	3	79.4
8-gene subset	+1	+1	+1	+1	+1	+1	+1	+1	+1	+1	+1	−1	−1	+1	−1	−1	+1	+1	0	−1	+1	+1	−1	−1	−1	−1	−1	+1	+1	0	+1	+1	+1	+1	29	3	2	85.3
9-gene subset	+1	0	+1	+1	+1	+1	+1	+1	+1	+1	+1	−1	−1	−1	−1	−1	0	+1	−1	−1	+1	−1	−1	0	−1	−1	−1	−1	+1	+1	+1	+1	+1	+1	31	0	3	91.2
10-gene subset	+1	+1	+1	0	+1	+1	+1	+1	+1	+1	+1	−1	−1	+1	−1	+1	+1	+1	+1	−1	+1	+1	+1	0	+1	−1	+1	+1	+1	+1	+1	+1	+1	+1	24	8	2	70.6
11-gene subset	+1	+1	+1	−1	+1	+1	+1	+1	+1	+1	+1	−1	−1	+1	−1	−1	+1	+1	0	−1	+1	+1	0	+1	−1	−1	+1	+1	+1	+1	+1	+1	+1	+1	26	6	2	76.4
12-gene subset	+1	+1	+1	+1	+1	+1	+1	+1	+1	+1	+1	−1	−1	−1	−1	−1	0	+1	−1	−1	+1	−1	−1	0	−1	−1	−1	−1	+1	+1	+1	+1	+1	+1	32	0	2	94.1
13-gene subset	+1	0	+1	+1	+1	+1	+1	+1	+1	+1	+1	−1	−1	−1	——1	−1	0	+1	−1	−1	+1	−1	−1	0	−1	−1	−1	−1	+1	+1	+1	+1	+1	+1	31	0	3	91.2
14-gene subset	+1	0	+1	+1	+1	+1	+1	+1	+1	+1	+1	−1	−1	−1	−1	−1	0	+1	−1	−1	+1	−1	−1	0	−1	−1	−1	−1	+1	+1	+1	+1	+1	+1	31	0	3	91.2
15-gene subset	+1	+1	+1	0	+1	+1	+1	+1	+1	+1	+1	−1	−1	0	−1	+1	+1	+1	0	−1	+1	+1	−1	−1	−1	−1	+1	+1	+1	+1	+1	+1	+1	+1	27	4	3	79.4

Table 11.3 (continued)

Gene subsets	Prediction of 34 test samples (no. 39–72)																																		Results of Classification			
	39	40	41	42	43	44	45	46	47	48	49	50	51	52	53	54	55	56	57	58	59	60	61	62	63	64	65	66	67	68	69	70	71	72	Correct	Incorrect	Unknown	Success rate %
16-gene subset	+1	0	+1	+1	+1	+1	+1	+1	+1	+1	+1	−1	−1	−1	−1	−1	0	+1	−1	−1	+1	−1	−1	0	−1	−1	−1	−1	+1	+1	+1	+1	+1	+1	31	0	3	91.2
17-gene subset	+1	0	+1	+1	+1	+1	+1	+1	+1	+1	+1	−1	−1	−1	−1	−1	0	+1	−1	−1	+1	−1	−1	−1	−1	−1	−1	−1	+1	+1	+1	+1	+1	+1	32	0	2	94.1
18-gene subset	+1	0	+1	+1	+1	+1	+1	+1	+1	+1	+1	−1	−1	−1	−1	−1	0	+1	−1	−1	+1	−1	−1	−1	−1	−1	−1	−1	+1	+1	+1	+1	+1	+1	32	0	2	94.1
19-gene subset	+1	0	+1	+1	+1	+1	+1	+1	+1	+1	+1	−1	−1	−1	−1	−1	0	+1	−1	−1	+1	−1	−1	0	−1	−1	−1	−1	+1	+1	+1	+1	+1	+1	31	0	3	91.2
20-gene subset	+1	0	+1	+1	+1	+1	+1	+1	+1	+1	+1	−1	−1	−1	−1	−1	0	+1	−1	−1	+1	−1	−1	0	−1	−1	−1	−1	+1	+1	+1	+1	+1	+1	31	0	3	91.2
21-gene subset	+1	0	+1	+1	+1	+1	+1	+1	+1	+1	+1	−1	−1	−1	−1	−1	0	+1	−1	−1	+1	−1	−1	0	−1	−1	−1	−1	+1	+1	+1	+1	+1	+1	31	0	3	91.2
22-gene subset	+1	0	+1	+1	+1	+1	+1	+1	+1	+1	+1	−1	−1	−1	−1	−1	0	+1	−1	−1	+1	−1	−1	−1	−1	−1	−1	−1	0	+1	+1	+1	+1	+1	31	0	3	91.2
23-gene subset	+1	0	+1	+1	+1	+1	+1	+1	+1	+1	+1	−1	−1	−1	−1	−1	0	+1	−1	−1	+1	−1	−1	0	−1	-1	−1	−1	0	+1	+1	+1	+1	+1	30	0	4	88.2
Sum of votes:	+23	+7	+23	+15	+23	+23	+23	+23	+23	+23	+23	−22	−22	−10	−22	−17	+7	+23	−15	−23	+22	−8	−15	−4	−19	−21	−13	−8	+20	+22	+23	+22	+22	+23				
Classified as:	+1	+1	+1	+1	+1	+1	+1	+1	+1	+1	+1	−1	−1	−1	−1	−1	+1	+1	−1	−1	+1	−1	−1	−1	−1	−1	−1	−1	+1	+1	+1	+1	+1	+1	34	0	0	100

Every gene subset is used to classify the 34 test samples. The predicted class for every sample is represented by a vote value [+1 for acute lymphoblastic leukaemia (ALL), −1 for acute myeloid leukaemia (AML), and 0 for unknown]. For the sum of votes, one adds up the vote values across all 23 gene subsets for every sample. If the sum of the 23 prediction votes is positive value (which indicates that there are more gene subsets favouring the ALL class than the AML class), the corresponding sample is classified as an ALL sample with the code of 1. If the sum of the 23 prediction votes is negative value (which indicates there are more gene subsets favouring the AML class than the ALL class), the corresponding sample is classified as an AML sample with the code of −1. In case of the sum of the 23 prediction votes is equal to zero, the corresponding sample is unclassified with the code of 0.

avoid having any repeating genes in a single gene subset. 242 subsets were evaluated with the objective function in the current iteration, and 10% of top performing subsets were used to reduce the search space. Only two top performing gene subsets were passed to the next iteration. Within the search space of 7129 genes for the leukaemia data, DGL global optimisation found 23 optimal gene subsets with different lengths from 1 to 23 genes, which formed two pyramidal hierarchy class predictors (shown in Table 11.2). Those gene subsets were assumed to be the best performing gene combinations for classifying the gene data sets used in this study. The selected gene subsets were then used in classifying the test samples in the leukaemia data sets. Table 11.3 summarises the classification results. Once the validation of all the 23 optimal gene subsets was completed, the proposed multi-subsets voting mechanism was adopted. One of the classification results (1 for class 1, –1 for class 2, and 0 for unclassified) was obtained by balancing the votes from the 23 gene subsets for the particular testing sample of interest. It is a process of counting votes to make a final decision on the class of the sample under test.

11.5 Discussion

It is worth observing that the established multi-subsets class predictor could be reduced in size through removing the first five or more unstable short gene subsets. The remaining subsets would still perform well, which is shown on the supporting website [29]. In general, the predicting strength may be improved. However, having those genes selected in the short subsets included may be significant to biologists as they could well be informative. Another interesting observation is that there are not many genes that play a more important role than any other gene. The genes 2642 and 4050 were the most frequently used genes being included 16 times. The gene IDs assigned by this study and real gene accession numbers from the original data sets are listed in the Table 11.4. Some previous research works proposed to find out many near optimal gene subsets through a well-tuned GA procedure and pick up top 50–200 most frequently appeared genes to construct a long gene subset as a predictor [7]. Although the performance of such a predictor was reasonably good, the large amount of computation might not be affordable or cost effective and might not be necessary.

For the leukaemia data, 219 (shown in Table 11.4) out of 7129 genes in the data set were selected by DGL for constructing the class predictor. Table 11.5 lists the genes appearing more than once in the leukaemia class predictor based on frequency rank. It is worthwhile to note that the gene 2642 (U05259_ma1) and the gene 4050 (X03934) both appear 16 times (their frequency is much higher than other's). A subset with only these two genes is able to classify 31 out of 34 samples in the leukaemia test data set and three samples remain as unclassified. When a subset of top four genes (2642, 4050, 2020, and 1) is

Table 11.4 The 219 genes selected by the leukaemia class predictor

IDs	Gene accession number	IDs	Gene accession number	IDs	Gene accession number	IDs	Gene accession number	IDs	Gene accession number
5501	Z15115	1506	L36051	2342	M90696	6136	U28749_s	1925	M31165
3320	U50136_rna1	4459	X67683	5251	D28791	4464	X68149	301	D25303
1068	J03040	1060	J02883	4139	X13956	714	D87443	1126	J04809_rna1
2020	M55150	6467	U29463_s	4720	X85134_rna1	1714	M14123_xpt2	3034	U31449
4782	X90908	2295	M85169	1834	M23197	5912	HG880-HT880	6940	Z30644
2348	M91432	2483	S73813	4751	X87342	4711	X84195	1594	L41147
4270	X54936	6910	U84388	6438	S77154_s	3839	U82320	3342	U51166
2039	M57471	4669	X81889	3414	U56814	3215	U43522	5384	U13022
4050	X03934	6939	Z30643	4224	X52001	2506	S77576	5064	Z15108
2642	U05259_rna1	1891	M28713	5949	M29610	3804	U80017_rna2	5692	D89377_s
1837	M23379	4916	X99657	4889	X98263	1900	M29273	6034	U50360_s
1488	L34357	6487	X75346_s	1056	J02843	5299	L07919	6435	U05012_s
5605	D29675	1442	L27479	6559	U41315_rna1_s	5609	X14085_s	628	D83784
3137	U38846	4950	Y07596	2648	U05875	6655	Z11518_s	4960	Y07846
3336	U50939	2128	M63379	5210	Z79581	6372	M81182_s	4908	X99268
2368	M93284	1934	M31642	5166	Z48804	2791	U14550	5882	HG417-HT417_s
2852	U18004	3906	U89278	3888	U86782	1211	L05512	2227	M76558
1725	M14636	3010	U30245	5134	Z35491	3068	U33818	3998	U96629_rna2
2531	S81221	3392	U53476	1834	M23197	3515	U62437	2004	M37763
2096	M61156	5906	X07618_s	4640	X80062	3854	U83303_cds2	4723	X85372
4991	Y09615	7129	Z78285_f	3189	U41813	6762	M21388	7021	M33318_r
2120	M62994	4453	X67155	6872	M92642	5826	HG3125-HT3301_s	2829	U16296
4492	X69908_rna1	4724	X85373	3118	U37283	1250	L08424	1513	L36645
307	D26067	4961	Y07847	2433	S34389	2416	M97639	3423	U57099
6368	M80397_s	2280	M83651	1740	M15841	1021	HG511-HT511	3642	U70732_rna1
3753	U79249	1	AFFX-BioB-5	5326	M13577	3322	U50315	5477	X71661

Table 11.4 (continued)

IDs	Gene accession number	IDs	Gene accession number	IDs	Gene accession number	IDs	Gene accession number	IDs	Gene accession number
4708	X84002	1362	L19067	4768	X89750	5451	X14766	4534	X74104
5655	U58046_s	6771	X87344_cds10_r	2469	S70348	5508	HG2157-HT2227	4572	X76105
1481	L33881	2090	M60749	6042	L10333_s	4410	X64643	643	D85376
2224	M76424	6681	X74874_rna1_s	4444	X66534	2327	M88282	3066	U33447
109	AC002115_cds4	2811	U15177	4252	X53742	4037	X02751	1229	L07077
5094	Z24727	988	HG4245-HT4515	5828	HG3187-HT3366_s	6639	U83598	1425	L25270
3565	U66048	4574	X76180	442	D45370	4278	X55666	4634	X79865
6441	S78873_s	4727	X85750	3299	U49187	4334	X59711	6416	S57153_s
2619	U03644	5673	D85425_s	6548	Z69030_s	5745	HG2261-HT2351_s	4452	X67098
3119	U37352	3191	U41816	2400	M95925	92	AB003698	3149	U39412
3056	U32944	1427	L25444	2378	M94167	6833	J00220_cds5	4063	X04434
2971	U27185	3565	U66048	3525	U63289	1385	L20348	3026	U31120_rna1
4339	X59812	1853	M25077	5452	X15422	1801	M21154	3780	U79287
5297	L07615	501	D50931	4127	X12901	3102	U36501		
2861	U18288	1387	L20773	5770	X52009_s	4251	X53587		
5247	D17532	4414	X64838	5342	M37712	6832	J00210_rna1		
2001	M37435	1630	L47738	6319	M60450_s	5651	D50477_s		
1584	L40410	6243	M24486_s	1945	M32315	2449	S76992		
4023	X01059	1143	J05213	2780	U13737	4189	X16667		

Table 11.5 The genes appear more than once in the leukaemia class predictor

Rank	Gene IDs	Frequency	Gene accession number	Gene description
1	2642	16	U05259_rna1	MB-1gene
2	4050	16	X03934	GB DEF = T-cell antigen receptor gene T3 delta
3	2020	6	M55150	FAH fumarylacetoacetate
4	1	6	AFFX-BioB-5	AFFX-BioB-5_at (endogenous control)
5	3565	4	U66048	Clone 161455 breast expressed mRNA from chromosome X
6	7129	4	Z78285_f	GB DEF = mRNA (clone 1A7)
7	2348	3	M91432	ACADM acyl-coenzyme A dehydrogenase, C-4 to C-12 straight chain
8	4991	3	Y09615	GB DEF = mitochondrial transcription termination factor
9	2852	2	U18004	HSU18004 Homo sapiens cDNA
10	3056	2	U32944	Cytoplasmic dynein light chain 1 (hdlc1) mRNA
11	5826	2	HG3125-HT3301_s	Estrogen receptor (Gb:S67777)
12	501	2	D50931	KIAA0141 gene
13	714	2	D87443	KIAA0254 gene
14	2327	2	M88282	T-cell surface protein tactile precursor
15	1250	2	L08424	Achaete scute homologous protein (ASH1) mRNA

used, 32 out of 34 samples can be predicted correctly with two remaining as unclassified. There are four genes (2642, 2020, 2348, and 3056) in the Table 11.5, which were identified by the previous researchers in their 50genes most highly correlated with the ALL–AML class distinction [5]. With the method of Golub et al., 29 out of 34 test samples could be classified correctly, while the DGL classified all of them correctly. Moreover, the DGL method, by selecting sets of genes based on their joint ability to discriminate, can identify genes that are important jointly, but do not discriminate individually. This indicates that the DGL method has potential in identifying genes that not only discriminate between the ALL and the AML but also distinguish existing subtypes without applying any prior knowledge.

11.6 Conclusion

A gene is a fundamental constituent of any living organism. The machinery of each human body is built and run with 50,000–100,000 different kinds of genes or protein molecules. With the completion of the Human Genome Project, one has access to large databases of biological information. Proper analysis of such huge data holds immense promise in Bioinformatics. The applicability of data mining in this domain cannot be denied, given the lifesaving prospects of effective drug design. This is also of practical interest to the pharmaceutical industry [21]. The success of DAN technologies and the digital revolution with the growth of the Internet have ensured that huge volumes of high-dimensional microarray expression data are available all around us. Data mining is an evolving and growing area of research and development. The problem is to mine useful information or patterns from the huge data sets. Microarrays provide a powerful basis to monitor the expression of tens of thousands of genes, in order to identify mechanisms that govern the activation of genes in an organism. Microarray experiments are done to produce gene expression patterns, which provide dynamic information about cell function. The huge volume of such data, and their high dimensions, make gene expression data to be suitable candidates for the application of data mining functions.

In this chapter, I have provided an introduction to knowledge discovery from microarray experimental data sets. The major functions of data mining have been discussed from the perspectives of machine learning, pattern recognition, and artificial intelligence. Soft computing methodologies, involving fuzzy sets, neural networks, GAs, rough sets, wavelets, and their hybridisations, have recently been used to solve data mining problems. They strive to provide approximate solutions at low cost, thereby speeding up the process. For the future research and development in microarray data analysis and mining, all the methods are useful tools. The role of soft computing in microarray gene expression study is very promising with the learning ability of neural networks to predict the searching potential of GAs and DGL and the uncertainty handling capacity of fuzzy sets.

DNA microarrays make it practical, for the first time, to survey the expression of thousands of genes under thousands of conditions. This technology makes it possible to study the expression of all of the genes at once. Large-scale expression profiling has emerged as a leading technology in the systematic analysis of cellular physiology. However, method development for analysing gene expression data is still in its infancy. The DGL optimisation uses a mathematical method based on orthogonal sets of numbers. By slicing the multi-dimensional parameter space with a horizontal plane of the objective function, with each parameter independent of the others, a peak is always surrounded by a slope. By finding all regions in which the objective function has values above that of the plane, one can narrow the search region. After finding the boundary of all the isolated regions where this occurs, the plane is raised again and the process repeated. OAs are immensely important in all areas of human investigation. In statistics, they are primarily used in designing experiments. An OA is an array of numbers constructed by utilising orthogonal Latin Squares, one can form an array of several dimensions that are orthogonal to each other and therefore allow the calculation of a resultant using many interdependent variables. Combining OA's sampling with function domain contraction techniques results in an optimisation with two desirable properties. Firstly, the number of function evaluations can be greatly reduced, and secondly, there is a guarantee of finding the global optimum solution. In this study, a carefully selected OA was successfully used for conducting an orthogonal search space sampling. By using an OA and other mathematical techniques, it is practical to develop a global optimisation program for cancer classification and validation on a desktop computer. The primary advantages of this technique are that the global optimum is always found, excellent solutions can be found with little prior knowledge, and the new objective functions can be created according to whatever combination of parameters are required.

The mathematical procedures used in this form of global optimisation are possible to apply to a variety of other previously unsolved problems relating to the resultant of dependent variables, including experimental design and manufacturing variations. There are many other approaches people have adopted, but until now (with the exception of scanning), they all depend either on a starting design, some form of local optimisation, or some random variation. Each method will usually give rise to different solutions. For gene subsets using a large number of genes, these are still the only methods possible. In contrast, the DGL optimisation described here is a methodical global method. The proposed pyramidal hierarchy of the predictor for classification can effectively improve the signal to noise ratio in mining the high-dimensional microarray data sets. While the research in cancer classification with microarray expression data is the first to benefit from this method, the mathematical procedures, DGL global optimisation, used in this study are also applicable to a variety of other unsolved problems related to linked multi-variable problems. The application of this technique will undoubtedly have implications well beyond cancer classification application.

It is still too early to predict what the ultimate impact of microarray will be on our understanding of cancer although the possibility of the accurate diagnosis of cancers based on microarray expressions has emerged. This innovative research truly brings to light one of the hardest problems yet, the ability to accurately classify medical neoplasm. The DGL method provides a precise diagnostic tool that can find the true global optima with questions relating to gene malignancy. Furthermore, genetic screening for diseases are playing an increasingly important role in preventative medicine; if we can detect the presence of disease or predict the malignancy through microarray expression data with a desktop computer, before clinical diagnosis, a more efficient and clear cut treatment plan can be formulated, eliminating the possibility of clinician bias. More importantly, an unbiased and digital data-based approach can be easily applied to distinctions relating to future clinical outcome, such as drug response or survival. In cancer research, fundamental mechanisms that cut across distinct types of cancers could also be discovered through mining microarray data by the DGL global strategies.

References

1. Bassett Jr, D.E.B., Eisen, M.B., and Boguski, M.S., (1999) Gene expression informatics—it's all in your mine, 21 (suppl.), *Nature Genetics*, 51–55.
2. Aittokallio, T., Kurki, M., Nevalainen, O., Nikula, T., West, A., and Lahesmaa, R., (2003) Computational strategies for analyzing data in gene expression microarray experiments, *Journal of Bioinformatics and Computational Biology*, 1(3), 541–586.
3. Zhang, S. and Gant, T.W., (2004) A statistical framework for the design of microarray experiments and effective detection of differential gene expression, *Bioinformatics*, 20(16), 2821–2828.
4. Alon, U., Barkai, N., Notterman, D.A., Gish, K., Ybarra, S. Mack, D., and Levine, A.J., (1999) Broad patterns of gene expression revealed by clustering analysis of tumor and normal colon tissues probed by oligonucleotide arrays, Proc. Natl Acad. Sci. USA, 96, 6745–6750.
5. Golub, T.R., Slonim, D.K., Tamayo, P., Huard, C., Gaasenbeek, M., Mesirov, J.P., Coller, H., Loh, M.L., Downing, J.R., Caligiuri, M.A., Bloomfield, C.D., and Lander, E.S., (1999) Molecular classification of cancer: Class discovery and class prediction by gene expression monitoring, Science, 286, 531–537.
6. Li, L., Darden, T.A., Weinberg, C.R., Levine, A.J., and Pedersen, L.G., (2001) Gene assessment and sample classification for gene expression data using a genetic algorithm/k-nearest neighbour method, Combinatorial Chemistry & High Throughput Screening, 4, No. 8, 727–739.
7. Li, L., Weinberg, C.R., Darden, T.A., and Pedersen, L.G., (2001) Gene selection for sample classification based on gene expression data: study of sensitivity to choice of parameters of the GA/KNN method, Bioinformatics, 17, No. 12, 1131–1142.
8. Horst, R. and Pardalos, P.M., (1995) Handbook of Global Optimization, Kluwer Academic Publishers, Netherlands.
9. Li, D. and Nathan, B., (1996) Global optimization advances multivariable thin-film design, Laser Focus World, No. 5, 135–136.
10. Li, D. and Smith, C., (1996) A new global optimization algorithm based on Latin Square theory, Proceedings of 1996IEEE International Conference on Evolutionary Computation, ISBN: 0-7803-2902-3, 628–630.
11. Han J. and Kamber, M., (2001) Data Mining: Concepts and Techniques. San Diego: Academic Press.
12. Mitra, S., Pal, S.K., and Mitra, P., (2002) "Data mining in soft computing framework: A survey," IEEE Transactions on Neural Networks, vol. 13, pp. 3–14.
13. Hand, D., Mannila, H., and P. Smyth, (2001) Principles of Data Mining. London: MIT Press.
14. Kantardzic, M., (2002) Data Mining: Models, Methods, and Algorithms. Hoboken, NJ: Wiley Interscience, IEEE Press.
15. Schena, M., Shalon, D., Davis, R.W., and Brown, P.O., (1995) "Quantitative monitoring of gene expression patterns with a complementary DNA microarray", Science, 270, 467–470.
16. Alizadeh, A.A., et al., (2000) "Distinct types of diffuse large B-cell lymphoma identified by gene expression profiling", Nature, 403, 503–511.
17. Brown, M.P.S., Grundy, W.N., Lin, D., Critianini, N., Sungnet, C., Furey, T.S., Ares, M., Haussler, D., (2000) "Knowledge-Based analysis of microarray gene expression data using support vector machines", Proceedings of National Academy of Sciences, 97, 262–267.
18. Deutsch, J.M., (2003) "Evolutionary algorithms for finding optimal gene sets in microarray prediction", Bioinformatics, 19, 45–52.
19. Khan, J., Wei J.S., Ringner, M., Saal, L.H., Ladanyi, M., Westermann, F., Berthold, F., Schwab, M., Antonescu, C.R., Peterson, C., Meltzer, P.S., (2001) "Classification and

diagnostic prediction of cancers using gene expression profiling and artificial neural networks", Nature Medicine, 7, 673–679.
20. "Special Issue on Bioinformatics", IEEE Computer, vol. 35, July 2002.
21. Mitra, S. and Acharya, T., (2005) Data mining: Multimedia, Soft Computing, and Bioinformatics, John Wiley & Sons Inc., Newark, ISBN:0471474886.
22. Draghici, S., (2002) Statistical intelligence: effective analysis of high-density microarray data. Drug Discov Today, 7(11 Suppl).: S55–S63.
23. Tou, J.T. and Gonzalez, R.C. (1974) Pattern Recognition Principles. London: Addison-Wesley.
24. Cho, S.B. and Ryu, J. (2002) "Classifying gene expression data of cancer using classifier ensemble with mutually exclusive features", Proceedings of the IEEE, vol. 90, pp. 1744–1753.
25. Wang, L. and Fu, X., (2005) Data mining with computational intelligence, Springer, Germany.
26. Li D, (2004) "Global Optimisation for Optical Coating Design", Proceedings of 2004 Conferences in Internet Technologies and Applications, ISBN 86-7466-117-3, Purdue, Indiana, USA, July 8–11.
27. Peng, S., Xu, Q., Ling, X.B., Peng, X., Du, W., and Chen, L., (2003) Molecular classification of cancer types from microarray data using the combination of genetic algorithms and support vector machines, FEBS Letters, 555, 358–362.
28. Liu, J.J., Cutler. G., Li, W., Pan, Z., Peng, S., Hoey T., Chen, L., and Ling., X.B., (2005) Multiclass cancer classification and biomarker discovery using GA-based algorithms, Bioinformatics, 21, No. 11, 2691–2697.
29. Li, D., (2006) http://www.scis.ecu.edu.au/Staff/staffinfo.aspx?staffid = donggual

Index

Printed in the United States of America